RECORD OF RELEASES FILED

MANAGING YOUR MEDICAL PRACTICE

is filed with all previously issued releases
and is current through:

RELEASE NO. 6 • JANUARY 1992

Questions About This Publication

For assistance with replacement pages,
shipments, billing or other customer
service matters, please call our
Customer Services Department at 1–800–833–9844
Outside the United States and Canada
please call .... (518) 487–3026
or fax .... (518) 487–3584
To place an order, call 1–800–223–1940
or contact your Matthew Bender representative.

FOR EDITORIAL ASSISTANCE, please call
    Beverly Lieberman at .... (212) 216–8629
        or
    Rina Cascone at .... (212) 216–8858

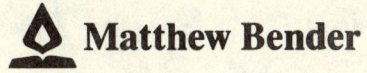

Times Mirror
Books

(Matthew Bender & Co., Inc.)   (Pub.372)

Managing Your Medical Practice

Charles R. Wold, C.P.B.C.

1992

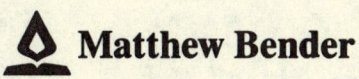
Matthew Bender

Times Mirror Books

Questions About This Publication

For assistance with replacement pages,
shipments, billing or other customer
service matters, please call our
Customer Services Department at 1-800-833-9844
Outside the United States and Canada
please call .... (518) 487-3026
or fax .... (518) 487-3584
To place an order, call 1-800-223-1940
or contact your Matthew Bender representative.

FOR EDITORIAL ASSISTANCE, please call
   Beverly Lieberman at .... (212) 216-8629
      or
   Rina Cascone at .... (212) 216-8858

Copyright © 1986, 1987, 1988, 1989, 1990, 1991, 1992
by MATTHEW BENDER & COMPANY,
Incorporated

No copyright is claimed in the text of U.S. and state
regulations, statutes, and excerpts from court cases quoted
within.

All Rights Reserved
Printed in United States of America

Library of Congress Catalog Card Number: 81-69350
ISBN: 0-8205-1372-5

MATTHEW BENDER & CO., INC.
EDITORIAL OFFICES
11 PEN PLAZA, NEW YORK, NY 10001-2006 (212) 967-7707
2101 WEBSTER ST., OAKLAND, CA 94612-3027 (510) 446-7100

(Matthew Bender & Co., Inc.)   (Rel.6–1/92 Pub.372)

"This publication is designed to provide accurate and authoritative information in regard to the subject matter covered. It is sold with the understanding that the publisher is not engaged in rendering legal, accounting or other professional service. If legal advice or other expert assistance is required, the services of a competent professional should be sought." — From a Declaration of Principles jointly adopted by a Committee of the American Bar Association and a Committee of Publishers and Associations.

When published as issued, works of the federal and state governments, including all statutes and decisions of the courts as well as all legislative and administrative histories, studies and reports, are matters in the public domain. As compiled, arranged and edited, however, such works and all other materials contained in this publication are subject to the foregoing copyright notice.

NOTE

The publisher's editorial staff wishes to state its awareness that physicians of both sexes use, as indeed they write, its treatises. We have done our best to use language that avoids gender distinctions. However, because clarity must be our prime concern, it has been necessary at times to use a singular pronoun.

Publisher's Editorial Staff

Diana T. Axelrod, J.D.	Director of Publishing
Barbara M. Robb	Editorial Director
Beverly R. Lieberman	Executive Editor
Rina Cascone	Publication Manager
Stefan R. Dziemianowicz	Staff Writer
Amy McDonald	Senior Medical Editor
Rose Aftergut	Indexing Manager

Editorial Services Staff

Donna Kusman	Editorial Services Manager
Paul Ralston	Editorial Supervisor
Michael A. Cantalupo	Copy Editor
Andrew S. Clarke	Copy Editor
James Kelly	Copy Editor
Kimberly Snead	Copy Editor

ABOUT THE AUTHOR

Charles R. Wold is the Chief Executive Officer of Professional Consulting Group, Inc., a financial and management consulting firm specializing in the medical area. Mr. Wold has worked with many physicians in private practice to help them with their financial affairs and day-to-day practice management. For the past 15 years, he has helped guide physicians through the rapid changes in the business of medical practice management and its emerging problems. Mr. Wold is currently president-elect of the Society of Medical–Dental Management Consultants (SMD), a national organization whose members provide objective and confidential consulting advice for the medical and dental professions and who do not accept fees or commissions from other sources except medical-dental clientele. He is a member of the editorial board of *Physician's Management,* a Certified Professional Business Consultant (C.P.B.C.), and a member of the Institute of Certified Professional Business Consultants (ICPBC). Mr. Wold is also a member of the National Society of Public Accountants and is enrolled to practice before the Internal Revenue Service.

LIST OF CONTRIBUTORS

Rebecca H. Anwar, Ph.D.

Chapter 16, Marketing Your Medical Practice

President of Hoover Anwar Associates, a firm that specializes in the development of marketing and management plans for health care organizations and professionals; member of the faculty of the Medical College of Pennsylvania; Associate Professor of Emergency Medicine.

Carl W. Brandt

Chapter 5, Computers in Health Care

Management consultant to medical practices and advisor to local post-secondary educational institutions that provide training programs for medical office administrators in the Minneapolis/St. Paul medical community; co-founder and past president of DISC Computer systems.

Earl L. Cook

Chapter 8, Risk Management and Insurance

President, Cook Pension Consultants, Inc.; past president, St. Paul Health Underwriters Association; recipient of the Distinguished Service Award from the International Association of Health Underwriters; Chartered Life Underwriter (CLU), American College of Life Underwriters, 1965.

David L. Hicks

Chapter 11, Pension and Retirement Plans

Founder, Hicks Pension Services; Chairman of the Board for all Hicks pension services affiliates in Fresno and San Luis Obispo, California, and in Honolulu, Hawaii; B.S. in Business Administration, California State University in Fresno; Chartered Life Underwriter (CLU), American College of Life Underwriters, 1971.

Edward Kelsay, J.D.

Chapter 12, Law for the Medical Practice

President, Ed Kelsay and Associates, Inc., a medical practice management consulting firm in Oklahoma City; Legal Counsel,

Oklahoma State Medical Association and Oklahoma Foundation for Peer Review; adjunct professor, Oklahoma School of Health; visiting lecturer, Department of Family Practice, Oklahoma University Medical School; malpractice loss-prevention manager; author of several books on the medico-legal aspects of medical practice management.

Joseph Miller

Chapter 8, Risk Management and Insurance

Life Member, Million Dollar Round Table (MDRT); Life Member, National Life of Vermont President's Club; Recipient of Summit Award, National Life of Vermont; B.B.A., Southern Methodist University, Dallas, Texas; Chartered Life Underwriter (CLU), American College of Life Underwriters, 1971.

Michael E. Mitchell

Chapter 8, Risk Management and Insurance

President, MICOR Insurance Brokers, a commercial brokerage in San Jose, California; past affiliations include Marsh and McClennan of Canada; Power and Dalziel, insurance brokers for the California Dental Association; Mark F. Hopkins, insurance brokers for the Santa Clara County Medical Society.

Kathryn I. Moghadas

Chapter 18, Managing Professional Liability Risk

President of Practice Management Solutions, Inc., Casselberry, Florida, a firm that specializes in health care management consulting; B.A., health care management, George Mason University, Fairfax, Virginia; certified registered nurse; member, Society of Medical/Dental Management Consultants.

Dorothy R. Sweeney

Chapter 2, Staff Recruiting, Development and Management

Vice President and Senior Consultant, The Health Care Group, Inc., Plymouth Meeting, Pennsylvania; President, Health Care Personnel Consulting, Inc.; Vice President and Senior Consultant, Health Care Consulting, Inc.; Vice President, Health Care Marketing Associates, Ltd.; Assistant Editor and Administrative Director, The Physician's Advisory; Editorial Consultant for

LIST OF CONTRIBUTORS

several medical practice management magazines and author of numerous journal articles.

(Text continued on page xi)

ACKNOWLEDGMENTS

No book can be written and published without the efforts and contributions of many people. My sincere appreciation and thanks to all who have contributed to the making of this book.

Special thanks to my mother, Bernadine Wold, who launched my writing career many years ago. Her experience as a business manager in a leading St. Paul internal medicine office qualified her to critique the manuscript not only for clarity but also for accuracy.

Special thanks are also in order for the Professional Consulting Group staff, who worked under a great deal of pressure in order to complete the various chapters on time. David Wold, Professional Consulting Group's Chief Financial Officer, graciously accepted additional responsibilities so the author could spend additional time working on the book.

This book certainly would not be possible if clients did not allow a consultant to review the most intimate details of their practices in order to sort out the strengths and weaknesses. To these many clients, thank you.

The contributing authors were selected for their expert knowledge and their willingness to share this knowledge with the readers of this book. The names of each contributor are listed on the contributor's page. Special thanks to Earl Cook, who called with some last-minute editing changes one day before leaving for China.

The people that I have worked with at Matthew Bender were extremely helpful. Their hard work in reviewing and editing the text has greatly enhanced it. Special thanks to Beverly Lieberman, Barbara Robb and Stefan Dziemianowicz.

Finally, special thanks must be given to my wife, Alice, who has given her full support to this project, despite the strains and the additional family burdens placed on her. Thank you, Alice, for your support and confidence.

PREFACE

Although a physician has many years of formal education, little if any of that education is devoted to business management. Yet physicians in private practice are faced with the monumental task of managing a large business. Any efforts they make to develop skills in this area are further hindered by the lack of informative books in this area. *Managing Your Medical Practice* was written to provide sound, readily accessible information that can help the private practitioner enhance the profitability of his or her practice and attend to the business details of a medical profession.

This book will be useful throughout a physician's career as a guide for running a medical practice and will provide answers to many if not all of the questions that arise during the management of a medical practice. We hope you will refer to it often, not only to find the solution to specific problems as they occur, but also to review and evaluate your practice's current systems and procedures.

Best wishes in your private practice.

Charles R. Wold

TABLE OF CONTENTS

[A detailed synopsis appears at the beginning of each chapter.]

Chapter 1	**Starting Your Medical Practice**
§ 1.01	Establishing a Business Plan
§ 1.02	Community Demographics
§ 1.03	Choosing Office Space
§ 1.04	Assessment of Space
§ 1.05	Creating a Layout
§ 1.06	Lease Arrangements
§ 1.07	Space Sharing
§ 1.08	Equipment Acquisitions
§ 1.09	Leasing Versus Purchasing
§ 1.10	Financial Modeling
§ 1.11	External Marketing
§ 1.12	Internal Marketing
§ 1.13	Checklist of Items to Be Considered When Starting a Practice
§ 1.14–§ 1.99	Reserved
§ 1.100	Bibliography
Appendix 1-A	Where to Find Help: Consultants for the Medical Office
Appendix 1-B	Patient Survey
Chapter 2	**Staff Recruiting, Development and Management**
§ 2.01	Types of Personnel
§ 2.02	Recruiting and Hiring
§ 2.03	Salary and Fringe Benefits
§ 2.04	Development of a Personnel Policy
§ 2.05	Creating a Procedure Manual
§ 2.06	Staff Management
§ 2.07	Employee Terminations
§ 2.08	Back-Up Personnel

TABLE OF CONTENTS

§ 2.09	Federal Laws Regarding Employment
§ 2.10	Checklist for Staff Recruiting, Development and Management
§ 2.11–§ 2.99	Reserved
§ 2.100	Bibliography
Appendix 2-A	Tests for General Office Skills
Appendix 2-B	General Outline of Job Descriptions for a Two-Doctor Practice

Chapter 3   Forms of Practice

§ 3.01	Different Forms of Practice
§ 3.02	Advantages of the Unincorporated Practice
§ 3.03	Advantages of Incorporating the Medical Practice
§ 3.04	Disadvantages of Single and Group Practices
§ 3.05	Profit Distribution in Groups
§ 3.06	Starting New Physicians in the Practice
§ 3.07	Valuing the Practice
§ 3.08	Checklist for Forms of Practice
§ 3.09–§ 3.99	Reserved
§ 3.100	Bibliography

Chapter 4   Office Systems

§ 4.01	Telephone Answering and Message Systems
§ 4.02	Appointment Systems
§ 4.03	Patient Flow
§ 4.04	Patient Records
§ 4.05	Dictation Processing
§ 4.06	Referral Information Systems
§ 4.07	Recall and Reminder Systems
§ 4.08	Follow-Up Systems
§ 4.09	Checklist for Office Systems
§ 4.10–§ 4.99	Reserved
§ 4.100	Bibliography
Appendix 4-A	Routing Slips

Chapter 5   Computers in Health Care

| § 5.01 | Management Information Systems |
| § 5.02 | Components of the Management Information System |

TABLE OF CONTENTS

§ 5.03	Data Processing Alternatives
§ 5.04	Planning for Automation
§ 5.05	Selecting a Management Information System
§ 5.06	Legal Considerations
§ 5.07	Computer Systems Checklist
§ 5.08–§ 5.99	Reserved
§ 5.100	Bibliography
Appendix 5-A	Sample Management Reports
Appendix 5-B	Sample Appointment Scheduling Reports
Appendix 5-C	Comparison of Service Bureaus and In-House Computer Systems
Appendix 5-D	Glossary of Basic Computer Terminology
Appendix 5-E	Request for Proposal

Chapter 6   Financial Management

§ 6.01	Budgeting and Financial Forecasting
§ 6.02	Financial Reports
§ 6.03	Accounts Payable
§ 6.04	Payroll
§ 6.05	General Ledger
§ 6.06	Choosing an Accountant
§ 6.07	Cash Flow Management
§ 6.08	Financial Management Checklist
§ 6.09–§ 6.99	Reserved
§ 6.100	Bibliography

Chapter 7   Credit and Collections

§ 7.01	Guidelines for Establishing a Credit Policy
§ 7.02	Written Collection Policy
§ 7.03	Collecting from Third Parties
§ 7.04	Collecting from Patients
§ 7.05	Monitoring Collections
§ 7.06	Collections Checklist
§ 7.07–§ 7.99	Reserved
§ 7.100	Bibliography
Appendix 7–A	Credit and Collection Policy
Appendix 7–B	Credit Letters

Chapter 8   Risk Management and Insurance

§ 8.01	Risk Identification
§ 8.02	Risk Prevention
§ 8.03	Insurance Coverage for the Practice
§ 8.04	Insurance Coverage for the Physician-Employee
§ 8.05	Risk Management Checklist
§ 8.06–§ 8.99	Reserved
§ 8.100	Bibliography
Appendix 8-A	Malpractice Avoidance Checklist

Chapter 9   Increasing Productivity Through Efficiency

§ 9.01	Productivity
§ 9.02	Value of Physician's Time
§ 9.03	The Work Week
§ 9.04	Production Goals
§ 9.05	Scheduling Work
§ 9.06	Facilities
§ 9.07	Utilizing Staff
§ 9.08	Staff Participation
§ 9.09	Incentive Program
§ 9.10	Ancillary Services
§ 9.11	Extramural Services
§ 9.12	Productivity Checklist
§ 9.13–§ 9.99	Reserved
§ 9.100	Bibliography

Chapter 10   Accounts Receivable Management

§ 10.01	Types of Systems
§ 10.02	Controls
§ 10.03	Third Party Billings
§ 10.04	Hospital Charges
§ 10.05	Miscellaneous Charges
§ 10.06	Accounts Receivable Management Reports
§ 10.07	Accounts Receivable Management Checklist
§ 10.08–§ 10.99	Reserved
§ 10.100	Bibliography
Appendix 10-A	Financial Transaction Forms for the Medical Office

TABLE OF CONTENTS

Chapter 11	**Retirement and Pension Plans**
§ 11.01	Pension and Retirement Plans
§ 11.02	Qualified Plans
§ 11.03	Types of Retirement Plans
§ 11.04	The 401(k) Plan
§ 11.05	Individual Retirement Plans
§ 11.06	Social Security Benefits
§ 11.07	Self-Employed and Partnership (KEOGH) Plans
§ 11.08	Disbursement of Funds and Benefits
§ 11.09	Checklist for Pension and Retirement Plans
Chapter 12	**Law for the Medical Practice**
§ 12.01	The Patient-Physician Relationship
§ 12.02	Consent for Medical Care
§ 12.03	Good Samaritan Laws
§ 12.04	Patient Information
§ 12.05	Medical Records
§ 12.06	Medical Record Preservation
§ 12.07	Collecting Debts
§ 12.08	Employment Applications
§ 12.09	Checklist for Law in the Medical Practice
§ 12.10–§ 12.99	Reserved
§ 12.100	Bibliography
Appendix 12-A	Patient Discharge Notices
Appendix 12-B	Acceptable Pre-Employment Inquiries Under EEO Guidelines
Appendix 12-C	Legislation Affecting Medical Practices
Chapter 13	**Medical Practice Mergers and Affiliations**
§ 13.01	Medical Practice Affiliations: The Options
§ 13.02	The Benefits of Combined Practices
§ 13.03	Consequences and Risks of Affiliation
§ 13.04	Is an Affiliation Right for You?
§ 13.05	Choosing Partners
§ 13.06	Initial Obstacles
§ 13.07	Establishing Time-Frames
§ 13.08	Restrictive Covenants
§ 13.09	Noncorporate Legal Agreements and Documents

TABLE OF CONTENTS

§ 13.10   Establishing the New Entity
§ 13.11   Public Relations
§ 13.12   Insurance Coverage
§ 13.13   Bail-Out Provisions
§ 13.14   Checklist
§ 13.100   Bibliography

Chapter 14   **Succeeding in a Prepaid Health Care Program**
§ 14.01   Prepaid Health Care Programs
§ 14.02   Reasons for Participating
§ 14.03   How a Prepaid Program Works: Pros and Cons
§ 14.04   Preparation: Evaluating Program Viability
§ 14.05   Federal and State Laws
§ 14.06   The Specific Contract
§ 14.07   Monitoring Profitability
§ 14.08   Checklist for Prepaid Health Care Programs
§ 14.09   Glossary of Terms in Prepaid Health Care
§ 14.100   Bibliography

Chapter 15   **Communication in the Medical Office**
§ 15.01   The Problems of Poor Communication
§ 15.02   Types of Communication
§ 15.03   Formulating Objectives
§ 15.04   Managerial Style
§ 15.05   Analyzing the Audience
§ 15.06   Structuring Your Message
§ 15.07   Putting a Message in Writing
§ 15.08   Making Presentations
§ 15.09   Effective Meetings
§ 15.10   Checklist for Office Communications
§ 15.100   Bibliography
Appendix 15-A   Daily Report
Appendix 15-B   Memorandum
Appendix 15-C   Meetings

Chapter 16   **Marketing Your Medical Practice**
§ 16.01   Why Physicians Need Marketing
§ 16.02   What is Marketing?

TABLE OF CONTENTS

§ 16.03	Developing a Marketing Plan
§ 16.04	Targeting Your Market
§ 16.05	Choosing Your Marketing Strategies
§ 16.06	The Practice Brochure
§ 16.07	Creating a Newsletter
§ 16.08	Public Relations
§ 16.09	Public Speaking
§ 16.10	Special Events
§ 16.11	Creating an Image
§ 16.12	Advertising
§ 16.13	Direct Mail
§ 16.14	Patient Education
§ 16.15	Patient Relations
§ 16.16	Professional Relations
§ 16.17	Marketing Checklist
Appendix 16-A	Marketing Resources

Chapter 17 **Understanding Medical Office Coding**

§ 17.01	Overview of Coding Systems
§ 17.02	Supporting Office Coding
§ 17.03	Using the CPT Text
§ 17.04	CPT: Medicine
§ 17.05	CPT: Surgery
§ 17.06	CPT: Radiology
§ 17.07	CPT: Pathology and Laboratory
§ 17.08	Modifiers for CPT Codes
§ 17.09	Other CPT Appendices and Index
§ 17.10	HCPC Coding
§ 17.11	Levels of Service
§ 17.12	Consultations
§ 17.13	Relative Value Indexes
§ 17.14	ICD-9-CM Diagnostic Coding
§ 17.15	Checklist for a Coding Library
§ 17.16	Tips for Proper Coding
§ 17.17	Coding Checklist

Chapter 18 **Managing Professional Liability Risk**

§ 18.01	Overview of the Malpractice Climate

TABLE OF CONTENTS

§ 18.02	Medical Records
§ 18.03	Communication
§ 18.04	Medication
§ 18.05	Treatment and Procedures
§ 18.06	Patient Rapport and Risk Management
§ 18.07	The Telephone and Risk Management
§ 18.08	Accounts Receivable and Risk Management
§ 18.09	Personnel
§ 18.10	Equipment
§ 18.11	General Quality Assurance Recommendations
§ 18.12	Handling Potential Litigation
§ 18.13	Managing Professional Liability Checklist
§ 18.14-§ 18.99	Reserved
§ 18.100	Bibliography
Appendix 18-A	Policy Proposal for Prescription Refills
Appendix 18-B	Medication Supplies Control Form
Appendix 18-C	Outline for Policy Manual
Appendix 18-D	Equipment Records

Index

CHAPTER 1

Starting Your Medical Practice

> **SCOPE**
>
> Starting a medical practice involves becoming versed in those aspects of management and business which can help insure success. It also involves learning about potential problems and how to resolve them. Prior to beginning a practice, there are a series of steps to be followed, including choosing the location, reviewing the demographics and locating financing. For the physician, choosing office space necessitates making a decision about the types of rooms needed, including specialized rooms in various fields of medicine. It means creating a layout and planning for size. The physician must also decide which medical equipment is necessary and whether it should be leased or purchased. This requires knowledge about the financial advantages and disadvantages of both methods of acquisition. When office space is chosen, lease arrangements must be made for that space. In order for such arrangements to be most beneficial, the physician needs to be informed about leasehold improvements, options on length of lease, and rights and responsibilities as a tenant. Should a doctor decide to share space with other physicians, a method for allocating costs must be worked out as well as termination arrangements should one or more doctors leave the group practice. Before opening the medical practice, a financial model must be drawn up to forecast income and expenses, and various items (such as tax identification numbers) secured. Both internal and external marketing ideas for attracting patients and keeping them should also be considered.

SYNOPSIS

§ 1.01 Establishing a Business Plan
§ 1.02 Community Demographics

- [1] Hospital Administrators
- [2] Industry
- [3] Third Party Health Coverage
- [4] Banks

§ 1.03 Choosing Office Space
§ 1.04 Assessment of Space
- [1] Specialized Rooms
- [2] Planning for Size

§ 1.05 Creating A Layout
§ 1.06 Lease Arrangements
§ 1.07 Space Sharing
- [1] Expenses to Be Shared
- [2] Termination Agreement

§ 1.08 Equipment Acquisitions
- [1] Equipment Needs
- [2] Cost of Items

§ 1.09 Leasing Versus Purchasing
- [1] Financing, Expensing, Tax Credits and Depreciation
- [2] Lease Arrangements
  - [a] Advantages
  - [b] Disadvantages
- [3] Determining Cost Differences

§ 1.10 Financial Modeling
§ 1.11 External Marketing
- [1] Advertising
- [2] Public Speaking and Seminars
- [3] Community Participation
- [4] Published Articles
- [5] One-to-One Contact
- [6] Miscellaneous Practice Builders

§ 1.12 Internal Marketing
- [1] Initial Patient Contact
- [2] Patient Visit
- [3] Patient Follow-Up

§ 1.13 Checklist of Items to Be Considered when Starting a Practice

§ 1.14–§ 1.99 Reserved

§ 1.100 Bibliography

Appendix 1-A Where to Find Help: Consultants for the Medical Office
Appendix 1-B Patient Survey

§ 1.01 Establishing a Business Plan

After a location for a medical practice is decided on, a business plan should be devised that takes into account the size of the practice and how the practice is to be managed.

The first question to be addressed is where the practice should be located. Once a decision is reached, each of the following questions will need to be considered.

- What type of space should be acquired?
- Should the space be leased or purchased?
- How much space? More than is needed initially or just enough to start?
- How much equipment should be acquired?
- Should the equipment be leased or purchased?
- What are the sources for new patients?
- How will the practice afford to purchase equipment and supplies and pay initial operating costs?
- How will accounts receivable be managed?
- What are the benefits of participating with certain third parties?

Because starting a practice can be a source of great tension, having a good business plan can minimize the stress and help to accomplish the goal of establishing a successful practice. This chapter is designed to assist the physician who is getting started. The text can be considered a road map to a successful practice.

(A list of business consultants who are skilled at answering questions the starting physician might have is provided in Appendix 1-A.)

§ 1.02 Community Demographics

Before making final business decisions on the location and size of the practice, you should consider community demographics such as the make-up of the population, the physician-patient ratio, the business character of the town, interaction between physicians and the hospital and the preferred third-party providers.

First determine the population of the community and its

(Pub.372)

surrounding areas as well as the average ages within the population and the per capita income. This information may be obtained by checking with government offices. Specifically, the state department of economic development can generally supply this data for every community in the state.

Next, check with the local medical society to learn the overall number of physicians in the area as well as the number of physicians in your specialty. These figures will allow you to calculate the ratio of people per doctor in that community. In 1983, nationwide, there were 462 people for each physician. The suggested ideal physician to population ratios as provided by the American Medical Association for the various specialties are as follows:

Specialty	Recommended population
Allergy	25,000
Anesthesiology	14,000
Cardiology	25,000
Dermatology	40,000
Gastroenterology	50,000
General and family practice	2,000
General surgery	10,000
Internal medicine	5,000
Neurology	60,000
Obstetrics and gynecology	11,000
Ophthalmology	20,000
Orthopedic surgery	25,000
Otolaryngology	25,000
Pathology	20,000
Pediatrics	10,000
Plastic surgery	50,000
Psychiatry	10,000
Pulmonary disease	100,000
Radiology	15,000
Thoracic surgery	100,000
Urology	30,000

Once you have obtained this information, visit the physicians who live in that community, both those within and outside of your speciality. Learn their perceptions of the need for more physicians.

(Pub.372)

STARTING YOUR MEDICAL PRACTICE § 1.02 [1]

MINNESOTA
Department of Energy
and Economic Development
900 American Center
150 East Kellogg Boulevard
St. Paul, Minnesota 55101

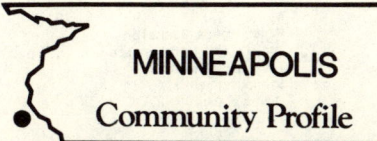

MINNEAPOLIS
Community Profile

COUNTY, CITY CODE NUMBER 27.28

CITY Minneapolis   COUNTY Hennepin   REGION 11
Distance from: Minneapolis/St. Paul   Duluth 160 miles S

POPULATION

	City	County	* SMSA
1960 Census	482,872	842,854	1,535,297
1970 Census	434,400	960,080	1,874,612
1980 Census	370,951	941,411	1,985,873
1983 Estimate	364,160	948,470	2,033,080
1984 est.	364,250	958,820	2,057,150

Source of Estimate: Metropolitan Council

INDUSTRY

Major Employers in Area:

Firm	Product/Service	Number of Employees	Union Initials	% in Union
3M Company	Tape/Abrasives Prod.	22,000		
Control Data Corporation	Terminal Products	17,550		
Honeywell, Inc.	Environmental System	17,000	Team.	
Northwestern Bell Telephone Co	Communications	10,400	CWA	70
Dayton Hudson Corporation	Retail	10,250	T/O/F/AGW	3
Sperry, Major Systems Division	Data Process. Equip.	10,100		
Northwest Airlines	Comm./Cargo Freight	6,692		
Norwest Bancorporation	Bank	5,100		
Fairview Community Hospitals	Hospital	4,800		
Northern States Power Company	Utility	4,471	UEW	
Cowles Media Company	Media	3,436		
Burlington Northern Railroad	Railroad	3,000		

* EMPLOYMENT

Labor Survey Date 1984 annual avg. nonagricultural wage and salary employment

Type of Employment: Number of Employees:

Manufacturing   256,600
Non-Manufacturing   915,400   Unemployment 4.8 % annual average

Total Labor Force   1,172,000   Available in Labor Force 1,236,407

The 1,172,000 figure is total nonag. wage & salary jobs (Mpls/St Paul SMSA)

(Pub.372)

* Manufacturing Occupations in Area
(Production and Clerical)

Occupation or Job Title	1984 Median Wage
Assembler, Exc. Electronic	$ 9.25 /hr.
Electronics Assembler	$ 7.35 /hr.
Machine Operator	$ 8.48 /hr.
Welder	$ 10.49 /hr.
Punch Press Operator	$ 9.21 /hr.
Machinist, Maintenance	$ 12.00 /hr.
Tool and Die Maker	$ 13.85 /hr.
Stenographer II	$ 7.21 /hr.

Source of Data

TRANSPORTATION

Rail Lines Soo Line; Burlington Northern; 5 main lines & 2 trunk lines
Frequency Unlimited
Reciprocal Switching yes   Distance to Main Line
Piggy-back Service yes   Passenger Service In St. Paul
* Truck Lines 27 headquartered in metro area; over 100 first   60 Terminals
class carriers
*12 Airports   Commercial Service yes   Charter Service yes   Jet Service yes
Nearest   Minneapolis-St. Paul Int'l
* Airlines 14 national/international; 10 local/regional
* Navigation Aids:
all FAA aids for International airport
* Runway 10,000 feet concrete
Distance to CBD 10 miles
* Bus — Inter City Greyhound, Jefferson, Zephyr   Intra City MTC
Navigable Water yes   Depth 9 feet
Highways — Interstate I-35, I-94 with I-694 and I-494 belt routes
    Federal 8, 12, 65, 169   State 55
Load Limits 9 tons

1984 COMMERCIAL/INDUSTRIAL TAXES PAYABLE 1985

Municipal Rate	$ 34.710	/$1000/assessed value
County Rate	$ 25.982	/$1000/assessed value
School Rate	$ 42.986	/$1000/assessed value
Misc. Rate	$ 5.181	/$1000/assessed value
Total Rate	$108.859	/$1000/assessed value

METHOD OF ASSESSMENT FOR COMMERCIAL/INDUSTRIAL PROPERTIES

Minnesota real estate taxes are based on market value. Market value is construed to be the price that a willing buyer would pay to a willing seller in a free market. A two-step formula is used for determining property taxes for commercial/industrial properties.
1. The first $60,000 of market value times 28% plus the remaining market value times 43% equals assessed valuation.
2. Assessed valuation times the total mill rate equals property taxes payable.

GOVERNMENT

Organization mayor council

	Regular Employees:	Part Time Employees:
Fire Department	458	volunteer
Police	684	volunteer
Sheriff		
City		

Refuse Service public   Master Plan yes   Annual Budget $
Industrial plans must be approved by: Insurance Rating class 3
Minneapolis Planning Department

UTILITIES

Municipal Water Source river   Storage Capacity 184,000,000 gallons
Pumping Capacity 200,000,000 gal/min   Total tapwater hardness   ppm
Average Demand 70,300,000 G/D   Peak Demand 155,000,000 G/D
Industrial Water Rate $.85 per 100 cubic feet.

SEWER Metropolitan Waste Control Commission 27.28
Capacity of Sewage Treatment Plant 350,000,000 G/D
Average Demand 216,000,000 G/D   Peak Demand 350,000,000 G/D
Sewer Use Charge:
$1.10 per 100 cubic feet.

ELECTRICITY
Electric Service Northern States Power Company
Contact 612-330-6255

GAS
Gas Service Minnegasco
Contact 612-372-4659

TELEPHONE
Telephone Co. Northwestern Bell Telephone Company

COMMUNITY SERVICES

Number of Hotels 27 Total Rooms 7,961   Number of Motels 8 Units 817
Hospital Beds 6,600 Nursing Home Beds 4,435 Doctors 4,700 Dentists 975
Nearest Hospital 13 in Minneapolis 33 in metro area

Number of Churches — Protestant 270 Catholic 32 Jewish 8 Other 5
Main Cultural Attractions & Festivals Guthrie Theater, Walker Art Center, Mpls Institute of Art, Mn Orchestra, Swedish Institute, Bell Museum of Natural History, Children's Theatre, Orpheum, Planetarium, Hennepin Ctr. for the Arts.

Parks and Playgrounds — Municipal 155 State ___ Private ___
Golf Courses — Municipal 5 Private 10 Tennis Courts 400 Swimming Pools ___
*Sports — College yes Professional football baseball hockey soccer

News Media — Papers 2 daily 8 weekly Radio Stations 25 AM 19 FM
Meeting Facilities — Total 225 Capacity of Three Largest 9,000 8,000 2,500
Retail Sales — County $ 8,012,831,219 (1983) City $
Per Capita Income — County $ 14,342 (1982)

Names of Banks/S&L/deposits for each Minneapolis bank clearings, as measured by Ninth District Federal Reserve Bank, averaged $8.2 billion per month in 1983.
*156 banks and 165 saving and loan branch offices; 7 home offices

Public Libraries — Local yes County yes Regional yes Bookmobile yes
Post Office first class Express Mail Service yes

Service Organizations: Membership
all major service organizations

EDUCATION

	Number	Enrollment	Grades Included
Elementary Schools	27	19,722	K-6
Junior High Schools	6	9,059	7-8
Senior High Schools	7	8,787	9-12
Parochial Schools	0	0	
Private Schools	0	0	

Pupil to Teacher Ratio — Elementary 26.6/1 High School 25.9/1
% High School going to College ___%   % College Graduates ___%
Nearest Area Vocational Training Institute Seven Metropolitan Area AVTI's
AVTI Training Specialty:
Wide variety of courses, contact city or AVTI for listings Distance ___ miles
Nearest Community College Minneapolis Community College Distance ___ miles
*Nearest University 4 year; 19 colleges and universities Distance ___ miles

(Pub.372)

CLIMATE 27.28

Coldest Month January
    Mean Daily Max 21 °F
    Mean Daily Min 3 °F

Number of days between killing frosts 166
Average Annual Snowfall 40 inches

Hottest Month July
    Mean Daily Max 83 °F
    Mean Daily Min 61 °F

Number of days above 90 degrees 17
Average Annual Precip. 26 inches

INDUSTRIAL SITES

Site No. Washington Ind. Park
Acres Available 200 acres
Site Owner Mpls. Comm. Dev. Agency
Option Held by Development Group no
Site Zoned yes   In City Limits yes
If not in city,   miles from city
Services at site:
    rail   sanitary sewer
    electricity   storm sewer
    gas   curb and gutter
    treated water paved roads

Site Northeast River Ind. Park
Acres Available 38 acres
Site Owner Mpls. Comm. Dev. Agency
Option Held by Development Group no
Site Zoned yes   In City Limits yes
If not in city,   miles from city
Services at Site:
    rail   sanitary sewer
    electricity   storm sewer
    gas   curb and gutter
    treated water paved roads

LOCATION SERVICES

Name of Local Development Corporation:
Minneapolis Community Development Agency

Chamber of Commerce Manager yes

COMMUNITY CONTACTS:

Donald Risk
Minneapolis Community Dev. Agency
331 Second Avenue S., Midland Sq.
Minneapolis, Mn 55401
612-348-7116

Business Information Department
Greater Minneapolis Chamber of
  Commerce
15 South Fifth Street
Minneapolis, Mn 55402
612-370-9164

INCENTIVES:
Minneapolis has 49 parochial/private schools with an enrollment of 9,213, grades K-12.

REMARKS:
* Seven County Metropolitan Area Statistics

Minnesota Department of Energy and Economic Development
Economic Development Division
900 American Center Building, 150 E. Kellogg Boulevard
St. Paul, Minnesota 55101   612-296-5022

Prepared 6/ 1/1985
Senate District:
57 thru 62
House District:
57a&b - 62 a&b

FIG. 1-1. This type of community profile information is generally available through state agencies, usually the department of economic development. Contact city hall or the local chamber of commerce. These offices will be able to direct you to the specific agency in the area that can provide population and employment statistics.

(Pub.372)

[1] Hospital Administrators

Meet with the local hospital administrators. They are business people who generally know whether another physician is needed in your area. Hospitals must have enough physicians on staff in order to survive. It is not uncommon for a hospital to assist a physician in launching a practice if the hospital needs a physician in a particular specialty. This might include both promotional and financial aid. Such aid has been provided by hospitals in small towns in which there is dire need of particular specialists, and by metropolitan area hospitals in order to bring more patients into their hospitals.

Community groups are another source of potential promotional and financial assistance in starting your practice. This is particularly true in areas where there are not enough physicians.

[2] Industry

It is also important to learn about the major employers in an area. This can be done by telephoning the chamber of commerce. It is financially safer to begin a practice in an area in which there is industrial diversification. If a community is dependent upon one major employer or industry, disaster can strike at any time. Layoffs will result not only in loss of income for the employees, but also in a loss of medical insurance benefits. For example, in one town in northern Michigan, one physician's collection percentage dropped from 95 percent to 60 percent in 12 months when a major employer left town.

[3] Third Party Health Coverage

Numerous types of third party health coverage are available to community residents. You will have to decide whether to become a participant in any of these plans or, if not, whether their competition will make establishing a practice difficult.

Health Maintenance Organization (HMO)—Open and Closed Panel: Health Maintenance Organizations attempt to control health care costs by rewarding physicians for cost effective utilization of medicine. This is done through a method of reimbursement called capitation through which a physician receives a set amount based on the number of patients in the practice. This is in contrast to the traditional fee-for-service method, which pays the physician for services performed.

A closed panel Health Maintenance Organization refers specifically to one in which enrolled patients must receive all of their care at that specific organization. Usually the physicians involved are employees of the HMO. Private practitioners are not involved with closed panel HMOs, and in any event, the patient does not have the option to see physicians outside of the specific organization. Sometimes consultants will work for closed panel HMOs. If this is the case, the consultants' fees are paid by the HMO out of the capitated income. The closed panel HMO will avoid referring business to physicians who are not its employees. The cost of referring a patient to a non-employee physician must be paid by the HMO out of the HMO's capitated income.

An open panel Health Maintenance Organization, commonly referred to as an IPA or Independent Practice Association, is a network of physicians (see below).

Preferred Provider Organization (PPO): The PPO is a new type of organization built on a network of private practicing physicians, hospitals and other health care providers. A PPO has open enrollment, which means that a physician new to a community has an opportunity to become a member of the PPO network. However, it is possible that a PPO would cease to allow new members, or only allow members on a limited basis, should it become beneficial for it to do so. PPO physicians are paid on a fee-for-service basis. The PPO has a tight peer review and requires that participating physicians work at a discounted fee. Patients who purchase insurance with a company affiliated with the PPO are given the option to use either the PPO network or physicians outside the PPO network. However, the PPO policies are generally structured to allow the patient to pay less when using PPO doctors.

Independent Practice Associations (IPA): IPAs are a network of private practitioners functioning as a group in a form of HMO medicine. Generally, an IPA has a third party that acts as a clearinghouse by taking the risk and receiving the capitated income. Members of the IPA are reimbursed on a fee-for-service basis. Usually, a portion of the fee for service is withheld from the physician and put into a risk pool. If the physician demonstrates cost-effective medicine and the IPA has economic success, the physician is rewarded financially through that pool. If the cost for treatment of the physician's patients is in excess of the average, he or she is generally penalized by not being awarded a share of the withholding. For the patient, the IPA is different than the PPO, since the patient may not seek medical services from physicians outside of the IPA network. IPAs compete more with the HMOs and generally have stricter cost containment policies.

Blue Cross/Blue Shield: The Blue Cross/Blue Shield program has been a major third party in health care for many years. Most physicians are aware of the Blue Cross/Blue Shield programs and many participate. Because patients with Blue Cross/Blue Shield coverage may go to participating or non-participating hospitals, the program resembles a PPO. Today, many of the Blue Cross/Blue Shield programs across the country have adopted and administer official PPO groups.

Other Major Private Insurers: In many areas, a particular industry dominates the employment market and, as a result, the insurance policy provided through that employer will dominate the health care field. If there is a major policy in the area where you decide to open a practice, you should review it for benefits and limitations.

Other third parties would include Medicare, Medicaid and small private insurers. You may be able to obtain from the hospital a breakdown of the percentage of business derived from each of the various third parties.

Pay particular attention to the HMOs, PPOs and IPAs. These organizations may be open or closed panels. For example, if a closed panel organization has 45 percent of the market share of population, you automatically lose that 45 percent as potential patients. If the organization is open panel, you need to know what type of potential discount they expect from you as well as the type of restrictions they will place on your medical practice. If a significant number of patients are covered under Medicare and Medicaid, it should be kept in mind that the government does not provide full coverage for services rendered; currently it is attempting to take full control of physician's fees and services in these areas.

[4] Banks

In a metropolitan area make appointments to visit a number of bankers. Most large banks have special procedures or departments to serve professionals. Your initial visits are not to secure financing, but to meet local businessmen, to get a sense of the current business climate and to learn about the bankers' experiences with physicians who have recently started practice.

After careful study of all the above considerations, you will have enough data to make an intelligent decision about selecting the location. Before you start your practice, you will be armed with both the positive and negative aspects of the particular community. The suggested worksheet below may be used to compare the various locations under consideration.

Comparative Worksheet of Locations Under Consideration

Community

Urban Area

Rural Area

Social Amenities

Near Friends

Near Relatives

Quality of Education System

Population

Per Capita Income of Physicians

Ratio of People per Doctor in your Specialty

Reception by Other Physicians (+ −)

Reception by Hospital Administrator (+ −)

Reception by Local Bankers (+ −)

Industrial Diversification

Market Share of Closed Panel HMOs and PPOs

§ 1.03 Choosing Office Space

A medical office should be located so that it is convenient, accessible and visible to the intended patient population.

If possible, the office space you choose should be near home and hospital, and if your practice includes primary care, then near nursing homes as well. This will allow you to make the most efficient use of your time. Ideally, the office should be a convenient distance from the homes of patients and places of business, and have adequate parking facilities. The office should also be accessible by public transportation.

As a professional, you will be referring patients to other health care providers, and it would be helpful if these were nearby. You will also be receiving referrals from health care providers and being in a convenient location will increase your chances for new patients.

Visibility is important. When you begin your practice, how will people see that you are there? Determine what type of signs you want at the office site, and also whether any restrictions are placed on the erection of signs by the building operators. Study the number of people who pass the office site each day.

§ 1.04 Assessment of Space

> When laying out a medical office the physician must keep in mind the scope of the practice and the anticipated patient volume. Considerations range from installing employee bathrooms; having an adequate number of patient waiting rooms; ensuring that halls are wide enough to accomodate a wheelchair; and providing additional rooms for special area needs. Since most new practices grow with time, it is wise to purchase an option on extra space or at least to negotiate flexible lease arrangement.

Although assessment of space needs will vary within medical specialites, the physician's basic needs remain the same. The following list identifies rooms or areas most physicians will use:

Examination Rooms: Physicians generally will need a minimum of two examination rooms per doctor. However, primary care physicians such as those in family practice, internal medicine or obstetrics will find three or four examination rooms more to their advantage. An inadequate number can result in an inefficient patient flow and less productivity, particularly when the office is busy. The size of a typical examination room is between 8' × 10' and 10' × 10' or approximately 80 to 100 square feet. Each room must be equipped with a sink and drain.

Laboratory: Most physicians will need some form of laboratory in which to draw blood and perform certain tests. Internists, for example, usually have large laboratories in order to perform more testing on the premises. A laboratory needs ample counter space,

(Pub.372)

cabinets and a sink, as well as space for refrigeration. A minimum of 60 square feet should be allocated for laboratory space.

X-Ray Room: Both primary care physicans and specialists will benefit from having x-ray equipment in their offices. An x-ray room requires leaded walls and special wiring. The size of the x-ray room should be at least 120 square feet. This should include room for an automatic processor and a darkroom to load the films.

Drug Room: It is advisable to have a locked room for storing drug samples and narcotics.

Changing Room: Practitioners in some medical specialties will find it beneficial to have a changing room, apart from the individual examining rooms. Examples would be radiology or gastroenterology, where patients are frequently moved around within the office for particular medical procedures.

Bathrooms: Most medical offices should have bathrooms within their suites, especially if one is not readily available nearby. Many medical offices are designed with bathrooms located near the laboratory to facilitate the taking of specimens. Bathrooms should be equipped with hand rails and with enough space to fit wheelchairs.

Consultation/Private Office: This room provides the physician with an area in which to talk with patients, do dictation, make phone calls and handle personal matters. A well-decorated and utilized consultation room also provides a positive environment for the patient. Some physicians also use their consultation room as an examination room and have the examination table and sink within the space. This is not an ideal situation, but can suffice if overall space is limited. The consultation room should be approximately 100 to 150 square feet; generally, 12 feet by 12 feet is optimum. This provides enough space for a desk, visitors' chairs, a credenza and book shelves.

Nurses' Station: Nurses or medical assistants need their own space in which to review charts, make entries and answer telephones. This area should be centrally located, but out of the way of traffic flow. A small station would require 60 to 80 square feet.

Reception Area: Patients waiting to be seen by the physician and staff should be provided with a comfortable area. To determine the

(Pub.372)

amount of space needed in the reception area, estimate the maximum number of patients who would be waiting in the office at any one time. Plan on having 15 to 20 square feet of space for each waiting patient. This area should have a counter on which patients can fill out forms. The waiting area should not be situated where the patient can see into examination or other professional rooms. In some medical specialties, it is useful to have waiting rooms for use by patients between procedures. For example, ophthalmologists may have an area in which patients wait until their eyes are dilated for further examination.

Conference Room/Library: In a larger practice a conference room for meetings of physicians and staff is extremely useful. The room can also double as a library and area for physicians to make phone calls or do other personal business, particularly where there is not enough space in each physician's private office.

Kitchen/"Break Room": This is an optional space in which staff can have their lunch or take a break, particularly if there is no other common area in the building.

Business Office: Every physician needs a business area in which to perform day-to-day activities such as appointment scheduling, insurance preparation and accounts receivable processing, to name a few. The minimum size of this room should be approximately 200 square feet. The size of the business area will depend on whether file space and storage space are within this office. If the overall space is small, the business area may be part of the reception area.

File Space: Be sure to allow enough space for business records. In addition to patient charts, there will be accounts receivable files and numerous other important business papers. A properly designed business area will include file space. However, certain records may be stored in the physician's private office.

Storage Space: Ample storage space is needed for both business and medical supplies. Storage space may be located within the business area, the medical rooms or in walk-in closets equipped with shelving.

Mechanical/Telephone Room: Generally, an office will require a space for the telephone box, circuit breakers and possibly a computer. In a large office building, this space is often shared within one area of the building. If this is not the case, this space must be planned for when determining the overall amount of space needed.

Hallways: It is important to remember that a fair amount of space can be taken up by hallways leading to different areas of the office. In planning the layout of an office, the hallways need to be wide enough for the easy passage of wheelchairs. Exterior hallways leading to the medical suite should be 8 feet wide, while hallways within the suite should be 4 feet wide. This generally consumes less than 15 percent of the total square footage.

Coat Closets: You should provide adequate space for the personal belongings of patients and employees, espcially if the practice is in a cold climate. Usually the belongings of patients are kept in a separate space from those of employees.

[1] Specialized Rooms

The following additional rooms should be considered by physicians in the various fields of medicine:

- Cardiologist—room for stress test equipment, EKG and Holter monitor equipment.
- Obstetrician—room for ultrasound and related equipment.
- Dermatologist—an area for dispensing medications.
- Gastroenterologist—endoscopy room and proctology room.
- Neurologist—a room for EEG and controls.
- Orthopedic Surgeon—rooms for cast fitting, whirlpool treatment and physical therapy.
- Plastic Surgeon—room for showing visual aids regarding cosmetic surgery. Consultation rooms may also be designed for this purpose.
- Psychiatrist—consultation rooms that are larger than rooms for other specialties and a group therapy room.
- Ophthalmologist—room for refracting and fitting contact and other lenses.
- Otolaryngologist—audio room for testing hearing.

- Oncologist—room for mixing and storing chemotherapy medications.
- Urologist—room for cystoscopy and radiography.

(For a summary of appropriate dimensions for generalized and specialized rooms, see Figure 1-2.)

Figure 1-2

GENERAL ROOM DIMENSIONS

Room type	Dimensions
Examination	8 × 10 = 80 sq. ft.
	10 × 10 = 100 sq. ft.
Laboratory	6 × 10 = 60 sq. ft.
X-ray	10 × 12 = 120 sq. ft.
Drug room	variable
Changing room (alcove)	4 × 5 = 20 sq. ft.
Bathroom	5 × 6 = 30 sq. ft.
Consultation room	12 × 12 = 144 sq. ft.
Nurses' station	60 to 80 sq. ft. (variable)
Reception area	15 to 20 sq. ft. per patient
Conference room/Library	variable
Staff kitchen	variable
Business office	200 sq. ft. minimum
File space	Variable
Storage	variable
Mechanical/Telephone room	variable
Hallways (interior)	4 ft wide
Hallways (exterior)	8 ft. wide

(Pub.372)

SPECIALIZED ROOM DIMENSIONS

Cardiologist: EKG Room	10 × 12 = 120 sq. ft. (minimum)
Obstetrician: Ultrasound Room	12 × 12 = 144 sq. ft.
Dermatologist: Ultraviolet Therapy	4 × 5 = 20 sq. ft. (minimum)
Gastroenterologist:	
Proctology and Endoscopy Room	12 × 15 = 180 sq. ft.
Neurologist: EEG Room	8 × 12 = 96 sq. ft.
Orthopedic Surgeon:	
Cast Room	12 × 12 = 144 sq. ft.
Whirlpool Cubicle	5 × 8 = 40 sq. ft.
Physical Therapy	variable
Plastic Surgeon: Consultation	12 × 16 = 192 sq. ft.
Psychiatrist:	
Consultation	14 × 16 = 224 sq. ft.
Group Therapy	16 × 18 = 288 sq. ft.
Ophthalmologist:	
Refracting and Fitting Room	10 × 12 - 120 sq. ft.
Otolaryngologist: Audio Room	11 × 12 = 132 sq. ft.
Oncologist: Chemotherapy	6 × 10 = 60 sq. ft.
Urologist:	
Cystoscopy with no Radiology	12 × 11 = 132 sq. ft.
Cystoscopy with Radiology	12 × 18 = 216 sq. ft.

[2] Planning for Size

How large or small will the initial practice be? A plan which addresses initial immediate needs will keep overhead low, have lower leasehold costs and lower monthly rental payment. In the long run, however, this may prove more expensive because it may hinder the growth of the practice and require a premature move to a new space. Therefore, planning the initial office may also require planning for growth.

Estimate how many physicians will practice in the office during the first term of the lease. If the practice becomes so successful that it outgrows the space, then clearly you will be in a position to afford additional space. The following ideas will help to maximize your future options:

- Take an option on adjacent space and have it incorporated into your lease.
- If you lease extra space, do not decorate or equip rooms in the suite which will not be used immediately.
- Secure an option to terminate your lease at various points of time. Alternatively, some landlords may agree to find additional space within the building or agree to terminate your lease if they cannot do so.

Once the the number and types of rooms needed have been determined, you will be able to start seeking a specific suite. If it is a space in a medical facility or a previous medical facility, then you will not need to worry about designing a layout. However, if this is not the case, you will first need to locate space and then sketch out a basic office layout.

§ 1.05 Creating a Layout

Sketching a detailed layout of an office on paper can help a physician to visualize optimal spacing in both pre-existing and yet-to-be-built facilities. Layouts should be sketched to scale, detail all unchangeable space such as walls and windows, and be understandable to the contractor.

Before meeting with a contractor or architect it is a good idea to prepare a layout of the office as it helps to focus your thinking and forces you to consider all options. An office layout is sketched on quarter-inch-square graph paper. First the outside perimeters of the walls are drawn to scale. Each quarter-inch square should represent one foot of space. Unchangeable space, such as walls, should be sketched in, along with the windows and the outside door.

Indicate the potential location for each room on the layout plan, keeping the laboratory and nurses' station near the examination rooms. Preferably the business office should be adjacent to the reception area. If possible, design the space with a private entrance. Both business furniture and equipment should be drawn on the layout in order to insure that adequate space will be provided for medical equipment.

After the initial plan has been completed, meet with a general

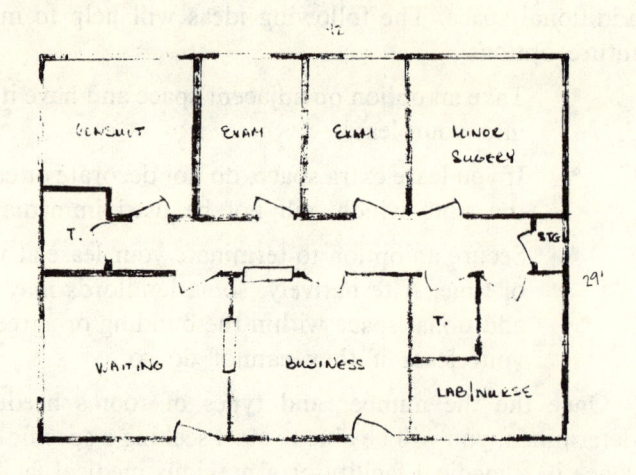

§ 1.06 MANAGING YOUR MEDICAL PRACTICE 1–20

FIG. 1-3. Sample office layout for a single physician practice. Note, as for Figures 1-4 and 1-5, that the layouts have been drawn to scale on graph paper, with each square equal to a distance of two feet. By laying out the office in this fashion, the physician will be able to give the architect a good idea of what is needed. Specific rooms can be also drawn to a larger scale, if necessary. Furniture can then be cut out on graph paper and moved around on the diagram to give the physician a better idea of placement of specific office furniture and equipment.

contractor or architect who has experience in the medical field and discuss the layout. Many medical office buildings will already have their own general contractor who will be extremely familiar with the layout design of medical practices. In such cases, it will not be necessary to use an architect. However, if the plan is to design an entire building, then it would be prudent to retain an experienced architect to prepare the final plan and oversee the entire project.

§ 1.06 Lease Arrangements

The lease for a medical office should detail physician rights and responsibilities as a tenant, the length of the lease, the cost, leasehold improvements allowed and any special contingencies regarding taxation, subleasing and options to renew or terminate the lease.

(Pub.372)

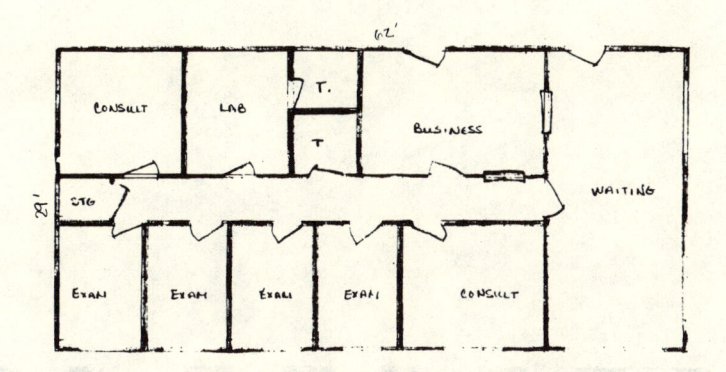

FIG. 1-4. Sample layout for a one- to two-physician practice. (See text accompanying Figure 1-3.)

Before signing any legal document, including an office lease, have your attorney review it. However, prior to contacting an attorney, there are a number of items you should be aware of.

The Length of the Lease: Generally, if landlords intend to make substantial improvements to a facility, they will seek a long-term lease. However, as a tenant, it is more beneficial for you to obtain a shorter term lease with an option to renew, and a provision to terminate the lease at various points.

The Amount of the Rental Charge: Today many leases contain escalation clauses rather than a fixed price. The escalation clauses may be based on increases in taxes and utilities or overall operating expenses. Some leases may contain a general cost of living increase. Obviously, a fixed lease price is the most advantageous, but if this is not obtainable attempt to set a limit on the potential tax, utilities or cost of living increases. Moreover an adjustable lease price that permits the rent to be revised on the basis of operating costs and taxes gives the landlord no incentive to operate the building efficiently.

Leasehold Improvements: A low monthly rent is not beneficial if you need to substantially improve the facility out of your own pocket. Because your right to use the property will terminate at the end of a lease, it is preferable to have the landlord pay for the

(Pub.372)

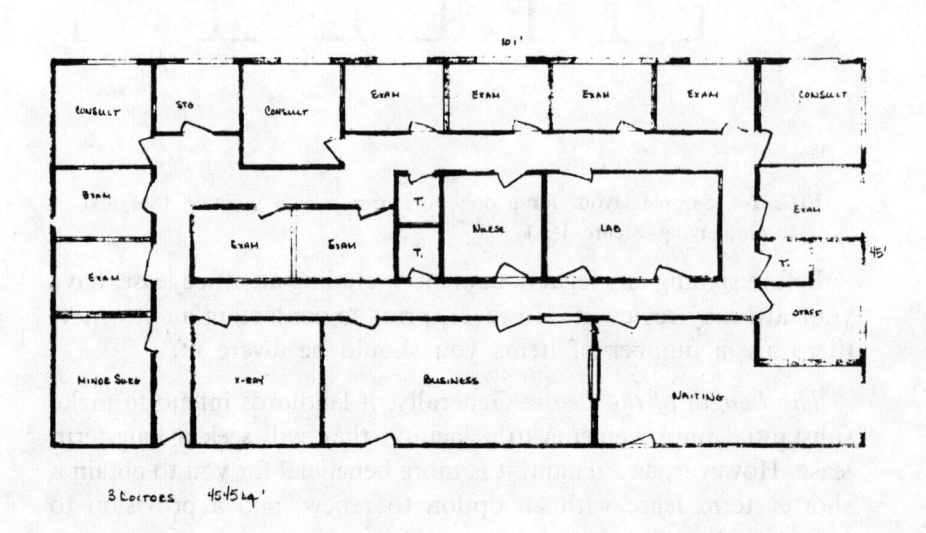

FIG. 1-5. Sample layout for a three-physician practice. (See text accompanying Figure 1-3.)

leasehold improvements. Generally, when a landlord does pay for leasehold improvements, the cost will be incorporated into the price of the lease. Nevertheless it is still more favorable to have the landlord pay for these improvements because it will not tie up your immediate cash or credit lines. Also, you will derive no tax advantage for paying for the leasehold improvements.

(Pub.372)

Rights as a Tenant: Most leases have certain restrictions on the use of the space. Make certain the lease permits the space to be used for medical practice. Also try to maintain the right to sublease the space in the event you wish to take on another physician or need to terminate the lease prematurely.

Responsibilities as a Tenant: Responsibilities range from paying rent on time to particular maintenance functions. However, the lease should make clear who will be required to do the maintenance on your particular suite and who will provide maintenance in any common building areas.

Special Provisions: If possible, there should be a clause incorporated into the lease which would automatically terminate the lease in the event of death or disability. This would prevent a substantial drain on your estate.

See Figure 1-6 for a comprehensive checklist of desirable lease provisions.

Figure 1-6

CHECKLIST FOR OFFICE LEASE

I. Items which should be in the lease:

— A warranty to practice medicine.

— A description of the facility and layout.

— Warranty of the facilities and condition of the facilities.

— A permission to alter facilities without having to restore them to their original condition at the end of the lease.

— Any guarantees of services to be provided by the landlord should be specified.

— The amount of rent payments, the time rent payments must be made and where the rent payments must be remitted.

— The condition the premises will be in (especially if not completed).

— A provision that there will be a warning granted before eviction.

(Pub.372)

§ 1.07   MANAGING YOUR MEDICAL PRACTICE   1–24

- A termination of the lease and a suspension of rent obligations if the building is damaged.
- The landlord should be responsible for maintenance or repairs.
- A provision relieving the tenant of fire liability.

II. The following options should be provided, if possible:

- Option to renew.
- Option to terminate.
- Escape clauses: death and/or disability.
- Leasehold improvement allowance.
- A right to sublease the premises.
- A right to share space.

III. Try to avoid the following provisions in the lease:

- Escalation provisions in the following areas:
  - Taxes
  - Utilities
  - Operating expenses
  - Cost of living
- Any clause that relieves the landlord of liability for damage due to falling plaster, broken pipes, plugged drains, etc.
- Any clause which continues the tenant's liability after the lease has expired.
- Any clause that automatically renews the lease unless you give a notice.
- Unlimited viewing of premise by landlord; limit this to the last 30 days of the lease.

§ 1.07 Space Sharing

Space sharing means sharing the practice and practice expenses in a way that is mutually satisfactory to all parties involved. Space and cost arrangements should take into account rent, advertising, telephone service, the use of office staff, equipment and supplies, and the

(Pub.372)

> division of accounts payable and receivable. Sharing can be done on either a fixed percentage or on a scale that varies depending on the percentage each physician brings in. Termination agreements should always be worked out with partners in advance.

Space sharing is becoming extremely popular. In such an arrangement, one physician is the principal lessee and subleases office space to another physician. A doctor beginning practice will find this an excellent way to minimize overhead expenses and reduce rental costs. Because most physicians do not use their offices continuously, there are certain times of day when the office will be available for use by others.

There are two basic methods for allocating costs in a space-sharing arrangement. One method is an actual cost split: that is, after physicians have been paid, they divide among themselves the actual costs encountered over a period of time. The second method is for a fixed rent to be charged by the lessors who can then achieve a gain or loss from their arrangement, based on the actual operating expenses. The latter arrangement is commonly used when an established physician shares space with a new physician or specialist and where the established physician already knows the overhead costs.

Both of the above methods may divide the cost on either a fixed or variable percentage basis. A fixed percentage is usually determined by the amount of anticipated use; a variable percentage is usually determined by some method of production measurement such as a percentage of the fees or a percentage of the collections. Space-sharing arrangements may range from the sublease of a few empty examination rooms to space sharing of all operating expenses.

For an example of costs divided for shared office space on a fixed and on a variable basis, see Figures 1-7 and 1-8.

Figure 1-7

SAMPLE OF FIXED PERCENTAGE
SPLIT OF OVERHEAD
ONE MONTH PERIOD

January
Shared Expenses

Rent and Occupancy	$1,800
Staff Salaries	2,500
Supplies	2,000
Telephone	400
Insurance	50
Equipment Lease	600
Total Shared Expenses	$7,350

Doctors A and B have agreed beforehand that Doctor A will pay 60 percent of the shared overhead and Doctor B will pay 40 percent of the overhead.

Doctor A's share: $7,350 × 60% = $4,410.

Doctor B's share: $7,350 × 40% = $2,940.

FIG. 1-7. A predetermined fixed percentage method of charging overhead could be used. For example, Doctor A could decide to lease Doctor B the office and staff for a flat $3,000 a month. This way Doctor A would benefit from many cost savings or pay alone any excess costs. Doctor B would be guaranteed a fixed cost under this scenerio.

Figure 1-8

SAMPLE OF VARIABLE PERCENTAGE SPLIT OF OVERHEAD ONE MONTH PERIOD

January Shared Expenses:

Rent and Occupancy Costs	$1,800.00
Staff Salaries	2,500.00
Supplies	2,000.00
Telephone	400.00
Insurance	50.00
Equipment Lease	600.00
Total Shared Expenses	$ 7,350.00
Doctor A's Net Charges	15,000.00
Doctor B's Net Charges	11,000.00
Total Net Charges	$26,000.00

Doctor A's percentage of Expenses: 15/26 or 57.7%
Doctor B's percentage of Expenses: 11/26 or 42.3%

Doctor A's share of Expenses ($7,350 x 57.7%)	$4,241
Doctor B's share of Expenses ($7,350 x 42.3%)	3,109
Total	$7,350

FIG. 1-8. Doctor A's percentage of expenses is 15/26, or 57.7 percent. The percentage is based on Doctor A's charges, $15,000 over the total charges, $26,000. Doctor B's percentage is 11/27 or 42.3 percent. This is based on the fact that Doctor B's charges are $11,000 divided by the total charges of $26,000.

[1] Expenses to Be Shared

In determining which expenses and services will be shared, the following items should be considered:

Name: Will the facility be under a joint name or will each practice be clearly distinguished as a separate entity with use of each name?

(Pub.372)

Marketing: Marketing expenses include efforts by the practice to bring in more patients, such as direct mailings, advertisements, Yellow Pages and other promotions. Will marketing expenses be shared or paid individually? Again, a determination must be made as to whether a shared practice will be presented individually or as a joint entity.

Office Rent, Utilities and Other Occupancy Costs: Generally, these items will be included. There may be a flat charge to the subtenant or a flat charge plus 50 percent of the utilities and other occupancy costs.

Equipment: Will the equipment be shared or will each practice have its own? Usually x-ray and laboratory equipment are shared as well as reception area furniture.

Telephones: Will each practice have a separate telephone line or will one line be shared? How will telephone costs be divided, or Yellow Page advertising?

Telephone Answering: Who will be responsible for answering the telephones? Will telephone coverage be handled separately within each practice? When the office is closed, will a joint answering service be used? If so, how will these costs be allocated?

Staff: Will each medical practice have its own staff or will there be one employer who subleases the employees? Will there be a third party retained to hire, manage and allocate staffing costs?

Supplies: Will each practice keep separate supplies or will supplies and costs be shared? This includes both medical supplies and office supplies such as letterhead paper, business cards, etc.

Patient Records: Will each practice maintain its own patient records or will patient records be commingled in a shared space? Will each practice have a separate charting system or will a uniform charting system be shared?

Accounts Receivable/Bookkeeping System: How will accounts receivable be maintained? Separately? Or will patient billing records be commingled? If accounts receivable are kept separately, will an overall bookkeeping system be used to facilitate the maintenance of the office records?

New Patient Allocation: There should be prior agreement among doctors on how new patients will be allocated. If a patient does not request a specific physician or has not been referred to one, an agreed-upon rotation will facilitate assignment of patient to doctor. A similar type of arrangement must be reached to acommodate walk-in patients.

[2] Termination Agreement

In addition to the above considerations, a termination agreement needs to be thought out at the time the original space-sharing agreement is set up. The following questions should be considered:

- Which physician must leave the facility?
- Which physician will retain use of the phone number? Will each of the doctors need to change phone numbers?
- Will there be any restriction on who may hire the key employees?
- If the practice is under a joint name, who will retain the name in the event of termination?
- If the equipment is shared, who will keep the equipment and how will the other physician be paid for the equipment?
- If the accounts receivable are commingled, who will be responsible for collecting payments, and how will each physician be remunerated?
- Who will keep patient records and what provisions will be made to make copies available to the other physician?

§ 1.08 Equipment Acquisitions

The physician should write medical equipment and furniture needs down on a master list. This can then be taken to a number of vendors for comparative shopping. Financing arrangements should also be worked out in advance.

The first step is to determine what equipment and furniture will be needed for your medical practice. We recommend that the initial list differentiate between medical equipment and business and furniture needs. The following sections provide a checklist containing a sample of probable equipment needs.

[1] Equipment Needs

Reception Area Furniture:

— Reception area chairs
— Tables
— Lamps
— Magazine racks
— Wall decorations, including prints or paintings
— Waste receptacle
— Telephone

Business Office Furniture:

— Secretarial chairs for employees
— Chairs for patients coming in for any type of consultation
— Desks, unless built-in counter space is available
— Standard pullout-type files for assorted business records
— Files for office charts
— Tape calculators (machines that can multiply, divide and store information, as well as add and subtract) for bookkeepers
— Typewriters (generally one for every two doctors)
— Waste receptacle
— Telephone
— Tables on which to place computer and printer if these are to be used
— Photocoping machine
— Postage machine
— Storage cabinet for supplies
— Transcribing equipment (i.e. dictaphones for the physician and transcribing equipment for the medical secretary)
— Wall decorations

Consultation Room:

— Desk and executive chair

___ Visitor chairs
___ Cabinet for private files
___ Bookshelves
___ Dictating equipment
___ Telephone
___ Calculator
___ Wall decorations

Examination Rooms:

___ Examination table
___ Desk chair
___ Doctor's stool and area for entries to be made
___ Hangers and clothing hooks
___ Mirror and supply cabinet
___ Wall decorations
___ Otoscope
___ Sphygmometer
___ Ophthalmoscope
___ Other medical instruments

Laboratory:

___ Refrigerator
___ Stools on which patients and/or technicians may sit while blood is drawn
___ Various supply cabinets
___ Small-size file for laboratory/business records
___ Telephone
___ Necessary laboratory instruments

X-Ray Room:

___ X-ray table
___ X-ray processor/developer

(Pub.372)

Nurses' Station:

— Counter space (built-in or added)
— Telephone
— Pigeon-hole cupboard for charts, charge and laboratory slips
— Rooms for storage and/or adequate shelving

Kitchen/Breakroom:

— Table and chairs
— Refrigerator
— Microwave oven
— Telephone

[2] Cost of Items

Once the initial list has been drawn up, assign a price to each item on the list. Often prices can be obtained directly from catalogues for business furniture and medical equipment. Subtotal each area of equipment. In starting a new practice, it is essential to keep costs low. Therefore, review the list carefully and cross off all items that are not immediately needed. Such items can be obtained later when either their use becomes more profitable or enough money has been earned to pay for them.

Using the pared-down list with prices for each item, examine the specific equipment and models of different manufacturers. In order to get the best possible price, it is better to deal with more than one vendor and to get bids from various representatives. By making bids to various vendors, you may receive discounts ranging from 30 to 50 percent. When possible, select local vendors because they may also be potential patients.

At this point, you will have to decide how equipment is to be financed. Equipment may be leased or purchased. Generally cash transactions can secure better deals on the equipment. There is a large markup on medical equipment and a variance in the initial price offered by different vendors.

§ 1.09 Leasing Versus Purchasing

A number of leasing and purchasing arrangements are available for medical office equipment. Consider depreciation, interest and tax investment credits when deciding whether it is wiser to purchase or lease specific items. Also consider the amount of time over which payments are amortized, since in some instances they can lead to a significantly greater cost than if the equipment were purchased outright.

Many physicians are misled into believing that leasing is better than purchasing because most big companies lease equipment. Sales people often state that while leasing may be slightly more expensive than purchasing, the tax advantages of leasing make it a much better deal. However, many sales people prefer leasing because the company they represent already has arrangements with lease companies, and they can close a sale extremely fast. Some companies have lease or subsidiary lease organizations and profit from leasing equipment, which creates an additional incentive to promote leasing.

Variable rate financing by banks, tax depreciation laws, expensing of capital assets and investment tax credit all add to the confusion. That is, once the proper equipment has been selected, the confusion over financing continues until the physician decides whether to buy or lease.

[1] Financing, Expensing, Tax Credits and Depreciation

Variable rate financing refers to loans in which the interest charge fluctuates based on current interest rate markets; it is typically based on the prime rate. Because the interest rate may vary, it is impossible to determine in advance both the specific monthly payment and number of payments. If the borrower prefers variable payments, the loan may be amortized over a specific period of time, in which event the repayment can go up or down, depending on the prime rate. If the borrower prefers a fixed payment, the number of payments will shorten or lengthen depending on the direction of prime rates.

Generally speaking, capital assets may not be immediately expensed. Most equipment is deductible over seven years. In addition, current laws provide for a tax credit, reducing a physician's tax dollar by 10 percent of the investment in capital assets. Although the government allows expensing of a limited amount of capital assets, the current deduction for which is limited to a maximum of 5,000 dollars, the physician who expenses capital under this rule may not take investment tax credit.

While depreciation is not deductible, the investment tax credit is a true incentive and provides an economic discount for the purchase of business equipment. Current depreciation laws allow for the following percentages to be written off for most business equipment:

Year	Percentage
1	15
2	22
3	21
4	21
5	21
TOTAL	100

[2] Lease Arrangements

A true lease is a method of financing, and is different from a monthly rental contract in which the renter is only obligated to continue with the lease on a month-by-month basis. A typical lease will have a buy-out agreement enabling the lessee to purchase equipment at the end of the lease at a certain savings.

[a] Advantages

The most important advantage of leasing is that a lease will not tie up the lessee's working capital and credit lines. By leasing equipment, the physician does not need to draw upon his or her investment capital or borrow money from the bank, thus leaving the credit available for other purposes.

In many cases, a lessor is able to pass an investment tax credit to the lessee, the physician. This will provide the doctor with a tax saving without having invested any cash in the equipment. Lease payments are currently deductible, and there is no need to keep detailed depreciation records and amortization schedules. Each payment on the lease is a tax-deductible expense.

Lease payments are a constant expense. Variable rates (based on the prime interest rate) are currently the rule with bank financing, and as a result, it is impossible to know the dollar amount of the

(Text continued on page 1–35)

payment each month or the exact term of the loan. The fixed payment of the lease is potentially a good investment if interest rates continue to exceed the assumed rate being charged by the lessor. In the past this has occurred when interest rates have skyrocketed. Occasionally, it may be possible to secure a lease at a below market financing rate because the lessor has not raised the initial rate, although interest rates have increased.

High utilization could cause equipment to depreciate more rapidly than anticipated by the lease company. When a lessor is determining the amount of lease price, the price must include what the life and value of the equipment will be when the lease terminates.

Occasionally, lease companies will provide a contract with "sliding" lease payments. This means lower lease payments in the early months that are helpful to the physician starting a practice.

Generally lease companies are more willing to work with a credit risk than are banks, and occasionally, a lease contract can be obtained, although financing is not available.

[b] Disadvantages

Generally, lease payments are based on interest rates higher than prevailing bank rates. Therefore the total cost for the equipment will be higher, and the lease company will require an additional final payment in order to purchase the equipment. Usually, there is also an advance down payment required.

There is a potential loss of investment tax credit because on leased equipment it is either not assured or unavailable to the lessee.

When leasing equipment, there is no depreciation tax deduction. It is possible, however, to have a depreciation write-off in excess of your annual cash flow. This write-off is possible both in the early years of the acquisition because of accelerated depreciation and expensing equipment, and in the later years because of a slower method of depreciation.

A larger discount from the vendor is usually offered when you purchase equipment outright.

[3] Determining Cost Differences

To compute the cost differences between the lease and bank

financing, a loan amortization book or a loan amortization calculator is needed. To determine the gross cost of bank financing, first determine the amount of payments needed to amortize the dollar amount of the loan over the amount of time and equal to the number of lease payments. (See sample calculation form in Figure 1-9.)

Determining the monthly payments enables you to make a quick calculation on the actual cash flow. Computing the tax consequence of the cost differences will require the assistance of an accountant. Suffice it to say, however, that while the timing of deductions can be different for a lease and a purchase, the overall advantages will be similar and more favorable with the purchase because the investment tax credit will be assumed. It is important not to be misled by misinterpretations of alleged tax advantages.

In summary, then, the decision to lease or purchase should be made on the availability of cash and credit. If ample credit is available through the bank, it will be more cost efficient to purchase the equipment.

Figure 1-9

QUICK CALCULATION OF LEASE VS. PURCHASE

(Example: $5,000 Copy Machine)

	Leased	Bank Financed
Monthly Payment	$126.96	$150.54
Number of Monthly Payments	× 60	× 36
Total Amount of Payments	$7,617.60	$5,419.44
Down Payment	+ 0	+500.00
"Buy-out" Cost	+ 500.00	+ 0
Gross Cost	$8,117.60	$5,919.44
Investment Tax Credit	− 0	−500.00
Net Cost	$8,117.60	$5,419.44

FIG. 1-9. In the example, the physician is looking at acquiring a $5,000 copy machine. The vendor has encouraged the doctor to lease, telling him the

(Pub.372)

monthly payments would be $126.96. At the end of the lease, the salesman tells the physician, he may purchase the copier for only $500. As an alternative, the salesman tells the doctor he may buy the machine for $5,000 cash. The doctor contacts his local banker who says he will finance it at 12.5 percent if the doctor puts a payment of $500 down. The banker informs the doctor that his monthly payments will be $150.54 and the loan will be paid up in three years. While an initial review indicates that it would be less costly for the physician to lease the equipment, saving him $500 down and $24 a month, the completion of the quick calculation form shows that the copy machine will cost the doctor almost $2,700 more if he leases it.

§ 1.10 Financial Modeling

Create a realistic financial model balancing anticipated revenue against expenses. This allows you to determine in advance how long it will take to pay off initial investments and whether it would be wiser to defer some until later.

Before you open your practice and obtain bank financing, it is important to create a financial model, divided into two sections: income and expenses. The income section will show anticipated charges and cash receipts on a month-to-month basis. The expense section will show anticipated capital expenditures and anticipated monthly operating expenses. This is not as simple as it sounds, because the new physician beginning a practice does not have the history on which to base such forecasts. Thus, it is prudent to be conservative on the income side, and careful not to leave out any items on the expense side.

Most physicians beginning practice anticipate greater revenues than actually occur in the early months, and generally fail to anticipate all of the operating expenses. As a result, an inadequate amount of working capital is obtained, which too often is the reason for business failure.

After an initial financial model is drawn up, meet with a management consultant or accountant specializing in the medical field who will have on hand a broad base of statistics from which a more precise financial forecast can be modelled. (See also Chapter 6, Financial Management, for detailed information on preparing forecast budgets as well as samples of financial models.)

(Pub.372)

§ 1.11 External Marketing

External marketing for a medical practice simply means seeking greater exposure in the patient community. It is done through advertising, public speaking and seminars, published articles, community participation and one-to-one contact with other health care professionals and members of the community. Always be on the lookout for external marketing opportunities that are consistent with the image the practice wishes to project.

In the context of practice-building, external marketing generally means active use of specific communications media to attract business to a practice. As with financial planning, you should plan out marketing strategies before opening a practice. Good strategies can be used to improve business for the rest of the practice's life.

[1] Advertising

Advertising is a major external marketing tool because it is both accessible and adaptable. You will have to decide which medium—radio, print, television, etc.—is most appropriate for your practice, and with whom your ad should be placed. A family practitioner, for example, might find a simple announcement in a community newspaper to be sufficient, while a large group practice offering a variety of specialties might find a larger and more diversified audience through radio. Advertising forces the physician to seriously consider who the preferred patient is, in terms of medical needs, income, etc. and what kind of services he or she should offer to give the practice a competitive edge.

Regardless of the medium you decide on, all advertisements should include basic information: location (perhaps any public transportation routes you are near as well), office hours, phone numbers (particularly if you have an answering service number different from the daytime practice number), the kinds of third party billings you deal with, payment arrangements and whatever else you wish to stress. Some common advertising mediums include:

Magazines and Newspapers: Although similar, ads for these two mediums often call for different formats. A newspaper ad should probably be brief. A magazine ad, on the other hand, can be more comprehensive. Likewise, the circulation size of publications in each of these categories will have a bearing on what you wish to say and how you say it. Consult with other physicians and the people with whom you place your ad for what they think would be a memorable and eyecatching ad format.

Yellow Pages: Yellow page ads are a must for all private practitioners. Advertisements should be placed under name, specialty and location headings.

Outdoor Advertising: Outdoor advertising traditionally takes the form of posterboards and painted boards. An advantage to outdoor advertising is that its location can be controlled to insure it is seen by a specifically targeted area.

Radio: A disadvantage with radio advertising is that you can wind up paying for exposure to a market where your services have little potential, since radio generally covers a large broadcast area. For a large practice or consortium of physicians, however, radio might offer ideal exposure.

Television: The average consumer spends many hours in front of the television set. However, a small practice will have to balance the expense of television advertising against the money to be made from the extra patients a commercial might attract.

Direct Mail: Direct mail is a popular form of target marketing that allows you to zero in on a specific segment of the population. It can take the form of an announcement that you are opening a new practice, changing your hours or adding a new physician to your group; a letter informing Medicare patients of a change in Medicare regulations and how it will affect them; or a clinic brochure or newsletter that can inform patients of services provided by your practice or work in which you and your colleagues are involved. The advantage of direct mail is that you are virtually mailing an advertisement to a select patient population. Mailing lists can be obtained from mailing houses, who may also offer to help you to create your mailings.

[2] Public Speaking and Seminars

Health care has become a topic of such interest that you will probably have no problem getting an audience for an informal discussion of topics of contemporary interest. Speeches and seminar topics should be geared to your audience. A speech at a business dinner, for instance, could focus on health risks for executives; at a sports club, the topic could be common athletic injuries; at a nursing home you might wish to concentrate on age-related topics; while in a housing development, family care would probably be more appropriate. Establish yourself as an authority on topics pertaining to your specialty.

[3] Community Participation

Community participation could entail volunteering to provide health care at locally sponsored events, doing public health screening for social agencies or counseling through church organizations. The idea behind community participation is that it introduces you to the members of your community and makes you visible to them.

[4] Published Articles

Articles on topics of interest to a variety of people can be placed with local newspapers or hospital newsletters. However, you need not go beyond your office. Copies made and left in your reception room are just as likely to reach the target audience.

[5] One-to-One Contact

The most influential people with whom you come in contact are the ones who will refer you to other patients. This includes both patients and health-related professionals whom you will get to know as you become a familiar face in your neighborhood.

If you are a specialist you should try to become known among the primary care physicians (they, in turn, will hope that you can provide them with referrals). By becoming known among fellow specialists you can often get referrals for overflow or coverage and by becoming known at the local hospital emergency room you might get outpatient referrals.

Don't limit your contacts to other physicians. Many patients ask other health professionals for physician recommendations. And, of course, staff should always be encouraged and rewarded for bringing new patients into the practice.

(Pub.372)

A lot of your contact building will be a natural function of your standing in the community. If you attend local club or citizen meetings and patronize shops in the town, you'll become known personally to many people as a regular and reliable member of the neighborhood.

[6] Miscellaneous Practice Builders

Always keep eyes and mind open for new and imaginative ways to promote your practice. The possibilities range from something as subtle as a stack of business cards kept at the reception desk to running shadow programs for schoolchildren to show them what the day-to-day life of a doctor is all about. If you are the beneficiary of a pharmaceutical company's advertising campaign, you may want to make free samples of products such as eyeglass fluid or soap available to patients at the end of a visit. The more accomodating you appear to patients, the more likely they are to recommend your services to others.

§ 1.12 Internal Marketing

Internal marketing involves the way you treat patients and associates. Every contact with patients, health care facilities and consultants should be thought of as a way of promoting the virtues of the practice. Courtesy and accomodation are essentials of good internal marketing.

Good internal marketing is a direct outgrowth of the efficiency of your medical practice and the courtesy you show your patients. Although internal marketing starts only after a practice is officially started, foundations for it should be laid in pre-established policies for running the practice. Without good internal marketing, external marketing is of little value.

[1] Initial Patient Contact

Internal marketing starts with the first patient contact. Generally, this is over the telephone, when the patient calls to schedule an appointment or obtain information. Your receptionist should be trained to be prompt and courteous in answering the telephone. The receptionist should always know where you are or where you can be located in the event that the call is an emergency. If the call is routine, the receptionist should know whether it is necessary to refer the caller to someone else. If the call is for an appointment the receptionist should get important patient information and supply the caller with necessary information about the practice, the appointment time and date, and what the patient should bring to the appointment. (For more information on how telephone calls should be handled by the staff, see Chapter 2, Staff Recruiting, Development and Management.)

[2] Patient Visit

The receptionist at the front desk should be familiar with the appointment book at all times so as to be able to greet patients coming into the office by name. After introductions are made and new patient information forms are completed, the patient should be shown where various rooms of the office are located while being brought in to see you. Your receptionist should have a prearranged policy for handling the patient in the event that you are running behind schedule.

You can put the patient at ease by explaining everything that is happening to him or her during the examination. You should give the patient your full attention and not allow telephone calls or other interruptions. Ask probing questions to investigate any patient problems but also listen carefully to the patient's description of his or her problem. In this way you may be able to determine not only the patient's immediate medical needs, but also any psychological or personality needs. If it is necessary to refer the patient to a hospital or to a specialist, explain why and supply the patient with all of the information he or she will need about location, preparation for any tests, length of stay and what forms to bring. You should only refer the patient to a specialist who will provide the same high level of service as you; if the patient is treated poorly by the specialist, it will be a negative reflection on you.

The staff should always try to minimize the paper shuffle for the patient. They should be familiar with popular insurance contracts in the area so they can advise a patient what he or she will be responsible for and which expenses the insurance company will reimburse, and they should be familiar with proper billing procedures for third parties and be able to maximize reimbursement from them. A patient should leave your office feeling that he or she can call you up at any time to discuss a problem or get information.

(Pub.372)

[3] Patient Follow-Up

You should follow up a new patient visit with a letter thanking the patient for selecting the practice, summarizing in layman's terms the diagnosis and treatment plan you have laid out, and inviting the patient to contact you for any clarification. If the patient was referred by someone else, you should also write that person a letter. If the referral was made by a patient, put a note in that patient's file to remind you the next time you see him or her. It is a good policy to periodically send out thank you letters to referring physicians telling them that you appreciate the confidence they place in you.

Referring doctors should receive a report on what happened to the patient as soon as possible. A delay in reporting back to the referring physician can cause embarrassment if the patient or a relative of the patient calls up to talk to the original physician about the results of your examination, only to find out that the primary doctor doesn't know them. Consultants' reports should be promptly dictated, typed and mailed. It is a good idea for you to make a personal telephone call to the referring physician as well so that, if the report is delayed, you can give the results verbally.

A recall system should be established to keep a record of followup services recommended for patients and to remind patients when they should come in for their next checkup. A 4" x 5" card file indexed by month is usually adequate for keeping such a record. Each time it is suggested that a patient come in for followup and the appointment is not immediately scheduled, record the patient's name, date of visit, recommended time of followup, recommended reason for followup and telephone number. Each month your secretary can pull cards from the recall system for that month and contact patients who have not already scheduled an appointment. When the patient is contacted, the secretary should say that you asked him or her to call the patient and schedule a followup appointment on the basis of the patient's last visit. This usually impresses patients with your efficiency and concern for them.

Followup can be carried out beyond the practice as well. It may be worthwhile to have office staff keep an eye out for announcements in newspapers about patients and their families so that congratulations, condolences, wedding cards, seasonal greeting

(Pub.372)

cards, etc. can be sent. You can also note down such things as vacation plans or patient hobbies in the patient's file and discuss them with the patient at his or her next visit. By doing so you let the patient know that what is going on in his or her life is important to you. You may even gain patients by impressing the spouse or parents with your concern for the whole family.

You should encourage patient feedback, comments and suggestions to give the patient the impression you are interested in knowing how you can better serve his or her needs. (A sample patient survey questionnaire is provided in Appendix 1-B.) Always be on the lookout for unusual ideas and unusual ways to provide service to patients that will single you out from the "norm" as an accomodating physician.

§ 1.13 Checklist of Items to Be Considered When Starting a Practice

Information about obtaining the necessary identification numbers is provided, as well as advice regarding important contacts to make before the practice is opened to the public.

— Tax Identification Numbers. The federal number is applied for on Internal Revenue Service form number SS-4, which is obtained from the local IRS office. The federal number is used for identification on bank accounts, third party payments and payroll taxes. Do not use your social security number in place of the tax identification number; this may cause the IRS to flag your tax return for an audit because certain income items by third parties will be reported directly to the IRS. In many states a state identification number is needed and possibly a separate state unemployment tax number. In other states the federal identification number is used and there is no need for a state number.

— Third Party Identification Numbers. These include the following:

— Medicare. Contact the local Medicare office to secure application for a provider number. Decide whether you will be a participating provider or a nonparticipating provider. The former receives payments directly from Medicare, but cannot charge the full fee if it exceeds Medicare's charges.

(Pub.372)

— Medicaid/Welfare. If you provide service to Medicaid patients, secure a provider number from the local Medicaid office, where you will also need to sign a contract. Bills for services are sent directly to the local Medicaid office, not to Medicaid patients. Medicaid determines the payments.

— Blue Cross and Blue Shield. To become a participating provider of services under Blue Cross and Blue Shield you will need to enter into a contract with the program and secure a provider identification program. The physician accepts the lesser of his or her fee schedule or the Blue Cross/Blue Shield customary fee.

— Other third party contracts and identification numbers. These include such health insurers as HMO, PPO, IPA or other private insurers.

— Drug Enforcement Administration (DEA) Number. In order to prescribe controlled substances, it is necessary to obtain a number from DEA. It usually takes a few months to obtain the number.

— Hospital Staff Privileges. Select and make application to join at least one hospital staff and more if in a metropolitan area.

— Bank Accounts. Open both a checking account and savings account for the medical practice, and obtain credit lines. Business income is deposited in the business checking account. Only business expenses are paid out of the business checking account. A separate personal checking account should be opened to pay nonbusiness expenses. Setting up the accounts this way simplifies bookkeeping and accounting. Order printed checks and a deposit book for the business account. The deposit book should contain carbon copies for the bank and the office.

— Set Up a Fee Schedule. Failure to establish a fee schedule will delay billings and interfere with the initial cash flow. (See Chapter 7, Credit and Collections, for more detailed discussion.)

— Current Procedure Terminology (CPT) Code Text. Secure the text of current procedure terminology, CPT, from the American Medical Association. These codes are used in establishing fee schedules, charge slips and all billing which includes most third parties.

— Relative Value Index Text. This index lists procedures and procedure codes, and assigns each procedure a relative monetary value for billing purposes. This book may be ordered from McGraw-Hill Book Company, P.O. Box 400, Heightstown, N.J. 08520.

— ICD.9 Code Text. Obtain the *International Classification of Diseases,* ninth revision, a book which lists the codes for all possible disease diagnoses. These codes are required on most third party billing forms. A list of common diseases and their ICD.9 code should be available in the office for quick reference. Clinical modifications may be ordered from: ICD.9CM, P.O. Box 991, Ann Arbor, MI 48106-0991; (phone: 313-769-1000).

— Telephone Company. Contact the telephone company to secure service and a telephone number. This needs to be done before letterhead, business cards, announcements, etc. are ordered, and before placing any advertisements.

— Yellow Pages. Decide how you wish to be listed in the telephone book and locate the publisher of the Yellow Pages. A review of these pages will indicate the type of listings physicians use in your community.

— Mailing List. Prepare a mailing list which includes friends, relatives, social and business contacts and local business owners. Then prepare an announcement of the commencement of your practice with dates of availability, office address and telephone number to send to people on the list. Some physicians place this announcement as an advertisement in the local paper. A press release may also be prepared and sent to local newspapers.

— Printed Supplies. Order business letterhead, envelopes, business cards and prescription pads.

— Business Insurance. Select an insurance agent to handle insurance for the medical practice. Frequently an insurance agent sponsored by local medical societies will offer a package policy. Proposals may be obtained from more than one agent for comparative purposes. (See also Chapter 8, Risk Management and Insurance, for more information on types of insurance.)

— Charting System. It is important to select the proper charting system because changing it later on will be difficult. One of the best types of chart files is the color-coded, side-tab file, which allows the chart to be established on an $8^1/_2 \times 11$ inch format and provides space for other documents such as hospital reports and medical correspondence. There are numerous types of charts available. Review the ones used by peers and review the standard chart formats offered by various supply companies. It is also possible to set up your own chart form and have it printed.

— Select a Billing System. This can range from a manual to a computer-based system. (See also Chapter 4, Office Systems, for more information on billing systems.)

— Answering Service. Arrange for a 24-hour answering service, one that has experience with physician needs. Call one of the offices using the service in order to hear the way in which the call is handled. (See also Chapter 4.)

— Coverage Arrangement. Alternate coverage for patients will alleviate the need to be on call 24 hours a day, every day. (See also Chapter 3, Forms of Practice, for a number of methods in which coverage may be arranged.)

— Purchase of Drugs and Professional Supplies. Meet with a medical supplier detail person who will assist in preparing a list of needed supplies. Generally, supplyhouses will provide detailed lists of professional supplies to physicians starting practice. Before purchasing supplies make a list of what is desired, then cross off anything that is not needed in the first few months.

— Necessary Office Supplies:
  — Pencils and pens
  — Staplers and staples
  — Paper clips

- Small scratch pads
- Large lined note pads
- Insurance forms (standard and forms for participating providers)
- Typewriter paper
- Scotch tape
- Glue
- Message pads for telephone calls
- Labels for mailing and files
- Large manila envelopes
- File folders
- Rubber bands
- Pencil sharpener
- Liquid typewriter corrector fluid and thinner

— External Marketing:
- Newspaper, magazine, radio, television and Yellow Pages advertising
- Public speaking and seminars
- Articles for community
- Volunteer work and community participation
- One-to-one contact with patients and referring physicians

— Internal Marketing:
- Office efficiency, courtesy and patient accomodation
- Explanation and information given in layman's terms
- Patient follow-up system
- Thank you letters
- Minimize patient's third-party coverage paper work
- Personal patient history files

(Pub.372)

§ 1.100 Bibliography

Anders, G. T., et al.: Marketing Concepts for Medical Practices. Missouri Medicine 79:589-592, Aug. 1982.

Anderson, D. C.: Focusing in Your Market. Group Practice Journal, Jan.-Feb. 1983, pp. 23-25.

Andreasen, A. R.: Nonprofits. Check Your Attention to Customers. Harvard Business Review 60:105-110, May-June 1982.

Balliett, G.: Getting Started in Private Practice. Medical Economics 7, 1978.

Barney, D. R.: Regulation of Health Services Advertising. Hospital and Health Services Administration, May-June 1983, pp. 85-110.

Baugh, T.: Consumer Research—A Valuable Tool in the Marketing of Health Behavior Change. Proceedings from Advances in Health Care Research. Snowbird, UT: Association for Consumer Research, April 1982.

Beck, L. C., et al.: Effective Marketing. Are you Keeping Pace? Pennsylvania Medicine 85:12-17, Jan. 1982.

Beck, L. C., et al.: Practice Management: Effective Marketing Good for Patients Too. Pennsylvania Medicine 85:50-53, June 1982.

Berkowitz, E. N. and Flexner, W.: The Market for Health Care Services: Is There a Non-Traditional Consumer? Journal of Health Care Marketing 1:25-34, Winter 1980-1981.

Breindel, C. L. and Breindel, J. T.: The Marketing of Obstetrics. Health Care Planning and Marketing 1: April 1981.

Brown, S.: Candid Observations on the Status of Health Services Marketing. Journal of Health Care Marketing 3:45-52, Summer 1983.

Brown, S. W. and Gaulden, C. F.: Attitudinal and Behavioral Characteristics of the Patient Activist. Proceedings from Advances in Health Care Research. Snowbird, UT: Association for Consumer Research, April 1982.

(Pub.372)

Bushman, T. and Cooper, P.: A Process for Developing New Health Services. Health Care Management Review 5:41-48, Winter 1980.

Clarke, R. N. and Shyavitz, L. J.: Market Research: When, Why and How. Health Care Management Review 5:29-34, Winter 1982.

Cooper, P. D.: What Is Health Care Marketing? Health Care Marketing—Issues and Trends. Germantown, MD: Aspen Systems, 1980.

Cushman, R. F. and Perry, S. R.: Planning, Financing and Constructing Health Care Facilities. Rockville, MD: Aspen Systems, 1983.

Doxtader, G. W. and Makela, C. J.: Health Care Consumer's Intention to Utilize a Medical Second Opinion. Proceedings from Advances in Health Care Research. Snowbird, UT: Association for Consumer Research, April 1982.

Flexner, W. A.: Guest Editorial. Health Care Marketing. Journal of Health Care Marketing 1:5-7, Fall 1981.

Friedman, E.: Doctor, The Patient Will See You Now. Hospitals, Sept. 16, 1981, pp. 117-128.

Gallegos, K.: A Sampling of Marketing Techniques. Medical Group Management 28:30-32, 34, 38, Sept.-Oct. 1981.

Hauser, L. J.: Market Research (Can You Afford Not to Have It?). Michigan Hospitals 18:13-15, 17, March 1982.

Hilestad, S. G. and Berry, R.: Applying Strategic Marketing. Hospital and Health Services Administration. 1980 Special II, pp. 7-16.

Lovelock, C. H.: Concepts and Strategies for Health Marketers. In Cooper, P. D. (Ed.): Health Care Marketing—Issues and Trends. Germantown, MD: Aspen Systems, 1980, pp. 19-28.

McLaughlin, C. P. and Littlefield, J. E.: Marketing in Practice Management. North Carolina Medical Journal, Jan. 1983, pp. 9-13.

Malkin, J.: The Design of Medical and Dental Facilities. New York: Van Nostrand Reinhold Co., 1982.

Merill, C. W.: House Calls Are My Extra Practice. Medical Economics, Sept. 3, 1984, pp. 189-192.

Merrill, C. W.: Toward a Flourishing Medical Practice: Analyzing and Meeting Marketing Objectives. Michigan Medicine, Nov. 1982, pp. 631-634.

Miaoulis, G., et al.: Marketing Strategies in Health Education. Journal of Health Care Marketing 1:35-44, Winter 1980-1981.

Rodgers, W. C.: Improving and Expanding Dental Patient Care: A Market Research Perspective. Journal of Health Care Marketing 2:34-40, Fall 1982.

Zimmerman, L. and Baker, J. A., Jr.: Marketing Guidelines for Medical Group Practice. Medical Group Management, July-Aug. 1979, pp. 38-42.

Appendix 1-A

WHERE TO FIND HELP: CONSULTANTS FOR THE MEDICAL OFFICE

American Medical Association
Practice Management Division
535 No. Dearborn St.
Chicago, IL 60610
(312) 751-6000

Institute of Certified Professional Business Consultants
221 No. LaSalle Street
Chicago, IL 60602
(312) 346-1600

The Society of Medical-Dental Management Consultants
7318 Raytown Road
Raytown, MO 64133
(816) 353-8488
1-800-826-2264

Society of Professional Business Consultants
221 No. Lasalle Street
Chicago, IL 60601
(312) 346-1600

The PM Group
Black & Skaggs Associates
1190 Camerica Bldg.
P.O. Box 1130
Battle Creek, MI 49106

Appendix 1-B

PATIENT SURVEY

(1) When you initially contacted our office either by telephone or stopping by:

— I was treated exceptionally well.

— I was treated very well.

— I was treated adequately.

— I felt as though I was inconveniencing the staff.

— The service was intolerable.

(2) In your telephone contact with our office, was your call handled promptly?

— My call was handled immediately.

— Quite promptly.

— Adequately.

— I was left on hold a very long time.

— I had to hang up and try again later.

(3) When you first entered our office, how did you feel about what you saw? (Your first impression)

— I was very impressed and pleased.

— Your office is pleasant.

— The office looks typical—about what I expected.

— The office was a bit dull.

— The office was really shabby.

(4) How were you treated by the staff?

— I was treated like a good friend.

— I was treated very nicely.

— I was treated adequately.

— I felt like I was an inconvenience.

— The staff was downright rude.

(5) The wait from when I checked in and when I was seen was:

(Pub.372)

- Exceptionally brief.
- Brief.
- About what I expected.
- Excessive.
- Much too long—intolerable.

(6) The quality of the reception room environment was:
- Very fresh.
- Comfortable.
- Adequate.
- Smelled like a doctor's office.
- Very stale and stuffy.

(7) The temperature in the office was:
- Very comfortable at all times.
- A bit cold.
- Very cold.
- A bit warm.
- Too hot.

(8) Did you feel the staff kept you well informed during your visit? Did you feel you knew what to expect next during your visit?
- I felt very comfortable with the information provided.
- It was adequate.
- I felt confused as to what would happen next.
- I felt very confused and uncomfortable.

(9) When you left the office did you feel you had adequate information as to the status of your health or condition?
- Everything was explained exceptionally well, including home care, prescriptions and what to expect.
- I felt well informed.

— Everything was adequately explained.
— I felt a bit baffled but didn't feel confortable asking questions.
— I felt totally confused and frustrated.

CHAPTER 2

Staff Recruiting, Development and Management

by

Dorothy Sweeney

> **SCOPE**
>
> A medical practice with good, competent and caring personnel will be a pleasant experience for patients, while the most efficiently run office with the wrong employees will be a disaster for patients, physicians and other staff. Good hiring techniques, combined with paying fairly and competitively for a job well-done, good communication, supervision, praise where warranted and criticism where needed, should assure you of obtaining and retaining quality people for your practice. Physician attention to staff performance assures that while quality employees remain, those who are not satisfactory or only marginally satisfactory will move elsewhere. Although the physician should be saddled with as few of the burdens of personnel and hiring as necessary, he or she must follow some commonsense guidelines from the outset and establish consistent routines that can be implemented and updated for the duration of the practice. The amount spent for staff salaries in a primary care practice is usually anywhere from 12 to 18 percent of gross receipts; an expenditure of this size requires the physician-owner's time and attention.

SYNOPSIS

§ 2.01 Types of Personnel
    [1] First Business Employee
    [2] Medical Assistant/Nurse
§ 2.02 Recruiting and Hiring
    [1] Creating a Pool of Applicants

    [a] Newspaper Ads
    [b] Private Employment Agencies
    [c] Public Employment Agencies
    [d] Schools
    [e] Family Members or Friends
    [f] Piracy
   [2] Screening Applicants
   [3] Initial Personal Interview
    [a] Application Form
    [b] Skill Testing
   [4] The Actual Interview
   [5] Review of Applicants Interviewed
   [6] The Second Interview
   [7] Reference Checking
   [8] Hiring
§ 2.03 Salary and Fringe Benefits
   [1] Wages
   [2] Fringe Benefits
   [3] Hours
   [4] Evaluation and Salary Increase
    [a] The Evaluation Process
    [b] Salary Adjustment
§ 2.04 Development of a Personnel Policy
§ 2.05 Creating a Procedure Manual
   [1] Job Descriptions
   [2] Specific Duties
§ 2.06 Staff Management
§ 2.07 Employee Terminations
   [1] Firing
   [2] Voluntary Termination
§ 2.08 Back-Up Personnel
   [1] Temporary Agencies
   [2] Experienced Part-Time Employees
   [3] Nurses
§ 2.09 Federal Laws Regarding Employment
§ 2.10 Checklist for Staff Recruiting, Development and Management
§ 2.11–§ 2.99 Reserved
 § 2.100 Bibliography
Appendix 2-A Tests for General Office Skills
Appendix 2-B General Outline of Job Descriptions for a Two-Doctor Practice

(Pub.372)

§ 2.01 Types of Personnel

A physician must consider hiring both professional medical and business office personnel. Employees hired first must be chosen wisely and paid well if the physician is to establish a base of reliable help. It is essential that the first employees hired get along with one another and work as a team.

The people you hire will perform most of the day-to-day work that keeps your practice running smoothly. These people fall into one of two groups: professional medical help and business office personnel. The criteria you use to select these employees helps set the tone for a general hiring policy.

[1] First Business Employee

Your choice of the first business employee can be critical to the well-being and long-term health of your practice. This person, if chosen wisely and well, will probably become the office manager as your practice grows and adds physicians, other office sites and additional staff employees. You should exercise special care when recruiting for this positiion because the person you choose generally relieves you of most subsequent hiring and personnel concerns.

The first business employee should be able to run all aspects of a medical practice. Someone with a mature outlook (which does not necessarily correlate with age) should be able to handle patients on the telephone and in person, scheduling appointments, billing, fee collection and insurance procedures. In addition, this individual will act as your representative in the commnunity as you build up a practice. This person should be conversant and experienced in third party insurance reimbursement, especially if the practice is just starting out, since physicians new to practice often have neither experience with the various requirements and procedures of the third party carriers nor the time or inclination to learn.

When a medical office is just opening, it is important to create the illusion that it has been operational for some time, even if the doctor is still completing training or other commitments. The first business employee should have a "presence" in the office that helps project an image of permanence and experience. He or she should ideally be hired and working a few weeks before the office officially opens in order to answer telephones, make appointments and organize

(Pub.372)

business systems and supplies. In addition, the employee should be available to handle any marketing or public relations efforts on behalf of the new practice. This may entail sending out letters and announcements, visiting referring doctors' offices or any other appropriate initial marketing efforts. When the official opening day arrives, everything should run smoothly if details were handled in advance.

The first business employee is an investment that will benefit the practice greatly, both immediately and in the future. This employee should be paid the going rate or slightly more from the beginning. (See § 2.03 for a discussion of employee wages and fringe benefits.)

[2] Medical Assistant/Nurse

Depending on your practice and working style, it may be appropriate to hire a part-time medical assistant, or nurse, to work with you during patient hours. If so, that employee should be hired to work only those hours. In the beginning, a full-time nurse or medical assistant is generally not needed.

If at all possible, the first business employee should also interview this nurse or assistant, since the two employees will need to interact well and work closely together. Such a meeting also initiates the policy of a full-time business employee functioning as the lay person in charge. This person can help you formulate a consistent hiring policy and assume much of the responsibilty for hiring and recruiting of future employees. Having such a person in your employ is especially important if you have a large and growing practice.

§ 2.02 Recruiting and Hiring

> Hire with the intention of creating a team that will run the practice, and therefore applicants should demonstrate not just job aptitude but also loyalty, intelligence, good judgment and enthusiasm. Finding the best people for your practice begins with a systematic procedure for recruiting and screening applicants.

The recruiting and hiring of employees should never be regarded casually. An effective recruiting process should find the best qualified and most conscientious people who can be integrated into a "team" to make your medical practice a good and caring place.

You should have a definite, prearranged recruiting process so that when a position vacancy arises, the appropriate people know the routine for filling it.

When an opening occurs, and before the interviewing begins, you should give thought to the type of person to be hired. Each business and medical employee must obviously have a basic level of intelligence and the ability to perform specific job functions. However, beyond that level both the employee's work performance and contribution to the office depend on certain intangible factors that play a greater role in establishing a team than IQ, typing speed, knowledge of bookkeeping or nursing credentials.

Six characteristics to look for in hiring any new medical office employee, starting with the most important, are:

- Loyalty
- Stability
- Enthusiasm
- Judgment
- Intelligence
- Technical ability

Too much emphasis is often placed on technical ability, as it is the most easily tested and readily discerned qualification. Although technical ability is necessary, the other characteristics must be present as well for a person to become a compatible member of a working team. They can be identified only by drawing out an applicant through a structured interview process.

[1] Creating a Pool of Applicants

There are many ways to find people interested in working for you, and as many as are practical should be used to create the largest group of applicants. A practice does not know where its "superstar" will come from, so word about the available position needs to get out to as broad a group of potential employees as possible.

[a] Newspaper Ads

The most reliable and cost-effective way to find good applicants is usually through well-drafted help wanted ads in local newspapers.

(Pub.372)

The want ad should convey an image of the practice. It is not cost-effective, in the long run, to economize by using the cheapest ad with the fewest words if it puts off the most qualified applicants. Headings, bold type, a border around the ad or extra white space around it are eye-catching ways to attract attention.

Compare the image each of these ads projects:

Secretary/Receptionist. Medical Office—Typing needed. Call Sue 234-5678.

SECRETARY/RECEPTIONIST

Growing suburban internal medicine practice needs experienced person to handle all correspondence. Experience needed in typing from dictation tapes. Some patient contact by phone and in person as a relief receptionist. Good salary and benefits. Call Sue at 234-5678.

In large metropolitan areas, ads should be placed in both city and local weekly neighborhood papers. An ad sometimes needs to run several consecutive weeks to be effective.

Opinion differs as to whether an ad should give a telephone number for an interested applicant to call or an address to which a resume should be sent. For most positions in a medical practice, listing a telephone number is more appropriate. Many qualified clerical people do not have resumes prepared, and requiring one could limit your group of applicants. More importantly, a telephone call can help you screen out those who may not have the personality to deal effectively with patients over the telephone.

[b] Private Employment Agencies

Although employment agencies can be a source of good applicants, many perform little or no screening. In their concern for obtaining fees some agencies of lesser quality will refer any applicant, qualified or not, in the hope that an employer will hire out of desperation. Employment agencies should be used as a means of getting the word out to qualified applicants, but candidates from those agencies should be subjected to the same screening and testing procedures as others.

If an employment agency applicant is chosen, be sure the fee structure is clearly spelled out; that is, who pays the agency fee, when the fee is due and what guarantee there is if the person chosen does not work out after a few months. Agency commissions are often very steep, ranging from 10 to 20 percent of a first year's salary. Do not be embarrassed to ask for clarification regarding the fee.

[c] Public Employment Agencies

Government-supported employment agencies, such as state unemployment or welfare offices, typically post job requirements for interested candidates but do not screen applicants. A public employment agency may help fill clerical or minimally skilled positions, but it is not usually recommended as a good source of quality employees.

[d] Schools

Many junior colleges offer two-year business courses, some of which specialize in a medical curriculum. Such schools can be excellent sources of applicants with basic skills but not much actual work experience. Students may have worked in an intern program under a doctor's direct supervision and they may have basic book knowledge as well as the enthusiasm to work in a medical setting.

These schools usually offer free placement service to their graduates. By registering with the placement service, you will be exposed to graduates who have combined scholastic training and business experience. These applicants need to be screened as well, but they are usually good candidates for your opening.

[e] Family Members or Friends

Considering family members or friends of either the doctor or staff to fill the position can cause problems. Although someone presently working in the office may have a good idea of the qualifications necessary for the job and the personality needed to "fit in," the working relationship between employees in a small medical practice is usually so close that hiring a friend or relative is likely create problems for several reasons.

There is the chance that the interviewing and testing processes will be short-cut and that the person's promised technical competence and/or personal qualifications may not be as critically evaluated as those of someone else applying for the position. There is also a greater likelihood that friends or relatives will form informal cliques among themselves. This can be disastrous for both employee morale and working efficiency in a small or moderate-sized office. If a member of the doctor's family is hired, there can be natural feelings of uneasiness among other staff that the new employee is reporting "back to the boss." Even if it is not true, it can adversely affect morale and is not worth the risk.

If the friend or relative fails to work out and has to be replaced, it can cause embarrassment to all concerned. With a deliberate and careful recruitment effort, you should be able to find equally good or better candidates without pre-existing ties to the practice.

[f] Piracy

Sometimes, in an effort to minimize a new employee's training period, a doctor will offer the position to someone already working in the same field in another doctor's office, a clinic or the local hospital, or perhaps to someone who used to work in another doctor's office or who covered for a few days while present staff members were out. Although a "pirated" employee may work out well, there are some important questions to ask before offering a job to someone presently employed in the same field. Why is that employee willing to leave the present job? Could it be that the present employer is unhappy and has suggested that the employee look elsewhere? Could it be that the person's qualifications and experience are not as good as they appear? Or does the employee have technical competence but a personality that is difficult to integrate into a team situation.

Recruiting another physician's employee may be successful if the entire recruiting process is strictly followed, and the applicant is treated as any other and given the same interview, tests and reference checks. In creating a large pool of excellent potential employees, everyone should be treated the same regardless of previous experience. Never short-cut the hiring process for any applicant.

[2] Screening Applicants

The hiring routine should require that all applicants go through an initial telephone screening. This will streamline the interview process somewhat, since not everyone who applies for the job should be given an in-person interview. Some will not meet the basic job requirements or have the proper personality; others will find the salary scale and hours unsatisfactory.

The doctor should not carry out the initial screening unless there is no one else to handle it. Involving the staff in the initial hiring process increases the chances of hiring someone compatible with the rest of the staff. Staff members will work closely with the new employee, hence their participation in the selection process can help forestall potential personality problems.

The manager or office employee who handles the screening should have full authority to decide who shall be invited for an in-person interview. Although there is a risk that a potentially good employee will be missed, the likelihood of creating a good working team by involving everyone in the process is sufficient that authority for this decision should be delegated.

The person doing the screening should prepare some basic questions to ask each caller. These question would obviously deal with past work experience, technical qualifications and the applicant's ability to meet the criteria the office has set. Some questions might be:

- Why does this job appeal to you? Why did you answer our ad?
- What past work experience do you have that would qualify you for this position?
- Our job may require that you be in early or stay late if our hours run over. Would this present any problems?
- While not wanting to pin down a specific figure, what salary range are you interested in for this position?

The same series of questions should be used for each person screened by telephone. Answers given to these questions will determine, in part, if an in-person interview should be granted.

Salary range should be discussed, but it should be kept fairly open and flexible. You need to have a pay range in mind, but it should not be an inflexible figure. Be open-minded enough to realize that an extra 10 dollars per week for an outstanding employee may be the best investment a practice can make.

The person doing the screening should be instructed to pay

attention to questions asked by the applicants during the telephone screening. Do you really want to employ someone who expresses more interest in vacation, holidays, lunch hour and timeliness of office hours than in on-the-job duties? An applicant's responses to questions and the questions he or she asks should be the basis for any further consideration.

The screening process should enable the doctor and staff to selectively narrow down the list of telephone callers to those candidates with the experience, technical ability and attitude necessary to fill the vacant position. The people chosen would then be taken to the next step in the hiring process, the initial in-person interview.

[3] Initial Personal Interview

The initial personal interview should be handled primarily by the same person who did the telephone screening. As with screening, the doctor need not be included in this stage of the interview process. Depending on the number of people involved, the interviews can be scheduled for successive mornings or afternoons as a matter of time efficiency. Interviewing is a difficult process, and the interviewer who tries to handle too many candidates in one session may pay less attention to the applicants who are the last to be interviewed. It is a good policy to schedule no more than three interviews in any one session.

[a] Application Form

Each person to be interviewed should be asked first to complete an application form. (See Figure 2-1.) The applicant's answers should be handwritten, since paperwork neatness and legibility are expected of medical office employees: a receptionist must fill in the appointment book carefully; an assistant must enter information on the chart; an insurance clerk may have to complete some parts of the claim forms by hand. Some of your employees will be required to write notes quickly and neatly in haste or under stress. Since sloppy handwriting can hamper the efficiency of the entire office, a neat and legible handwritten application can serve as the first job-related employment test.

You can tailor the application form to each applicant by deliberately omitting lines and check-off boxes. This forces the applicant to write sentences describing education and work experience, and is another means by which you can ascertain relevant work characteristics of each person interviewed.

In addition to questions about past work experience and education, it is important to ask about an applicant's outside activities and interests. This gives the interviewer something else to discuss besides work when trying to draw out the applicant.

Figure 2-1

APPLICATION FOR EMPLOYMENT

DATE _____
NAME _____ TELEPHONE # _____
ADDRESS _____ SOC. SEC.# _____
IN CASE OF EMERGENCY NOTIFY:
_____
           (Name)
_____
       (Address)   (Telephone #)

EDUCATION: Please list schools attended, years attended and major fields of study. List any degrees received.

WORK EXPERIENCE: List the names and addresses of all your former employers, beginning with the most recent. Please indicate your starting and leaving salary, the reason you left and the name and phone number of your immediate supervisor at each position. Continue the list on the reverse side, if necessary.

What salary would you expect for this position? _____

How would you get to work? _____

Date employment can begin _____

Would you object to being bonded? _____

Outside Interests, Activities, Etc. _____
_____
_____

[b] Skill Testing

Job-related skill tests should be given for virtually all positions that are conveniently testable, such as secretary, bookkeeper and

(Pub.372)

clerk. The skills required for certain other positions, such as a nurse or technician, are very difficult to test except on the job.

A variety of self-designed tests can be administered as job-related skill tests. If most typing for the job will be done from dictation tapes, present a short tape for the applicant to transcribe in letter format. This allows you to test for ability as well as neatness.

An actual bookkeeping chore can be assigned as a job-related test; for example, totalling a page from a check register and preparing an income statement. You can even build in some errors to see how observant the applicant is. Role-playing situations can help you to see how an applicant would handle a busy front desk. Spelling tests are often very telling in the hiring of file clerks.

Tests are a legal and valid measurement of an applicant's ability, as long as they are job-related. With some thought the doctor and staff can design job-related tests to help screen out less qualified applicants in the hiring process. Appendix A includes a variety of sample tests to be used as guides in developing your own tests.

[4] The Actual Interview

Interviewing is never easy, even for someone who does it routinely. Both parties are likely to be on guard, and the applicant is often nervous. An interviewer needs to develop a good rapport with the applicant to discover the "real person." If a casual chat serves that purpose, it should be used to help draw out the candidate. The interview should be the means through which a potential employer learns something about the individual's personality, motivation and general enthusiasm, those intangible factors which often make the difference between a marginal employee and a real "superstar."

Opinion differs regarding the best style of interviewing, but the indirect and unstructured kind is probably the best for assessing a candidate's intangible assets. In this type of interview, the interviewer asks open-ended questions to judge the applicant's ability to express his or her thoughts clearly. Some examples of open-ended questions include:

- Why are you interested in changing jobs now?
- Why did you respond to our ad?
- What do you like best about your present job?

(Pub.372)

- What job duty of yours do you enjoy least?
- What is your present job (or your boss) like?
- What factors in this described job appeal to you?
- Where do you see yourself five years from now in your professional career?

Salary is a natural topic for discussion in the initial interview. Since the potential employee's desired pay range will have been discussed over the telephone and given on the application form, it can serve as a starting point for discussion. Flexibility is advised. You should be seeking the ideal employee who will become a valued member of your working team; a somewhat higher than planned salary might be a bargain for obtaining that person.

For a practice without an office manager, where the general staff conducts parts of the initial interview, the discussion about salary should be left to the doctor when he or she meets the applicant. Too many complications can arise if the staff is involved in a salary discussion with a peer level employee.

The interviewer must be careful not to ask questions that could be construed as discriminatory. Questions about an applicant that are not directly related to job duties, education or work experience should not be broached. While it is permissible to ask a candidate's date of birth, a hiring decision based on an applicant's age could be considered discriminatory. It is not necessary, or advisable, to inquire about the applicant's number of children and their ages, a spouse's occupation, or anything that may be considered discriminatory because of sex, race, religion or age. Most applicants are open and honest during interview sessions, but common sense should be exercised so that offensive and discriminatory questions are not asked.

Immediately after meeting with each applicant, the interviewer should jot down impressions while they are still fresh.

[5] Review of Applicants Interviewed

After all the initial interviews have been completed, you or the person you have entrusted to do the interviewing should review the application forms, notes and skill-test results to choose "finalists."

While care and attention must be given to objective test results and previous work experience, perhaps greater emphasis should now be placed on those previously-mentioned intangible factors. Consider which person best fits into the working relationship among your present staff and whether this applicant can become part of the "team."

Your manager or senior assistant should be authorized to choose the finalist candidates. Since the manager and other staff will work closely with the newly-hired employee, you must have confidence in their selections.

Applicants not chosen for second interviews should immediately be notified in writing. The letter, which should be very short and courteous, should thank the applicant for coming in for the interview, and wish him or her good luck in the job search. It is much easier to do this in a letter than by telephone, and basic fairness calls for such letters to be sent promptly so applicants are not left wondering about their prospects.

[6] The Second Interview

The second interview should include both the doctor (or doctors, in a group practice) and the manager or assistant who did the preliminary work. It need not be as long or in-depth as the first interview since its purpose is essentially to reappraise personality and character traits and to confirm first interview impressions. It has already been ascertained that the applicant has the necessary technical skills.

The job can be explained again with the doctor asking relevant questions about former work experience. Since interviewing is a two-way street, the applicant should be encouraged to ask the doctor questions about the practice to decide if he or she really wants the position being offered.

At the end of each interview, the applicant should be informed that others are to be interviewed as well and that that you will need a day or two to make the final decision. Even if there is a clear choice, no job offer should be made at this interview. The doctor and staff will want to compare notes so that a joint hiring decision can be made, and an important part of the recruiting process, the reference check, will have to be carried out.

[7] Reference Checking

As part of the second interview, finalists should be told that references with their present and/or last previous employers will be checked. You may assure them that you will delay calling a present employer until the applicant has a chance to forewarn a supervisor, but you must insist on taking the step. If the applicant is sincerely interested in the job you offer, his or her present employer will need to be told sooner or later, so any objections should be invalid. The reference check is simply too important to skip and your ultimate rule should be that no one will be hired for any job unless and until it is done.

Reference checking is best done by telephone, and usually on a peer-to-peer basis; for example, if the last employer was listed as a doctor or business executive, then you should make the call; if the person listed was a manager or supervisor, the office manager or assistant should make the call. Discussion on a peer basis tends to be more honest and open in the event that embarrassing matters come to light.

The reason for using the telephone for all reference checks is that a former employer will rarely put something unfavorable about a person in writing. Skillful questioning, however, can elicit answers and revealing hesitations or voice inflections. An answer given over the telephone can be pursued further if it is vague or uncertain, an opportunity not afforded by a written references.

A series of reference questions should be prepared. (See Figure 2-2.) Some should be checked against answers the applicant gave on the application form as a means of assessing his or her basic honesty. Questions about an applicant's potential for personality conflicts with other workers or supervisors are valid and important to the smooth functioning of your practice. Questions about money-handling and bonding are important if the applicant will perform those functions for you. Probably the most important question to ask is if the reference would rehire the person you are inquiring about; even a slightly hesitant or negative response should be pursued further.

Personal references have little or no bearing on an applicant's ability to do the job. In certain instances a potential employer might wish to check school records, but that is usually unnecessary since

(Pub.372)

present or previous work experience is by far the most reliable source of reference information.

If an applicant is a woman coming back into the work force after being home to raise a family or someone who has been out of the job market for some time, reference checking may be a tricky matter since past work experience is no longer timely. In such instances, stability, judgment and similar characteristics might be checked through volunteer work the applicant has performed for churches, schools or civic organizations.

Figure 2-2

EMPLOYMENT REFERENCE QUESTIONS

(1) How long was the person employed by you?

(2) What was his/her starting salary? Salary at termination?

(3) When did this person leave your employment? Why did he/she leave?

(4) What were his/her duties? Were these duties performed to your satisfaction?

(5) Were you satisfied with his/her work habits? Were assignments completed on time?

(6) Were there any personality conflicts with others in the office? How did he/she get along with supervisors?

(7) Did he/she demonstrate any leadership abilities? Do you think he/she could be considered for a position where he/she would supervise others?

(8) Was he/she punctual? Was absenteeism a problem?

(9) Did family or personal matters reflect in work performance?

(10) Did this person handle money for you? Was he/she bonded?

(11) What did he/she do best? Worst?

(12) Would you rehire this person?

[8] Hiring

The person you finally choose should be promptly telephoned and offered the job at the salary agreed upon, and a mutually acceptable starting date should be decided upon. As soon as that person accepts the offer, a short, courteous note should be written to the other finalists thanking them for their interest. They should also be told that their applications will be kept on file for any future openings. Since one never knows when an opening will occur, these people may be excellent possibilities for another job position in the practice.

Most employees should be hired for a probationary period, usually a three-month interval in which both the employee and the practice can decide if the situation should be made permanent.

An assessment should be made at the end of the three-month period. The doctor or office manager should discuss strengths and weaknesses with the employee and solicit his or her comments. If both parties are satisfied, the new employee should be given permanent status. Otherwise the relationship should be terminated for the good of both the practice and the employee. Termination at the end of a probationary period is far less traumatic than after someone has become a permanent employee.

§ 2.03 Salary and Fringe Benefits

> A fair and competitive package of wages and fringe benefits is necessary to attract and keep good employees. Benefits include various types of personal insurance, paid holidays and a policy for sick days, personal days and vacation. A regular routine for evaluating an employee's work and awarding of merit increases in pay should be established.

While many experts say that money is not a prime motivator of quality employees, a fair and competitive wage is necessary to obtain and retain employees. A fair starting salary, annual merit evaluations and a competitive fringe benefit package is essential for a medical practice to maintain quality personnel. Your practice must be able to compete with larger institutions and industry for good employees.

[1] Wages

It is difficult to put an exact salary figure on any position in a medical practice, since the duties for each position vary from practice to practice and different regions of the country use different wage scales. In grouping what physicians should be paying for staff salaries, a good measuring device is what the practice is paying for staff salaries as a percentage of its gross receipts.

The Society of Medical-Dental Consultants 1987 survey gives the "average" cost for staff salaries in the following specialties:

Specialty	Percentage of Gross Receipts
Allergy	19.3
Anesthesiology without CRNA	4.3
Anesthesiology with CRNA	18.5
Cardiology	14.9
Dermatology	16.9
Family Practice	20.6
Gastroenterology	24.7
Internal Medicine	17.1
Neurosurgery	16.3
Obstetrics/Gynecology	15.4
Ophthalmology	13.5
Orthopedic Surgery	14.6
Otolaryngology	16.3
Pediatrics	19.0
Plastic Surgery	11.0
General Surgery	12.0
Urology	12.4

Many hospitals make wage surveys available to physicians to be used as a guide to pay scales for employees. In addition, Chambers of Commerce, labor bureaus and various industries all publish salary statistics. While these are helpful reference tools, most practices should not use them as the final word on setting a salary. Employers who release these statistics are usually larger than a private practice, and have higher salary levels. (For example, hospitals often need to pay higher wages in order to attract employees for shift work, weekend and holiday duties, etc.)

Physicians should determine salaries based on factors such as the employee's position in the practice, what percentage of gross receipts goes toward the payroll, what other physicians' offices in the area are paying and what the practice can afford.

[2] Fringe Benefits

In today's environment, fringe benefits are almost as important as salary. If your practice is to stay competitive in obtaining or retaining employees, it must offer a fairly standard set of fringe benefits, including:

Health Insurance: Paid Blue Cross/Blue Shield or other comparable health insurance is common. Single, rather than family, coverage is provided for those who need it. (If an employee is covered under a spouse's policy, the coverage is not provided.) Major medical insurance is often provided, especially in an incorporated practice when it is provided as part of a corporate group package.

Other Insurance: Depending on the physician's preferences, long-term disability insurance and life insurance may be provided, although they are not as common as basic health insurance.

Vacations: Usually, no vacation time is awarded until the employee completes six months of service, after which time he or she is entitled to one week. Thereafter, a typical scale is as follows:

- 1 to 5 years: 2 weeks
- 5 to 10 (or 15) years: 3 weeks
- over 10 (or 15) years: 4 weeks

The amount awarded for years of service varies with the wishes of the physician(s), size of the practice and custom of the area.

Sick Days: Most practices base the number of paid sick days on years of service. For simplicity and clarity, it is best to match the number of paid sick days with the number of vacation days. Thus, paid sick days normally provided are:

- up to 6 months: 0 days
- 6 to 12 months: 5 days
- 1 to 5 years: 10 days
- 5 to 10 (or 15) years: 15 days
- over 10 (or 15) years: 20 days

Since sick days should only be used for an employee's illness, it is recommended that unused sick days neither be paid for nor allowed to accumulate from year to year. Any abuse of sick days should be reflected in the employee's salary evaluation.

Personal Days: A number of practices allow employees who have completed at least one year of service several personal days in each calendar year. These days are usually discussed in advance and used however the employee wishes.

Holidays: Most medical practices are closed and offer paid holidays for:

New Year's Day
Memorial Day
Fourth of July
Labor Day
Thanksgiving
Christmas

Of course, local customs and physician preferences may add to this list.

Fringe benefits should be provided for all full-time employees, that is, employees working at least 35 to 40 hours a week. However, it is important to provide vacation, sick days and holidays for regular part-time employees too, since many quality employees work less than full time in nursing, clinical and clerical activities. Regularly scheduled part-time employees should receive proportionately less fringe benefits than a full-time employee. An employee working three days each week, for example, would be entitled to three-fifths of the fringe benefits. Occasional employees, such as "temporaries," are not entitled to any fringe benefits at all, and only full-time employees are entitled to insurance.

[3] Hours

Federal and state laws limit the number of hours a person may work without receiving overtime pay. The rule, simply stated, is this: An employee must be paid time and one half for over 40 hours of work in a so-called work week. A promise of compensatory time off given in a different work week will not count.

Unless the work can be done by no other person, very few employees in a medical office are exempt from wage and hour laws. An office manager, for example, would be exempt only if over 80 percent of the time required of him or her is actually spent managing the office. Routine duties such as bookkeeping, filing or work at the reception desk would not count toward employee exemption. Even a registered nurse would not be exempt from overtime pay unless the bulk of the work can be performed only by an RN—which is not usually the case in most medical practices.

Although such a policy appears to run contrary to the professional attitude required of medical personnel—that is, patients must be serviced even if the work hours stretch beyond the norm—it is the law, and it is actively enforced by wage and hour audits. It is unprofessional to say that employees should leave as soon as their hours are up even if patients still need to be seen; at the same time it is necessary for you to comply with wage and hour laws.

To protect yourself against any charge of wage and hour rule violations brought either by an audit or a disgruntled employee, employees should fill out a time sheet each week that states the number of hours they have worked. (See Figure 2-3.) This sheet becomes the basis for preparing payroll checks, with hours up to 40 paid at straight time and hours over 40 paid at the time and one-half rate. Larger practices may find it feasible to install a time clock to maintain proper records.

A word of warning: Be sure not to create a false set of economics by getting so concerned about keeping each employee's hours under forty in each week that necessary work is not accomplished.

Figure 2-3

SAMPLE EMPLOYEE TIME-SHEET

Employee: _____
Week of: _____

Number of hrs. worked:
Mon. Tues. Wed. Thurs. Fri. Sat. Sun.

____ ____ ____ ____ ____ ____ ____

Total Hrs: _____
Signature: _____

Payroll: Number hrs. straight time: _____
Number hrs. at 1 1/2: _____
Total hrs. worked: _____

[4] Evaluation and Salary Increase

One of the most significant employee motivators is consistent and valid evaluation, with salary increases based strictly on merit. An employee who knows that good job performance will be rewarded by an evaluation and pay increase based on merit is more likely to perform well than an employee who knows everyone will get the same increase, regardless of performance.

Employees will probably not be motivated if all you offer is a cost of living raise, in which once again everyone receives the same percentage of increase in salary. Awarding marginal employees the same increase as the better employees is unfair. This flat increase often arises from the doctor's belief that it is easier to implement and that uniform salary increases will spare employees' feelings.

[a] The Evaluation Process

Each employee's performance needs to be evaluated at least once a year, either on the anniversary date of hire or else on a set date when everyone's performance is reviewed and salaries are adjusted. It is often more effective to do this only once, and thus assure that nobody is missed in the process.

Evaluations should be handled by the doctor(s) and the office manager (if there is one). The employee's strengths and weaknesses should be discussed, and the employee should be given time to share his or her thoughts about the job duties and practice in general and make suggestions for improvements or changes in procedures. An evaluation session should be a good two-way discussion that enables both parties to exchange ideas.

[b] Salary Adjustment

As part of the evaluation process, there should be a discussion about salary adjustment. An efficient method is to budget at the beginning of the year the amount of staff salary increases you can afford. That amount should then be apportioned to the employees strictly on a merit basis: the best employees would thus receive a good increase; average employees would receive an average increase; marginal employees would receive little or no increase in wages. This apportionment should be communicated to each employee so that the people know they are receiving an increase based on merit for a job well done. If an employee realizes that poor performance will directly affect salary, then one of two things will happen: the employee will improve his or her performance, in the hope of receiving a higher raise; or the employee will face the fact that there is no future in the practice and move on. Either option will prove beneficial to the practice.

Evaluation sessions take time from a busy practice and require planning and thought, yet they motivate good employees and create a good working relationship.

§ 2.04 Development of a Personnel Policy

A written personnel policy should be given to every new employee. It should cover all aspects of being an employee of the practice, including wage and benefit specifications and grounds for disciplinary action or dismissal. Employees should sign a statement to the effect that they understand the policies and will abide by the terms.

All too often confusion, dissatisfaction and a feeling of unjust treatment of employees develops from lack of a formal personnel policy. Typically, when a physician starts a practice, he or she will prefer not to consider ll of the potential problems and hope to solve each problem as it arises. Because the physician generally starts out with only one or two employees, he or she may feel there is no need to develop a formal policy regarding what holidays will be given, what vacation pay will be given, when salary reviews will be done, etc.

Unfortunately, failure to adopt a comprehensive policy can lead to bad feelings among employees and between the employees and physician. Before the first employee is hired, a personnel policy should be developed. It is recommended that this be a written policy that can be copied and given to each new employee. As the practice grows, amendments and addenda may be added. Figure 2-4 provides a suggested framework for a comprehensive office personnel policy.

Recently, it has been a trend among state courts to treat employee personnel policies as binding employment contracts. Owing to recent cases pertaining to personnel policies, physicians should learn how to protect themselves against exposure to potential litigation problems and have their personnel policy periodically reviewed by legal counsel ensuring that it does not put the employer in a dangerous position.

The introduction section of the personnel policy should contain the explanation that information contained in the personnel policy is a general statement of the employer's current policy and procedures. Generally, the introduction includes a specific statement to the effect that the employer reserves the right to terminat the employment relationship at will, and that the employment relationship between the organization and the employee is not for any fixed term. In addition, the employer should reserve the right to modify and interpret the policy at his or her sole discretion.

Figure 2-4

PERSONNEL POLICY MANUAL

Forward

In this section, state:

- The importance of reading the policy.

- Whom the employees should seek out for clarification of the policy. This would generally be the office supervisor (although in a small office this may be the doctor).

- The importance of the employee keeping the policy on hand and referring to it for questions about office policy.

Introduction and Welcome

This section should include:

- An emphasis that the policy is for both new and long-term employees.

- An explanation that the policy is intended to outline the benefits, privileges, duties, rules and responsibilities for each employee.

- Encouragement of suggestions and constructive criticism.

- An emphasis on office policy, i.e., to give the best possible service and care to patients.

Orientation and Training

This section should include:

(Text continued on page 2-25)

- The length of time new employees are on probation (typically, three months).
- A statement to the effect that during probation the employee's work will be carefully evaluated and assessed.
- A general statement that the employee will be given training and guidance. Whom the employee should seek out to ask questions regarding procedures should be stated.
- An explanation of the process of review at the end of the probation period.
- An explanation of the policy regarding termination during the probation period, contrasted to the policy of termination after the probation period.

Organization and Management

The "chain of command" of the practice should be illustrated and should include the employee's immediate supervisors and whom he or she should go to with problems. Employee suggestions should be encouraged in this section. The purpose and frequency of office management meetings should be covered.

Office Hours

The routine office hours and hours in which the employee is expected to be at work should be listed. The policy regarding overtime expectations when the office is running behind schedule should also be stated.

Breaks

This section should cover the office policy on breaks, including lunch hours and any coffee or rest breaks permitted during the working day. Usually a 15-minute break is granted in the morning and a 15-minute break in the afternoon for full-time employees. In situations where employees need to be covered during their break, the order of priority should be discussed.

Personal Appearance

In this section, cover:
- The importance of looking neat.
- The policy on medical wear (uniforms or jackets).

- The importance of personal cleanliness in a medical office.

Attitude

In this section, emphasize the importance of a courteous, friendly, helpful attitude in dealing with patients.

Telephone

The following items should be covered under the policy of answering the telephone:

- The importance of having a friendly, helpful and considerate attitude when answering the telephones.
- Answering the telephone promptly.
- Properly identifying oneself.
- Transferring calls.
- The importance of accurate answers.
- The importance of following a call through to conclusion and not leaving the patient's problems unsolved.
- The policy regarding putting patients "on hold."
- The policy on personal calls.
- The policy on long distance calls.

Security

In this section, a policy on office security should be discussed. For example, the last person in the office for the day should be sure that the files and doors are locked, that machines are turned off, etc.

Confidentiality

The importance of keeping all items learned from the patient or from the patient's records in the strictest confidence should be emphasized. Employees should be informed that a discussion of confidential information with anyone other than an authorized person in the office for reasons other than office purposes will be considered an invasion of privacy and grounds for termination. The policy on material leaving the office should be discussed in this section. The importance of not leaving confidential information on an employee's desk at the end of the day or while a visitor is in the office should be discussed.

(Pub.372)

Payroll

This section should cover:

- When and how employees will be paid.
- Withholdings from the employee's check (e.g. FICA, State and Federal Income Taxes, etc.).
- Time records required from employees, such as time cards.

Miscellaneous Benefits

This section of the policy should outline miscellaneous employee benefits, such as:

- Employee pension plan.
- Employee profit-sharing plan.
- Bonus programs.
- Hospitalization or medical insurance.
- Life insurance.
- Disability insurance.
- Uniform allowance.
- Holiday bonuses.

Holidays

The following items should be covered in this section:

- The formal holidays which will be considered paid holidays. (Usually, this would include New Year's Day, Labor Day, Memorial Day, Thanksgiving Day, Fourth of July and Christmas Day.);
- Whether there is a waiting period to be paid for holidays.
- Whether there is pay for a holiday when it falls on a nonworking day.
- Whether the employee needs to work the days immediately preceding and following a holiday or have a proved absence to receive holiday pay.
- Whether or not part-time or temporary employees receive holiday pay.

Vacations

In this section, you should discuss:

- The amount of vacation time the employee accrues each year.
- Specifically when the employee is eligible for vacation time.
- The policy on unused vacation time.
- The policy on scheduling vacations.
- The policy on vacations when a conflict occurs.
- Whether or not part-time employees accrue any vacation time.

Education

The policy regarding job-related formal education should be discussed here, including:

- Who is eligible to take days off for professional education.
- Whether days off for continued education will be paid or unpaid.
- Whether the employee or employer will be responsible for paying tuition.
- By whom the employee should have educational time approved.

Sick Pay

The policy on sick pay should cover such issues as:

- At what time a person becomes eligible for sick pay.
- At what rate sick days occur.
- Whether sick days can be accumulated from one year to the next.
- Whether employees will be paid for unused sick pay.
- Whether part-time or temporary employees are eligible for sick pay.

Maternity Leave

Federal law requires that women unable to perform their job because of pregnancy be treated at least as though on sick leave. To comply with this, the office must make maternity allowances as liberal as sick day allowances. It is also possible to allow an unpaid

(Pub.372)

leave of absence for pregnant women, in addition to the available sick time.

Worker's Compensation

Since worker's compensation insurance is required and since this is an employee benefit, this coverage should be mentioned in the personnel policy, along with statements that:

- The policy is in place and employees are covered.
- The employee must immediately report all accidents, regardless of the extent of the injury, to the personnel director if he or she is to be eligible for benefits.

Jury Duty

Since it is necessary to grant a leave of absence for employees who have been summoned for jury duty, items to be covered in this section should include:

- The importance of immediately notifying the supervisor in the event that the employee is summoned for jury duty.
- How an employee will be paid during time spent on jury duty. (Typically, the employee will receive his or her regular pay.)

Family Emergencies

The employee should be instructed to contact the supervisor to discuss the circumstances of any family emergency that will absent the employee from work or disrupt the employee's work. Consideration should be given to the employee, depending on the nature of the emergency.

Funerals

The policy on funerals should cover:

- When a leave of absence will be permitted, i.e., depending on the person's relationship to the deceased (parent, parent-in-law, brother, sister, son, daughter, husband, wife, etc.).
- The maximum leave of absence permitted.
- Whether the absence will be paid or unpaid.

(Pub.372)

- Whom the employee should contact to report the necesary absence.

Absenteeism

This section should cover:
- The importance of notifying the supervisor of an anticipated absence as soon as possible.
- Whom the employee should notify regarding an absence.
- Whom the employee should notify in the event the office is closed, such as in the evening or on the weekend.
- The inclement weather absentee policy.

Performance Review

This section should address:
- The frequency with which an employee will be reviewed. (Typically, this would be at the completion of the probation period and on a semi-annual basis thereafter.)
- When the reviews will occur. (Typically, on the employee's anniversary date or at an annual time when all employees are reviewed.)
- Who will be doing the reviewing and participating in the employee conference.

Salary Reviews

Items to be covered in this section include:
- Frequency of salary reviews.
- Whether or not salary increases are automatic or based on merit.
- Factors considered in a salary review; i.e, performance, job position, responsibility, employee participation, tenure, inflation, etc.;
- With whom the employee should discuss salary satisfaction or dissatisfaction.

Disciplinary Action

Employee behavior or conduct that can result in disciplinary action should be outlined. Disciplinary action can take the form of unpaid leave of absence or termination. The list outlined in the

(Pub.372)

personnel policy would not be exclusive, but would point out areas of potential problems, such as:

- Discourtesy to patients.
- Use of profane language.
- Needless obstruction of work service and facilities.
- Failure to perform assignments or follow instructions.
- Interference with other employees' performance.
- Insubordination.
- Concealing defective work.
- Absence without proper notice.
- Leaving a work station without permission or coverage.
- Habitual tardiness or absence.
- Deliberate actions against the office policy.
- Intoxication on office premises.
- Unauthorized or illegal possession or use of narcotics or other drugs, or being under the influence of illegal drugs while on the premises.
- Divulging confidential information.
- Damaging or defacing office equipment or property.
- Failure to report an injury or accident concerning a patient, employee or visitor.
- Willful violation of safety regulations.

Termination

This section should cover the procedure for resignation or other termination of employment. Items to be considered are:

- Who should be advised when an employee decides to resign.
- Whether or not a written resignation must be submitted (this is recommended).
- The amount of notice required for an employee to avoid losing accrued benefits.

(Pub.372)

- "Housekeeping tasks" to be done at the time of termination:

    Turning in of keys or special equipment.

    Whether or not an exit interview is to be conducted.

    Arrangements for forwarding the last paycheck.

    Notification of insurance companies to discontinue an employee's policy or to continue contracts at the employee's expense.

    Securing a permanent address to which the W2 income tax statement may be sent.

Statment of Acknowledgement

A statement of acknowledgement should be part of the personnel policy. It should acknowledge that the employee has received and read the policy and agrees to abide by the rules as presented. The statement should be detached, signed and returned to the employer.

§ 2.05 Creating A Procedure Manual

> An office can protect itself from the confusion caused by an unexpected employee termination or absence by developing and updating a procedure manual. The completed manual can then be used as a guide for new employees and referred to at a performance review to measure how well an employee has fulfilled his or her duties.

Different from the personnel policy manual, which states rules and benefits, a procedure manual is the "how-to" book of a medical practice. It sets out how each job within the practice functions and how the practice handles items such as scheduling, telephone answering, billing, third-party insurance and fee collection. It should serve as a reference guide for existing employees and as an excellent training device for new employees.

A common employee excuse for not writing down a procedure is "we know how to do all the jobs." That may be true, but the practice that permits this to happen finds itself in a predicament when knowledgeable employees leave and take with them information about how the practice runs.

Admittedly, a procedure manual is difficult to write, simply because a busy practice often does not have enough time to develop one. Nevertheless, each employee should be responsible for initially writing out the portion of the procedure manual that relates to his or her job. The collection of drafts should then be put together by the office manager or senior assistant to form an effective working tool.

A copy of the completed manual with all forms used in the business side of the practice should be kept as the definitive "how-to" guide. The procedure manual should be reviewed and updated at least annually, or whenever any significant changes take place in a practice. Once the manual is written, updating should be the responsibility of an office manager or specific senior assistant.

[1] Job Descriptions

The first step in developing a procedure manual is to develop job descriptions. Every position in the medical office requires a job description that outlines both primary and secondary responsibilities. These job descriptions should be reviewed and changed as job duties change; a job description is usually outdated after it has been in effect for one year or more.

Each employee should make a list of those duties performed daily, routinely or occasionally at his or her position. A list should also be made for those jobs performed as back-up to a supervisor or on specific occasions. These lists should be collated by the office manager (or senior assistant) so that he or she not only creates a formal job description for each position, but also recognizes how each job and each person relates to the others. One of the best introductions to running an office for a new office manager is to create, edit and revise job descriptions.

If the practice creates a new position, a job description should be created for it before any ad is placed or any prospective employee is interviewed. This job description becomes the basis for describing the job to applicants and for hiring the appropriate person.

In addition to providing a framework for the procedure manual, the job descriptions can also be used:

- By the employee for reference.
- By the supervisor to determine the allocation of jobs among employees and to determine the importance of all the jobs being performed.

(Pub.372)

- As a part of the permanent personnel record of the employee. Job descriptions can be helpful in conducting employee reviews and in determining salary levels. If a new description is done annually, it can be compared with that of the preceding year as a method of determining the employee's responsibilities and changes in responsibilities.

Several sample job descriptions are provided in Appendix 2-B. However, job descriptions will differ with each practice.

[2] Specific Duties

Once the job descriptions are prepared, the procedure manual can be developed with specific descriptions of how to perform each job. For example, the medical secretary would describe the exact equipment used, how to use the equipment, where to pick up tapes, the schedule by which they are transcribed and the style of letter the physician prefers, along with a sample.

§ 2.06 Staff Management

> Setting up a chain of command helps to keep lines of communication open between management and employees. Employees who feel management is listening to their recommendations and criticism, and who are given feedback on their contributions at periodic staff meetings and one-to-one meetings with the doctor or supervisor, are more likely to have the morale necessary for a good team attitude.

Following the creation and implementation of an office system, personnel policy and procedure manual, another area needing attention is communication. A common example is an employee's failure to know who is his or her direct supervisor. In medical practices with more than one physician, the employees quickly learn which physician will give them the answer they desire. This leads to the impression that no one is managing the office, especially if physicians contradict one another.

The first step in avoiding this problem and assuring effective communications is to set up a proper chain of command. A simple flow chart illustrating each person's place in the office routine and whom they answer to, from the part-time workers up to the physician in charge, can be copied and given to each new employee. It should show how everyone in the office interrelates and give the employee the information necessary to determine to whose attention a problem should be brought.

Once a chain of command is developed, the employees will be clear as to the identities of their supervisors. Keeping effective communications open between the staff and management then becomes the responsibility of the supervisors. The physicians in charge of or involved in the management, along with each of the supervisors, should adhere to several principles:

Listen to Employees: Actively listening to employees involves listening for understanding and listening without prejudice or rehearsing a response. Physicians and managers working in a rushed or hectic atmosphere who attempt to pass off a problem or concern by only half-listening or half-responding only further confuse an employee. There are several ways to listen:

Ineffective Style—The doctor or manager who never asks an employee's opinion or discovers if the employee understands directions. This listener gives orders without considering the employee's ideas and creates job dissatisfaction.

The Listens-But-Does-Not-Hear Style—This manager will give the impression of listening because he or she appears to be concentrating on the person doing the talking; however, the manager in fact is preoccupied and does not hear what is being said, and never acts on an employee's suggestion.

The Do-Two-Things-At-One-Time Approach—This person glances at letters or telephone messages or writes notes while another is speaking.

An effective manager or supervisor must learn to listen to employees. Listening takes practice.

Give Feedback to Employees: It is easy to give feedback in a pleasant employee situation, such as a good employee evaluation. But in an unpleasant situation—for example, an evaluation of a marginal employee—the manner in which feedback is given can affect the employment situation.

Feedback should be constructive to the employee and used to confront a problem rather than to attack a person. To be credible, criticism and feedback needs to be realistic and specific, and given through clear examples. The use of nonspecific phrases, such as "you always," and "all the time" makes feedback less effective.

Hold Office Staff Meetings: One of the best ways to open the lines

(Pub.372)

of communication is to hold regularly scheduled staff meetings. Depending on the size of the practice, the philosophy of the physicians involved and the situations in the office, these meetings could be held every four to six weeks.

Everyone should attend these meetings, including part-time people (even if it means asking them to come in and paying them on their day or time off). Office managers should chair the meeting and create an agenda.

Some of these meetings could be "staff only" meetings, that is, without the doctors. At these sessions, employees are often more open.

Finally, one or two meetings per year should be medical in nature. At these meetings the doctor can discuss a particular procedure, describe something new in the practice specialty or give some basic medical information appropriate to the lay staff.

§ 2.07 Employee Terminations

An employee's voluntary or involuntary resignation can be difficult in a small medical practice. An established policy regarding reasons for dismissal is necessary.

For a variety of reasons, an employment situation may at times not work out. This can lead to dismissal by a supervisor or voluntary termination.

[1] Firing

Firing an employee is never a pleasant experience, but unfortunately the necessity occurs in most business situations. Incidents of firing should certainly be kept to a minimum if good hiring, regular evaluation sessions and good communication are carried out. However, employees who give a less than satisfactory performance and show no sign of improvement will not benefit the practice.

To protect the practice from possible charges of unfair or discriminatory practices, all employee problems should be recorded in individual personnel folders. Whenever a disciplinary problem is discussed, a complaint is lodged or a violation of rules is noted, a statement to that effect should be inserted in the employee's folder, along with the date and the initials of the physician and/or supervisor.

(Pub.372)

This notation should be preceded by a meeting with the employee to discuss the apparent problem, and the employee should be informed that a notation will be made in the personnel folder. Warnings, putting employees on probation or other evaluations should prompt one-on-one discussions between the employee and his or her direct supervisor or, in a small practice, with the doctor.

When terminating employment is the only solution, it is usually best done in a private session at the end of the week, although there is no "right time." A check for the last pay period, including any severance pay, should already be prepared and given to the employee so that the termination is effective immediately.

The final meeting should also be summarized on the employee's record, with the proper notations and signatures recorded. Keys, identification cards or other items owned by the practice should be collected, and the dismissed employee should be given the opportunity to retrieve any personal items.

[2] Voluntary Termination

Voluntary terminations are emotionally less painful, but generally create more problems for the office, since they often involve the loss of a valuable employee. To protect yourself against terminations without notice, a policy on voluntary termination should be spelled out in the personnel policy manual.

(See § 2.04 for a discussion of what items should be covered in the personnel policy under termination. These items should be reviewed prior to the employee's leaving.)

Many states require that a separation notice be filed with the state in the event of termination. This helps the state determine whether or not the employee is eligible for unemployment compensation and whether or not there is a dispute between the employer and employee over the circumstances surrounding the termination. Questions regarding this procedure can be answered by your local unemployment department.

§ 2.08 Back-Up Personnel

A medical practice, large or small, can be disrupted when an employee is unexpectedly absent, particularly during heavy work periods. Temporary workers or part-time professional medical employees are often an effective short-term stopgap.

(Pub.372)

In a medical office critical attention should be given to those times when the office needs extra help. This could be during vacation time or when the office is particularly busy. At those times the practice needs extra personnel to help carry it through until the work load or staffing is back to normal.

A variety of sources can supply you with the people you need, and any well-run and efficient office should have a set routine to follow whenever a personnel shortage occurs.

[1] Temporary Agencies

Temporary workers from an agency that has a health care division can be very helpful. Also if there is a working relationship with a particular agency, you can request the same employee and thereby avoid having to retrain the temporary worker each time you use the agency.

The temporary agency handles all of the employee's personnel records and tax information, with the practice paying a set fee to the agency. Although this is higher than a normal hourly rate for the particular job, it relieves the practice of a number of potential problems.

[2] Experienced Part-Time Employees

When several medical practices are located in a single complex, the offices often create a pool of temporary people to be called upon as needed. Temporary employees would be on the practice payroll, but because of their irregular part-time status would not be eligible for any fringe benefits.

[3] Nurses

For a practice in need of a Registered Nurse (RN) or a Licensed Practical Nurse (LPN), temporary agencies with health-related divisions may be consulted. However, it is often possible to contact the nursing supervisor at a nearby hospital first. This informal network is aware of nurses who want to return to the job market on a short-term basis.

§ 2.09 Federal Laws Regarding Employment

Every physician should be familiar with and periodically review federal legislation against unfair or discriminatory hiring and employment practices. Penalties imposed by the law, civil law suits and poor publicity are possible consequences of remaining unaware of such laws.

Physicians must be careful in the recruitment and selection of employees to avoid violation of any federal or state laws. This means complying with the major pieces of legislation listed below, even if the office is small enough to be exempt. Common sense handling of the entire recruiting and selection process should avoid any legal problems.

Title VII of the Civil Rights Act of 1964, as amended by the Equal Employment Opportunity Act of 1972: This law applies to all employers who regularly employ 15 or more employees (including management employees). Basically, it prohibits discrimination on the basis of a person's race, religion, color, sex or national origin except where a race, religion, color, sex or national origin is a bona fide occupational qualification (for example, hiring a woman as a women's locker room attendant). Title VII also makes it unlawful to foster possible discrimination in the help-wanted ads on the basis of race, religion, color, sex or national origin.

The 1978 ammendment to this law prohibits discrimination because of, or on the basis of pregnancy, childbirth or related medical conditions, and provides that pregnant women will be treated the same for all employment related purposes, including the receipt of benefits under fringe benefit programs, as other persons not so affected. The Equal Opportunity Commission (EOC) regulations basically rule that a pregnant employee must be treated as a disabled employee when pregnancy affects job performance. If employees are allowed to use sick or vacation leave for disability, the same privilege must be allowed to pregnant employees. If disabled employees continue to accrue seniority during such leave, a pregnant employee must be entitled to the same.

Sexual harassment as it relates to employment is prohibited under the act. Sexual harassment is deemed related to employment if it is a basis for employment or employment decisions, interferes with the individual's work performance, or creates an offensive working situation. Sexual harassment could include unwelcome sexual advances, requests for sexual favors or other conduct of a sexual nature.

Civil Rights Act of 1866: This act was originally passed to prevent abuses of the newly freed slaves. The United States Supreme Court ruled in 1866 that the act precluded discrimination in employment on account of race or color by private employers. It is an important law today because it applies to all employers, not just to those having more than 15 employees.

Equal Pay Act, 1963: This act requires all employers to provide equal pay for men and women performing equal work in jobs that require equal skill, effort and responsibilities.

Age Discrimination in Employment Act of 1967, as amended in 1978: This act prohibits employment discrimination against persons between the ages of 40 and 70, except where age is a bona fide occupational qualification.

The Fair Labor Standards Act: This law provides that employees in other than a supervisory capacity (i.e., those spending more than 80 percent of their time supervising) must be paid time and one-half for hours worked in one week over 40 hours. Compensatory time cannot be taken within the same week. This law is probably violated more times in a medical practice than in any other type of work, as doctors ignore paying overtime when hours run late or emergency work or work on patients requires the staff to stay late.

The current minimum hourly wage is $3.35. Under certain circumstances, a lower wage rate may be approved. In order to attract and keep top employees, salaries in the medical office should exceed minimum standards and be based on prevailing community averages.

Wage and hour audits by the Department of Labor of employee payroll records are being made with greater frequency among smaller employers. Establish a written policy that overtime is paid for employees' time worked beyond 40 hours a week, and follow it to the letter.

The Consolidated Omnibus Budget Reconciliation Act of 1986 (COBRA): On April 7, 1986, President Reagan signed into law the Consolidated Omnibus Budget Reconciliation Act of 1986 (CO-

BRA), which amended the Internal Revenue Code of 1954, the Age Discrimination in Employment Act of 1967 (ADEA), the Employee Retirement Income Security Act of 1974 (ERISA), the Social Security Act and the Public Health Service Act. Except for a few special cases, this federal budget bill significantly affects employee benefit plans of all employers who employed 20 or more persons during the preceding calendar year and who maintain a group health benefit plan.

Basically, the bill requires employers to offer, in writing, a continuation of group health coverage to employees who have terminated employment or who have had their hours reduced so that they are no longer eligible for health coverage under the employer's group health plan. Continuation in these two events must be offered for a period of not less than 18 months following the event. Employers must also offer in writing continuation of group health coverage to dependant spouses and children in the event they lose their coverage under the group health plan due to the employee's death, divorce or cessation of dependent child coverage under the terms of the group health plan (e.g. when the child attains the maximum age limit).

Any eligible employers who fail to comply with this federal legislation will not be permitted to take the federal tax deduction normally allowed for expenses paid or incurred by employers for any group health plans they maintain. In addition, "highly compensated" employees will not be allowed to exclude from their gross income for tax purposes the amounts contributed by an employer to accident and health plans on their behalf. Employers who fail to provide adequate notice to employees and/or dependants may be liable for reimbursing them at a rate of up to $100 per day.

The bill also requires employers to offer, *in writing,* their group health plans as primary coverage to Medicare-eligible individuals who are still actively at work (age 65 and over) with no upper age limit. The same offer must be made to active employees' spouses who are age 65 and over. These requirements are commonly referred to as "Medicare Secondary" rules.

The "Medicare Secondary" rules of the bill became effective May 1, 1986. The Continuation of Coverage Provisions apply to plan years (as defined by ERISA) beginning on, or after, July 1, 1986. Special rules apply regarding the effective date of the continuation of coverage provision for group health plans maintained pursuant to collective bargaining agreements between employee representatives and one or more employers which were ratified before the date of the enactment of the Federal legislation.

- Purpose and Effective Date

In general, COBRA continuation of coverage is effective for "plan years" beginning on or after July 1, 1986. "Plan year" refers to the definition started under ERISA. COBRA gives employees the right to continue group health coverage after termination of employment at group rates, rather than the more costly individual rates. Continuation of coverage must also be offered to widows, divorced spouses, spouses of Medicare-eligible employees and dependent children. Coverage under the continuation provision must last for at least 36 months, depending on the status of the person entitled to continuation of coverage. Employers may require that the person continuing coverage pay for the coverage, even if active employees are not otherwise charged for such coverage.

- Who is Affected?

All employers who maintain a group health plan are affected by COBRA continuation of coverage except:

- any employer maintaining a group health program who employs fewer than 20 employees on a typical business day during the preceding calendar year (although some states have adopted COBRA rules for employers of less than 20 people);
- the United States government or the government of the District of Columbia or agencies thereof; or
- any church, convention of churches or association of churches which is exempt from taxation under the Internal Revenue Code.

The term "group health plan" means any plan of, or plan contributed to by, an employer to provide medical care (as defined by IRC 213(d)) to his or her employees, former employees or the families of such employees or former employees, directly or through insurance, reimbursement or other means (insured and self-funded plans). Weekly income and long-term disability benefits are *not* included under the term "group health plan."

State and local government group health plans which receive funds under the Public Health Service Act must also allow continuation of coverage.

- What COBRA Requires of the Employer

1. Notification of Election Rights

Employers are required to provide written notice of continuation of coverage election to all covered employees and their spouses at the the time they come under plan coverage. When a plan first becomes subject to the continuation of coverage provision, notice of the plan's continuation coverage option must be sent to employees and spouses currently covered by the plan.

(Appendix 2-C is an example of a form that can be used for Notification of Continuation of Coverage Rights.)

2. Notification Upon Occurrence of a Qualifying Event

The employer is required to notify the carrier of the group health plan when one of the following "qualifying events" occurs:

- the employee dies;
- the employee terminates his or her employment (for reasons other than gross misconduct of the employee) or the employee's hours are reduced so that he or she is no longer eligible for coverage under the group health plan; or
- the employee becomes entitled to benefits under Medicare.

The plan administrator is:

- the person specifically so designated by the terms of the instrument under which the plan operates; or
- the "plan sponsor," where there is no designated administrator.

The term "sponsor" refers to the employer or, in the case of a plan established by multiple employers or employee organizations, the association committee, board of trustees or similar group of representatives of the parties who establish or maintain the plan.

(Rel.3–2/89 Pub.372)

Notification must be made within 30 days of the occurrence date of the "qualifying event."

The plan administrator must notify the employee and/or dependents affected by such termination within 14 days of the date on which he or she receives notice from the employer. This should be a notice, in writing, mailed to the last known address of the employee and/or dependents. The employee and/or dependents has a 60-day period during which he or she may elect to continue coverage. The 60-day election period begins on the date coverage under the plan terminates, or on the date the employee and/or dependent receives notice of his or her right to continue coverage under the group health plan, whichever is the later of the two.

Appendix 2-D is a sample Continuation of Coverage of Election Form which employers can use as a guide for providing notification and election of continuation to employees and/or dependents when a "qualifying event" occurs. Appendix 2-D also contains a form cover letter stating the premium required, the address to which the premium would be mailed, the premium due date, the period during which the premium must be paid and notification that the election must be made within 60 days. The notification must be mailed out within 14 days of the date of receipt of the notice of the "qualifying event."

When an affected employee and/or dependent elects to continue coverage, the insurance carrier must be sent a copy of the completed election form (in lieu of a carrier-provided form) to ensure continuation of coverage under the group policy.

3. What Type of Coverage Must be Offered?

Under the continuation provision, coverage must be identical to the coverage provided for similarly situated individuals under the group health plan to whom a "qualifying event" has not occurred. The coverage must be extended for at least the period beginning on the day of the "qualifying event" and ending not earlier than the earliest of the following occasions:

(a) in the case of termination of employment or reduction in hours, the date which is 18 months after the date of the "qualifying event";

(b) in the case of any "qualifying event," other than those described in (a), the date of which is 36 months after the date of the "qualifying event";

(c) the date on which the employer ceases to provide any group health plan to any employees;

(d) the date on which coverage ceases under the plan by reason of failure to make timely payment of any premium required under the plan with respect to the individual continuing coverage;

(e) the date on which the individual continuing coverage first becomes, after the date of the election:

    (i) a covered employee under any other group health plan;

    (ii) entitled to benefits under Medicare;

(f) (in the case of an individual who is the spouse of a covered employee) the date on which the spouse remarries and becomes covered under a group health plan.

If an individual's period of continuation of coverage expires, as stated in (a) or (b), the plan must notify and, during the 180-day period ending on such expiration date, provide to the individual the option of enrollment under a conversion health plan otherwise generally available under the plan.

4. Who Pays the Premium for Continuation of Coverage?

The plan may require payment of premium by the individual continuing coverage for any period of continuation of coverage, except that such premium shall not exceed 102 percent of the applicable premium for such a period and may, at the option of the individual continuing coverage, be made in monthly installments. (Even though the act allows 102 percent of the premium, most carriers will charge the same premium for active employees.)

- What COBRA Requires of the Employee

Each employee or dependent covered under a group health plan is responsible for notifying the plan administrator of the occurrence of any of the following "qualifying events":

- the divorce or legal separation of the covered employee from the employee's spouse; or

- a dependent child ceasing to be an eligible dependent under the applicable requiremenets of the plan.

The plan administrator must notify the employee and/or dependent of his or her rights for continuation of coverage within 14 days following the date the plan administrator receives the notice from the employee and/or dependent.

The Immigration Reform and Control Act of 1986: This law was designed to hinder the employment of illegal aliens. It requires that *all* employers:

- have employees fill out their part of the Form I–9 when they start work;
- check documents establishing the employee's identity and eligibility to work;
- properly complete the form I–9;
- retain the form for at least three years (if the employee is employed for more than three years, a copy of the form must be retained for one year after the person leaves employment);
- present the form for inspection to a United States Immigration and Naturalization Service officer or a Department of Labor officer upon request. The departments are required to give three days advance notice.

Employers are required to have this form on file for any employee hired after November 7, 1986. These forms should be prepared and maintained on file for all employees hired after that date. Fines for violation range from not less than $250 for the first violation to more than $10,000 for each unauthorized employee or subsequent violations. (See Appendix 2-E for as copy of the I–9 form.)

§ 2.10 Checklist for Staff Recruiting, Development and Management

A checklist of things to consider when devising a personnel policy is provided.

— Hiring

    — Determine need

    — Create pool of applicants

STAFF RECRUITING § 2.10

- Screen applicants
- Test applicants
- Interview applicants
- Check references
- Select and hire employee(s)

— Salary and Fringe Benefit Consideration
- Prevailing wages
- Position and responsibilities
- The practice budget
- Health insurance
- Disability insurance
- Life insurance
- Vacations
- Sick days
- Personal days
- Holidays
- Periodic evaluation of salaries and benefits

— Items To Be Considered for Inclusion in Personnel Policy
- Forward
- Introduction and welcome
- Orientation and training
- Organization and management
- Office hours
- Breaks
- Personal appearance
- Attitude
- Telephone
- Security
- Confidentiality

- Payroll
- Miscellaneous benefits
- Holidays
- Vacations
- Education
- Sick pay
- Maternity leave
- Worker's compensation
- Jury duty
- Family emergencies
- Funerals
- Absenteeism
- Performance review
- Salary review
- Disciplinary action
- Termination

- Development of Procedure Manual
  - Develop a job description for each employee
  - Review the job descriptions for comprehensiveness, redundancy and efficiency
  - Prepare a detailed "how-to" typed description of each duty listed in the job descriptions
  - Collate and assemble data in a central manual
  - Review annually and update with any changes in procedures

- Staff Management
  - Set up a chain of command
  - Develop a printed flow chart to be given to employees so that they will all know the chain of command in terms of communication

- _ Listen to employees
- _ Give feedback to employees
- _ Conduct periodic staff meetings
- _ Conduct periodic individual interviews with employees

_ Give new employee
- _ Personnel policy
- _ Procedure manual
- _ Office key
- _ Form I-9
- _ Form W-4
- _ Insurance applications
- _ Applicable state forms

_ Terminations
- _ Request resignation
- _ Conduct exit interview and attempt to gain an insight into practice problems
- _ Have employee turn in keys and any other equipment issued by the practice
- _ Get the employee's forwarding address for paycheck and W2 income tax statements
- _ Notify employee and insurance companies of termination and discontinue employer payment of premiums. Employee may wish to pick up the coverage for a period of time out of his or her own pocket.
- _ File separation notice with the State Unemployment Department if necessary and give a copy to the employee
- _ Have employee complete COBRA continuation of coverage

_ Check compliance with Federal Employment Laws
- _ Title VII of the Civil Rights Act of 1964 as amended by the Equal Employment Opportunity Act of 1972

(Rel.3–2/89 Pub.372)

- The Civil Rights Act of 1866
- The Equal Pay Act of 1963
- Age Discrimination and Employment Act of 1967 as amended in 1978
- Fair Labor Standards Act
- The Consolidated Omnibus Budget Reconciliation Act of 1986 (COBRA)
- The Immigration Reform and Control Act of 1986

§ 2.100 Bibliography

Aluise, J. J.: The Physician as Manager. Boivre, MD: Charles Press, 1979.

Cattan, H.: Medical Practice Management. Medical Economics, 60, 1977.

Cotton, H. and Martin, N.: Aid for the Medical Assistant: Managing the Doctor's Office. Oradell, NJ: Medical Economics Books, 1975.

Division of Medical Practice: The Business Side of Medical Practice. Chicago: American Medical Association, 1973.

Golden, A. S.: An Inventory for Primary Health Care Practice. Cambridge, MA: Ballinger Publishing Co., 1976.

McCormick, J., et. al.: The Management of Medical Practice. Cambridge, MA: Ballinger Publishing Co., 1978.

Mitzber, N.: The Health Care Supervisor's Handbook. Germantown, MD: Aspen Systems Corp, 1978.

Pressman, R. M. and Siegler, R.: The Independent Practitioner: Practice Management for the Allied Health Professional. Dow Jones-Irwin, 1983.

Rubin, I. H., et. al.: Improving the Coordination of Care: A Program for Health Team Development. Cambridge, MA: Ballinger Publishing Co., 1975.

Sloan, R. M. and Sloane, B.: A Guide to Health Facilities: Personnel Management. St. Louis: C. V. Mosby, 1977.

Wise, H.: Making Health Teams Work. Cambridge, MA: Ballinger Publishing Co., 1974.

(Text continued on page 2–45)

Appendix 2-A

TESTS FOR GENERAL OFFICE SKILLS

BOOKKEEPING SKILLS

Instructions:

This test will be used to evaluate your skill in the fundamental bookkeeping/accounting functions required for this position. The test is not difficult but it does require concentration and awareness on your part.

This is a page from the month's expenses; a page of checks written. Column 1 is correct and should be your base. Please do the following:

(1) Total the columns, making corrections if necessary to prove expenses for the month of January.

(2) Find the ending bank balance.

(See Figure 2-5.)

(Pub.372)

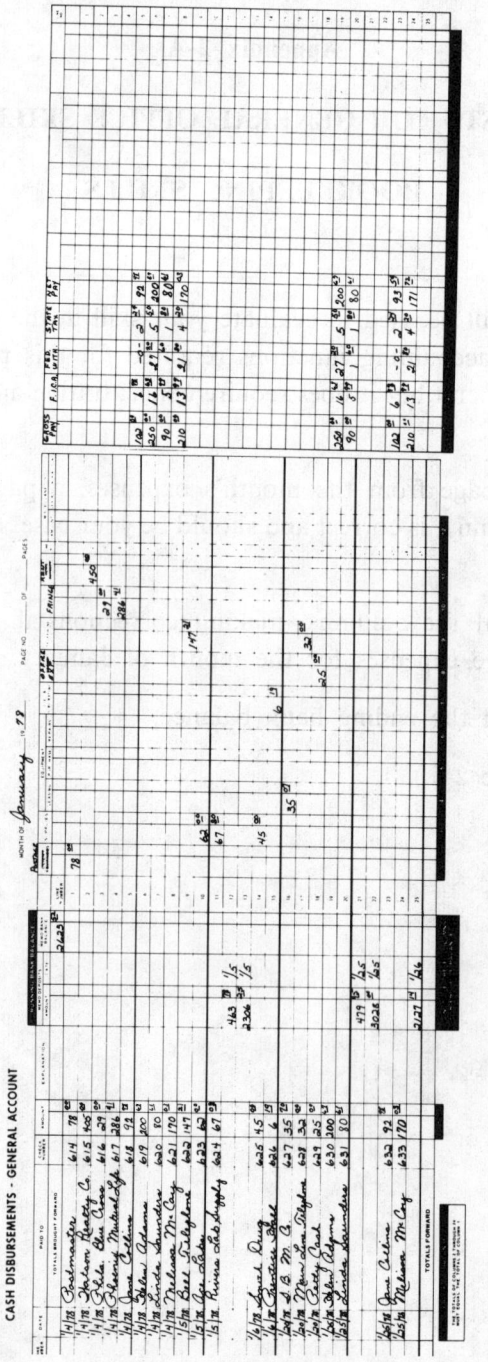

FIG. 2-5. A page from a general account ledger to be used for bookkeeper skills test.

RECEPTIONIST'S POSITION

Instructions:

The following situation could very easily happen in a medical office. If you were the receptionist, how would you respond to this situation?

Thursdays and Fridays are very heavy office-visit days. The day begins at 5:30 A.M. and continues until 7:00 P.M. On these days doctor and patient demands on you are much greater. Because you are situated out front, your work day is often disrupted to greet patients, answer both doctor and patient questions and, in some instances, act as cashier. What would you do in a situation in which you have a patient standing at the cashier window and a patient who has just entered the office and your phone is ringing? Give your opinion on how to handle this situation in the most professional way.

TRANSCRIBER/TYPIST

Instructions:

This is not a test for speed, but for neatness and correct letter format. If you make a mistake in this letter, please correct it. When completed this letter should be ready for mailing.

John F. Greene, 7860 North Regency Street, Philadelphia, PA 19001

Dear Mr. Greene We welcome you to our practice and look forward to seeing you at your first appointment at ten A.M. on Wednesday April 8.

As background information prior to your appointment we enclose our Patient Information Booklet. We strongly urge our patients to read this booklet prior to their first appointment. It explains our practice philosophy as well as our thoughts on insurance and payment at the time of your appointment.

Again, welcome to our practice. We look forward to seeing vou on April 8th. Sincerely Dr. William F. Morgan

(Pub.372)

App. 2-A   MANAGING YOUR MEDICAL PRACTICE   2-48

SPELLING TEST FOR A CLERK

Instructions:

Here are just a few frequently misspelled words. See if you can locate all of the errors.

Attendance ___
Benefitted ___
Bullatin ___
Defendent ___
Fictitous ___
Guarentee ___
Interferred ___
Maintenence ___
Miscellanous ___
Occassionally ___
Occurrence ___
Priviledge ___
Psychietry ___
Questionairre ___
Recipient ___
Simultaneous ___
Sizeable ___
Tangable ___
Undoubtly ___
Withholding ___

(Pub.372)

Appendix 2-B

GENERAL OUTLINE OF JOB DESCRIPTIONS FOR A TWO-DOCTOR PRACTICE

Check-Out Receptionist
- Collect all in-office payments.
- Post all office charges and payments.
- Reconcile daysheet.
- Prepare bank deposit.
- Do miscellaneous office duties as needed, including filing.

Hours: 7:30 A.M.-3:30 P.M.

Check-In Receptionist
- Pull and prepare charts for the day.
- Greet patients.
- Register new patients as needed.
- Answer telephones.
- Surgical scheduling.

Hours: 7:30 A.M.-3:30 P.M.

Scheduling
- Telephones—primary.
- Maintain office schedules.
- Prepare daily patient list.
- Manage recall system.
- File.
- Miscellaneous office duties as needed.

Insurance/Billing/Collection
- Office billing.
- HMO billing.
- Hospital and surgical billing.

(Pub. 372)

- Insurance form preparation as needed.
- Collection procedures.

Hours: 10:00 A.M.—5:30 P.M.

Office Manager

Financial:
- Prepare proposed annual budget.
- Approve all expenditures.
- Prepare review and analysis of monthly statements, all special financial studies, reports, etc. requested.
- Liasion with accountants.

Personnel:
- Recruiting, hiring and firing.
- Supervision, including salary review and proposed salary adjustments and evaluation.
- Maintain records of vacations, sick leave, etc.
- Organize regular office meetings and set agendas.
- Determine and change personnel assignments and job descriptions as needed.

Supplies:
- Order all supplies, medical and clerical.
- Maintain supply records, pricing studies, etc.

Professional and Corporate:
- Monitor fringe benefit programs.
- Supervise pension and profit sharing funds (as liaison between advisors and doctors).
- Coordinate with attorney and accountant on corporate details.

Collections:
- Supervise systems for delinquent account follow-up.
- Handle difficult collection matters.

Audit Controls:

(Pub.372)

- Review and supervise internal systems for handling cash, recording mail receipts, writing checks, etc.
- Follow-up audit control systems devised by accountants.

Insurance:
- Handle and recommend all office corporate insurance coverage.

Office Facilities:
- Assure proper maintenance of present office; order new equipment; obtain supplies and services.
- Be responsible for all aspects of office maintenance and coordination with landlord.
- Investigate and act as agent for doctor in office building ownership, development of plans for office changes, etc.

Handling Personal Business for Doctors:
- Act as business agent for doctors in all areas where their time can be saved for medical work.

Medical Secretary
- Transcription and typing for all physicians, including dictation tapes, copywork, and use of word processor.
- Back-up telephone coordinator relating messages and instructions between doctors, patients, and hospital. Scheduling hospital admissions or tests as may be required.
- All-practice filing: correspondence, lab slips, test results and personal correspondence for physicians.
- Assistance or back-up as may be required at front desk area.

Receptionist
- Main check-in receptionist for all physicians' hours. Answer all telephones and make all appointments. Patient escort duties as may be required during office hours.
- Back-up responsibility as cashier, taking payments, hand-

ling insurance and billing as may be required.
- Scheduling of any tests or procedures that may be required.

CHAPTER 3

Forms of Practice

> **SCOPE**
>
> Whether to work alone or in a group medical practice and whether that practice should be incorporated are decisions that many physicians make several times in the course of a career. The choice must be based not only on personal preference but also on what is practical at different times of life. Single practice provides total control over running the business and collecting and investing profits and offers tax and investment incentives not available to corporations. However, it does not provide the same security and cost-efficiency usually associated with an incorporated partnership. Although working in a group practice does entail a loss of privacy and certain shared liabilities, it also provides easy access to consultation and a more dependable patient flow, and it alleviates the pressure of coverage. An incorporated or group practice may have to be more meticulous and precise in its record keeping, with regard to profit sharing and valuation of the practice, but for that reason it is often possible to be more farsighted and to plan for contingencies such as tax shelters or retaining profits in the practice that may not easily be done by the single practitioner.

SYNOPSIS

§ 3.01 Different Forms of Practice
    [1] Single Practitioner
    [2] Incorporated Practices
    [3] Group Practices
        [a] Simple Partnerships
        [b] Incorporated Group Practices

§ 3.02 Advantages of the Unincorporated Practice
§ 3.03 Advantages of Incorporating the Medical Practice
   [1] Budgeting
   [2] Scheduling of Fiscal Year
   [3] Retaining Profits in the Corporation
   [4] Limited Liability
   [5] Flexible Benefit Plans (Cafeteria Plans)
   [6] Insurance Benefits
   [7] Tighter Financial Controls
§ 3.04 Disadvantages of Single and Group Practices
   [1] Single Practice
   [2] Group Practice
§ 3.05 Profit Distribution in Groups
   [1] Equity vs. Productivity
   [2] Criteria for Profit Distribution
§ 3.06 Starting New Physicians in the Practice
§ 3.07 Valuing the Practice
   [1] Valuing Assets
   [2] Valuing Liabilities
   [3] Preset Buy-Sell Agreements
§ 3.08 Checklist for Forms of Practice
§ 3.09–§ 3.99 Reserved
§ 3.100 Bibliography

§ 3.01 Different Forms of Practice

Among medical practice options are the single practice, the professional association or corporation (P.A. or P.C.), the simple partnership and the incorporated partnership. Each has its own particular limitations and benefits.

Once you have decided where you would like to work, you must decide whether you want to establish your own medical practice or, if an invitation has been extended, work in a group practice. If you value privacy and being able to work at your own pace, a single practice may be right for you. However, if you are a new practitioner, the cost- and risk-sharing benefits of a group practice may be more economically feasible. There are many types of single and group practices.

[1] Single Practitioner

The simplest form of practice is the single practice. The single practitioner has no associates, can make decisions without consulting partners or a board of directors, and accepts sole responsibility for successes and mistakes.

(Text continued on page 3–3)

A single practitioner may turn a medical practice into a proprietorship or a professional association, also called a Professional Corporation. A doctor practicing as a sole proprietor declares all income from the practice and deducts all business expenses (including employee payroll and liabilities) on his or her personal income tax return.

Income is determined by the gross income less expenses. Since practice income and personal income are the same for this type of practitioner, the amount the physician takes out of the practice (or draws) has no bearing on income taxes. Although payroll taxes withheld from employees must be deposited in the usual way (see Chapter 6, Financial Management), the physician pays no employee taxes personally, because he or she is self-employed.

The single practitioner must pay income taxes quarterly with estimated tax vouchers (form 1040ES). Since a sole-proprietor physician is not considered an employee, the physician pays no FICA tax. However, a self-employed physician is required to pay a self-employment tax equal to 11.3 percent of the first $39,600 of income.

[2] Incorporated Practices

A practitioner may wish to work alone, yet incorporate his or her practice. However, once the physician forms a professional association, he or she must fullfil a number of roles.

As the owner of the corporation, the physician is a stockholder. As a stockholder, the physician is responsible for electing a board of directors. In this type of corporation, the board of directors usually consists of the physician, who is also the director. As a director, the physician must elect a president, vice president, secretary and treasurer. Again, the physician fills all of these roles. As president and chief executive officer of the corporation, the physician is responsible for hiring a physician employee to carry out the day-to-day patient care. Thus the practitioner becomes an employee of his or her own practice. (For a flow chart on corporate structure, see Figure 3–1.)

By becoming an employee of the corporation, a physician who incorporates his or her practice must be paid a salary, from which FICA and federal, state and local taxes are withheld. The

Corporate Flow Chart

```
        ┌─────────────────┐
        │  Stockholders   │
        │    (owners)     │
        └─────────────────┘
                 │
        ┌─────────────────┐
        │ Board of Directors │
        └─────────────────┘
                 │
        ┌─────────────────┐
        │    Officers:    │
        │    President    │
        │  Vice President │
        │    Secretary    │
        │    Treasurer    │
        └─────────────────┘
                 │
        ┌─────────────────┐
        │ Physician Employees │
        └─────────────────┘
                 │
        ┌─────────────────┐
        │  Office Manager │
        └─────────────────┘
           │           │
    ┌──────────┐  ┌──────────────┐
    │ Medical  │  │  Business    │
    │  Staff   │  │   Staff      │
    └──────────┘  └──────────────┘
```

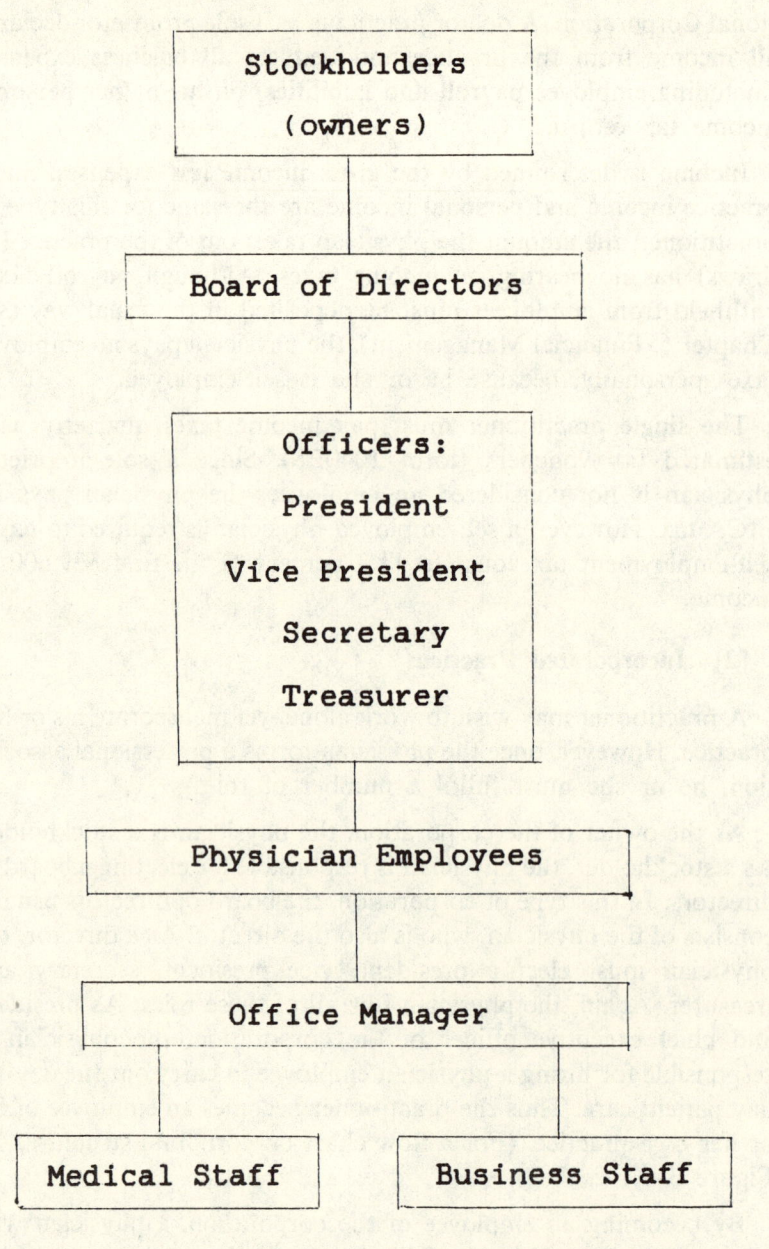

FIG. 3–1. Flow chart showing the chain of responsibility for the most basic corporate structure.

(Pub.372)

corporation must pay payroll taxes on the physician's salary, such as the employer's share of FICA, federal unemployment taxes and state unemployment taxes. In many cases, worker's compensation insurance premiums must be paid on the physician's salary. Since taxes are withheld, most physicians do not need to make estimated income tax payments if their practice is incorporated. Instead of filing a Schedule C (Form 1040), the physician simply attaches a copy of his or her W2 form to Form 1040.

Gross income and practice expenses are not reported on the physician's personal income tax return, but on a corporate income tax return. Because the corporation is considered a legal entity, a separate income tax return, Form 1120, must be filed annually. If the corporation has net income, it may be necessary to pay corporate income taxes. (A medical corporation can generally reduce taxable income to a minimum by increasing deductible expenses, such as physicians' bonuses; but if income exceeds deductible expenses, the result is a net income, taxable as corporate income.) Distributions other than salary by the corporation to the physician are generally considered dividends; dividends are not deductible by a corporation but are income (and therefore taxable) for the physician.

Most physicians who incorporate their practice do so with the intent of establishing a corporate pension and/or profit sharing plan. By doing so, they generally become administrators of the plan, trustees of the trust and participants in the plan. Under these circumstances, pension and profit sharing payments may not be made on dividend distribution. (For a flow chart on how pension and profit sharing plans are administered, see Figure 3-2.)

Physicians incorporating their practice must keep meticulous records. At the very least a professional association must keep minutes of stockholder meetings and board meetings. Significant decisions, such as officer salaries, pension and profit sharing contributions and corporate loans must be recorded. Bank resolutions must be made to open an account or take out a loan. Many practitioners find these requirements burdensome.

[3] Group Practices

The major reason physicians practice in a group is to share

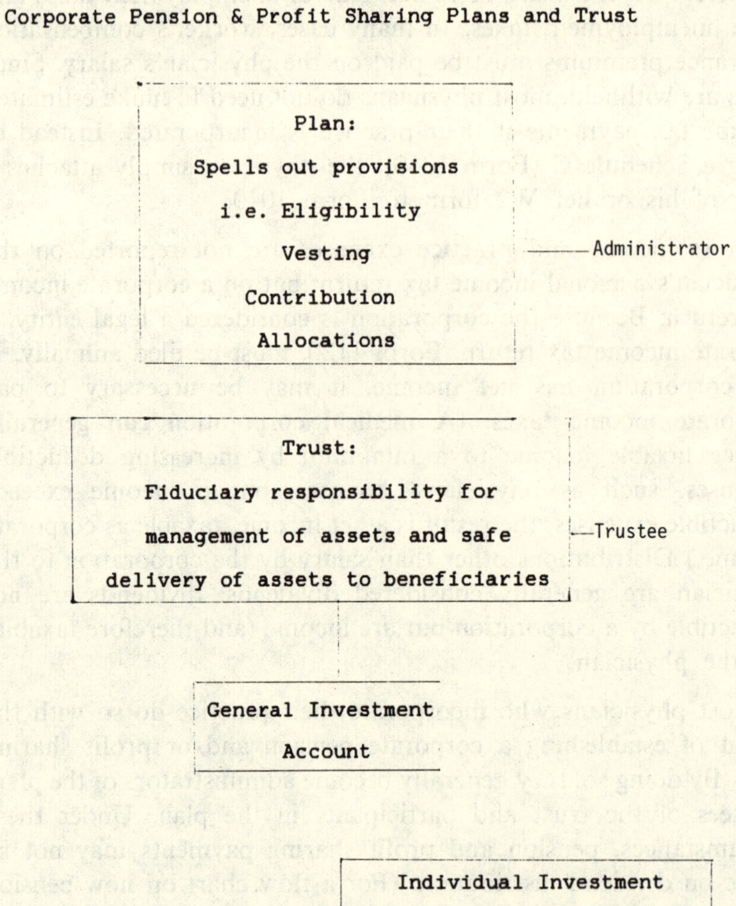

Corporate Pension & Profit Sharing Plans and Trust

```
┌─────────────────────────┐
│         Plan:           │
│   Spells out provisions │
│     i.e. Eligibility    │
│         Vesting         │────── Administrator
│       Contribution      │
│       Allocations       │
└─────────────────────────┘

┌─────────────────────────┐
│         Trust:          │
│ Fiduciary responsibility for │
│ management of assets and safe │──── Trustee
│ delivery of assets to beneficiaries │
└─────────────────────────┘

        ┌───────────────────┐
        │ General Investment│
        │     Account       │
        └───────────────────┘

        ┌───────────────────┐
        │Individual Investment│
        │     Accounts      │
        └───────────────────┘
```

FIG. 3–2. Chart demonstrating how a corporate pension and profit sharing plan is administered for an incorporated practice.

(Pub.372)

coverage (e.g., malpractice insurance). However, some physicians are becoming involved with groups because they feel the future of medicine is not with the single practitioner but with the larger group.

Group practices can range from a space-sharing arrangement to a formal partnership or corporation. With a space-sharing arrangement, each physician may maintain a sole proprietorship, or P.A., in which each doctor sees his or her own patients, bills them and collects from them for services rendered. Expenses are generally paid to a central account and distributed appropriately to the various doctors. When one physician covers for another, the attending physician generally bills the patient, even if the covering physician made the rounds. As compensation, the attending physician either pays the covering physician or performs a reciprocal service.

[a] Simple Partnerships

A physician who wishes to enter a more formal business arrangement with other physicians may decide to form a medical practice partnership. With a partnership, there is one practice. The partnership bills all of the patients and the partnership pays all expenses. Profit from the partnership is divided among the doctors according to agreed upon compensation formulas.

The partnership files a partnership income tax return, but pays no tax on the partnership income. Instead, the partnership income is allocated to personal income (in accordance with the partners' compensation agreement) and reported on the personal income tax form. A sample Schedule K–1 is provided in Figure 3–3.

With a partnership, certain tax benefits "flow through" to the partners. These benefits include investment tax credit, depreciation and contributions. Although obtained for a single entity—i.e., the practice—these benefits can be allocated individually to each member of the practice.

Some physicians form partnerships in which some of the partners are P.A.'s (Professional Associations), because they may wish to be eligible for corporate benefits such as corporate pension plans and medical reimbursement plans. Due to the potential for abuse in such an arrangement, the government has established strict regulations governing partnerships of professional associations. If you are

SCHEDULE K-1 (Form 1065) Department of the Treasury Internal Revenue Service	**Partner's Share of Income, Credits, Deductions, etc.** For calendar year 1984 or fiscal year beginning _____, 1984, and ending _____, 19___	OMB No. 1545-0099 **1984**

Partner's identifying number ▶   Partnership's identifying number ▶

Partner's name, address, and ZIP code   Partnership's name, address, and ZIP code

A Is partner a general partner (see page 3 of Instructions for Form 1065)? ☐ Yes ☐ No
B Partner's share of liabilities (see page 10 of Instructions for Form 1065):
   Nonrecourse . . . . $ _____
   Other . . . . $ _____
C What type of entity is this partner? ▶

D Enter partner's percentage of: (i) Before decrease or termination   (ii) End of year
   Profit sharing . . . . ____%   ____%
   Loss sharing . . . . ____%   ____%
   Ownership of capital . . . . . ____%   ____%
E IRS Center where partnership filed return ▶

F Reconciliation of partner's capital account:

(a) Capital account at beginning of year	(b) Capital contributed during year	(c) Ordinary income (loss) from line 1 below	(d) Income not included in column (c), plus nontaxable income	(e) Losses not included in column (c), plus unallowable deductions	(f) Withdrawals and distributions	(g) Capital account at end of year

	(a) Distributive share item	(b) Amount	(c) 1040 filers enter the amount in column (b) on:
Income (Loss)	1 Ordinary income (loss)		Sch. E, Part II, col. (d) or (e)
	2 Guaranteed payments		Sch. E, Part II, column (e)
	3 Dividends qualifying for exclusion		Sch. B, Part II, line 4
	4 Net short-term capital gain (loss)		Sch. D, line 4, col. f. or g.
	5 Net long-term capital gain (loss)		Sch. D, line 12, col. f. or g.
	6 Net gain (loss) from involuntary conversions due to casualty or theft		(See Partner's Instructions for Schedule K-1 (Form 1065))
	7 Other net gain (loss) under section 1231 . . .		Form 4797, line 1
	8 Other (attach schedule)		(Enter on applicable lines of your return)
Deductions	9 Charitable contributions: 50% ____ 30% ____ 20% ____		See Form 1040 instructions
	10 Expense deduction for recovery property (section 179)		(See Partner's Instructions for Schedule K-1 (Form 1065))
	11a Payments for partner to an IRA		See Form 1040 instructions
	b Payments for partner to a Keogh Plan (Type of plan ▶ ____)		Form 1040, line 27
	c Payments for partner to Simplified Employee Pension (SEP)		Form 1040, line 27
	12 Other (attach schedule)		(Enter on applicable lines of your return)
Credits	13 Jobs credit		Form 5884
	14 Credit for alcohol used as fuel		Form 6478
	15 Credit for income tax withheld		See Form 1040 instructions
	16 Other (attach schedule)		(Enter on applicable lines of your return)
Self-employment	17a Net earnings (loss) from self-employment . . .		Sch. SE, Part I
	b Gross farming or fishing income		(See Partner's Instructions for Schedule K-1 (Form 1065))
	c Gross nonfarm income		(See Partner's Instructions for Schedule K-1 (Form 1065))
Tax Preference Items	18a Accelerated depreciation on nonrecovery real property or 15-year or 18-year real property		Form 6251, line 4c
	b Accelerated depreciation on leased personal property or leased recovery property other than 15-year or 18-year real property		Form 6251, line 4d
	c Depletion (other than oil and gas)		Form 6251, line 4i
	d (1) Gross income from oil, gas, and geothermal properties		See Form 6251 instructions
	(2) Deductions allocable to oil, gas, and geothermal properties		See Form 6251 instructions
	e (1) Qualified investment income included in line 1 above		(See Partner's Instructions for Schedule K-1 (Form 1065))
	(2) Qualified investment expenses included in line 1 above		(See Partner's Instructions for Schedule K-1 (Form 1065))
	f Other (attach schedule)		(See Partner's Instructions for Schedule K-1 (Form 1065))

For Paperwork Reduction Act Notice, see Form 1065 Instructions.   Schedule K-1 (Form 1065) 1984 considering forming or becoming a member of such a partnership, you should first seek competent legal and accounting advice.

A partnership of professional associations involves a number of P.A.'s. An advantage of such an arrangement is that each physician can maintain personal control over his or her professional association. However, there are many disadvantages, not the least of which are the cost of additional accounting and legal

Schedule K-1 (Form 1065) (1984)			Page 2
(a) Distributive share item		(b) Amount	(c) 1040 filers enter the amount in column (b) on:

Investment Interest
- 19 a Interest expense on:
  - (1) Investment debts incurred before 12/17/69 — Form 4952, line 1
  - (2) Investment debts incurred before 9/11/75, but after 12/16/69 — Form 4952, line 15
  - (3) Investment debts incurred after 9/10/75 — Form 4952, line 5
- b (1) Investment income included in line 1 (not (1) above) — (See Partner's Instructions for Schedule K-1 (Form 1065))
  (2) Investment expenses included in line 1 (not (1) above) — (See Partner's Instructions for Schedule K-1 (Form 1065))
- c (1) Income from "net lease property" included in line 1 (not (1) above) — (See Partner's Instructions for Schedule K-1 (Form 1065))
  (2) Expenses from "net lease property" included in line 1 (not (1) above) — (See Partner's Instructions for Schedule K-1 (Form 1065))

Foreign Taxes
- 20 a Type of income — Form 1116, Check boxes
  b Name of foreign country or U.S. possession — Form 1116, Part I
  c Total gross income from sources outside the U.S. (attach schedule) — Form 1116, Part I
  d Total applicable deductions and losses (attach schedule) — Form 1116, Part I
  e Total foreign taxes (check one): ► ☐ Paid ☐ Accrued — Form 1116, Part II
  f Reduction in taxes available for credit (attach schedule) — Form 1116, Part III
  g Other (attach schedule) — Form 1116 Instructions

Other
- 21 Other items and amounts not included in lines 1 through 20g and 22 and 23 that are required to be reported separately to you. — (See Partner's Instructions for Schedule K-1 (Form 1065))

Property Eligible for Investment Credit
- 22 Regular Percentage
  - Unadjusted basis of new recovery property: a 3-Year — Form 3468, line 1(a); b Other — Form 3468, line 1(b)
  - Unadjusted basis of used recovery property: c 3-Year — Form 3468, line 1(c); d Other — Form 3468, line 1(d)
- Section 48(q) Election to Reduce Credit (Instead of Adjusting Basis)
  - Unadjusted basis of new recovery property: e 3-year — Form 3468, line 1(e); f Other — Form 3468, line 1(f)
  - Unadjusted basis of used recovery property: g 3-year — Form 3468, line 1(g); h Other — Form 3468, line 1(h)
- i Other (see instructions for Schedule K-1 (Form 1065) in the Instructions for Form 1065) — (See Partner's Instructions for Schedule K-1 (Form 1065))

Property Subject to Recapture of Investment Credit
- 23 Properties: A | B | C
  a Description of property (State whether recovery or nonrecovery property. If recovery property, state whether regular percentage method or section 48(q) election used.) — Form 4255, top
  b Date placed in service — Form 4255, line 2
  c Cost or other basis — Form 4255, line 3
  d Class of recovery property or original estimated useful life — Form 4255, line 4
  e Date item ceased to be investment credit property — Form 4255, line 8

FIG. 3-3. Schedule K-1 is an information return given to each member of a partnership and filed by the partnership. The partner completes his personal income tax return (Form 1040) with the information provided on the K-1. The K-1 is an information return only, and need not be attached to the partner's personal income tax return.

fees and the possibility of investigation by the IRS as to the propriety of the partnership arrangement.

[b] Incorporated Group Practices

Perhaps the most formal type of group practice is the incorporated group P.A., in which participating physicians enjoy the economy and benefits of a corporate practice. A group medical corporation differs substantially from a partnership of different corporations (a partnership in which some physicians have formed P.A.'s). A group corporation functions as and is considered to be a single entity. All of the physicians become employees of that entity, in contrast to partners or subcontractors. Careful consideration must be given to which expenses are paid by the P.A. and which expenses the employer (i.e., the incorporated practice) must pay out. Common problem areas include business cars, professional dues and continuing education costs. If the corporation is liable for expenses in these areas, the employee physician may not take a deduction for them as out-of-pocket costs.

Incorporated single practices and incorporated and unincorporated group practices should consider drawing up the following legal documentation and agreements:

Articles of Incorporation: These documents, which are the same for incorporated single practices and incorporated group practices, are filed with the secretary of state. They establish the corporation. The articles of incorporation spell out the type of corporation chosen by the practice and its purpose. Although articles of incorporation are considered a formality by most physicians, they are the actual proof that the corporation exists. Generally, attorneys make the articles and purpose of the corporation as broad as possible to insure that the corporation can be used for a variety of business purposes.

By-laws: By-laws spell out the official corporate protocol. The by-laws, like the articles of incorporation, are prepared during the creation of the corporation. Generally, attorneys will attempt to make the by-laws as broad as possible to permit great flexibility within the corporation.

Bill of Sale (Equipment Transfers): Generally, if a practice incorporates ownership of the equipment and other assets, it may transfer ownership from the proprietorship to the corporation. The

(Text continued on page 3–11)

previous owner, i.e. the physician, generally receives stock for this contribution of equipment and other assets.

Buy-Sell Agreement: These agreements spell out the terms under which a departing physician will be compensated for his or her interest in the business. Much like a "prenuptial" agreement, these documents should be settled on and drafted at the time the group is established, before any problems arise.

Employment Agreement: This official document spells out the terms of physician employment, including whether the physician is a full-time employee, whether he or she is allowed to work anywhere else or for anyone else, what the compensation arrangement is, the agreed-upon length of employment, expenses the corporation and/or the employee is responsible for, vacation, sick day and disability agreements, etc.

Wage Continuation Contracts: The wage continuation contract is a method of compensating a physician for his or her interest in the corporate accounts receivable. A cash-basis corporation pays taxes only when money is collected, so it does not pay income tax on the accounts receivable. A physician who terminates his or her employment with the group always does so a few months before all of the accounts receivable he or she has a share in are collected. The wage continuation agreement permits the corporation to pay the accounts receivable out to the physician and receive a deduction for those payments.

Minutes of the Stockholder Meetings: Written records recording the significant items of discussion and decisions made at the stockholder meetings must be kept. A stockholder meeting must be held to elect a board of directors, and the minutes must record the results of these and other elections.

Minutes of Director Meetings: Written records of significant items discussed and decisions made at each board meeting must be kept.

Waiver of Meeting Notice: Generally, corporate laws require that stockholders and board members be notified of their respective meetings. The notification rule may be avoided if the stockholders and board members sign a waiver of notice. Normally, these documents are used in the medical office to avoid any question of whether or not proper notice was given.

Benefit Plans: Documentation should be provided for each of the benefit plans listed below, if they are adopted.

Pension and Profit Sharing Plans: Such plans are governed by rigid laws designed to protect employees from unscrupulous employers and trustees. Complete legal documentation of these plans must be created when they are first adopted. Since 1974, frequent amendments have been made and, as a result, most physicians must have their plans reviewed at least annually and proper amendments drafted.

Disability Plans: You or your practice should adopt a disability plan if you wish to take advantage of tax deductible premium payments for the corporation. Such plans are formalized with documentation.

Flexible Benefit Plans: If a flexible benefit plan is adopted to take advantage of miscellaneous deductible items, it must be formalized in writing. In recent years, laws governing these flexible benefit plans have changed and amendments have been added to keep them up to date.

Death Benefit Plans: The corporation may pay a deceased employee's surviving beneficiaries up to $5,000 in death benefits. The employer can deduct the payment, which is not taxable to the decedent or the decedent's estate.

Life Insurance Plan: The corporation may wish to adopt a group or other type of life insurance plan for employees. If such a plan is adopted, it should be a formal written plan.

Medical Insurance Plan: Many offices provide health insurance to employees. This plan, like the life insurance plan, should be documented in writing.

§ 3.02 Advantages of the Unincorporated Practice

The advantages of working in an unincorporated practice include the fact that there is no need for formal bookkeeping and no need to withhold or pay FICA and other payroll taxes for the physician and family members employed by the practice. In addition, reporting of all practice income is done on the personal income statement and investment tax credits will be available.

The trend to incorporate medical practices has slowed down as a result of laws directed at equalizing the tax benefits between incorporated and unincorporated businesses. There are numerous advantages to a practice remaining unincorporated and many physicians choose to run their practices as proprietorships or partnerships.

Proprietorship is the natural state of a practice. A business that is just starting up is a proprietorship until steps are taken to create a corporation. As a result, a proprietorship may be started without any legal or accounting costs. (However, a substantial number of businesses started without accounting or consulting advice either fail or never experience financial rewards.)

Incorporation requires that official records of stockholder meetings and board meetings be prepared periodically. To insure that the records are properly prepared, an incorporated practice generally must employ an attorney on an annual basis. An unincorporated practice does not require as formal a bookkeeping system as a corporation. It is not necessary for a proprietorship to have a balance sheet for tax purposes, whereas the books of a corporation must be balanced accurately each fiscal period and an account made of all the money coming in and going out, along with all other assets, liabilities and equity.

Since a single practitioner in an unincorporated practice is considered self-employed, rather than an employee, no salary or withholding taxes need be paid on the physician's draw. This reduces or avoids altogether the possibility of incurring a penalty for improper or late withholding deposits. In lieu of withholding, the self-employed physician must make quarterly income tax estimates. Since a corporation is a separate entity and must pay income taxes, a sole proprietor avoids any risk of dual taxation. All income and expenses are reported on the physician's personal return, and taxes are paid accordingly.

The physician in an unincorporated practice may enjoy the full benefits of depreciation on equipment owned by the practice. A physician starting a new practice who makes a substantial initial investment may reduce his or her tax liability by receiving depreciation deductions in excess of the actual cash outlay.

In the event of an audit, the IRS may pay careful attention to whether income and expenses were properly reported on the physician's individual and corporate returns. A corporation solves this problem by having proper documentation but, since there is only one entity involved with a proprietorship, this issue is eliminated for the unincorporated practice. Since all business expenses are deductible on the proprietor's income tax return, the paperwork and documentation needed to show reimbursement of the physician is also eliminated.

§ 3.03 Advantages of Incorporating the Medical Practice

The advantages of incorporating a practice include good budget management and financial control; limited liability for the actions of other stockholders; taking non-taxable benefits in exchange for salary deductions; and deducting premiums for employee insurance.

For many years the major advantage to a physician in establishing a corporation was the tax deduction allowed for pension and profit sharing plans. Once a P.A. is incorporated, the physician may make substantial contributions to pension and profit sharing plans that the corporation can deduct. These contributions are not considered physician income (and thus not taxable) since they cannot be withdrawn until the physician's retirement. In addition, the earnings on the investments are not taxable.

Physicians whose practices are not incorporated may take partial advantage of pension laws by establishing a Keogh Plan, the maximum annual contribution for which is $15,000. However, in 1983, legislation that attempted to equalize the Keogh and corporate retirement plan deductions was passed. This has led many professionals to conclude that the professional association is dead since the physician can now achieve substantial deductions for noncorporate retirement plans. However, some of the benefits available to the incorporated practice are still unavailable to the unincorporated practice.

(Text continued on page 3–15)

[1] Budgeting

Many physicians cannot anticipate the ups and downs in cash flow in a medical practice, and a good or bad collection month upsets their personal finances or significantly affects their budgeted quarterly income tax estimates. Physicians who have incorporated their practices, however, receive a fixed salary like other employees and, as a result, receive a net salary check each month. Because the amount they receive is predictable, personal financial management is simplified.

Each paycheck has FICA (until maximum limits are met), federal and state income taxes withheld and applied toward income tax liability. As a result, the physician generally does not need to make quarterly tax estimates of his or her personal funds and suffers a tax bite no worse than that for other employees.

[2] Scheduling of Fiscal Year

Although the IRS does not like physicians to have corporate fiscal years that differ from the regular calendar year, an established corporation with its fiscal year already approved and that filed an election to maintain it can continue with that fiscal year. New corporations have the right to pick a fiscal year that ends in October or November.

In the past, a fiscal year was an excellent tax planning tool for physicians that enabled them to predict their calendar year income. The current law, however, requires minimum payouts to physicians by December 31, in order to prevent tax problems. As such, the tax advantage of the fiscal year has been diminished.

An important exception to this rule is the physician on a fiscal year plan whose practice income is increasing. In this situation, the physician can defer income taxes on growing income, since the minimum payout distributions are based on the previous year.

[3] Retaining Profits in the Corporation

Income from the corporation which is distributed to stockholders is considered a dividend. It cannot be deducted by the corporation, and it is taxable income for the stockholder. This double tax can erode a substantial portion of corporate and personal income and should be avoided.

A physician in a high tax bracket, who has taken advantage of other corporate tax shelters, may elect to retain profits in the corporation (for which income tax may be substantially lower). Funds accumulated in the corporation may be invested in stock and other income-producing investments; dividend income on stock owned in a corporation is not taxable through a special dividend exclusion. If money accumulated in a corporation is kept below $250,000, an excess accumulated earnings tax is avoided. Furthermore, by holding the cash in the corporation, the physician may eventually achieve capital gains through the sale of the practice or its liquidation.

[4] Limited Liability

Incorporation generally frees stockholders from personal liability for actions of the corporation. Because of the personal nature of the practice of medicine, special laws governing medical corporations have been established.

Thus, a doctor who is found liable for an act of malpractice will not be shielded from liability merely because he or she is a stockholder in a medical corporation. If there are other shareholders in the corporation, however (for example, other physicians or members of the physicians family) these shareholders will not be personally liable.

In contrast, in a partnership all partners are liable for the action of other partners, whether or not they are directly involved.

Other types of liability, such as public liability (a liability any business is exposed to, such as a client tripping in the reception room or pinching a hand in a door), do not "flow through" to the stockholders or owners, as they would in a proprietorship or partnership.

[5] Flexible Benefit Plans (Cafeteria Plans)

Flexible benefit plans provide options to employees (including the physician employee) for selecting taxable and non-taxable fringe benefits. With use of a cafeteria plan, an employee may select a salary reduction in exchange for benefits such as medical reimbursement, dental reimbursement or day care reimbursement. When an employee selects a non-taxable benefit, it reduces the employee's gross income, and thus the employee's taxes. The employee also pays no FICA tax on such a benefit. In addition, the employer's federal and state taxes are lowered.

As a result of an employee electing non-taxable benefits, an employer may avoid paying:

- Employer share of FICA tax.
- Federal unemployment taxes.
- State unemployment taxes.
- Workers' compensation premium.
- Pension payments.
- Profit sharing payments.

Under the current law, a stockholder (usually the physicians of the group) may select non-taxable benefits of up to 25 percent of the cafeteria plan's benefits.

[6] Insurance Benefits

Incorporation allows the physician to use certain types of insurance for tax-favored treatment. The physician who offers medical insurance for employees, for example, can deduct the premiums. Although it is recommended that all full-time employees be provided with medical insurance, it is possible for the physician to provide medical insurance for a select group of employees (i.e., only the employees under the physician's direct supervision).

Disability insurance, like health insurance, may be offered to a select group of employees. By having a disability and reimbursement policy, the physician-employee may be reimbursed on a tax-free basis for disability premiums. However, while premiums are deductible if paid by the corporation, benefits paid in the event of a disability are taxable to the recipient. It is recommended that consideration be given to this issue at the time the need for disability insurance is analyzed. It should also be realized that the average policy holder will pay more in premiums than he or she will collect from disability insurance.

Life insurance may also be provided as a fringe benefit. Unlike medical insurance or disability insurance, life insurance must be offered on a group basis. The first $50,000 of term insurance offered to the employee is not taxed. The amount in excess of $50,000 is taxed at what are considered favorable tax rates. An employer is allowed to provide different levels of life insurance to different employees, depending on categorization. No one categorization may fall below $5,000 of the category preceding it: for example, physicians could receive $50,000, nurses $45,000 and office employees $40,000. With a little imagination, though, creative insurance representatives can design many such categories to lower the amount of insurance necessary for some office employees.

[7] Tighter Financial Controls

Incorporating a medical practice requires the tightening of financial controls. Since a P.A. is a separate entity, its records must be kept separate from the physician's personal records. The physician may not intermingle personal expenses with business expenses or draw money in a haphazard manner. The physician will be on a monthly salary from which income taxes are withheld. As a result, peaks and valleys in the physician's income are minimized or eliminated altogether.

Incorporation guarantees the physician's taxes will be kept up to date. Furthermore, the physician in an incorporated practice generally avoids having to worry about paying estimated income taxes. By committing to a pension plan, the physician is forced to put money away for retirement. Since the corporation puts the money into the plan directly, the physician is not tempted to use the money for personal reasons.

§ 3.04 Disadvantages of Single and Group Practices

Although the single practitioner has total responsibility for the business and professional sides of the practice, he or she has no back-up coverage or immediate forum for professional consultation. In addition, the single practitioner cannot take advantage of time and cost-sharing plans or risk diversification to the same extent as a group.

Although the professional duties of a single and a group practitioner are similar, the business duties may not be. You must weigh the benefit of having total control over your practice against the amount of time you wish to devote to its non-medical aspects before you choose a single over a group practice.

[1] Single Practice

Single practitioners are their own bosses. They have no conflicts with associates, since there is no question of who is in charge, and they can make their own decisions regarding financial matters, hiring, personnel policies, continued education, when to make hospital rounds, when to use the office, etc. The solo practitioner has maximum flexibility in both the business and professional sides of the practice.

One of the major conflicts a single practitioner avoids is deciding how to distribute profits. The single practitioner also bears entire responsibility for any deicision that results in reduced profit. In many cases, the physician takes a cut in profit for a benefit he or she might not be able to take advantage of in a group situation. For example, a physician who wishes to take continuing education classes in Hawaii or who wants a more expensive company car may not be able to get them if the members of his or her group will not share the cost.

In a professional sense, the single practitioner is responsible for his or her actions alone. After working to build an outstanding reputation, the single practitioner need not worry that it will be endangered by an associate's unprofessional conduct.

[2] Group Practice

The most frustrating aspect of a single medical practice undoubtedly is the pressure of having no back-up coverage. A single practitioner who wishes to build his or her practice is often constantly on call. Although occasionally the practitioner may refer coverage out to another doctor or to a group of doctors or hospital residents, he or she knows that care for a patient is ultimately a personal responsibility. A well-run group practice, however, provides efficient coverage. With a group practice, physicians are relieved of patient care for nights, weekends and vacations and have the knowledge that patients are being taken care of by someone from their practice.

Most physicians are periodically confronted with problems that call for professional discussion. Unusual symptoms, diagnosis and treatment are better handled with consultation, and having colleagues to discuss them with is convenient and, in some cases, a confidence builder.

A well-run group can reap economic benefits not available to the single practitioner. By splitting shifts, a group practice can maximize utilization of office facilities: for example, two physicians can work in the office while the other two make hospital rounds. The same efficiency can be extended to use of staff and equipment. A computer system, for example, is far less expensive when four doctors are paying for it but only two need terminals at any given time. By consolidating purchases, a physician group may get better discounts than would an individual practitioner.

The image projected by the group practice has always been one of continuity while that of the single practitioner appears to be more precarious. It is becoming increasingly difficult for the single practitioner to compete with the large HMO's and group practices. It is far easier for an independent practice association (IPA) to discharge a single practitioner from membership than to discharge a major group serving a large portion of the community. In addition, risk diversification makes it unlikely that a single practitioner will be able to participate in capitation programs on a fiscally sound basis.

§ 3.05 Profit Distribution in Groups

For the good of the group, a fair method of profit distribution must be agreed on in advance. Criteria may include equity, productivity, tenure, certifications, time worked and attempts to contain costs. Profits can be distributed in part through compensation packages.

One of the most delicate issues of group practice and perhaps the major reason for the dissolution of some group practices is economics. It is essential that a group practice have a fair, just and agreed upon profit distribution system to assure continuity and stability of the group.

[1] Equity vs Productivity

Perhaps the simplest form of profit distribution is to split the profits equally. This may work well in a situation where practitioners are equally trained, have similar patient loads and produce equal amounts of work. Conflict quickly arises, however, when one physician produces more than the others and feels the others are taking advantage of his or her capabilities.

A profit distribution formula based on productivity is popular. This type of formula determines a physician's share of the profit by determining a ratio of production over the total clinic production. If, for example, the physician did $20,000 worth of business and the total clinic production was $100,000, he or she would receive 20 percent of the profits. However, some physicians are uncomfortable with a production-only method of profit distribution; they feel it makes the group too competitive for patients and eliminates the incentive for inter-office referrals.

Figure 3-4 is a sample of a profit distribution based on productivity for a four doctor clinic. The example uses a profit of $32,000 and illustrates how each physicians' charges for the period affects his or her share of profit.

Figure 3-4

SAMPLE OF PROFIT DISTRIBUTION BASED ON PRODUCTIVITY

CHARGES FOR JUNE:	DOLLAR	% OF TOTAL
DOCTOR A	$ 25000.00	37.31%
DOCTOR B	20000.00	29.85%
DOCTOR C	10000.00	14.93%
DOCTOR D	12000.00	17.91%
TOTAL	$ 67000.00	100.00%

DISTRIBUTION

DOCTOR	A	B	C	D	TOTAL %
SHARE PROFIT	37.31%	29.85%	14.93%	17.91%	100.00%
SHARE	11939.00	9552.00	4778.00	5731.00	32000.00
DRAWS	−8000.00	−6000.00	−3000.00	−3000.00	− 20000.00
KEOGH	−1200.00	−900.00	−450.00	−450.00	−3000.00
TOTAL	$2739.00	$2652.00	$1328.00	$2281.00	$9000.00

[2] Criteria for Profit Distribution

Some physicians feel other items of importance must be considered in the profit distribution. They include:

- Equity in the practice.
- Productivity.
- Cost containment.
- Tenure.
- Office management.
- Board certifications.
- Days worked.

Once the elements important to the physicians in the group are identified, the formula can be established. For example, assume a

(Pub.372)

three physician group wishes to place a 10 percent value on equity, a 10 percent value on years of service and an 80 percent value on production. Assume further that each doctor owns an equal share of the practice, and that Doctor A produced $25,000 and has been with the practice for 15 years, Doctor B produced $20,000 and has been with the practice for 10 years, and Doctor C produced $10,000 and has been with the practice for 2 years. If the practice profit for the period was $26,000, it would be distributed as illustrated in Figure 3–5.

Each physician's share of profit is received via a compensation package. A practice which distributes compensation through an entire package, in contrast to a draw or a salary, avoids further problems in group economics. For example, car, continuing education and entertainment expenses paid for by the practice might be allocated to the appropriate physician and be considered part of the compensation package. In this way, all items considered part of the compensation package are added back to the taxable profit of the practice when the total amount available to the physicians is calculated. The following example illustrates how to determine the available profit once compensation packages have been determined.

Profit after Compensation Packages

Corporate taxable income	$ 1,200.00
Physician salaries	150,000.00
Physician pension & profit sharing contributions	37,500.00
Physician disability insurance premiums	3,000.00
Physician life insurance premiums	1,500.00
Physician car expenses	8,500.00
Physician entertainment	500.00
Physician continued education	3,000.00
Profit available for distribution	$ 205,200.00

A profit distribution system that is considered fair by all the

PROFIT:		$ 26000.00
EQUITY SHARE @ 10%		2600.00
YEARS OF SERVICE SHARE @ 10%		2600.00
PRODUCTIVITY SHARE @ 80%		20800.00

VALUES

	PRODUCTION	YEARS OF SERVICE	EQUITY
DOCTOR A	25,000/55,000 OR 45.45%	15/27 OR 55.56%	33 1/3%
DOCTOR B	20,000/55,000 OR 36.36%	10/27 OR 37.04%	33 1/3%
DOCTOR C	10,000/55,000 OR 18.19%	2/27 OR 7.40%	33 1/3%
TOTAL	100%	100%	100%

DISTRIBUTION OF PROFIT

DOCTOR	A	B	C	TOTAL	
EQUITY %	33.3%	33.3%	33.3%	100%	
YEARS OF SERVICE %	55.56%	37.04%	7.40%		
PRODUCTIVITY %	45.45%	36.36%	18.19%		
EQUITY $	866.67	866.67	866.66	2600.00	(10%)
YEARS OF SERVICE $	1,444.56	963.04	192.40	2600.00	(10%)
PRODUCTIVITY $	9,453.60	7,562.88	3,783.52	20800.00	(80%)
TOTAL PROFIT	11,764.83	9,392.59	4,842.58	26000.00	

IF PROFIT HAD BEEN SPLIT ON AN EQUAL BASIS, IT WOULD BE AS FOLLOWS:

DOCTOR A	$	8666.00
DOCTOR B		8666.00
DOCTOR C		8666.00

FIG. 3–5. Compare the actual distribution of profit on the basis of the agreed upon criteria with the distribution that would have occurred through equal shares.

members of the group is essential for continuity and cohesiveness of the group. The initial formula should consider philosophical factors, not just economics. Various components of the practice should be weighed, based on their importance to the physicians.

Once implemented, a profit distribution system should remain in effect for a fiscal period of at least 12 months. Each year, the group may wish to look at the formula to determine if changes in the practice or in medicine in general warrant additional changes. It is not uncommon, however, for a practice to use the same profit distribution formula for many years.

§ 3.06 Starting New Physicians in the Practice

> When hiring a new physician the other physicians in the group must make many decisions and discuss them with the new physician. These decisions include restrictive covenant and moonlighting policies, vacation and fringe benefit payments such as disability and insurance, payment for continuing education and professional dues, coverage arrangements and hospital or nursing home work, appointment-making and staff support, availability of facilities, ownership of medical records, allocation of charges and the option of buying into the practice.

Whether you are a single practitioner or a member of a group, the decision to to bring a new physician into the practice entails a host of other decisions. The established physician or physicians should take the initiative to anticipate problems that can occur with hiring a new physician and take steps to head them off. A number of items should be considered before a practice recruits a physician and formal policies regarding these items should be established before prospective physicians are interviewed.

Restrictive Covenants: A restrictive covenant is designed to prevent the new associate from leaving the practice and becoming a competitor. Generally, a restrictive covenant prohibits the new physician from practicing medicine in the same vicinity as his or her former employer (i.e., your practice) for a reasonable amount of time following termination. A typical restrictive covenant might require that, in the event of termination, a new associate not practice medicine within a three mile radius of the current medical practice for three years. The other physician(s) would ask for this type of provision to prevent the new associate from leaving once senior physicians have introduced him or her to patients, referring physicians, hospital contacts, etc.

Because restrictive covenants, by their nature, restrict the freedom of the employee, they must be considered "reasonable" in the eyes of the law or they will be unenforceable. Any restrictive covenant should be reviewed by experienced legal counsel before it is implemented.

Many doctors do not have restrictive covenants, as they feel that the physician should only remain in the group if it is beneficial to both parties. Furthermore, they feel that because medicine is a service business, a young physician should not be exploited. However, as private practice becomes more competitive, restrictive covenants of one type or another are becoming more common in the physician contract. Capitated clinics find a restrictive covenant unnecessary since, under the rules of most types of such coverage, patients must stay with the group and cannot follow any one physician.

Vacation: Generally, the amount of pressure in the practice and specialty is used as a guideline to determine the amount of vacation time reasonable for a new physician in his or her initial term. What is common for the area is usually used as a guideline.

Sick Pay or Disability Pay: Decide how long the practice will continue a salary in the event of illness or disability of the participating physician. To avoid unreasonable hardship to the practice, keep this to a minimum for a new physician.

Continuing Education: Consider how much time to allot to the new physician for continuing education and professional meetings. Since a physician has to complete a certain number of hours of formal continuing education to maintain his or her license, it is normal to allow the necessary time off.

Compensation: As mentioned in § 3.05, a compensation plan should be established for a practice. Depending on the practice potential and the need for another physician, it may be possible to compensate the new physician without a loss of money for the practice, since it is expected that the new physician will be able to generate at least enough income to pay for his or her own salary and share of the overhead.

A number of points should be considered. First, the compensation should be thought of in terms of a "compensation package" that includes salary, bonuses, pension and profit sharing contributions, and miscellaneous fringe benefits such as life, health and disability insurance. To assure the physician of his or her opportunity with the practice, it is generally necessary to pay a base salary or guarantee. A bonus plan should be incorporated into the compensation agreement to create additional practice building incentives and to compensate the new physician for extra work. The typical bonus plan allows the physician to receive a bonus when production exceeds the new physician's share of overhead, compensation and a 10 percent override.

Professional Liability Insurance: It is standard for the practice to pay malpractice insurance premiums. The exception is when a physician works on a part-time basis or is involved with a number of different clinics. In multi-specialty groups, the insurance premiums may be included as part of the compensation package to account for large differences in the premium for each practitioner. (For example, a family practitioner who does not do surgery and obstetrics pays far less insurance than an associate who performs these services. He or she may wish to pay individually rather than split the cost of insurance premiums equally.)

Professional Dues and Journal Subscriptions: Some dues and journal subscription costs are shared. Others are best paid by the individual physician.

Transportation: Most physicians need a car to conduct their practices. The practice can either provide the car or require the physician to provide his or her own car. In either case it is common for the practice to reimburse the physician for expenses involving the car. This is frequently included in the compensation package.

Hours: It is important to outline the hours the new associate will be expected to work.

Coverage Arrangements: In many practices, coverage is split equally among the physicians in the group. Other groups provide senior physicians with less of a burden in this area. Small groups may have coverage arrangements with other physicians or physician groups. Special problems can arise when the physician has a specialty different from other physicians in the practice.

Hospitals and Other Facilities: The time the physician must allocate for working at and providing coverage for specific hospitals, nursing homes and other facilities should be discussed.

Appointment Scheduling and Allocation of New and Established Patients: Generally, efforts must be made when a new physician joins a practice to get patients to establish a relationship with him or her. Before the new physician joins the group, his or her qualifications should be promoted through newsletters, announce-

(Pub.372)

ments, etc. Consider bringing the physician on shortly after senior physicians go on vacation so that patients must meet the new physician.

Staff Support for the New Physician: The assistants or nurses available to the new physician should be discussed. While this issue should be generally based on the productivity of the physician, conflict can arise since hiring new staff means an additional expense for the practice.

What Part of the Facility Will Be Available to the New Physician? How will the practice absorb the new physician? Will there be enough examination rooms available for the new member of the practice? If not, and physicians must work split shifts, who will work which shift?

Ownership of Medical Records: Generally, medical records are the property of the clinic rather than of the individual physicians. This should be made clear.

Moonlighting: Generally, moonlighting should be prohibited so that the new physician will concentrate effort on the practice and on building a patient following. All revenues generated by the physician should be submitted to the clinic.

Accounts Receivable: Generally, a new physician is paid immediately, even though billings may take one and a half to three months to collect. When this is not clarified, new physicians sometimes think they have ownership in the accounts receivable. Generally, an employed physician does not obtain equity in the accounts receivable until he or she purchases them or is "given" them by the employer as a form of compensation. The amount the associate physician must pay for accounts receivable and the terms of purchase are spelled out when the associate becomes a partner of the practice. An exception to this procedure is if the associate agrees to forgo a salary for a certain period of time at the beginning to achieve immediate equity in accounts receivable.

Allocation of Charges: If the clinic works on a productivity basis, it is very important to determine how charges are allocated when more than one physician works with a particular patient. Physician credit for charges should be clarified. Problem areas usually include such things as coverage, prenatal care and deliveries, and ancillary services.

Moving Expenses: If the physician is moving from a considerable distance, the practice might pay for moving expenses, or a portion thereof.

Ownership and Future Buy-In: It should be made clear from the beginning whether the associate physician will be able to buy into the practice. If the right to buy-in is an option, specify when it can be exercised. The basic formulas used to value the practice should be discussed initially to avoid any future conflict or misunderstanding (see § 3.07).

Future Profit Distribution: The earning potential and method of profit distribution for the new physician, once he or she becomes an "equal," should be outlined to insure philosophical compatability among practice members.

Length of Notice of Termination: A 30- to 90-day notice clause prior to termination is typical. Whether the contract should automatically be renewed should be discussed. Many employment contracts automatically renew every 12 months unless expressly terminated by one of the parties. This provision is created in order to keep the agreement in effect in the event that a new contract is not signed by the time the old contract expires.

Once the senior physician or physicians in the group have discussed these items among themselves, they can discuss them with the new associate. The prospective associate should be invited to the clinic to see the facilities, meet the staff and visit the various hospitals serviced by the practice. Ideally, the prospective associates could spend several days with the senior physician to get a feel for the practice.

At the meeting with the associate it should be the senior practitioner's responsibility to mention all of the items listed above. Once a tentative oral agreement has been reached, the senior physician can issue a letter to the prospective associate outlining all of the terms agreed upon. If the prospective associate agrees with these terms, the letter should be sent to the practice attorney for the drafting of an employment contract. These basic steps will expedite "signing up" a new associate and eliminate some lengthy meetings with the prospective associate and attorneys.

§ 3.07 Valuing the Practice

> When a change of membership in the practice occurs, a valuation is usually necessary. Both assets and liabilities must be determined. Assets would include supply inventories, accounts receivable, equipment and furniture, goodwill and miscellaneous items such as investments and bank accounts. Liabilities would include taxes, accounts payable, leases and outstanding loans. For the sake of convenience, some practices use a prearranged formula for evaluating practices on an annual basis.

There are many instances in which it is necessary to have a monetary value for the practice:

- When a new associate enters the practice.
- When a senior physician retires.
- Complete sale of the practice.
- Permanent disability of a practice owner.
- Death of a practice owner.

Unfortunately, there is no secret formula for doing a quick practice evaluation. Value must be determined on an individual basis, and it is ultimately determined by the marketplace.

[1] Valuing Assets

The four principal assets the buyer and seller must consider when valuing a practice are:

Equipment and Furniture: The initial starting point for valuing equipment and furniture is the practice depreciation form. These records should list all equipment at cost, the depreciation deducted and the remaining book value. The records should be reviewed to assure that all equipment and furniture items are included. If sloppy records have been kept in the past, it may be necessary to do a complete equipment and furniture inventory.

When placing a price on equipment and furniture, you must consider both the low distressed sale value, or the price you would get if you were to liquidate the practice and sell the equipment piece by piece; and the replacement cost value, or the maximum amount required to replace the piece of equipment with inflated dollars (a higher figure than the original cost). Usually an equipment supplier can provide both of these figures. For purposes of a sale, equitable valuation is usually the midpoint between book value and cost (see Figure 3–6).

Supply Inventories: An inventory of all medical and office supplies should be made. Outdated and worthless items should be left out and current inventory should be valued at cost. Most medical practices do not do inventory routinely. Furthermore, inventory generally changes on a day-to-day basis. When valuing the practice, a final inventory should be made and compared to the initial inventory, and appropriate adjustments should be made.

Accounts Receivable: The accounts receivable of the practice are generally a substantial asset. They should be broken down into those accounts paid by patients and those in which direct third party reimbursement is involved. Private fee values should be based on the experience of the practice. If the practice has a liberal write-off policy and poor collection follow-up, there may be a low collection percentage and a lower value to the accounts receivable. In general, private accounts receivable can be valued as follows:

    Book value of accounts receivable
- All accounts which have not received payment for six or more months
- Accounts at the collection agency
= Collectible accounts receivable
- 15 percent collection and time use of money
= Accounts receivable value

Accounts receivable owed by third parties such as Medicaid must be valued according to the payment terms agreed upon by the third party. Some practices have poor bookkeeping in these areas that makes calculating the face value of accounts receivable complicated, since uncollected amounts were never written off. The value on these accounts must be determined by looking at the outstanding claims to the carrier (i.e., the third party), what the contract calls for as payment and the carrier's payment history. Once these items are determined, the accounts receivable can be valued as follows:

    Book value of accounts receivable

Asset Valuation
(Not Including Accounts Receivable)

	Cost	Adj.	Book	Estimated Market
Cash	2,500		2,500	2,500
Medical Equip (Cost)	50,000			
Accum. Depr.		(20,000)		
"Book" Value			30,000	40,000
Office Furniture (Cost)	15,000			
Accum. Depr.		(5,000)		
"Book" Value			10,000	12,500
Security Deposit	2,500		2,500	2,500
Total Assets	70,000	(25,000)	45,000	57,500

FIG. 3–6. An asset valuation in which the cost, adjustment and book columns represent the practice depreciation form: cost is the amount originally paid for an item; the adjustment is the amount of depreciation; the book value is the cost minus the accumulated depreciation. The estimated market value is calculated as the midpoint between the item's original cost and book value. It is considered a fair sale value that takes into account the cost of replacing the piece of equipment or furniture.

- Amounts previously disallowed
- Amounts to be discounted as per third party agreement
- Claims pending for over six months
= Collectible amount of accounts receivable
- 10 percent for collection and handling
= Value of accounts receivable

Goodwill: Goodwill of the practice is an intangible asset, hence the most difficult item to value. The goodwill of the practice includes, for example, the fact that all of the systems in the practice are in place and functioning, that staff has been hired and trained, patient flow, etc.

(Text continued on page 3–33)

In areas where there is a physician shortage, the value for goodwill may be negligible—i.e. in certain areas of the country in which a particular specialty is highly needed any qualified physician may start a practice and have an immediate following. In many areas of the country, though, the value of goodwill increases as a result of a physician surplus in those areas—i.e., physicians purchasing a practice are willing to pay more for goodwill (a functional practice with established patient flow) than they have in the past. Because HMO's and hospitals are also beginning to buy private practices in some areas, the practice price increases even more. Both the buyer and seller must remember that when transferring the ownership of a practice, the value of goodwill is related to the profitability of the practice. If the buyer is able to make more money by purchasing the practice than would otherwise be available to him or her there is, indeed, value to goodwill.

In recent years, more and more physicians have signed restrictive covenant agreements that prohibit them from terminating their employment with the practice and going out and competing with their employer. Such restrictions add goodwill to the practice and prohibit an employee physician from terminating the practice and taking a large volume of patients with him.

Recent practice sales throughout the country show the following trends* in goodwill as measured by a percentage of production:

Cardiology	22%
Dermatology	29%
Family practice	27%
Internal medicine	20%
Obstetrics/Gynecology	26%
Ophthalmology	40%
Orthopedics	27%
Pediatrics	34%

In addition to the four principle assets mentioned above, some practices must evaluate the following assets:

Real Estate: If the practice owns a building that is being sold with the practice, it must be considered separately. The only way to get a

---
*Source: The Health Care Group, Bala Cynwyd, PA 19004

§ 3.07[1] MANAGING YOUR MEDICAL PRACTICE 3-34

reasonable value on a building is to have a "fee appraisal" done. A fee appraisal is different from the usual type of market analysis done by realtors or brokers who include their commission fee in the value.

One of the following three approaches can be taken in a fee appraisal of the value of a building:

(1) The Income Approach: In this approach, the value of the property is based on the return on the investment in the property. This approach measures the incomes of the property against the various expenses such as interest and maintenance.

(2) Replacement Cost: This approach analyzes what it would cost to purchase the land and construct a new building. A depreciation factor is used in recognition of the fact that a new building would be more valuable.

(3) Market Analysis: This approach attempts to review other similar buildings in the vicinity which have recently been sold to determine a selling price.

Lease and Leasehold Improvements: In many cases, it is necessary for a tenant to make substantial leasehold improvements in a facility before the practice can begin. Because the leasehold improvements are ultimately "owned" by the landlord, they are a form of occupancy cost. Undepreciated leasehold improvements are in effect an asset, not unlike prepaid rent.

When determining the value of the leasehold improvements, the initial cost of the leasehold improvements is divided by the number of months of the lease term. That figure times the number of months left in the lease equals the value of the leasehold improvements.

Cash and Securities: If the practice has any cash in a checking account, savings account, money market account, etc. or any other investments such as stocks or bonds, these items would obviously be put at face value.

Other: Miscellaneous assets should be looked at with caution and the appropriateness of their being in a medical practice should be questioned.

(Rel.3–2/89 Pub.372)

[2] Valuing Liabilities

Once the total assets of the practice have been valued and totaled, practice liabilities must be determined and subtracted from total assets:

Payroll Taxes: Every pay period payroll taxes are withheld from employees' salaries. Depending on their size, payroll taxes must be deposited within three days to three months. Payment of these taxes is strictly enforced by the IRS. Unpaid taxes are considered a liability.

Accounts Payable: Every functioning practice has accounts payable, or the amounts due to the various creditors for items purchased through accounts (often on credit). These include all unpaid statements along with all of the items purchased and delivered but not yet billed for. In a large medical practice, the accounts payable can be substantial.

Equipment and Other Loans: Most practices are in debt for equipment, leasehold improvements or even loans used to subsidize periods of unprofitability. Obviously, the amounts due on any such loans must be determined and considered a liability.

Lease Commitments: Many businesses lease rather than purchase equipment. When the practice has signed a lease, payments must be made until the end of the lease, which is a liability for the purchaser if the lease is bought before payments are completed.

Once all of the assets and liabilities have been determined, the value of the practice is determined simply by subtracting the total liabilities from the total assets.

[3] Preset Buy-Sell Agreements

To facilitate the buy-out of physicians in the event of death, disability or retirement, many practices enter into buy-sell agreements in which the value of the practice is determined according to a preset formula. These agreements are made to expedite the exchange of the practice with a minimum of legal conflicts. To avoid a conflict in the event of the untimely breakup of a group, many practices use one of two methods:

(1) Each year a value is assigned to the practice by the current owners. The owners must agree on the value

assigned each year, otherwise the previous year's valuation is used. Since no one knows who the buyer or seller will be at the time the value is placed, the value is arrived at objectively.

(2) An agreement is made so that in the event someone wishes to leave the practice, the other physician(s) has the first option to buy out his or her share for the agreed upon price. Since the person initiating the transfer may end up buying or selling the practice, he or she must determine a fair price.

§ 3.08 Checklist for Forms of Practice

A comprehensive list of points to keep in mind is given.

__ Types of practice
  __ Single practitioner
  __ Professional association (P.A., P.C.)
  __ Space-sharing partnership
  __ Incorporated partnerships

__ Advantages of unincorporated practice
  __ Total control
  __ No legal or accounting costs
  __ Informal bookkeeping
  __ All business income reported as personal income
  __ Fewer tax liabilities
  __ Investment tax credits

__ Advantages of corporation vs. single practice
  __ Budgeting
  __ Dividend exclusions
  __ Limited liability
  __ Flexible benefit plans
  __ Insurance benefits:
    __ Life

— Disability
— Medical insurance
— Tighter financial controls

(Text continued on page 3–37)

— Legal documents for a corporation
  — Articles of incorporation
  — By-laws
  — Bill of sale (equipment transfers)
  — Buy-sell agreement
  — Employment agreement
  — Wage continuation provisions
  — Pension plan
  — Profit sharing plan
  — Disability plan
  — Flexible benefit plan
  — Life insurance plan/death benefits
  — Medical insurance plan
  — Minutes of stockholder meetings
  — Minutes of director meetings
  — Waiver of meeting notice

— Hiring new physician into partnership
  — Restricting covenant, moonlighting
  — Hours, vacation
  — Sick pay/disability
  — Continuing education
  — Compensation
  — Professional liability insurance
  — Professional dues and journal subscriptions
  — Transportation, fees
  — Coverage, hospital arrangements, allocation of charges
  — New patients
  — Availability of facilities
  — Ownership of medical records
  — Accounts receivable

(Pub.372)

- Future profit distribution
- Terms of termination
- Profit distribution in groups
    - Productivity
    - Equity in practice
    - Seniority
    - Office management
    - Days worked
    - Certification
    - Cost containment
- Valuing the Practice
    - Assets
        - Equipment and furniture
        - Supply inventory (professional and office)
        - Accounts receivable
        - Goodwill
        - Building
        - Lease and leasehold improvements
        - Prepaid rent
        - Cash and securities
    - Liabilities
        - Payroll taxes
        - Accounts payable
        - Equipment and other loans
        - Lease committment

§ 3.100 Bibliography

Brown, S.: The Statewide PPO that Couldn't Miss—But Did. Medical Economics, Oct. 15, 1984, pp. 64–67.

Ritterband, A. B.: Why We've Never Gone Wrong on a New

Associate. Medical Economics, Aug. 6, 1984, pp. 149–162.

Scherger, J. E.: Small Practices Won't Survive? Don't You Believe It! Medical Economics, Oct. 15, 1984, pp. 33–36.

CHAPTER 4

Office Systems

> **SCOPE**
>
> The physician who wishes to provide the best possible medical care in an economical and efficient manner must use the best office systems available. Almost every aspect of a practice can be thought of in terms of a system: the way telephones are answered; the way information on each patient is gathered and stored; the way appointments are scheduled; the way that the time of the patient and physician is spent in the office; and the way that follow-up examinations and test results are handled. When the physician makes an effort to organize patient services and to accommodate patient needs, it communicates concern for patients and assures delivery of orderly and professional care.

SYNOPSIS

§ 4.01 Telephone Answering and Message Systems
 [1] Telephone Messages
 [2] Priority System
 [3] Answering Machines and Services
  [a] Answering Machines
  [b] Answering Services
 [4] Buying/Renting a Telephone System
§ 4.02 Appointment Systems
 [1] Appointment Books
 [2] Computerized Appointment Systems
 [3] Timing Appointments
 [4] Wave System
 [5] Delays and Miscellaneous Considerations
§ 4.03 Patient Flow
 [1] Preparation
 [2] Examination
 [3] Ancillary Services
 [4] After the Examination

    [5] Referral and Hospitalization
§ 4.04 Patient Records
    [1] Patient Information Forms
    [2] Assignment of Benefits Form
    [3] Routing Slip
    [4] Medical History
    [5] Chart Notations
    [6] Systematic Filing
§ 4.05 Dictation Processing
    [1] Portable vs. Desktop Equipment
    [2] Transcription
§ 4.06 Referral Information Systems
§ 4.07 Recall and Reminder Systems
§ 4.08 Follow-Up Systems
§ 4.09 Checklist for Office Systems
§ 4.10–§ 4.99 Reserved
§ 4.100 Bibliography
Appendix 4-A Routing Slips

§ 4.01 Telephone Answering and Message Systems

> The initial contact most patients have with the medical office takes place over the telephone. A well-thought out telephone answering policy should be designed and implemented in the office. Message slips, telephone systems, answering service and answering machines are all items that the physician with a busy and growing practice should consider.

The office telephone is the liaison between doctor and patient. Telephones that are not answered promptly, prolonged busy signals, lost messages and curt receptionists are not only bad practice but they can also lead to malpractice and professional liability lawsuits.

A telephone policy should be implemented and every employee made familiar with the policy at the start of his or her employment. Ideally, the telephone should be answered after one ring, and in no case should it be allowed to ring more than three times. If necessary, the person handling the telephone may put the caller on hold, but only after confirming that the situation is not an emergency. The caller must always be treated with the utmost respect.

(Pub.372)

[1] Telephone Messages

The person who answers the telephone will be either the receptionist or medical asitant. Do not assume that he or she will automatically know how to handle various types of calls. Some calls must be transferred from a receptionist to a medical assistant, nurse or physician, and patient charts will have to be pulled so that the physician or assistant will be familiar with the patient's history when responding to questions.

If the physician or medical assistant is not available to take the call, specific information will have to be recorded. The information may vary depending on the doctor's field, but essentially, information should always include:

- The caller's complete name, spelled accurately.
- A telephone number at which the caller may be reached (if necessary, more than one number should be recorded, along with the time the caller will be at that particular number).
- The reason for the call, i.e., a medical problem, a business call or a personal call.
- Whether the call is an emergency.
- If it is a business call, the business association and company the caller is representing.
- The specific message.
- Who referred the patient to the office, especially if the caller is a new patient.

[2] Priority System

Any employee who answers the telephone should be trained to know the priority of calls. In a medical office, the priority would range from the most important, a medical emergency, to a call from a salesman. The medical assistant or receptionist should be able to tell whether or not the problem is an emergency and, if the physician is not immediately available, be able to advise the caller whether to report to the office, go to the hospital or wait for a return call from the physician.

In addition to training an assistant or receptionist in how to handle emergency calls, you should design a protocol he or she can give an emergency patient, whether or not you are in your office at the time.

At the other end of the spectrum, a telephone call from a sales representative should routinely be recorded and referred to the doctor at his or her convenience. How calls in between these two extremes are to be handled depends on the nature of the call, your attitude and the attitude of the caller. Typically, calls from family members, the office accountant or attorney can be handled satisfactorily by a return call from the physician within a few hours. The relationship between these callers and the physician is such that if the call requires immediate attention the caller will say so, in which case the call should be put through to the physician.

The medical assistant or receptionist may be able to handle calls regarding medical problems with low priority. In addition, your office can implement a system designed to handle calls for medication refills. When medication that may need to be refilled is prescribed, the patient's name, the type of medication and the circumstances allowing refill should be recorded. Then, when a call for a prescription refill comes in, the medical assistant will be able to immediately check the prescription refill file and either give permission, pass the call to the physician or request that the patient return for another office visit.

[3] Answering Machines and Services

Medical problems can and often do occur outside of office hours and on weekends. This makes a 24-hour a day answering service a necessity for a physician in private practice. There are basically two choices: the answering machine and the answering service.

[a] Answering Machines

The main advantage of an answering machine is that you can control exactly what message is given and, barring mechanical failure, rest assured that the telephone will be answered 24 hours a day, 365 days a year.

An appropriate message for an answering machine would be as follows:

"Thank you for calling Dr. Robert's office. Our office is currently not open. If you have an emergency, you may reach Dr. Roberts at 123–4567. If you have an emergency and are unable to reach Dr. Roberts, proceed immediately to Bellview Memorial Hospital's emergency room, located at 495 Smith Street. The emergency room is open and staffed with a physician 24 hours a day. The emergency phone number is 123–4567. Dr. Robert's office is open from 9:00 A.M. to 5:00 P.M., Monday through Friday. If you would like to schedule an appointment or discuss a non-emergency matter, please call us anytime during these hours. We would be pleased to hear from you. Thank you for calling".

Notice that this message gives the patient crucial information first and then routine information. It is informative and does not require that the patient "talk to a machine."

[b] Answering Services

The alternative to the answering machine is the answering service. Unfortunately, good answering services are hard to find. Even finding a competent answering service does not permanently solve the problem, as a good answering service can quickly slip as a result of employee turnover.

When selecting an answering service, speak to other physicians in the area and find out what service they are using. Also speak to the hospital with whom you are affiliated, since hospitals sometimes provide answering services for their physicians. This may be your best choice, since the hospital deals with the same types of problems as a physician's office deals with and has a medical staff to evaluate the seriousness of a call.

Once you have developed a list of potential answering services, contact them and ask for information regarding cost, how they answer the phone, and whether or not they are available 24 hours a day, 365 days a year. Question them on how they recruit staff and the minimum qualifications for their operators. Find out the actual mechanics of subscribing to the answering service, such as whether or not special equipment or a special telephone line will need to be installed in your office.

Once you have obtained this information, randomly call some of the offices using a particular telephone service during a time you know the service will be picking up calls. Act like a patient and see how the service handles the call: whether or not they answer the telephone quickly and give the proper information is the best barometer for the quality of service.

Once you decide which answering machine or service is appropriate for your office, program it or leave instructions for when it is to be used. An answering service should be instructed, for example, to pick up calls after the telephone has rung three times. This will protect the office in the event the staff forgets to check out with the answering service at the end of the work day. A telephone answering machine can be set the same way.

Once the office has checked out with the telephone service, the service should be instructed to answer the telephone on the first ring. Ideally, the answering machine should be set to answer the telephone after the first ring. Periodically monitor your answering service by calling your office on off hours as though you were a patient calling. This will give you insight as to how calls to your office are being handled during the off hours. If you discover a problem, register a complaint, and if the problem is not solved, don't hesitate to change services.

[4] Buying/Renting a Telephone System

Not too long ago, having a telephone system installed in the office was a simple matter. However, increased competition, anti-trust suits and federal deregulation have made obtaining a telephone system much more complex. There are currently three options available regarding telephone equipment:

(1) Renting a telephone system. This was standard until a few years ago, and if a new telephone system has not been installed recently, or you have not made changes in your service for the past few years, this is probably the way your telephone system is handled.

(2) Leasing. This is like a rental situation, but less expensive. However, it generally commits the lessor to a particular piece of equipment for a longer period of time.

(3) Purchase. Generally, purchasing the telephone system is your best choice. This is because even though a rental system may theoretically be changed any month, as a practical matter the system will not be changed due to

(Pub.372)

high installation and removal costs. By purchasing equipment, the cost may be amortized over five years. Generally, this will result in a lower price not only after the equipment is amortized, but also during the period of amortization.

When selecting telephone equipment, do not be mesmerized or overwhelmed by companies that promise their telephones will do just about everything but see your patients. As a practical matter, you should follow two rules when selecting telephone equipment:

- Get what you need. Remember, you are buying a telephone system to perform an important function in your office. Do not waste money on gimmicks that look great but are unnecessary.

- Get dependable service. Pick a system that is known for quality and minimum down time. Make sure the vendor of the equipment has a competent maintenance department that can provide immediate service in the event of a system failure. Also make sure the vendor takes full responsibility for a downed system and coordinates any problems between the equipment failure and line problems with the telephone company.

§ 4.02 Appointment Systems

The appointment book should be the "control tower" of the medical office. Whether kept manually for a small practice or on computer for a number of cooperating physicians, the office appointment system should keep track of all office hours and all services provided. Timing of appointments is determined largely by the amount of time it takes a physician and assistants to perform specific procedures, and by the amount of time it takes a patient to fill out forms and provide necessary information. The most efficient way of scheduling patients so that the physcian can be productive without having to work under stress or waste a patient's time is entirely up to office policy. However, every appointment system should be flexible enough to accommodate emergency patients, walk-in patients and other "squeeze-ins."

In the past, patients in need of physician's services could stop by and see the physician at any time without an appointment. This was not an efficient system for either the patient or the physician, especially if several patients came at one time; it often resulted in

(Pub.372)

patients having to wait a long time and the physician having to work under great stress. With today's increased competition in the medical area, and with the high value of both the physician's and patient's time, it is crucial that your practice implement an efficient appointment system.

[1] Appointment Books

An appointment system may be either manual (the traditional appointment book) or automated (computerized). In the medical industry, the appointment book is the most commonly used system. The "week at a glance" type of appointment book is generally the best, since it can usually accommodate more than one physician or department. The advantage of a week at a glance model appointment book is that it allows enough room for a receptionist or assistant to schedule appointments without having to turn the page to find available appointments that week, or turn only a few pages to find available appointments for that month.

[2] Computerized Appointment Systems

An automated or computerized appointment system has a number of advantages:

Integration: In a large practice with an on-line computer system, a number of different users can be working with the appointment schedule at the same time. When an appointment slot fills up, it is automatically displayed on each computer terminal. More than one person can use this type of system at the same time without having to fight over the appointment book.

Neatness: An appointment book can become messy if a number of changes need to be made, but it is easy to change appointments on a computerized system.

Time Saving: At the end of the day (or at the beginning of the day of the appointments), the computer can print out a work schedule for each physician and charge slips for each patient to be seen the following day. Under a manual system, work schedules need to be typed from the appointment book and charge slips need to be prepared by hand.

Internal Control: Computerized appointment scheduling can keep track of all the patients who should have been in and had charges, and report back any patients who were scheduled but had no charges entered into the computer.

Volume: Whereas a manual system may entail the use of multiple appointment books for a large practice, a computer system provides virtually unlimited "columns" or space available to make appointments.

There is one major disadvantage to computerized appointment scheduling: down time. If, for some reason, the computer is disabled, the office will neither know who is coming in nor be able to schedule future appointments. As a result, the office will appear to be disorganized. For this reason, it is essential that a back-up system be in place. At the end of each day, for example, the staff should print out a listing of appointments for at least the next two weeks. That way, if the computer breaks down, the bulk of the appointment scheduling will be available on hard copy and the appointment clerks will be able to make do. Any mistakes detected once the computer is operational again will need to be corrected and confirmed with the patient involved.

[3] Timing Appointments

Regardless of the type of appointment system used, certain problems in scheduling will occur in any medical office. Every physician works differently, and the amount of time needed to perform certain procedures will vary with the individual. It is therefore necessary to "customize" a schedule for each physician so that problems can be anticipated and handled without jeopardizing efficiency of services.

Some procedures require a set amount of time. This should be based on the amount of time you feel is needed to get the job done satisfactorily. In addition, you should periodically "test" your skills to determine whether or not the procedure can be performed in a shorter amount of time. In the beginning, for example, you may wish to schedule a set amount of time for a procedure, but once you become more efficient and experienced, you may be able to cut the time by as much as 40 or 50 percent. Be careful not to fall into the trap of slowing down the procedure to fill the appointment.

Some procedures, such as a physical examination, require patient contact with both the physician and ancillary staff, such as laboratory and x-ray technicians. The appointment schedule should be coordinated so that you are seeing another patient while the patient is with one of the assistants. Under these circumstances, each portion of the overall examination must be evaluated in time frames so that the appointment secretary will not over- or underbook you. Many internists prefer to have patients come in for routine laboratory and x-ray tests prior to being seen by the physician. This eliminates having to move the patient around from station to station on the day of the examination and also assures that test results will be available for evaluation at the time the patient is seen by the physician.

Patient convenience and comfort are of paramount importance when setting up appointment schedules. If a patient has to fast the night before certain tests are performed, for example, he or she should be given priority scheduling for the first time slot in the morning.

[4] **Wave System**

It is impossible to determine the exact amount time needed for many procedures: some will take five or ten minutes, others may need twenty, and all will depend on the individual patient. Neither does the appointment secretary have any way of knowing exactly how long many of these office procedures take, and he or she will typically schedule appointments based on an average amount of time per patient. If the average visit runs 12 minutes, the secretary will schedule an appointment every 12 minutes. This can disrupt your schedule if the first three patients are five-minute appointments and the last three are 20-minute appointments.

A "wave system" of scheduling is designed to eliminate this problem and maximize the use of a physician's time. With a wave scheduling system, all of the patients to be seen during the hour are scheduled at the beginning of the hour at the same time. The physician constantly has a patient available to work on under this system and is generally caught up at the end of each hour. But while this is an efficient system for the physician, it is generally not well received by patients, who sometimes are upset to learn that five other patients are scheduled to see the doctor at the same time they are. Furthermore, if the five-minute patient is the last patient to be seen, he or she may end up waiting 55 minutes to see the physician. This is a negative practice builder.

The best solution to this problem is to adopt a hybrid, or modified, wave system. Under a modified wave method, the average number of patients per hour and the range of time each is expected to spend with the physician is determined. Assume, for example, that Dr. Nickels sees an average of six patients per hour and time spent with the patients ranges from seven to twenty minutes. Under this method, a patient should be scheduled every seven minutes. This will ensure that the physician will always have a patient ready to be seen. From the patient's point of view, each patient has a specific time designated (i.e., there will be no duplicate appointment times) and, barring unusual circumstances, no patient should have to wait more than sixteen minutes to see the physician.

[5] Delays and Miscellaneous Considerations

If you arrive late at the office for your first appointment or underestimate the amount of time it will take, it may put you behind schedule for the entire day. This happens occasionally, and most patients are willing to accept it on a limited basis; few, however, are willing to accept waiting a few hours every time they go to see the physician. This indicates to them that the physician is too busy for his or her patients and has little respect for their time. The notion that the successful physician is always two or three hours behind schedule was discarded years ago and is not likely to be resurrected.

In the event a delay or hospital emergency prevents you from getting to the office on time, contact your appointment secretary to report the delay and give an estimated time of arrival. The receptionist should then inform waiting patients that you have been delayed due to an emergency, and tell them how many hours behind schedule you are. The patients should be treated hospitably and offered use of the telephone, since they may need to inform their own next appointments of the delay. If the physician is going to be delayed for a long period of time, the patients should be offered the opportunity to reschedule their appointments at another time or to leave the office and come back.

When scheduling appointments, be sure to allow enough time for patients to complete any necessary registration forms. A new patient generally has more forms to complete and should be instructed to come to the office before his or her scheduled appointment. For example, if a patient is scheduled to see you at 8:00 A.M., and completing necessary forms is expected to take seven minutes, it is recommended that the patient be told his or her appointment time is 7:53 A.M. Although giving such precise times may seem unrealistic, many patients feel that an appointment time is an estimate, rather than an actual time. (This is especially true if the physician is chronically off-schedule, either because of overwork or failure to respect the appointment book.) Giving such a precise time implies to the patient that your office is time-conscious and intends to be punctual. Patients will sometimes assume that an 8:00 A.M. appointment means "about" 8:00 A.M., and they may show up late on the assumption that the doctor will be behind or does not pay exact attention to time.

Another problem that disrupts appointment schedules is the emergency and walk-in patient. Although emergencies are unpredictable, your office may be able to anticipate the amount of emergency and walk-in patients on a given day the same way a restaurant determines the amount of a particular entree to have on hand. Once the average number of emergencies and walk-ins is determined, time on the appointment schedule can be budgeted to handle them. Except for emergencies or circumstances requiring immediate attention, priority should be given to patients with appointments. Walk-in patients will understand they may need to wait and will appreciate the fact that they will be seen at all.

A busy physician may begin by leaving a week open each month, a day open each week and an hour each day. Based on practice statistics, the exact amount of time left open in each of these periods should be adjusted. If, for example, the average day requires half an hour of time for walk-ins and emergencies, a half-hour should be left open each day instead of an hour.

§ 4.03 Patient Flow

What happens in the office during a patient's appointment is of great importance to your professional image. Large or small, a well-run office should have a system of patient flow with which all employees are familiar. A good patient flow system begins with anticipation of the daily appointment schedule and the ordering of any tests that will need to be done outside of the office before the patient visits; an examination during which salient points about the patient's problem and medical history are obtained; routing of the patient to various assistants for ancillary tests, if necessary, and strict accounting of all tests performed; checking out and settlement of accounts; and information for the patient who needs to be referred to a consulting physician or hospital. An appointment schedule should always be structured in such a way that the physician can work on more than one patient at a time and still provide satisfactory care.

Everthing that happens between the time the patient enters the office for his or her appointment until the time the patient leaves the office is extremely important, from the standpoint of both public relations and efficiency. The flow through the office should make the patient feel expected and welcome, and should manifest a well-organized office. The patient's opinion of the physician will be greatly influenced by whether or not the entire office and staff seem organized, efficient and hospitable. Moreover, the smoother an office is run, the greater its productivity is likely to be.

[1] Preparation

At the end of each day, after the last patient is seen, or at the beginning of each day, before the first patient is seen, the appointment secretary should review the schedule for the upcoming day and prepare a list showing the time of the appointment, the patient's name and the procedure to be performed on the patient by each provider. A copy of this list should be prepared for you and for each person who will provide care for the patient.

The medical chart of each patient to be seen should be pulled. Any "flags" on the chart should be noted and acted upon. (A sample of a "flag" on a chart would be a reminder that the patient is delinquent in payment and should see the person who handles fee collection before leaving the office that day; for a sample delinquent payment flag, see Figure 4–1.)

Your office should be laid out so that the receptionist can see arriving patients. He or she should anticipate each patient's arrival and greet the patient by name and with a cheerful smile. New patients should be given new patient information forms to complete and established patients should be asked if there has been any

§ 4.03 [1]   MANAGING YOUR MEDICAL PRACTICE   4–14

CHART FLAG

Clinic _____   Chart Number _____   Account Number _____

Patient _____
         (Last)   (First)   (Middle)

☐ Account sent to collections on _____ amount _____
☐ Bankrupt
☐ Do not see patient without talking with Credit Department.

Form 2

FIG. 4–1. The chart flag can be used to remind the physician's office that the patient has an outstanding account. A charge slip with the patient's name and account number should be attached to the chart. If the patient receives Medicare and outside laboratory work will be ordered, a slip should be prepared to be attached to the specimen for forwarding to the outside lab. With a pegboard billing system, it may be appropriate to pull the financial ledger cards for each of the patients to be seen and have them arranged in the order in which patients are scheduled.

(Pub.372)

change in their address or third-party coverage since their last visit. If the patient is covered by a third party that requires identification at each visit (e.g. Medicaid), the receptionist should request such identification and record the account numbers and eligibility dates directly from the card. Once these bookkeeping tasks are accomplished, the patient should be invited to take a seat in the reception area.

As noted above, a new patient should be told to arrive at the office slightly ahead of the appointed time to complete any forms. Ideally, the patient will be ready to be seen at his or her appointed time and you will be ready to see the patient. The medical assistant should pick up the patient chart, charge slip and other data, proceed to the reception area at the appointed time, and greet the patient. The medical assistant should introduce himself or herself to the patient (it is also recommended that the staff wear name tags) and lead the patient to the appropriate station, generally the examination room or consultation room. The patient should be informed by the medical assistant of what is to happen next. If the patient is to be seen by the physician, he or she should be instructed to wait, and if the patient needs to disrobe and put on a gown for an examination, the assistant should instruct the patient to do so.

If the patient is new, it is recommended that he or she remain clothed for your first meeting in the consultation room. This allows the patient to meet with you on an "equal," face-to-face basis. Although this may seem like a waste of time, it usually makes a patient feel more confident and comfortable with a physician and helps the physician to view patients as people rather than as medical problems.

[2] Examination

Once the initial introduction procedures have been taken care of, the examination may begin. At this point, you should ask specific questions relating to the patient's problem. If you are giving the patient a physical examination, you should ask questions from a medical history questionnaire. Some physicians feel it is important to conduct the interview themselves so that they can obtain additional information from body language and facial expressions. Other physicians feel the patient is sometimes more comfortable speaking with the assistant and that more information can be obtained that way.

For routine procedures, such as physical examination, the office staff will know how much time is to be spent on the interview and what additional tests and procedures will be performed, and will be able to anticipate patient flow accordingly. In other situations, you must determine at the end of your information-gathering whether a diagnosis can be made or additional tests need to be performed. Additional tests range from those which can be immediately performed at the office, to those which can be done at the office but at a later date, to those which can only be done in facilities outside the office.

If you make the diagnosis and decide upon the course of treatment, you should discuss this with the patient at this time. Explain to the patient, in layman's terms, what the problem is and the recommended treatment. Ask questions of the patient and take time to answer any of the patient's questions carefully.

Check off all procedures performed and your diagnosis on the patient's routing slip (see § 4.04[3]). You should also chart all of the procedures performed and check to see if all procedures performed by the assistants have been recorded. Entries into the medical history should then be signed or initialed. The routing slip should be removed from the chart at this time and given to the patient, along with instructions to check out and give the routing slip to the receptionist.

When you leave the examining room, take the chart with you and place it in a central location where it can be picked up and filed by the receptionist. Each examining room should have a tray or slot in which to place the patient's chart when the patient is waiting to be seen by the physician or physician's assistant.

It is convenient to have a signal system on the door or near each examining room to indicate the status of the room: i.e. "patient waiting to see doctor," "patient receiving ancillary services," and "examination complete." This type of system alerts everyone to what is happening in the room and its availability, and prevents a patient from being "forgotten."

(Pub.372)

[3] Ancillary Services

If during the course of the initial examination, you decide additional tests such as x-rays or laboratory tests must be conducted, inform the patient and tell him or her who will perform the test. Check off the ordered procedures on the routing slip, chart what you have done so far, tell the patient where to go and proceed to your next patient.

Large practices may have different people at various stations to perform tests. In some, for example, each doctor has a personal assistant and, in addition, the clinic or practice employs a technician to draw blood and conduct lab tests and a technician to take and process x-rays. In such an environment, it would be the medical assistant's duty to bring the patient to the appropriate technician, along with the chart and routing slip showing the procedures requested by the physician. The medical assistant would also "flag" the room as to its status. In this case the room would be flagged to indicate that it is not available for other patients because the patient occupying the room is at the lab having blood drawn. In a smaller office without technicians, it may be the assistant's job not only to take the patient to the lab but to perform the ancillary tests as well.

Once the ancillary service is performed, the assistant or technician can move the patient back to the examining room, and flag it to indicate that the patient is back and ready to be seen by the physician by placing the chart, routing slip and test results (if available) in the chart slot or tray. You should complete the examination at this point and discharge the patient when done. With coordinated team work and adequate facilities, you can keep moving from examining room to examining room, performing necessary work without having to wait for patients to be placed in rooms or for rooms to be prepared.

[4] After the Examination

After you have completed the examination, instruct the patient to give the receptionist the routing slip upon checking out. The receptionist should be alert to the patient forgetting or deliberately avoiding checking out. As each patient leaves, the receptionist should take the routing slip, review it for obvious errors and see if

§ 4.03 [5]   MANAGING YOUR MEDICAL PRACTICE   4–18

the patient has been instructed to make another appointment. If you have indicated the need for a follow-up appointment, the receptionist should remind the patient at this time and the next appointment should be recorded in the appointment book, on the routing slip and on an appointment card which is given to the patient.

The receptionist should then add up the total charges for that day and ask if the patient would like to make a payment. If the patient makes a payment, it should be recorded on the routing slip and a copy of the routing slip given to the patient for his or her receipt. In many cases, insurance does not cover office visits. If insurance is involved, though, the patient should be asked to sign the insurance form and the assignment of benefits on the insurance form. If the patient does not wish to make a payment at the time, he or she should be given a copy of the routing slip, with the explanation that it is a statement of charges, along with an envelope for future payment purposes. The patient should then be cheerfully thanked for coming to the office.

(For a flow-chart on a typical routine for seeing the patient through the office, see Figure 4–2.)

[5] Referral and Hospitalization

In cases where you refer the patient to a consulting physician or to the hospital, it will be necessary for you or your assistant to talk to the patient before he or she leaves. A smooth system should be set up to handle each of these situations.

In the event the patient is being referred to a consulting doctor, it is best for the assistant to sit down with the patient and schedule the appointment. The assistant should give the patient instructions on the location of the consulting physician's office along with the name, address and telephone number. If the patient needs to prepare in any way for the consultation—for example, by fasting—the assistant should explain this. The patient should be told how much time to allow for the consultation and when you will have the results to discuss with him or her. The patient should then be given a referral slip containing the information about the consulting office and introducing him or her to the consulting physician.

In the event the patient is to be hospitalized, the assistant should contact the hospital to make necessary arrangements and instruct

PATIENT FLOW CHART

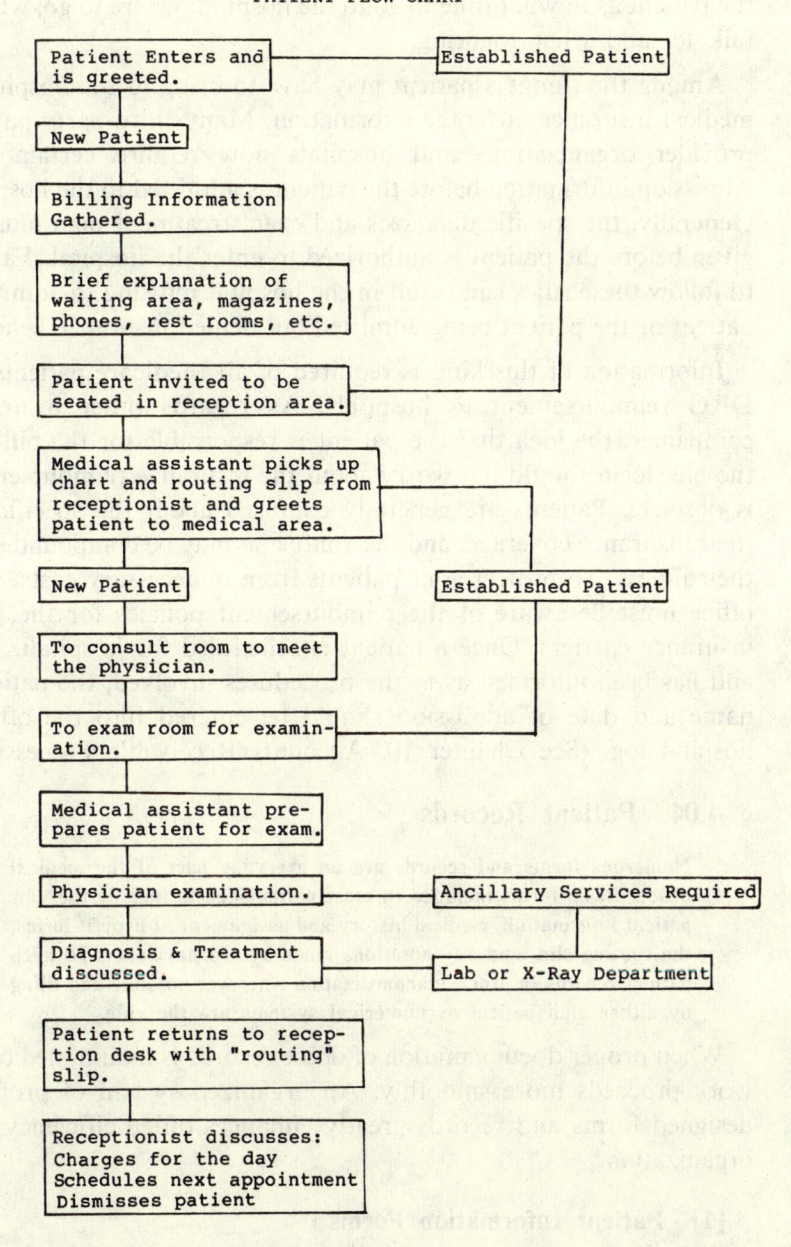

```
┌─────────────────────┐         ┌─────────────────────┐
│ Patient Enters and  ├─────────┤ Established Patient │
│ is greeted.         │         │                     │
└──────────┬──────────┘         └─────────────────────┘
           │
┌──────────┴──────────┐
│ New Patient         │
└──────────┬──────────┘
           │
┌──────────┴──────────┐
│ Billing Information │
│ Gathered.           │
└──────────┬──────────┘
           │
┌──────────┴──────────┐
│ Brief explanation of│
│ waiting area, magaz-│
│ ines, phones, rest  │
│ rooms, etc.         │
└──────────┬──────────┘
           │
┌──────────┴──────────┐
│ Patient invited to  │
│ be seated in        │
│ reception area.     │
└──────────┬──────────┘
           │
┌──────────┴──────────┐
│ Medical assistant   │
│ picks up chart and  │
│ routing slip from   │
│ receptionist and    │
│ greets patient to   │
│ medical area.       │
└──────────┬──────────┘
           │
┌──────────┴──────────┐         ┌─────────────────────┐
│ New Patient         │         │ Established Patient │
└──────────┬──────────┘         └─────────────────────┘
           │
┌──────────┴──────────┐
│ To consult room to  │
│ meet the physician. │
└──────────┬──────────┘
           │
┌──────────┴──────────┐
│ To exam room for    │
│ examination.        │
└──────────┬──────────┘
           │
┌──────────┴──────────┐
│ Medical assistant   │
│ prepares patient    │
│ for exam.           │
└──────────┬──────────┘
           │
┌──────────┴──────────┐         ┌─────────────────────┐
│ Physician examin-   ├─────────┤Ancillary Services   │
│ ation.              │         │Required             │
└──────────┬──────────┘         └─────────────────────┘
           │                    ┌─────────────────────┐
┌──────────┴──────────┐         │ Lab or X-Ray        │
│ Diagnosis &         ├─────────┤ Department          │
│ Treatment discussed.│         │                     │
└──────────┬──────────┘         └─────────────────────┘
           │
┌──────────┴──────────┐
│ Patient returns to  │
│ reception desk with │
│ "routing" slip.     │
└──────────┬──────────┘
           │
┌──────────┴──────────┐
│ Receptionist discus-│
│ ses:                │
│ Charges for the day │
│ Schedules next      │
│ appointment         │
│ Dismisses patient   │
└─────────────────────┘
```

FIG. 4–2. The medical office should have an orderly procedure for conducting new and regular patients through an office visit. All office personnel should be familiar with this system.

(Pub.372)

the patient as to what time to go to the hospital, where to go, who to talk to, and what to bring.

Among the things a patient may have to bring to the hospital is medical insurance coverage information. Many third-party payers, provider organizations and hospitals now require certain pre-admission information before the patient is admitted to the hospital. Generally, the specific diagnosis and exact treatment plan must be given before the patient is authorized to enter the hospital. Failure to follow these rules can result in the hospital refusing to admit the patient or the patient being admitted but denied insurance benefits.

Information of this kind is required of all Medicare patients for DRG reimbursement to hospitals. As regards other insurance companies, the idea that the patient is responsible for the bill and the physician should not worry about the insurance reimbursement is obsolete. Patients are generally confused about the specifics of their insurance coverage, and the confusion may be compounded by their illness. To protect your patients from unnecessary costs, your office must be aware of the reimbursement policies for the local insurance carriers. Once a patient is scheduled for hospitalization and has been informed as to the procedures involved, the patient's name and date of admission should be entered into the office's hospital log. (See Chapter 10, Accounts Receivable Processing.)

§ 4.04 Patient Records

Numerous forms and records are an everyday part of the medical office. Basic forms included in most patient charts include the new patient information, medical history and assignment of benefit forms, the routing slip, and any notations made by the physician. To keep patient records in order, standardization wherever possible and filing by either alphabetical or numerical systems are the rule.

When proper documentation of office records is maintained office work proceeds more smoothly. An organized system of properly designed forms and records greatly enhances office efficiency and organization.

[1] Patient Information Forms

The new patient information form should be filled out by all new patients and updated whenever an item on the form changes. The receptionist should give the form to the patient at his or her initial

§ 4.04[1]

visit, and see that the patient completes it in a time period specifically set aside for this purpose (see § 4.03[1]). Each time the patient visits thereafter, the receptionist should ask if there have been any changes.

The following items should be included on the patient information form:

- The patient's complete name.
- The patient's complete address and mailing address.
- The party responsible for the bill in the event the patient is a minor or otherwise not responsible for the bill.
- The name and telephone number of the person to be contacted in the event of an emergency.
- The patient's primary insurance coverage, including:
  Insurance company
  Company address
  Telephone number
  Policy number
  Group number, if applicable
  Insurance sponsor, if applicable.
- Name of employer.
- Employer address and telephone number.
- Patient's social security number.
- Patient's birth date.
- Patient's sex.
- Marital status.
- Spouse's name.
- Spouse's employer.
- Address and telephone number of spouse's employer.
- Statement of patient's intent to pay bill. An example would be:
  I prefer to:
  _____Pay my bills at the time of services.
  _____Pay my bill upon receipt of statement.
  _____Make credit arrangements with the credit manager.

(Pub.372)

- Patient's signature and date.
- Whom may we thank for referring you to our office?

Information gathered on the new patient information form is entered into the billing system. The actual form is generally kept with the patient's chart.

(For an example of the patient information form, see Figure 4–3.)

[2] Assignment of Benefits Form

The assignment of benefits form should be completed by the new patient at the initial visit, or when an established patient changes insurance companies. Offices occasionally incorporate this form into the new patient information form; however, it is a good practice to keep this as a separate form, since you may have to send a copy to the insurance company.

The assignment of benefits forms is a master form that assigns all of the patient's third-party medical benefits for services performed at the physician's office directly to the physician's office. This is advantageous to the patient, since it routes the check directly to the physician's office without having to pass through his or her hands. Under these circumstances, the patient need only pay that portion of the bill that is part of the deductible or coinsurance, or that is not covered by the insurance. Occasionally, a patient who has assigned benefits to the physician mistakenly pays the bill, with the result that the physician is paid twice for services. As a policy, you should make prompt refunds when this happens; if the patient is expected to pay promptly, the office should abide by the same rule.

As part of the assignment of benefits form, a statement should be appended authorizing the physician's office to provide information to the third party. The following is an example of an assignment of benefits form with such authorization:

I hereby authorize insurance payments to be made directly to the Smith Clinic, (address of office). I further authorize a release of any medical information necessary to process the claim and payment of benefits to myself or the party who accepts assignment.

_____

Patient's Signature

Patient Registration

(Confidential information necessary for your file)

Patient's Name (Last)	(First)	(Initial)	Age	Marital Status	
Person responsible for payment of account (Last)		(First)	(Initial)	Relationship to Patient	
Address		City	State	Zip	Home Phone
Employer's Name		How Long	Address		Business Phone
Spouse Employed by			Who referred you to this office?		
Insurance or 3rd party coverage	Policy or Identification Number		Date of Birth	Social Security Number	

Please check the appropriate line

_____ I will pay my balance in full at time of service.

_____ I will pay my balance in full upon receipt of first statement.

_____ I will make payment arrangements with the Credit Manager prior to services being rendered.

Signature of Patient _____ Date _____

FIG. 4–3. A basic patient information form.

(Pub.372)

Patients who do not authorize the assignment of benefits will have to sign a form authorizing you to release records to the insurance carrier. If this form is not signed, you will not be able to bill the insurance company directly. Generic release of records forms that authorize the physician's office to send necessary records to another physician or clinic are available.

(See Figure 4-4 for a sample patient registration form with attached assignment of benefits form.)

[3] Routing Slip

The next essential form to be designed is the routing, or charge, slip. The purpose of this form is to organize the method of recording charges and diagnoses for each patient encounter with the physician and/or other members of your practice. The routing slip should include information such as:

- The clinic name.
- The doctor's name(s).
- The account number.
- The patient's name.
- The date.
- The referring doctor (if any).
- A list of all common procedures performed by the office along with the CPT code, a place to make a checkmark, and a place to mark a fee; a fair amount of space should be allowed to fill in uncommon procedures, codes and fees.
- A list of common ICD9 codes and a place to put checkmarks next to them.

The patient's name, account number, date and referring doctor information should all be entered onto the routing slip, and the slip attached to the patient's chart before the patient is seen by the physician. For additional control, routing slips can be put in numerical sequence by appointment so that at the end of the day all slips can be accounted for. Any missing slips would indicate lost charges that need to be traced.

As the patient and the patient's chart move through the office, the physician, medical assistant or technician checks off procedures

FIG. 4–4. This comprehensive patient information form also carries a provision for the assignment of third-party carrier benefits to the physician.

as they are performed. At the end of the patient encounter, the diagnosis is listed.

A properly designed and utilized routing slip is a tremendous worksaver. In addition to providing control of lost charges, it provides other advantages:

- It contains the complete financial information to be entered into the patient's billing records for private billing and third-party billing. Without the use of a charge slip it is necessary for bookkeepers to extract this information from the patient's medical history file.

- It reduces the amount of lost or misplaced charges, since the bookkeepers need not pull the patient's medical records for the purposes of billing.

- Since the form is completed as activity occurs in the office, it provides the receptionist with immediate information as to which procedures were performed on the patient and what charges were made. This gives the receptionist an opportunity to ask the patient for a payment.

- The actual charge slip, when made in duplicate, may be used as the patient's first statement and given to the patient at the time services are rendered.

- The charge slip, when used in duplicate, may be used as a "super bill." All of the information, i.e. the CPT and ICD9 codes, are illustrated on the form. This information, when attached to a standard insurance form or a specific insurance form, provides all of the medical information needed by third parties. The charge slip itself generally serves as documentation that services were performed.

- The forms may be "batched" for posting purposes. The total charges for the batch can be independently added up and compared with the total postings by the computer or the totals shown on the day sheet.

(For examples of routing slips, see Appendix 4-A.)

[4] Medical History

Whether it is to be completed by the patient, or by the physician or a staff member during an interview with patient, all medical offices should have a medical history form. This form insures that all essential or potentially essential questions will be asked of the patient. Having all of this information on a single form makes it easier to consult.

Certain health questions are rudimentary to all health care professionals; others may be salient to a particular specialty. Standard patient history questionnaires that allow for this range of information are available through various suppliers.

The medical history form should be a part of the patient's permanent chart. The patient's name, account number and date should all be listed at the top. The size of the form should be compatible with the patient's medical file, in most cases a standard $8-1/2 \times 11$ inches.

Many different types of medical charts have been used in physician's offices, but most consultants agree that the best chart for efficiency, versatility, storage and retrieval is the basic side-tab chart designed to accommodate $8-1/2 \times 11$-inch paper. In this format, each patient's chart has a number of different sections. The flexibility this type of chart allows increases its adaptability and acceptability among different physicians. Generally, the new patient information form and the medical history are tabbed to the left side of the chart, while the right side of the chart has sections for physician and staff notes, lab reports, consultant reports and general correspondence. In addition the chart may have a section for tests such as the EKG.

Although it would be convenient to have the patient's x-rays with his or her chart, the size of x-rays generally prohibits this. It is therefore necessary to file x-rays in a separate area. Standard x-ray envelopes filed in "pigeon holes," six inches apart, makes retrieval of the x-ray files easiest.

[5] Chart Notations

Physician and staff notes on most charts are handwritten. The reasons for this are that handwritten charts may be immediately completed at the time the patient visits the office, reports are not subject to delay if the secretary is absent, and expensive secretarial time is eliminated. The major disadvantage of handwritten chart notes, however, is that notes taken in haste during an examination or in a situation where the physician's mind is more on the patient than on the chart are often illegible. As a result, chart information is sometimes worthless to another physician or staff member because it is incomprehensible. In some instances, even the physician who makes the notations may be unable to decipher, at a later date, entries that were not carefully written. Another disadvantage of handwritten notes is that they tend to be brief, at times so brief that they are incomplete.

Dictating charts generally results in a more readable, transferable and complete chart. However, a potential problem with the dictated chart is that it may become unnecessarily wordy. Another disadvantage of dictated notes for the medical chart is the cost involved and potential delays or errors in transcription.

Handwritten charts are recommended for a the new physician on a tight budget. It is also recommended that the physician take the time to make sure the notes are recorded neatly and legibly. As the practice grows the physician can change from writing to dictating notes. The modern pocket-size dictator should become the constant companion of a busy physician.

The transition from handwritten notes to typed notes need not require a change in the charting system. The medical secretary transcribes dictated notes directly onto chart labels that are placed in the chart in the same area where the physician would have written the notes. In the event a copy of the chart is needed for a consultant, insurance company, etc. it can be photocopied. It is recommended that you review any transcribed notes for accuracy and initial them.

The patient's chart should be completed at the time of examination. Don't make the mistake of not recording notes on a patient's chart immediately on a busy day. It is easy to fall into this trap, with the idea that you can catch up later when you have more time. However, it is also easy to let this situation get out of hand, to the point where you have fifty or more charts on your desk needing dictation. The result is usually inaccurate and incomplete charts, or lost and missing charts.

[6] Systematic Filing

Side shelving is recommended for storing file charts: it minimizes the amount of space required for patient charts and allows charts to be filed from floor to ceiling, if necessary. Charts with side tabs and color coding can minimize the potential for loss and misplacement.

There are two basic systems for filing charts: alphabetical and numerical. Alphabetical filing has been favored traditionally by smaller offices, while larger clinics tend to file by number.

The main advantage of numerical filing is that similar names are not placed next to each other in the file and so honest mistakes are made less often. In addition it is believed that errors tend to be less frequent in filing when dealing with numbers rather than alphabetical characters, as people tend to know numerical sequences better than alphabetical sequences. In addition, color coding was once available only for numerical systems.

The major disadvantage of numerical filing is that each patient's chart must be cross-referenced alphabetically to the patient's name. This requires additional time in setting up the chart and an additional step each time the chart is pulled. In pre-computer days, it was necessary to have a manual card file on Rolodex indexing every patient by name and chart number. Today the computer can store all of this information and make access easier, and a microfiche backup can be made for down time on the computer.

The advantage of the alphabetical filing system is that it does not require any cross-referencing: charts may be filed alphabetically by patient names. Many color-coding systems for alphabetical filing are currently available. Whether numerical or alphabetical, a color-coded system greatly reduces the chance of misfiled charts and improves a file clerk's chances of finding a misfiled chart.

The main disadvantage of the alphabetical filing system is that, in the event you provide service to many patients with the same name, it is necessary for your assistant to pull each of the charts with that name until the proper one is identified.

The decision to implement an alphabetical or numerical system should be based on the size or potential size of your practice and whether or not the practice has or will have a computer. Generally, an alphabetical system is best for a smaller clinic. Although difficult, it is always possible to switch from an alphabetical system to a numerical system if your practice grows to such a size that redundancy in patient names makes retrieval cumbersome.

(Pub.372)

§ 4.05 Dictation Processing

> Portable cassette dictating units have largely replaced handwritten notes and desktop dictating units because of their sophistication and convenience. Use of a dictating unit implies the need for a person in the physician's office or an outside service to transcribe tapes. Because the slightest mistake in transcription can make a major difference in meaning for diagnostic purposes, dictation units should be chosen for their fidelity in sound reproduction, and the physician should always review transcripts for accuracy.

Dictation processing plays a major role in the medical office, so it is important that you have an efficient, streamlined system. Consider the following uses of dictation:

- General correspondence.
- Thank you letters to referring patients and physicians.
- Follow-up reports to referring physicians.
- Insurance reports.
- Patient charts.
- Recording hospital, nursing home and other away-from-the-office charges.
- Recording messages to your staff while away from the office.

Good dictation processing requires good dictating equipment. A system with poor fidelity makes the medical secretary's job much more difficult and increases the number of errors in transcription and the number of questions about garbled words or phrases. When selecting dictating equipment, pay attention to the fidelity and not to buttons, beeps or windows available on the system.

[1] Portable vs Desktop Equipment

The two basic models of dictating equipment are the desk and the portable units. Cassettes are currently the standard, and come in three basic sizes: the standard cassette, the mini-cassette and the micro-cassette. The mini- and micro-cassette are growing in popularity. The difference between them is that the mini-cassette has a fifteen-minute-per-side limit, whereas the micro-cassette has a thirty-minute-per-side limit. The standard cassette has the advantage of using longer playing tapes and the versatility to be used on home recorders, but the equipment involved is generally much larger and more cumbersome than for smaller types of cassettes. The most popular cassette today, the mini, can be used in small portable units as well as with many desk models.

Desk model dictating equipment is slowly becoming obsolete. Today's modern portables have all of the features of the desk model, but only take up about as much space as the desktop model's microphone. The small size of the portable unit allows you to carry dictating equipment around to record charges, histories, notes and correspondence at any time of the day.

Physicians who find it impossible to keep track of a portable dictating unit tend to prefer the desk models. These units can be made "portable" with the use of a telephone answering machine to receive dictated material. You can set up a private line within the office, attached to an answering machine, and use this line to call in dictation at any time of the day or night.

[2] Transcription

Dictated information has to be transcribed into a permanent form by someone able to work transcribing equipment. Transcribing equipment should have certain basic features. Like the dictating equipment, it should have high quality fidelity. In addition the unit should have earphones so that the material can be transcribed confidentially; a speaker switch for occasional use when it is necessary to play the tape for more than one person to hear; and, especially important, a foot pedal to stop and start transmission, since the secretary's hands will be on the typewriter keyboard. It should be possible to speed up, slow down and stop the tape to adjust playback to a rate at which the secretary can transcribe.

You should review all transcribed material for accuracy. Minor errors in spelling or interpretation (e.g. "hypotension" for "hypertension") could result in major changes in the meaning of a medical record or letter. You should initial all properly transcribed material only after you have taken the time to review it.

Small offices typically use secretarial services to avoid the initial cost of transcribing equipment and to compensate for not having a person capable of doing medical secretary work. Many such services are available, some specializing in the medical field. In addition some hospitals set up a division of their medical secretaries to do work for private physicians. Outside transcribing services generally have a pickup service for physician tapes or use a call in system in which a physician calls in, identifies himself or herself, and gives the dictation.

While the dictation service may be effectively used for a new practice or in times of overload, generally it is more economical and easier to control transcribing services which are performed in-house.

§ 4.06 Referral Information Systems

An organized system of thanking people who refer patients to your office should be set up to maintain good public relations. The system should distinguish the various sources from which referrals come, and should include putting memos into patient charts reminding the physician to thank patients for their referrals and a schedule for sending out signed thank-you letters.

It is important to have an organized system for keeping track of referrals and for thanking people who make them. Otherwise, failure to express your appreciation will be considered a lack of respect, and failure to provide referring doctors with examination results may be interpreted as incompetence.

A good system does not require a lot of effort. Each new patient coming into the clinic should complete the new patient information form, part of which inquires, "Whom may we thank for referring you to our office?" Your receptionist should prepare a master sheet on which the answer to this question can be categorized: a section of the report should show patients; another section should show specific physicians who refer patients; another section should focus on advertising; and another section should show miscellaneous referral sources. Each time a new patient is referred to the office, a mark should be made in the appropriate column.

Another place where referrals should be kept track of is on a thank-you letter list. The referral source's name and the patient referred to the office would be listed and at the end of each week, letters would be sent to referral sources on the list for that week's new patients. If you are just starting a practice and have the time, you might write personal thank you letters to these patients. As your practice becomes more busy, your secretary can type individual form letters for you to sign.

(Pub.372)

If the new patient was referred to you by another patient, a memo recording the referred patient's name and the date he or she appeared in your office should be put in the referring patient's chart. If any obvious relationship between the two patients is known, this also should be recorded. This way when the referring patient next visits the office, you will see the note and make it a point to personally thank the patient for making the referral. This is in addition to the thank you letter that would have been sent at the time the referred patient was in.

The better computer systems can facilitate this type of information processing. Many have a section in which the referring information can be entered. At the end of the month, the computer can generate a report showing the volume and dollar value of various referrals. The word processing features of many of the computers present obvious advantages in generating thank-you letters. Whether your office is on computer or not, however, a good system for keeping track of and thanking referrals should be implemented and maintained.

§ 4.07 Recall and Reminder Systems

A simple recall system should be set up to insure that patients make necessary follow-up appointments. A telephone call from the office not only gets more patients to make appointments but is also an impressive way of showing concern for patients.

Most efficiently run businesses use a recall and reminder system for keeping in touch with clients. Recall and reminder systems serve two basic purposes in the physician's office. First, they give the office a greater control of future activity, thereby increasing the quality of services provided; second, they serve as a practice builder.

Like other systems in the office, a recall and reminder system should be designed with simplicity in mind. The first step is to outline basic information on a 4 × 5-inch index card. The patient's name should be at the top of the index card, followed by:

- The patient's telephone numbers.
- The patient's physician, if there is more than one physician at your practice.
- The date of the patient's last visit to the office.

(Pub.372)

- The reason for the recall or reminder.

A filing tray, indexed by months, is used to hold these cards. Offices on computer may find software that will store recall and reminder information.

With regard to controlling future activity, the recall and reminder system should be used to record any follow-up needed on patients. If you rely on the patient to follow up with an appointment, you soon learn that patients generally do not return if they are feeling good, even if you told them to check back with you at a specific date. On the other hand, patients contacted by the office are highly likely to make the follow-up appointment. They are generally impressed that you had the time and concern to follow up, and in most cases they will think twice about switching physicians, since you obviously have such excellent control over their case.

Once you have a basic system set up, it is a matter of recording all salient information on the index card. The card is then placed in the slot for the month in which the patient is to be contacted. Each month the index cards for that month are pulled by the medical assistant and the patient is called. Armed with the information on the index card, the assistant is able to speak intelligently with the patient, give the date that he or she was last in, and the reason it is important for the patient to return. The assistant should explain to the patient that he or she is being called as a result of the physician requesting the follow-up. Because of negative connotations, the word "recall" should never be used.

§ 4.08 Follow-Up Systems

> The simplest follow-up system is a postcard that can be mailed to inform patients that test results are negative, or that they are positive and therefore another appointment needs to be scheduled. The timeliness of the follow-up depends on the urgency of the test. Follow-up should also be used to inform referring physicians of test results for the clients they refer to another practice.

A simple system insures proper follow-up for certain items for which the office is responsible: specifically, when tests such as throat cultures or pap smears are taken at the office, a record of the tests should be entered into a follow-up system. Normal procedure is to contact the patient with negative results requiring no follow-up testing, or to reschedule the patient for additional testing or follow-up in the event of a positive test.

(Pub.372)

Another time a follow-up system is needed is when the patient is referred to a consulting physician. In this case it is normal for the consultant not to report results directly to the patient, but rather contact the primary physician.

Unless the procedure is part of a routine examination, a patient is generally very anxious to hear the result. Routine lab test results can be given on a post card filled out with the patient's name and address on one side and a place for the test results on the other side. The card should be filed by week, alphabetically. If negative test results come in the card should be pulled from the file, results of the tests should be marked, and the card sent to the patient. If the results are positive and require a special follow-up, such as a call from the physician, the card should be pulled and given to you along with the patient's chart and telephone number. You can then contact the patient and give proper instructions.

At the end of each week cards remaining in the tray for that week should be examined to find out why the test results have not been returned.

For the "non-routine" type of services which call for follow-up (e.g. a report from a consulting physician), a system should be set up to record the patient's name, the reason for follow-up and who should make the follow-up. These sheets should be reviewed at the end of each day to make sure proper follow-up has been made, and that patients have not been left "hanging." Even if your office is small enough that follow-up is largely something you can remember, you should implement a system to avoid occasions where a patient's results may "slip through the cracks."

§ 4.09 Checklist for Office Systems

This section recaps all the various systems necessary to run an efficient medical office.

__ Telephone Answering Policy:

    __ Telephone never to ring more than three times before being answered

    __ Message slips with general caller information

    __ Priority routing of calls

__ Answering Services:

(Pub.372)

§ 4.09　　MANAGING YOUR MEDICAL PRACTICE　　4–36

- __ Create tape message for machine
- __ Answering service:
  - __ Establish pickup policy
  - __ Check on service periodically
- __ Telephone Systems:
  - __ Rent
  - __ Lease
  - __ Purchase
- __ Appointment Systems:
  - __ Appointment book vs on-line computer
  - __ Customize schedule according to work rate
  - __ "Wave" vs "modified wave" scheduling
  - __ Allow for delays, emergencies, walk-in patients
  - __ Allow time for new-patient information
- __ Patient Flow:
  - __ Establish patient flow chart for employees
  - __ Become familiar with each day's appointments in advance
  - __ Process patient insurance forms, etc.
- __ Examination:
  - __ Patient history
  - __ Referral for additional tests
  - __ Diagnosis
  - __ Routing slip
  - __ Flagging charts
  - __ Flagging examination rooms
  - __ Ancillary tests
  - __ Referral to specialist or hospital
- __ Check Out:
  - __ Routing slip to receptionist
  - __ Take care of delinquent payments

(Pub.372)

- Routing slip as receipt of payment
- Schedule next appointment
- Patient Records
  - New-patient forms
  - Assignment of benefits form
  - Routing or charge slip
  - Medical history form
  - Dictation notes
- Filing:
  - Side-shelved, tabbed manila folders
  - Alphabetical, numerical and color-coded systems
- Dictation Processing:
  - Portable vs. desktop model
  - Transcribing equipment
  - In-house vs. outside transcription services
- Referral Information System:
  - New patient information form
  - Inter-office list of referrals
  - Mailing list for thank-you letters
  - Notation in patient chart
  - Personal vs. form thank-you note
- Recall and Reminder Systems:
  - Index cards vs. on-line computer
  - General information on reason for recall
  - Attribute telephone call to doctor's concern
- Follow-Up:
  - Information on negative test to patient
  - Information on positive test to patient with future appointment scheduled
  - Test results sent to referring physician

(Pub.372)

§ 4.100 Bibliography

Cotton, H.: Medical Practice Management. Oradell, NJ: Medical Economics Co., 1977.

Huffman, E. K.: Medical Records Management. Birwyn See: Physicians Record Co., 1981.

Liebler, J. G.: Managing Health Records. Administrative Principles. Germantown, MD: Aspen Systems Corp., 1980.

McCormick, J., et al.: The Management of Medical Practice. Cambridge, MA: Ballinger Publishing Co., 1978.

Sloane, R. M. and Sloane, B.: A Guide to Health Facilities: Personnel Management. St. Louis: C. V. Mosby, 1977.

Sullivan, R. J.: Medical Record and Index Systems for Community Practice. Cambridge, MA: Ballinger Publishing Co., 1979.

Appendix 4-A

Routing Slips

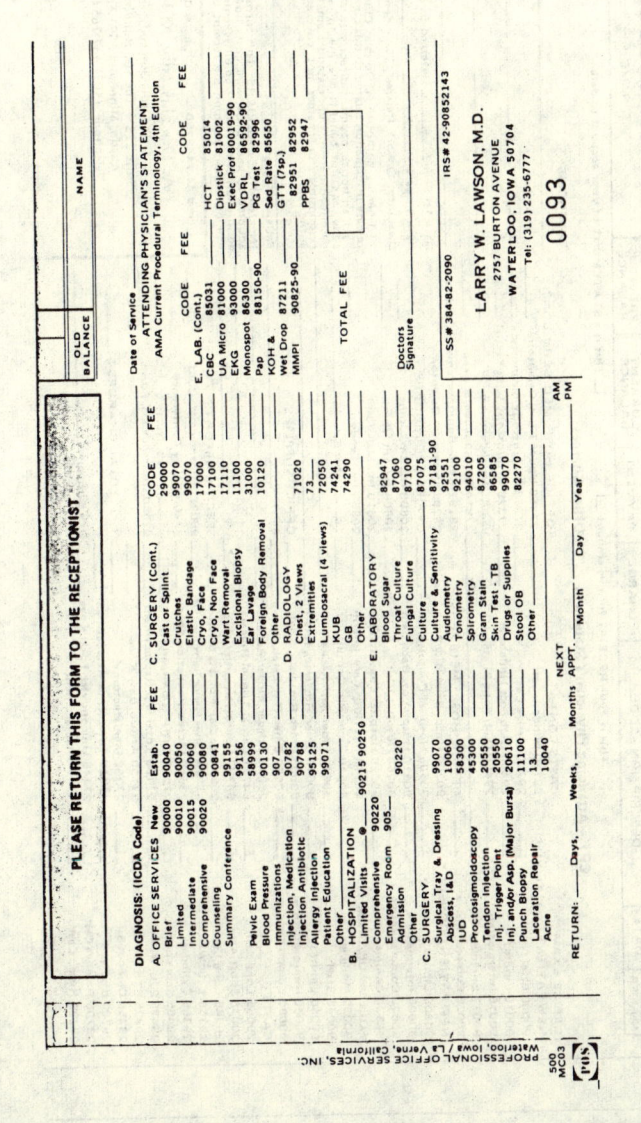

FIG. 4-5. A routing slip that calls for ICDA, or ICD-9 code. Note the slots left open for fee designations that make this a useful charge slip.

(Pub.372)

110

RECEIPT NUMBER	DATE	DESCRIPTION - CODE	CHARGE	PAYMENT	CURRENT BALANCE	PREVIOUS BALANCE	NAME

This is your **RECEIPT** for this amount ↑ — ↑ This is a **STATEMENT** of your account to date

CPT —Attending Physician's Statement **Office Charges**

OFFICE EXAM
NEW PATIENT INITIAL VISIT
90000 Brief ______
90010 Limited ______
90015 Intermediate ______
90017 Extended Service ______
90020 Comprehensive ______
NEW PATIENT CONSULT.
90600 Limited ______
90605 Intermediate ______
90620 Comprehensive ______
90630 Complex ______
FOLLOW UP EXAM
90030 Minimal ______
90040 Brief ______
90050 Limited ______
90060 Intermediate ______
90080 Comprehensive ______
CASTS
29065 Long Arm ______
29075 Short Arm ______
29345 Long Leg ______
29355 L. L. Walker ______
29365 Cylinder ______
29405 Short Leg ______
29425 S. L. Walker ______
29435 PTB ______
29455 Cl. Foot Bil. ______
29700 Bivalve ______
29705 Remove Cast ______
29720 Repair Cast ______

CASTS CONT.
29730 Window Cast ______
29740 Wedge Cast ______
29450 Club Foot Unilateral ______
29455 Club Foot Bilateral ______
______
OFFICE, HOSP., MED. SERV.
90200 Hosp, Brief H & P ______
90605 Hospital Consultation ______
90610 Hosp.- Low Back pain ______
90260 Hospital Visit ______
90620 Hospital Consultation ______
90215 Init. Hosp. Care - Interm. ______
90510 Emer. Rm Consult. ______
90540 Emer. Rm - Recheck ______
90515 Emer. Rm - New, Interm. ______
90505 Emer. Rm - New, Brief ______
90560 Emer. Rm - Estab., Interm. ______
26055 Trigger Finger Repair ______
64721 Carpal Tunnel Release ______
64727 Neurolysis with C.TR ______
25611 Radial #-pins & plaster ______
64718 Ulnar Nerve Transposition ______
23655 Closed Reduction Shld. ______
27244 ORIF Hip Fracture ______
27130 Total Hip Replacement ______
27130 Arthrotomy Knee ______
27332 Meniscectomy ______
27447 Total Knee Replacement ______
27446 Unicondylar Total Knee Replacement ______

OFFICE, HOSP., MED. SERV. CONT.
27456 Upper Tibral Osteotomy ______
27373 Arthroscopy-diagnostic ______
27378 Arthroscopy with Partial ______ Meniscectomy ______
27814 OR Bimalleolar Frac. ______
28292 Keller Bunionectomy ______
28296 Metatarsal Osteotomy ______
OFFICE PROCEDURES
20600 Inj. Sm. Joint ______
20605 Inj. Int. Joint ______
20610 Inj. Maj. Joint ______
20550 Inj. Tendon ______
______ Other ______
______
OFFICE SUPPLIES
99070 ______
______
______
SPECIAL REPORTS
99032 Attorney Off. Conf. ______
99200 Office Conference ______
______ Rehab. Nurse ______
99080 Insurance Co. Form ______

TOTAL CHARGES $______

Dr's Signature:______

DIAGNOSIS:
______
______
______
______

Date 1st Seen______ Referred By______
Date Surgery______ Proc.______
Disability: ☐ Work Related ☐ Accident ☐ Other

1) I hereby authorize A. Douglas Lilly, M.D. to release information related to this claim.
2) I authorize payment directly to A. Douglas Lilly, M.D. of benefits due me for services as described herein. I understand I am financially responsible for charges not covered by this authorization.

Patient's Signature ______

INSURANCE CARRIERS: This form has been adopted to keep paperwork costs down. If any additional forms or itemized bill is requiring they will be completed upon the receipt of $25.00.

I.D. # 41-1449250 Lic. # 017649-7
A. Douglas Lilly, M.D.
Orthopedic Surgeon
Suite 228 – The 100 Building
Austin, Minnesota 55912
Telephone: (507) 437-7654

FIG. 4–6. A slightly different routing slip. Notice how routing slips can be tailored for the needs of the individual medical office.

FIG. 4–7. A different routing slip.

App. 4-A   MANAGING YOUR MEDICAL PRACTICE

DESCRIPTION	CODE	FEE	DESCRIPTION	CODE	FEE	DESCRIPTION	CODE	FEE
OFFICE EVALUATIONS			**INJECTIONS**			**RADIOLOGY**		
NEW PATIENT			Depo Medrol 120 mg	90766		Thoracic Spine 2V	72070	
Limited Service	90010		Diphtheria Tetanus	90702		Toes 2V	73660	
Intermediate Service	90015		Flu Vaccine	90767		Wrist 3V	73110	
Comprehensive Service	90020		Gamma Globulin (per c.c.)	90768		Unlisted Radiology	76499	
Initial W/C Visit	90025		Kenalog (Im) 40 mg/c.c.	90770		**PHYSICALS**		
ESTABLISHED PATIENT			Mantoux	90789		FAA I	90631	
Limited Service	90050		Penicillin 1.2 units	90774		FAA II	90632	
Intermediate Service	90060		Penicillin 4.8 units	90776		FAA III	90633	
Comprehensive Service	90080		Polio Vaccine	90713		I.C.C.	90640	
Subsequent W/C Visit	90065		Smallpox	90711		Evaluation	90636	
LABORATORY PROCEDURES			Steroid Injection	90766		Executive VI	90638	
Blood Sugar	82947		Tetanus	90703		Executive VII	90628	
CBC	85031		Typhoid	90714		Executive VIII	90627	
Cholesterol Blood	82465		Typhus	90716		Executive IX	90630	
Diff.	85007		Yellow Fever	90717		Executive X	90626	
GC Culture	87081		**DRUGS AND SUPPLIES**			Immigration	90634	
Gram Stain	87205		Ace Large	99036		Insurance	90639	
Guaiac	82270		Ace Small	99033		Radiation	90635	
Hemoglobin Electrophoresis	83020		Analgesic	99010		General Physical	90642	
HGB	85018		Butazolidin Alka.	99007		Pre-Placement I	90637	
Test	86300		Dressing/Burn Kit	99049		Pre-Placement II	90643	
Pap	88150		Finger Splint	99041		Pre-Placement III	90644	
Platelets	85580		Keflex 250 mg.	99017		Pre-Placement IV	90645	
Potassium	84132		Neosporin Ointment	99019		Pre-Placement V	90646	
Pregnancy Test	82996		Norgesic Forte	99022		**MISC. PROCEDURES**		
Protime	85610		Norgesic (Plain)	99021		EKG	93000	
Rheumatoid Battery Profile	82305		Parafon Forte	99023		EKG Masters	93017	
Sed. Rate	85650		Penicillin VK	99026		EKG Stress	93015	
Serology	86592		Sulamyd 10% drops	99028		Audiometry	92551	
SMAC	80019		Tylenol 3	99030		Copies Medical Records	99087	
SMA 12	80012		Wrist Splint Brace (Short)	99045		Corneal Curettage	65435	
Throat Culture	87060		Motrin	99055		Ear Irrigation	69210	
Tissue Pathology	88300		Clinoril	99057		M/L Report	99080	
TSH	84443		Miscellaneous Drugs	99084		Proctoscopy	45300	
T3	84480		**RADIOLOGY**			Pulmonary Function	94010	
T4	84441		Ankle 3V	73610		Retainer	99083	
U.A. (Cult/Sen. & Colony)	87086		Cervical 5V	72050		I.V.	36400	
U.A. (Dip)	81000		Chest 1V	71010		Court Testimony	99940	
Uric Acid	84550		Chest 2V	71020		Appt. Failure Ins. Exam	90647	
WBC	85048		Elbow 2V	73070				
Wet Mount	87210		Finger 3V	73140				
Wound Culture	87070		Foot 3V	73630				
Unlisted Lab Procedure	87999		Hand 3V	73130				
INJECTIONS			Knee 2V	73560				
Allergy, One Injection	90718		Knee 3V	73570		C.D.	99901	
Allergy, Two Injections	90719		Lumbar Spine 3V	72100		E.D.	99905	
Allergy, Three Injections	90724		Lumbar Spine w/obliques 5V	72110		I.D.	99904	
Bicillin 1.2 Units	90759		Shoulder 2V	73030		**TOTAL CHARGES**		
Cholera	90788		Skull 3V — 4 Films	70260				

OFFICE COPY

FIG. 4–8. A routing slip used by a different practice.

(Pub. 372)

DATE	CODE	TYPE OF EXAM	TIME
PATIENT NAME		BIRTHDATE	PHONE
STREET	CITY	STATE	ZIP
INSURANCE COMPANY	POLICY NUMBER	DICTATE	

PROCEDURE	✓	CODE
OFFICE VISIT—NEW PATIENT		
New Complete Exam		90020
Extended Service		90017
Office Call		90015
OFFICE VISIT—EST. PATIENT		
Brief		90040
Office Call		90060
Extended Office Call		90070
Comprehensive Office Call		90080
INJECTIONS		90720
Cholera		B
Flu		E
Gamma Globulin		A
Measles		G
Mumps		H
Pneumovax		F
Typhoid		C
Tetanus Toxoid		J
		90782
Allergy		B
B-12		L
Delestrogen		E

PROCEDURE	✓	CODE
Delatestryl		F
Demerol		J
Depo Medrol		A
Depo Prover A		C
Depotestadiol		Y
Depotestosterone		G
Myo Christine (Gold)		M
Penicillin		H
Tigan		K
Mantoux Test		86580
LABORATORY		
Alkaline Phos.		85540
Acid Phos.		84060
Blood Sugar		82948
Cholesterol		82465
Diff		85007
Dig/Lanoxin Level		82643
Dilantin Level		84045
HDL		83715
Hematocrit		85014
Hemoccult		82270
Hemoglobin		85018

PROCEDURE	✓	CODE
Lipids Profile		83700
Liver Profile		80011
Mono Test		86300
Platelet Count		85580
Potassium		84132
Profile II		80019
Pro-time		85610
Sed Rate		85650
Selective Profile		80004
T-4 (TO Mayo T & F)		84251
T-4		84441
TSH (Tomayo)		84443
Throat Culture		87060
Triglycerides		83705
Uric Acid		84550
Urinalysis		81000
WBC		85048
X–RAY–975		
Chest (2 Views)		71020
Chest (1 View)		71010
L.S. Spine		72100
OTHER SERVICES:		

PROCEDURE	✓	CODE
EKG		93000
Holter Monitor		93274
CHEMOTHERAPY		90790
Adriamycin mg.		
Bleomycin mg.		
Cytosa R (Cytosine) mg.		
Cytoxen I.V. mg.		
5 FU mg.		
Methotrexate mg.		
Velban mg.		
Mitomycin mg.		
Oncovin mg.		
IV Tubing		99070
OTHER PROCEDURES		
Ear Wash		69210
Nutrition Consult		06100
Nutrition Follow up Visit		06100A
Procto		45300
Stitches Removed		90040
Stress Test		93015

DIAGNOSIS	✓	CODE
CARDIOVASCULAR		
Angina Pectoris		413
Aortic Insufficiency		424
ASHD		414.0
Cardiac Arrhythmias		427.
Cardiac Valvular Disease		753.2
Chest Pain		786
Chest Wall Pain		786.5
Congestive Heart Failure		428
Edema		782.3
Hypertension		401.
Hypotension, Postural		458.
Myocardial Infarction		410
Mitral Valve Prolapse		424
Myocardiopathy		425
Pericarditis		423.9
Peripheral Vascular Disease		443.9
Pulmon. Thrombo Embolism		415.
Phlebitis		451
Varicose Veins		454.9
GASTRO–INTESTINAL		
Abdominal Pain		789
Anal Fissure		565.0
Appendicitis		540
Bowel Obstruction		560.9
Cholecystitis		575.
Cholelithiasis		574.
Cirrhosis of the Liver		571
Colon Polyp		211.3
Constipation		564
Diarrhea		558.9
Diverticulitis		562
Dysphagia		787.2
Enteritis		558.9
Exposure to Hepatitis		V07
Gastritis		535
Gastro Intestinal Bleeding		578.9
Gastroenteritis		558.9
Hemorrhoids		455
Hepatitis Infectious		070
Hernia — Hiatal		551.3
Hernia — Inguinal		550
Pancreatitis		577
Peptic Ulcer		533.9
Rectal Polyp		569.0

DIAGNOSIS	✓	CODE
Spastic Colon		564.1
Ulcer, Gastric		531
Ulcerative Colitis		556.
GENITO–URINARY TRACT		
Amenorrhea		626.0
Benign Prostatic Hypertrophy		600
Cystitis		595
Dysmenorrhea (Painful)		625.3
Fibroid (Tumor, U terus)		218.9
Hematuria		599.7
Menopause Syndrome		627.2
Prostatitis		601
Renal Calculus		592
Renal Failure		586
Urethritis		597
Urinary Tract Infection		599.0
Vaginitis		616
HEMATOLOGIC DISEASE		
Anemia, Unspecified		285
Anemia, Iron Def.		280
Anemia, Pernicious		281.0
Leukopenia		288.0
Myelo Fibrosis		289.8
Polycythemia Vera		238.4
Thrombocytopenin		287.1
NEURO–PSYCHIATRIC SYSTEM		
Alcoholism		303.9
Anxiety State		300.0
Cerebrovascular Insuff.		437.1
CVA — Acute		436
Discogenic Disease		722
Headache		784.0
Headache, Migraine		346.
Headache, Tension		306.81
Hyperventilation		786.01
Neuropathy, Unspecified		357.9
Parkinsonism		332.0
Seizure Disorders		780.0
Syncope		780.2
Vertigo		780.4
Weakness, General		780.7

DIAGNOSIS	✓	CODE
ONCOLOGY		
Bladder		188
Brain		191
Breast		174
Cervix		233
Colon		153
Esophagus		150
Gallbladder/Bile Duct		156
Hodgkins Disease		201
Kidney		189.0
Liver		
Lung		162
Lympho, Leukemia		204
Lymphoma		202.8
Melanoma		172.9
Multiple Myeloma		203
Myelogen, Leukemia		205
Ovary		183
Pancreas		157
Prostate		185
Rectum		154
Stomach		151
Testes		186
Thyroid		193
Unknown Primary		199.1
Uterus		182
OTHER DIAGNOSIS		
Allergic Reaction/Medication		995.2
Cellulitis		682.9
Conjunctivitis		372.
Crohn's Disease		555
Epistaxis		784.7
Fever of Undetermined		780.6
General Physical		V70.9
Herpes Simplex		054
Herpes Zoster		053
Laceration		
Loss of Appetite		783.0
Lupus Erythematosus		695.4
Lymphodenopathy		785.6
Radiculitis		729.2
Tendinitis		726
Urticaria		708
Weight Gain, Unknown		783.1
Weight Loss, Unknown		783.2

DIAGNOSIS	✓	CODE
PULMONARY DISEASE		
Allergic Rhinitis		477
Asthma		
Bronchitis		490
Chron. Ostruct. Pulmon. Dis.		496
Common Cold		460
Infectious Mononucleosis		075
Otitis, Externa		380.10
Otitis, Media		382
Pharyngitis		462
Pleural Effusion		511.9
Pleurisy		511
Pneumonia		486
Sinusitis		473.9
Strep Throat		034
Upper Respiratory Infect.		465
RENAL, METABOLIC, ENDOCRINE		
Diabetes Mellitus		250
Hypercholesterolemia		272
Hyperlipemia		272.4
Hyperthyroidism		242
Hypoglycemia		251
Hypothyroidism		244
Non-Toxic Goiter		241.9
Obesity		278
RHEUMATOLOGY		
Ankylosing Spondylitis		720
Bursitis		727.3
Carpel Tunnel Syndrome		354
Coccydynia		724.79
Degenerative Arthritis		715
Gout		274
Low Back Pain		724.2
Myositis		729.11
Neuritis		729.2
Osteoporosis		733
Paget's Disease		731.0
Polymyalgia Rheumatica		725
Reiter's Syndrome		099.3
Rheumatoid Arthritis		714
Shortness of Breath		786.0

FIG. 4–9. The back of a comprehensive routing slip listing common diagnoses and diagnostic codes.

CHAPTER 5

Computers in Health Care

by

Carl Brandt

> **SCOPE**
>
> The collection and manipulation of data is a time-consuming and labor-intensive activity that has grown with increased government regulation, emphasis on reducing the costs of medical care and the role played by third party insurers. Data processing systems can take on many of the tedious and cumbersome tasks involved in practice information management and provide the quality information needed for decision making. The success or failure of a computer system, however, is directly dependent on how it is used by the medical practice. For that reason, the selection of a computer system begins with an examination of the practice's goals. Among other things, you should consider what office functions—billing, organizing patient files, handling insurance payments, etc.—can be handled by computer; whether you want an in-house or service bureau system; how computer software and hardware will be organized; what kind of service can be expected from the computer vendor; and whether computer capabilities can be expanded to match the expected growth of the practice. For any purchase of this magnitude, a great deal of advance planning and research must be undertaken before a decision is made. Once a decision has been made to install a computer system, it must receive the commitment of all parties involved (physicians, administrators, office personnel, computer vendor personnel) to make it successful.

SYNOPSIS

§ 5.01 Management Information Systems

- [1] Business Needs Addressed by a Management Information System
- [2] Benefits of the Management Information System

§ 5.02 Components of the Management Information System
- [1] Accounts Receivable Management (ARM)
  - [a] Patient/Responsible Party Maintenance Functions
  - [b] Master File Maintenance
  - [c] Data Transaction Entry
  - [d] Insurance Processing
  - [e] Billing
  - [f] Collection Management
  - [g] Management Reports
  - [h] Generating Custom Reports
  - [i] Referring Doctor/Referred to Applications
  - [j] System Utilities
- [2] Appointment Scheduling
- [3] Patient Recall
- [4] Word Processing
- [5] General Accounting Ledger
- [6] Payroll
- [7] Accounts Payable
- [8] Medical Records
  - [a] Problems in Definition
  - [b] Subfunctions of Medical Records Capacity
  - [c] Miscellaneous Applications

§ 5.03 Data Processing Alternatives
- [1] Automated Pegboard System
- [2] Batch/Mail-In Service Bureau
- [3] On-Line/Real Time Service Bureau
- [4] In-House Computer System
- [5] Sources of System Purchase

§ 5.04 Planning for Automation
- [1] Assessing Practice Needs
- [2] Request for Proposal (RFP)
  - [a] Drawbacks to the Request for Proposal
  - [b] Use of the RFP in the Selection Process
- [3] Use of a Consultant
  - [a] Selecting a Consultant
  - [b] Disadvantages of Using a Consultant

§ 5.05 Selecting a Management Information System

        [1] Selecting the Company
        [2] Selecting the Software
            [a] Access
            [b] Security and Confidentiality
            [c] Backup Procedures
        [3] Selecting the Hardware
            [a] Operating System
            [b] Operator Vocabulary
            [c] Common Mistakes
        [4] Service, Support and Maintenance
            [a] Hardware Maintenance
            [b] Software Maintenance
            [c] Maintenance Contracts
            [d] Ongoing Educational Training
            [e] Software Documentation
            [f] Installation, Conversion and Training
§ 5.06 Legal Considerations
§ 5.07 Computer Systems Checklist
§ 5.08–§ 5.99 Reserved
§ 5.100 Bibliography
Appendix 5-A Sample Management Reports
Appendix 5-B Sample Appointment Scheduling Reports
Appendix 5-C Comparison of Service Bureaus and In-House Computer Systems
Appendix 5-D Glossary of Basic Computer Terminology
Appendix 5-E Request for Proposal

§ 5.01 Management Information Systems

> Government regulations, the proliferation of alternative health care strategies and the purchase of health insurance by employers have all increased competition in the health care industry and put pressure on practitioners to supply expert, cost-efficient medical care. A management information system can organize all information a practice needs to keep a competitive edge, perform routine administrative tasks with greater efficiency and enhance the overall professionalism of the practice.

Changes in the health care industry such as alternative health care delivery systems, government regulation, employer purchase of health care, the expanded role of the hospital, increased health care costs and increased competition among providers have shifted the emphasis on data processing's functions from billing and insurance

(Pub.372)

to management information systems. Physicians are now expected to stand watch not only over their own performance, but also over the entire health care system to ensure that each patient receives proper, cost-effective care. Measuring cost-effectiveness requires sophisticated management of financial information.

[1] Business Needs Addressed by a Management Information System

Employers have watched costs for employee health care benefits rise at a rate faster than for any other business expense. This has led them to become actively involved in managing the health care of their employees through preventive care, wellness and self-insurance programs. The group buying power of these employers also puts increased pressure on the health care provider to offer cost-effective services. Furthermore, the pressures employers, government regulations and alternative health care programs have placed on hospitals has motivated them to change their emphasis and, in many instances, place additional controls on the physicians who practice in them. The pressure from all these factors has increased the competitive nature of health care.

The health care delivery system has shifted significantly from fee-for-service to prepaid care programs, including health maintenance organizations (HMOs) and preferred provider organizations (PPOs). A practice's participation in one or many of these programs generates additional claim filing and billing, making more paperwork and requiring more manpower. In addition, a practice must be able to evaluate its production costs and recovery to determine the wisdom of participation in such programs.

The reduction in fee-for-service patients has reduced the number of statements mailed to patients but increased the number of claims submitted to insurance programs. Standard insurance forms have been losing ground in recent years; the trend has been for each insurance program to develop its own submission requirements. In addition, electronic claims submission has gained popularity among major carriers. These factors have created the need for a data processing system that can efficiently produce the various forms and media for submission. Practices have emphasized this in their selection of data processing systems for the last ten years.

Practice management based on business principles requires the ability to analyze trends and compare data for production, revenues, payroll, word processing and financial planning. As automated means for doing this become available, the data processing system becomes a more useful management tool. But it is a good tool only if it can provide the information required to make complex decisions about staffing, participation with insurers and marketing targets. System flexibility that permits manipulation of the data is extremely important for making sure the system can keep up with the rapidly changing medical environment.

[2] Benefits of the Management Information System

When used for an information management system data processing can:

- Enhance ability to control office operating expenses.
- Allow the practice to comply with billing and insurance filing requirements.
- Enhance the professionalism and increase the flexibility of the billing and insurance departments.
- Improve credit and collection performance.
- Enable the office to control finances more closely.
- Upgrade staff positions as personnel become data managers rather than data gatherers.
- Enable the office to incorporate practice development techniques by monitoring referral sources and patient census.
- Enhance decision making by providing detailed management reports for use in practice development, staffing and negotiations.
- Improve patient care by facilitating research and patient recall.

§ 5.02 Components of the Management Information System

Before buying a management information system, you should have in mind which information you want to automate. This eliminates the unintentional purchase of equipment with superfluous functions. Systems are available for almost all types of information including (1) accounts receivable management; (2) appointment scheduling; (3) patient recall; (4) word processing; (5) general accounting; (6) payroll; (7) accounts payable; and (8) the keeping of medical records. You should decide if these functions will save your practice time, money and space before purchasing them.

The best management information system for a medical practice is the one which best meets the practice's specific needs. You must decide which information you want to automate before you implement a management system.

[1] **Accounts Receivable Management (ARM)**

An accounts receivable management system is designed to assist physicians, administrators and staff in improving not only office efficiency and productivity, but also the quality of medical care. Basically, the ARM system creates and maintains data base files for all patient and responsible party demographic and billing information used in the preparation of patient statements, insurance forms, management reports and accounts receivable.

[a] **Patient/Responsible Party Maintenance Functions.**

This component of an ARM system allows the user to enter and change patient demographic and billing information for the purposes described above. For example, whenever a program needs information about a patient, such as date of birth or address, it can be found in the data stored in the patient/responsible party demographics file.

The amount of information contained in the patient/responsible party data base files varies in scope from one data processing product to another. It is important that information needs be identified in advance to permit evaluation of an ARM system's capacity to maintain them. The general purpose of an ARM system is to collect and collate as much information about a patient/responsible party as possible for a broad range of specific management information needs. For example, the emphasis placed on marketing in the health care industry requires that a practice have extensive information related to the demographics of its patient population if it is deciding to open a satellite facility. One way in which a custom report generator or data base manager does this is by separating out patient populations according to zip code.

[b] Master File Maintenance

Master files are the foundation of an ARM system's ability to be adapted to fulfill information needs of a specific practice. If, for example, you want to define a custom ICD-9 diagnosis file unique to the practice, the diagnosis master can be used to create a file of diagnostic codes the practice uses on a day-to-day basis. The system then uses these descriptions when printing insurance forms, etc. Other types of files associated with a practice's master file include information related to individual physicians; hospitals or facilities where the doctors practice; a service code/CPT code master; and insurance company information.

[c] Data Transaction Entry

This function allows you to enter charges, receipts and journal entries in a patient's account. The method varies from system to system. However, the primary consideration in this area is maximizing operator efficiency and maintaining the integrity of the financial information. As an example, a data processing system that utilizes a "batch" method of operator input can enter a large volume of information for all patients at once, as opposed to entry of this type of information on an account-by-account basis.

The transaction information processed by the data processing system should provide a complete audit trail of all transactions to help prevent balancing and posting errors. An audit trail is also used to maintain a permanent record of all transactions entered.

Data entry functions should provide multiple methods for entering charges, such as batch entry, account-by-account entry or time of service charge entry which permits a statement to be generated at the time the patient leaves the office.

The amount of information that can be entered into an account for financial transactions varies from system to system. A practice considering buying this type of system should analyze specific needs to make sure the information it collects can be entered into the data processing system. Again, as the need for management information increases, a practice should consider whether its system can adequately enter information such as admit/discharge diagnoses, date of injury, prior authorization numbers for insurance filing purposes, facility where the service was rendered and other miscellaneous transaction data necessary to process a statement or insurance claim.

Recently, there has been a trend in ARM systems to enter service charges by occurrence. This enables you to enter transaction information associated with a specific encounter. Worker's Compensation claims, for example, usually require the medical practice to report the date of injury information associated with the encounter.

Another key factor in selecting an accounts receivable system is whether or not the data processing system maintains the financial integrity of the information. This means scrutinizing the posting and balancing methods employed in the data entry process used by the system.

[d] Insurance Processing

The insurance processing functions are one of the major time-saving features of an ARM system. However, they are often overlooked because most buyers assume a data processing system automatically has this capacity.

Typically, these functions enable a practice to automatically prepare insurance forms. Insurance processing capability varies with local, state and federal requirements, and it is important that a data processing system be able generate both the insurance claims unique to each practice and meet the varying claims filing requirements unique to the practice's health care community.

The capacity to submit a multitude of insurance form types should be a prerequisite for the data processing system selected. Forms for different insurance carriers should be available or the data processing system should be able to custom design insurance claims given unique insurance filing requirements. Many data processing products only allow a practice to generate one or two standard claim forms. If this is the case, you should investigate the possibility of adding additional insurance claim-filing functions to the system and their cost to the practice.

Many accounts receivable systems can use a custom insurance claim form generator which will design insurance claims forms to your specifications. Although some states have moved for a standard insurance claim for all major insurance carriers to be submitted on an industry-wide basis, in other states each insurance company uses different claim forms and requires different information.

Another function associated with an ARM system's insurance processing capacity is the ability to produce insurance claims on an exception rather than automatic basis. This is particularly useful in dealing with a patient's specific request. Many accounts receivable systems do not allow a practice to re-itemize or re-request an insurance claim. In addition to re-requesting an insurance claim, the accounts receivable management system should be able to request an itemized statement that details all transactions posted to a patient's account.

Traditionally, insurance processing functions only allowed a practice to enter claims by guarantor or responsible party. A trend in the computer industry, however, is to file entries by patient versus guarantor/responsible party. Similarly a subscriber in name, who in some cases is different from the responsible party, can be attached to the patient's insurance.

Another trend in the data processing industry is submitting insurance claims electronically. The demand for this capability is increasing, given the high cost of handling paper claims. Consequently, a practice should evaluate the accounts receivable system's capability to submit insurance claims by diskette claim submission, nine-track tape submission and/or telecommunications. It should be noted that electronic claims submission varies from state to state. A practice should evaluate the ARM system's ability to handle the unique circumstances associated with each health care community under its aegis.

[e] Billing

These functions should allow the user to calculate and print statements on a daily, weekly or monthly basis.

The term "cycle billing" is used to describe a data processing system's capability to prepare patient statements. Cycle billing allows the office to process statements on a predetermined set of cycles in a given month. This capability is useful not only because it spreads out the workload associated with printing and handling statements, but also because it has proven successful in evening out the cash flow of a practice.

The billing function should be able to prepare statements on a demand basis. If payment is collected at the time of service, you will probably want to generate a demand statement and insurance claim at the time the patient leaves the office. This capability is also useful if a patient loses a statement or needs an extra copy to file with a secondary insurance carrier.

The billing function should enable the practice to generate the specific type of statement it uses for billing purposes and produce a variety of billing statements (standard itemized statement, superbill format, mailer, etc.). Incorporation of a custom statement generator allows the practice to custom design its particular patient statement.

[f] Collection Management

An ARM system's collection management features vary greatly from system to system. The primary purpose of this function is to facilitate credit and collection activity. The collection management functions found in most data processing systems include the ability to:

- Age reports by patient.
- Age reports by specific billing type (e.g., insurance carrier) which, bascially, breaks out subsets of the practice's total accounts receivable balance.
- Generate collection agency reports to monitor the collection activity of accounts referred to a professional agency.
- Generate standard or customized letters to delinquent patient accounts.
- Monitor terms and payments.
- Access finance or rebilling charges on accounts given a specified age of the account balance.
- Record on-line collection notes to monitor the direct contact with a patient and/or insurance carrier.
- Print automatic collection notices on patient statements.
- Monitor collection activity by specific operator and/or person designated to conduct credit and collection activity.
- Generate reports on an exception basis for account balances over a specified aging category or size of account balance.

- Automatically collect letters generated subsequent to patient statement mailings.
- Generate customized messages on a patient's statement for unique collection purposes.
- Supply automatic credit flagging on patient/responsible party demographic files that can be viewed by all personnel in the practice.

The tools for credit and collection provided by an ARM system enhance the long-term financial viability of the practice. In some cases practices that have automated have been able to pay all or a portion of their system costs from their improved credit and collection activity.

[g] Management Reports

The emphasis placed on management information influences the decision of many physicians to automate their practices. An ARM system's reporting capability is best evaluated by first analyzing the practice's management information needs and comparing them with the management reporting capability of the ARM system.

[i] Generating Reports. The majority of the data processing systems place a heavy emphasis on producing so-called "standard" reports. These standard reports should be evaluated and compared to the management information needs of the practice. If the report produced is of limited value for your practice, it should not be purchased. Likewise, if the system's data base storage capability is limited, or the information it contains is not easily accessible, then the accounts receivable management system has limited reporting capability.

[ii] Maintaining Financial Integrity. Another key factor in assessing management report capability is whether the system can maintain the financial integrity of the practice's accounts receivable. The assumption that "computers never make mistakes" is an easy trap to fall into when many of the routine manual accounts receivable balancing techniques are a simple byproduct of an accounts receivable system. To evaluate the financial integrity of an accounts receivable system, determine whether or not the balancing and reporting routines require the business office staff to balance to the computer generated accounts receivable totals. Otherwise, many system and human errors may go undetected.

The system should be able to generate a complete audit trail of all transactions entered. These transaction "edits" become the permanent documents maintained by the practice. Many balancing concepts introduced with the "one-write" manual accounts receivable pegboard system can also be applied to the automated accounts receivable system. (For a complete discussion of pegboard accounts payable systems see Chapter 10, section 10.01.) The system should require that the data entered be routinely balanced. An automated accounts receivable system usually requires that an internal "control log" be maintained. This log is compared against the daily transaction reports generated by the computer system. If some type of balancing technique is recommended by the computer vendor the majority of accounts receivable errors can be eliminated and the financial integrity of the data processing system maintained.

[iii] Management by Exception. Another management reporting capability to evaluate is whether or not the "management by exception" approach is used in the processing of reports. This enables physicians, administrators and personnel to view management reports on an exception basis. For example, most data processing systems generate an aging report by patient and/or responsible party for all accounts which have a balance owed to the practice. However the management by exception approach would enable a practice to specify a subset of the total accounts receivable balance (i.e., Medicare patients) to analyze the aging of those accounts for which Medicare is the primary insurance carrier. This type of reporting capability enhances your ability to focus in on a special concern or problem which you may be facing.

[iv] Miscellaneous Considerations. Other considerations for evaluating a data processing system's reporting capabilities include:

- General design and layout of the management reports.
- Ease of interpretation.
- Ability to conduct comparative analyses based on current and previous data.
- Frequency of producing management reports (i.e., daily month to date, and year to date analysis).
- Financial integrity of reports produced.

Another major trend in the management reporting capability of data processing systems is the ability to "view" data versus printing hard copy. Many standard management reports can be displayed on a terminal as opposed to printing them out on paper. This can be a major step toward the ultimate goal of having a paperless management information system.

(Appendix 5-A includes several illustrations of management report functions.)

[h] Generating Custom Reports

This function allows the practice to access specific data base information for management reports on an "exception basis." It usually allows the operator to select specific data base criteria and to design the format in which this data is presented. The information can be printed out as a report or used to print mailing labels or custom letters as part of the word processing function.

The custom report generator should be easy to operate. Many custom report generators require an operator to have a far greater knowledge of general computer principles than most people are willing to take the time to learn or have an interest in learning.

[i] Referring Doctor/Referred to Applications

This type of program enables the practice to monitor patients referred by a physician and/or referred to a specific physician for treatment. It also permits monitoring of sources of patients and/or the number of patients referred to a specific specialist. It can be invaluable in marketing the services of the group practice.

The referral function should be able to print reports that relate to the number of patient encounters and the dollar values associated with treating those patients. Many systems provide the capability to match a referring physician and/or patient referred to a physician by specific location. In this way, the practice can refer patients demographically, such as to a specific medical group, professional building or group of physicians designated as a referral pool. Medical group practices affiliated with or who perform services for HMOs will find this type of reporting capability beneficial for monitoring their patient population as it relates to referral authorizations.

[j] System Utilities

System utility functions are designed to facilitate the end-user's use of the data processing system. Often these functions are overlooked during the selection process, generally due to a lack of knowledge concerning how a data processing system is managed. Functions commonly described as system utilities include:

- Backup of data base records.
- Print maintenance functions (i.e., statement preparation, processing of daily, monthly and year-to-date reports).
- System security (i.e., operator password maintenance application security).
- Routine maintenance of the computer system.
- Data removal.

Specific software features regarding each of these components can be found in § 5.04[2], Request for Proposal.

[2] Appointment Scheduling

Management of time with regard to scheduling appointments, locating charts, developing charge slips and other tasks associated with registration of patients can be improved through the basic management information system. Many of the accounts receivable management system products currently available incorporate appointment scheduling as a component of their standard system. Other vendors provide the appointment scheduling package as an "add-on" component to the ARM system. This permits a little more flexibility because it does not force a practice that does not want to have appointment scheduling into purchasing it because it is incorporated in the base package. If appointment scheduling is a secondary component of the system, it should be possible to integrate it into the base accounts receivable system so that the data base can be shared for the two functions.

Items to consider when determining whether or not an appointment scheduling package can benefit your practice include:

- Staffing considerations as they relate to the current manual appointment scheduling system.
- Whether the physical environment of the reception desk allows the placement of terminals and/or a printer.

- Defining the unique appointment scheduling criteria for the practice and for each physician and whether it can be applied to an automated appointment scheduling package.
- Medical records filing method (i.e., alphabetical versus numerical).
- Whether decentralized or centralized appointment scheduling is used.
- Identification of tasks currently performed by reception desk personnel as they relate to obtaining patient/responsible party information, developing a medical record, filing and refiling medical record charts, obtaining patient authorization signatures and other tasks associated with maintaining the reception desk.

In addition to assisting the reception desk in the tasks listed above, a good appointment scheduling system can also generate management reports for determining the effective use of the doctors' time. Cancellations versus "no-show" appointments, number of walk-ins versus prescheduled patients, etc., are all types of information that can be used to increase office efficiency and productivity.

(Appendix 5-B provides sample appointment scheduling reports.)

[3] Patient Recall

A recall system can have a significant impact on ability to generate new business from the existing patient population. Basically, patient recall is a system of reminders to call or send a letter or postcard to a patient who needs to schedule a future appointment based on his or her medical history. As an example, a chronically ill patient may require periodic examinations. A patient recall system assists you in making sure that this type of patient is routinely monitored. Similarly, if you provide annual physical examinations, you could use a patient recall system to remind patients they need to schedule an appointment for their annual physical.

Many recall systems incorporate word processing to develop user-defined recall letters or notices. This provides access to the ARM system's data base to print mailing labels or to develop "mail-merge" lists. Obviously, word processing capability can increase the flexibility of the patient recall system. However, most recall systems without word processing still allow users to compose their own letters or recall messages.

Other examples of how patient recall can be used to the benefit of the practice include:

- Marketing new services provided by the practice.
- Printing telephone lists to facilitate contact with patients, as opposed to sending out a recall letter or message.
- Incorporating a custom report generator to send out recall notices by specific medical condition or a previous service rendered to the patient.

[4] Word Processing

As the demand for streamlined recordkeeping is realized, word processing is expected to become an extremely cost effective tool in the practice setting. Word processing can be used in numerous areas in the medical office:

- Transcription of medical records.
- Transcription of referral letters, insurance reports and other correspondence.
- Integration with the accounts receivable management system for custom letters related to marketing, credit and collection, research patient recall, and other forms of correspondence sent directly to a patient.
- Research papers, articles and other documentation.
- Keeping medical records.

The word processing capacity offered by vendors can vary in its ability to meet a practice's needs. As a general rule, word processing packages are directly dependent on operating systems used by the computer hardware. Word processing packages are widely used in all business environments and, generally speaking, there is a word processing package that can meet the specific needs of any medical practice.

Other criteria for evaluating a word processing package are:

- Ease of use and operation.

- Integration with other software applications.
- Quality of the documentation and any other user training tools (tutorials, instruction diskettes, etc.).
- Number of work stations per software license fee.
- System dependent utilities, such as creating data base files and/or removing data base records from the word processing application.

[5] General Accounting Ledger

This package should be a financial reporting application designed to meet the needs of a specific medical group practice. Internalizing the general accounting ledger as part of the management information system can also help reduce ongoing accounting costs.

The general ledger program creates and maintains files of all financial transactions, including additions to and subtractions from specific disbursement accounts. These accounts are recorded in a chart of accounts. Furthermore, the financial reporting functions of a general ledger system allow you to make comparisons regarding income and expenses and generate reports by department specialty and provider. Similarly most general accounting ledgers allow you to develop comparative year-to-date reports, along with proposed budgets or cash flow reports.

Basic reports, such as detailed ledger balance and income statements, are the essential byproducts of most general accounting ledger applications. Other reports, such as the accountant's working trial balance report, the monthly general ledger detail report and the year-to-date general ledger report, are all essential reporting requirements of a general ledger system.

The addition of a custom financial report generator allows the user to design additional reports or modify reports to meet the specific needs of the practice. It provides maximum flexibility in the development of financial statements for the practice without the significant expense of customizing an income statement.

Other considerations in purchasing a general ledger accounting application are general ease of operation and whether it simplifies the work of the operator.

[6] Payroll

Payroll calculation, printing of checks and generating appropriate tax reporting documents (i.e., W-2 forms) can reduce accounting costs.

[7] Accounts Payable

This application provides the capability to maintain business records for the costs incurred in producing revenue. An accounts payable program creates and maintains files of invoices, credit memos and refunds for purchases and credits from vendors, functions designed typically to assist in controlling cash disbursements and payables. Most accounts payable systems should include a checkwriting capability, along with several key management report programs, such as:

- Open vouchers by vendor.
- Aged open vouchers.
- Cash requirement reports by week.
- Voucher aging by vendor.
- Vendor activity on a daily, monthly and year-to-date basis.
- Open vouchers on payment hold.

As noted, the check writing function should include a check register, checks and a trial payment report. The trial payment report is useful in budgeting and cash flow management.

It is essential that an accounts payable system include some form of accounting control log. An example is a program in which data is entered in batch format and each invoice is assigned an individual control number relating to a specific batch. The actual checks should also have specific control numbers. The combination of these features provides for an excellent tracking mechanism within the accounts payable application.

[8] Medical Records

This is a difficult area to discuss, since what constitutes a medical record varies with the data processing system. The capacity to organize medical records can range from maintaining miscellaneous health information on a patient to elimination of any hard copy of medical records.

[a] Problems in Definition

One of the major questions not resolved in this area is whether or not the computerized medical record is practical and, in most cases, whether its cost can be justified by the medical group. Computer professionals in the health care industry estimate that storing medical records takes between 10 to 100 times more data storage than the typical billing and collection management functions of a data processing system. Another item related to mass storage is the ability to correctly "size" the system based on the number of medical records unique to each specialty and office environment. Strong consideration should also be given to assessing the ability to back up this data and ensure its security, confidentiality and integrity. Given the large volume of data, the method of backing up large data base files is also an issue.

Given the lack of definition of what constitutes a computerized medical record, there is a controversy over the lack of a standardized coding scheme that can be used by the medical community. Either suppliers of medical computer systems must develop their own coding schemes, or end users must type out medical records in longhand. This, obviously, does not achieve the desired result, which is the ability to analyze free-form data from any angle at the touch of a button. Information processing is extremely time-consuming, given the large data base requirements for a medical records application. Consequently, a coding scheme is necessary for standardization and to maximize data searches. The responsibility for developing an acceptable coding scheme appears to rest with the medical community.

As stated earlier, a medical group must also be able to cost justify the medical records application. It appears that increased labor costs, coupled with the higher cost of computer mass storage, could increase operating costs, rather than lower them after computerization. If computer stored medical records do not improve collection, implementation of a computerized medical record would indicate that it makes the practice less profitable.

[b] Subfunctions of Medical Records Capacity

Since a completely automated medical record has not yet been developed, several data processing firms have slowly introduced subsets of a medical records application:

- Medication profiles by patient to permit development and maintenance of records related to the patient's medication history and to enable the physician and designated office personnel to view and record this information without having to pull the medical record.

- Diagnostic/special procedure reporting capability that permits development and maintenance of records related to a patient's laboratory/x-ray history or other special diagnostic tests associated with patient treatment.

- Self-administered patient history profiles to be used at the initial patient office visit for the physician to review and incorporate into the medical record.

- Access to a remote data base, such as the American Medical Association's GTE Telnet via a standardized communications protocol; this type of accessibility enables the physician to utilize remote data bases not only for diagnostic functions but also for research and development.

- Diagnostic software applications; there has been a surge in the development of diagnostic software for physicians. The software tends to be designed specifically for a medical specialty or health care condition. Many of these applications can be added to a data processing system without significant cost and typically will not be integrated with the other data processing functions of the system.

[c] **Miscellaneous Applications**

Many other data processing applications can be of benefit: for example, a spreadsheet software package for developing financial models for the practice, or a software application that can assist in monitoring vacation, sick leave, performance review and salary administration. Such applications tend to be "need specific;" that is, most vendors who specialize in the health care community would not have all of the data processing applications listed above and a secondary source for these types of applications would have to be consulted. If two vendors must be consulted, it is beneficial to determine whether or not an arrangement can be made with both to facilitate the use of these applications.

§ 5.03 Data Processing Alternatives

> Once you establish your needs, you must choose the most efficient type of data processing system. Data processing alternatives range from the relatively simple automated pegboard, to the time-shared or batch processing service bureau, to the purchase of an in-house computer system. Each system must be investigated with regard to the amount of vendor responsibility for processing and system maintenance.

There are several ways to automate a business. In general, variations of each of these major data processing alternatives are available for the health care industry.

[1] Automated Pegboard System

This method uses a traditional one-write manual pegboard system to serve as the primary accounts receivable record for all accounts receivable transactions. The original documents are then used for data entry purposes in an off-premises computer system (either on a service bureau or time-shared basis).

The automated pegboard evolved as the result of limitations inherent in the manual pegboard system, such as its inability to gather key management information to generate reports and collate data for the automatic preparation of insurance claim forms. In its true definition the automated pegboard only uses computer processing techniques to produce some simple and very basic management reports.

The automated pegboard system has a number of advantages:

- It improves general management reporting capability over the traditional manual pegboard system. It can produce basic management reports, such as physician production summaries and simple aging reports.

- In some circumstances, the automated pegboard system can produce an insurance claim form on a monthly basis. However, these forms are usually restricted to the major insurance carriers.

(Pub.372)

- It can produce a statement using a microfiche record and permit access to mail room service provided by the computer vendor.
- It produces a permanent record of the ledger card, which is maintained off the user's premises.
- The partial automation of the pegboard system requires office personnel to enhance their utilization of the manual pegboard system.

The automated pegboard system also has a number of disadvantages:

- This type of system does not overcome the inherent inefficiencies of maintaining a manual pegboard ledger card system. The repetitive, time-consuming tasks associated with maintaining the ledger card system (i.e., pulling and refiling ledger cards) are not reduced through automation.
- Management reports are generally very basic and the system provides little or no opportunity to customize them.
- Since the information is entered off the premises and processed by a third party (i.e., the vendor or time-sharing facility), there is usually a significant time delay in receiving the reports.
- It is expensive to implement, given the fact that output generated by this type of system is usually a simple byproduct of more sophisticated levels of data processing.
- You must rely on a third party to enter information and accept the financial integrity of the transaction information entered.

[2] Batch/Mail-In Service Bureau

One of the first data processing products offered to the health care community, the batch or mail-in service bureau product is computer time shared, or offered, by a data processing company. All information, including patient/responsible party demographics and billing information (payments, charges, etc.) are collated by the office staff and forwarded to the service bureau vendor for data entry. The computer processing company proofs, enters and validates the information, which is subsequently returned to the practice via paper reports. The company assumes total responsibility for the data entry of the information provided and usually charges a computer processing fee, plus an additional fee for data entry.

The advantages of this type of system are as follows:

- It is more highly sophisticated than a pegboard system, which results in significant improvement in management reporting capability.
- It is responsible for all data entry tasks assumed by the computer vendor.
- All computer processing functions are provided by the computer vendor (i.e., mail room service).
- It automatically prepares insurance claim forms for major third party carriers.
- It automatically prepares patient statements with a degree of flexibility as it relates to the frequency of processing statements.
- The user can request (for a fee) additional management reports beyond the standard reporting capability provided by the vendor.

The disadvantages are as follows:

- Generally speaking, this form of automation is expensive.
- Office personnel are required to continually transpose information, such as patient demographics, and maintain other methods of recording information to serve as data entry documents for the service bureau. This can be very time consuming and cumbersome, given the volume of data processing information being processed.
- The user loses control of information entered into the system. The practice is forced to maintain duplicate sets of records to ensure the integrity of the information being processed.
- The system relies heavily on paper "hard copy" output for information. Reliance on paper output is typically cumbersome and very time consuming.

- The design and features of a mail-in service bureau product typically are very generic to meet the needs of a wide range of medical practices.

- The system cannot provide information for other data processing applications (payroll, general ledger, word processing, etc.).

- As practice productivity increases, the cost of the mail-in service bureau generally increases proportionately. The related inefficiencies necessitated within the office to maintain the product become greater.

- Management information is generally more sophisticated than that produced by the automated pegboard. Most by-exception or specialized reports are produced at a cost to the medical practice.

- Since all of the information is entered off premises, there is usually a delay from the time the information is forwarded to the computer vendor to the time the information is returned to the practice.

[3] On-Line/Real Time Service Bureau

The term "on-line/real time" means that the medical practice can communicate directly with the computer system via a terminal and communications modem (telephone linkage). This form of data processing uses a company's data processing system for a fixed fee plus the cost of communications equipment and computer hardware. The office assumes the responsibility for entering all information into the computer system and the service bureau provides the software and computer processing capability.

The concept behind on-line/real time is that the information entered is typically validated at the point at which it is entered, rather than by a paper copy or edit of all transaction errors, as in the case of a batch or mail-in computer product.

The advantages of on-line/real time data processing are as follows:

- The practice regains control of the data entry functions without assuming the responsibility of the data processing management functions provided by the computer vendor.

- There is no capital expenditure for computer software and the computer hardware is usually provided on a lease or rental basis.

- Production problems are eliminated because the management reports, statements and insurance forms are processed by the service bureau.

- The degree of sophistication as it relates to management reporting typically increases with an on-line service bureau product.

- The system eliminates time delays from the point at which the data is entered and information is processed and received by the practice.

- System output can usually be printed via a remote printer; thus, some management reports and other system output can be produced at the office location. The information entered into the system is generally far greater than with the other forms of data processing previously discussed.

The system shares many disadvantages with the batch/mail-in service bureau system:

- It is generally more expensive because it requires on-site telecommunications and computer hardware (although the cost for a communications line has significantly decreased over the last several years).

- On-line service bureau products are generally subject to significant periods of "down time." During this down time the user does not have direct access to the computer system, and this usually results in a loss of productivity and efficiency.

- The general design and capability of the product is generic so that it meets the needs of a wide variety of health care practitioners. Usually, the system must be customized to meet the specific needs of the practice.

- It is unable to provide solutions for other data processing applications.

(Pub.372)

[4] In-House Computer System

In general, service bureaus that provide products and services to the health care community are experiencing difficulty competing with the popularity of in-house computer systems. As market forces affect service bureau products, in many instances it has become more economical for practices to purchase their own data processing system. The term "in-house" system is generally used to refer to a computer system used by a single medical group.

An in-house system may be purchased or leased and is maintained at the office facility. It may be a packaged or custom system. A packaged system is usually one whose software has been developed on a "generic" basis and which can be utilized by a wide variety of health care practitioners.

Custom software, in its truest form, is a software package specifically developed for a specific practice. However, these definitions are not black and white, and a variety of products fit into the gray area between them.

Computer experts and medical administrators agree that custom software is not practical and should be viewed only as a last resort if all packaged software proves unsatisfactory. It is not uncommon for professional programmers to spend two to three years developing a software package. In addition to a significant front-end cost to develop the custom software package, there are also significant ongoing support costs that users tend to underestimate. In addition, after the initial investment, the product may not work.

An in-house computer system presents a number of advantages:

- The practice is the sole user of the in-house system.
- The system provides maximum management reporting capability.
- You can expand the data processing system to include other applications with the addition of software (e.g., word processing).
- It can maintain data processing costs over a three to five year time period.
- It has a larger data base records capability than a service bureau system.

- It can manage the data base for custom report generation.
- You can customize software applications, given the unique environment of your medical practice.

The disadvantages of an in-house computer system are as follows:

- It entails a large up-front investment, although many computer vendors offer a lease program.
- Hardware and software become obsolete and must be replaced at your expense.
- Without proper maintenance, there is a potential for loss of the data base.
- Hardware and/or software may be underutilized, depending on the size and needs of the practice.
- The system internalizes routine data processing tasks assumed by a service bureau (i.e., printing, mail room processing).
- You cannot customize or add applications that are needed but incompatible with the existing computer system.
- Customized programming for a specific and unique application compatible with the system is often expensive.

All of these disadvantages are easily overcome with the selection of a vendor who provides ongoing support, including research and development, hardware and software maintenance and initial/ongoing training programs.

[5] Sources of System Purchase

The term "turnkey" vendor signifies a computer vendor who becomes the sole source of products and services purchased by the medical group, including hardware and software and hardware and software support services. The ideal vendor provides a turnkey product and service line and is experienced in the health care industry. The exception is the computer vendor who develops a software application specifically for the health care industry, but who does not sell or provide maintenance for the hardware components.

The software distributor is another source of purchase. The software distributor has entered into an agreement with a software developer to serve as a marketing/sales representative for the software developer. The distributor may or may not sell the computer system on a turnkey basis. Consequently, the medical group practice may have to do business with several vendors, even though the computer system was purchased through one distributor.

Another source from which to purchase an in-house system is the retail computer stores who market multiple software and hardware packages. Typically, the retail outlet does not have vertical market expertise in the health care industry, although in some cases they may have an arrangement with a specialist who has experience in the medical community.

(Further discussion related to the importance of selecting a computer vendor is provided in § 5.05, "Selecting a Management Information System." For a comparison of service bureaus and in-house computer systems, see Appendix 5-C.)

§ 5.04 Planning for Automation

> Before selecting a computer system you should determine the short- and long-term needs of your practice and write them down in a formal request for proposal. The request for proposal should be used to help narrow down the list of computer vendors to a handful whose products can then be compared on the basis of user feedback and on-site demonstrations. Use of a consultant in the selection process has advantages and disadvantages that must be weighed in advance.

As a result of the changes in the health care industry and the increased importance of accurate and reliable management information, only those practices with the means of making timely decisions are in a position to survive and prosper. In the past, consultants and administrators based the purchase of a computer on the expense of a billing system. Although cost is an important consideration when selecting a computer system, the specific data processing needs of the practice are more practical criteria.

Successful integration of automation systems and information demands advance planning. The planning process should be a team effort, and involve the key personnel who will use and/or be affected by the system ultimately decided on. (See Figure 5–1 for a schematic illustration of the information system planning process.)

(Pub.372)

```
                    GOALS AND
                    OBJECTIVES

     CURRENT            CURRENT
     SYSTEMS            COSTS
                                      COSTS/
                              COMPARISON   BENEFITS      INFORMATION
                                           ANALYSIS      SYSTEMS PLAN
     USER               PROJECTED
     REQUIREMENTS       BENEFITS

     POTENTIAL          PROJECTED
     SYSTEMS            COSTS
```

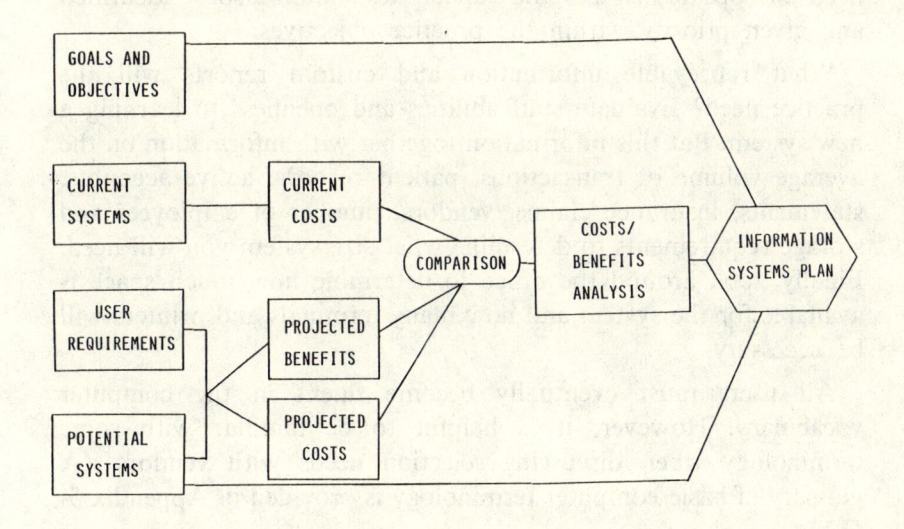

INFORMATION SYSTEMS PLANNING PROCESS

FIG. 5-1. This flow chart shows how the information systems planning process should proceed from the theoretical to system implementation.

[1] Assessing Practice Needs

The practice must determine its short-, mid- and long-term goals and objectives. It is important, when selecting a data processing system, to speculate what the practice will be like in three to five years. How many practitioners will be part of the practice and in what specialties? What influence will major factors such as third party insurers, employers and patient demographics have on a practice? By setting goals in these areas, you can plan the means for achieving them.

Once goals have been established, you should develop a list of the information or end products needed to monitor them. For example, in identifying a need to better manage delinquent accounts, you

(Pub.372)

should determine whether a letter system and aging is adequate or if flexible reminders, "chart flags" and other tools are needed. The need for specific services and capabilities should also be identified and given priority within the practice objectives.

What retrievable information and custom reports will the practice need? Evaluate staff abilities and openness to learning a new system. Put this information together with information on the average volume of transactions, patient records, active accounts, statements, insurance claims, vendors, number of employees and storage requirements to determine what size system you will need. Finally, look around the office to determine how much space is available for the system and how many terminals and printers will be necessary.

All users must eventually become fluent in the computer vocabulary. However, it is helpful to be familiar with some terminology when discussing selection needs with vendors. (A glossary of basic computer terminology is provided in Appendix 5-D.)

[2] Request for Proposal (RFP)

The traditional request for proposal (RFP) is the statement of the practice's data processing needs written as a formal document. This is one of several tools that enable the buyer and vendor to formally get to know one another during the selection process. The RFP should specify the software application and hardware needs of the practice. Many also specify service, support and general maintenance requirements.

[a] Drawbacks to the Request for Proposal

Even though RFPs are valuable, they can also be an obstacle in the decision-making process. The common problems associated with traditional RFPs are:

- RFPs tend to be unrealistic with regard to the immediate and future needs of the practice. If the RFP is viewed as a "wish list," the vendor will be frustrated in completing it.
- If the RFP is too specific as it relates to the statement of needs, especially in the area of software features, the selection of a computer system tends to focus on features rather than on all aspects of the system.

- RFPs, by their very nature, are costly to develop.
- The RFP tends to drag out the selection process due to the time commitments associated with developing the RFP and the vendor response.
- RFPs tend to be difficult to evaluate.
- From a vendor's perspective, it is difficult to interpret the RFP due to its complexity and because, in most cases, the vendor does not have an opportunity to visit the office personally. Consequently, response to the RFP tends to be vague so as not to alienate the practice. In addition, if the RFP is lengthy, the general response received from the vendors will be of equal length. Again, this makes it difficult for the practice to evaluate the RFP.

[b] **Use of the RFP in the Selection Process**

Many of the problems associated with an RFP can be resolved if you think of it as a tool to help guide you through the selection process.

The part of the selection process whereby the practice identifies the vendors it would like to receive proposals from is called the request for information. You can develop a list of potential vendors by soliciting input from practices currently utilizing a data processing system; contacting the medical organizations in your area for recommended systems; and, in general, evaluating the leading vendors in your state or region of the country. This narrows the list of potential vendors. The request for information process should include general background information about the practice. This part of the RFP costs very little to prepare.

Begin developing your RFP by itemizing your needs. Remember to be realistic in identifying the requirements and, if possible, itemize requirements based on immediate versus future needs.

Based on the information requested from each vendor, select four to six vendors whom you feel are most likely to fulfill your requirements. Invite each of them to visit your facility so they have the opportunity to get a good feel for how the practice operates—this enables them to respond to your RFP based on firsthand exposure to the practice. It also gives the vendor the opportunity to be specific in responses and, if necessary, to include examples related to the statement of need. It also allows you to become familiar with the vendor and, in most cases, determine whether you would like to continue with the vendor in the selection process.

Schedule on-site visits to practices currently using the vendor's products. Inform the vendor that you would like to visit a practice similar in nature to yours (i.e., approximately the same size and the same specialty) to see the computer system "in action" and get feedback on its capability. To minimize the disruption associated with on-site demonstrations, let the vendor arrange them.

Based on the steps taken, select a minimum of three vendors whom you would like to have receive your RFP. These vendors will now be in a position to complete your RFP in a realistic manner. You should also demand return of the RFP without delay.

Evaluate the completed RFPs received. Based on this evaluation, schedule a demonstration at the vendor's facility. This part of the process enables you to review the software and it provides a forum for clarifying responses in the RFP directly with the vendor. This is also a good opportunity to formulate opinions relative to the company and its ability to support your computer system. At this point in the selection process, you and the potential vendors have had the opportunity to get to know one another and are in a position to cooperate in implementing a computer system for the practice.

Re-evaluate the proposals and make a decision. Once the decision is made, inform the vendors not selected and do not give in to their counterproposals. The practice has psychologically committed to the vendor of its choice and any subsequent offers by the other companies will only deter you from final implementation. If a vendor makes a counterproposal offering a more attractive deal, ask why it was not proposed initially.

Begin negotiating your purchase agreement with the selected vendor.

A sample RFP is found in Appendix 5-E. The document is very thorough and provides an evaluation matrix not only for the software and hardware but also for the vendor completing the RFP. However, please note that this RFP should only be used as a model for developing an RFP specific to your practice.

MULTIPLE ROLES OF THE CONSULTANT

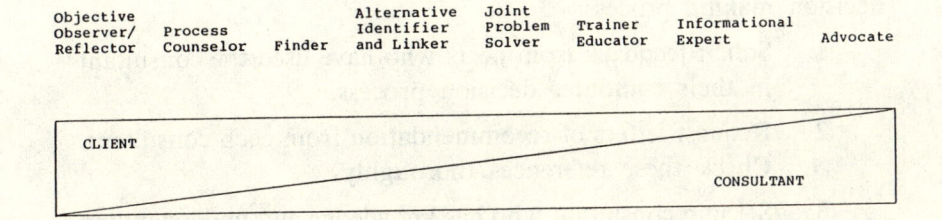

Objective Observer/ Reflector	Process Counselor	Finder	Alternative Identifier and Linker	Joint Problem Solver	Trainer Educator	Informational Expert		Advocate

CLIENT ———————————————————— CONSULTANT

LEVEL OF CONSULTANT ACTIVITY IN PROBLEM SOLVING

Nondirective ———————————————————————————— Directive

Raises questions for reflection	Observes problem-solving process and raises issues mirroring feedback	Gathers data and stimulates thinking inter-pretives	Identifies alternatives & resources for client and helps assess consequences	Offers alternatives & partici-pates in deci-sions	Trains client	Regards, links, & provides policy or practice decisions	Proposes guidelines persuades, or directs in the problem-solving process

FIG. 5-2. This diagram illustrates interaction between the client and the consultant. Ideally, as the consultant becomes more qualified and assumes a more directive role, he or she should relieve the client of many problem solving activities.

[3] Use of a Consultant

Planning is the key to successful implementation of a data processing system. A consultant can assist you in gathering, collating and evaluating information for making a data processing decision. Consultants can serve many roles and it is your responsibility to determine the specific role of the consultant in the planning/decision-making process. (See Figure 5-2.)

A computer consultant can be an asset to the practice in the decision-making process. However, to maximize utilization, the consultant should also be required to "follow up" after the purchase and installation of the computer system to ensure a smooth implementation. He or she can address specific questions and/or concerns during implementation and ensure the computer system is used to its maximum potential.

(Pub.372)

[a] Selecting a Consultant

Selecting the consultant can be a difficult process. However, if the following steps are taken, you will find a consultant to assist in the decision making process:

1. Solicit feedback from peers who have used the consultant in their computer decision process.

2. Request letters of recommendation from each consultant. Check these references thoroughly.

3. Select a consultant who has knowledge and understanding of the health care field.

4. The consultant should also have a level of expertise in the computer industry. He or she must keep up with computer technology to be able to advise clients on which system best suits the practice.

5. Based on the consultant's role definition, obtain a proposal from the consultant to perform the services you have defined.

[b] Disadvantages of Using a Consultant

There are several disadvantages to using a consultant when selecting a computer system:

- Generally speaking, most computer consultants lack vertical market expertise in the health care field. A consultant who lacks vertical market expertise tends to focus on the computer hardware at the expense of assessing the needs of the practice as it relates to software applications.

- Lack of role definition or changes in the role during the selection process can dramatically affect the decision making process.

- Higher costs are associated with the decision-making process when a consultant is used. The rule of thumb is that it adds 2 to 10 percent of the cost of the system to use a consultant. As an example, if the system selected costs $50,000, the consultant's fee will be $1,000 to $5,000.

- Given the lack of role definition, a consultant may not be in a position to make specific recommendations.

(Pub.372)

§ 5.05 Selecting a Management Information System

> When choosing a computer system, it is essential to buy from a vendor with a proven track record in the health care system who will stand behind the product. The vendor's software applications should be the main criteria for choosing the system. They should directly address the needs of the practice as recorded in the request for proposal. When choosing software applications, it is important that they be accessible and protected with a backup system. Hardware should be compatible with the software, and its operating system should allow multiple or single access as the practice desires. Hardware should be able to grow and expand with the practice. It should be established in advance whether the vendor or a third party will supply maintenance and upkeep of the system, and whether the vendor instructs the staff in the full and proper use of the system so that the practice can enjoy a maximum return on its investment.

The medical computer market is highly competitive, and each vendor will claim to have the best system. However, each system has strengths and weaknesses that must be evaluated. When evaluating these options, always refer back to the practice needs and goals as assessed in the RFP.

The four main areas to evaluate when selecting a management information system are the company, the data processing applications (software), the computer equipment (hardware) and the service provided. A problem in any of these areas can render the entire system ineffective.

[1] Selecting the Company

Key factors to evaluate in selecting a vendor include the vendor's expertise, clientele, longevity and professional recommendations. The company that has a team of experienced medical specialists, programmers and service representatives developing and maintaining its products is more likely to provide a high quality, usable product than a company that has adapted a general business system for a medical practice. Nothing can replace the experience of managing an active practice as a prerequisite of a medical management information system. The value of a medical background is also important for maintaining the system through changes and the development of new features for future needs.

Be sure to investigate the company through its clientele. How many installations are operating? Where are they located? How long has the company used the system? Is it satisfied? A site visit to a practice using the system can add a realistic dimension to the selection process. Be sure to ask about service and response to trouble calls. Studies indicate that many common computer problems can be traced to inadequate implementation, planning and execution. Does the company provide a complete implementation plan? Is it practical?

An evaluation by a computer specialist can be very useful if you have any doubts about the system, but be sure the specialist is a bona fide expert. Many consultants, accountants and attorneys who consider themselves experts have limited experience. Be sure that the consultant does a thorough evaluation and does not just render an opinion based on previous situations.

The company should be willing to stand behind its products. Look for guarantees and warranties. The system may be warranted for up-time (the time the computer is operational), for response to trouble calls and for the capabilities of the system.

Finally, check into the company's financial position and staying power, but do not be misled into thinking that the largest companies have the best products or are the best choice. Many smaller firms have developed excellent systems. However, it is critical that the vendor you choose be able to provide you with ongoing service.

[2] Selecting the Software

The parts of the data processing system that are applied to specific functions to meet the needs of the user are known as the application software. To select software appropriate for the practice, practice needs must be identified.

[a] Access

The language the software is written in is important for two major reasons. First, it should be compatible with all the software that will be used. Second, it should be a standard language for the industry. This enables other programmers to work on the system, if necessary.

A document known as the source code is also needed for programming. The source code is closely guarded by vendors. However, should the vendor no longer be able to service the system, the source code must be made available. This is accomplished through a custodial agreement, which entitles the end-user to access and use of the source code should warranted circumstances prevail.

Another basic software feature is random data access, a memory that can be both read from and written into easy-to-understand plain English directions and formats. Full-screen editing is generally preferrable to prompt and response because the operator can move at a faster pace. Most operators are more comfortable with full-screen because it is similar to written copy.

[b] Security and Confidentiality

A medical practice management information system should have three primary categories of security: (1) physical protection, (2) data manipulation protection, and (3) system integrity protection. Based on these three levels of security, you can evaluate whether the security protection provided in the software is adequate for your setting. Not every practice needs all three levels, as the type of security is directly dependent on the type of employee handling the computer system (i.e., operator versus programmer) and the physical environment of the practice. Generally speaking, the software applications should provide at least the following levels of security:

- Operator access to the system.
- Application protection by operator.
- Function protection by operator.
- Operator protection by hardware.

As an example, an operator can be assigned multiple levels of security that prohibit access to a specific application or function via a designated terminal. If payroll were part of the management information system, the software should be able to limit access to this application by operator, by application and by terminal. In other words, a particular terminal can be designated as the only device through which an operator with proper security can access a specific application on the computer system.

You should also implement data processing management procedures such as periodic spot checks on the system or simply making sure each person in your office takes a regular vacation to further prohibit data corruption. Most embezzlement schemes require the

(Pub.372)

embezzler to be physically present in the office, and they can usually be identified when he or she is not. In summary, computers often provide better controls than most manual systems, but every office should practice some essential preventive measures.

[c] Backup Procedures

Another often overlooked feature of any software package is the method of backing up the computer's data base to ensure protection and preservation of the data. Backup is a means of saving the programs and data to retain a recent version in the event of destruction or loss of the current data.

There are several types of backup media, each with advantages and disadvantages. (See Figure 5-3.) Backup procedures should be simple and short enough to ensure that they are done frequently, preferably on a daily basis.

Method	Advantages	Disadvantages
Hard disk to hard disk	Fast transfer rate of data	High cost; requires two identical hard disk drives
	Availability of removable hard disk drives to facilitate archiving	Lack of more than one backup medium
	Very reliable	Storage of medium off premises; difficult to store
Hard disk to floppy diskette	Low cost; most economic	Requires large number of diskettes
	Easy to store off premises	Slow transfer rate
	Most common method for small computer systems	Cumbersome and time-consuming
	Certified magnetic medium	Media is susceptible to environmental changes
Hard disk to tape option: cartridges or cassettes	Becoming very popular and usually offered as part of a standard computer configuration	Expensive; higher cost Software applications may not include this backup method
	Fast rate of transfer	
	Ability to store large volumes of data on a cassette or tape	
	Certified magnetic medium	

FIG. 5-3. Table of various system backup options with a brief listing of each option's advantages and disadvantages.

[i] Backup Methods. The method in which a computer system backs up its data can vary from vendor to vendor. There are, primarily, two backup techniques employed by most vendors: (1) complete disk copy and (2) file backup. The disk copy is an exact duplicate of all data on the disk, regardless of a specific data file. This form of backup actually verifies the physical integrity of both media: that from which the information is read and that to which it is copied. It allows for media detection of any damage to the surface of the disk before it accepts any information. One of the major advantages of this type of backup system is its speed when compared to the file backup method.

File backup is accomplished by reading the contents of a specific file and saving it on a backup medium (tapes, cassettes or diskettes). This technique also verifies the integrity of the file itself and alerts the user to any problem discovered in attempting to read it. One of the primary advantages of a file backup technique is that it can identify potential problems at the time the file is actually verified.

Some computer vendors employ a selective file backup method whereby only those files that have been updated or changed since the last complete backup are backed up. Although this method reduces the actual time spent backing up media on a daily basis, when a total recovery becomes necessary each incremental backup of those files has to be reloaded as of the last full tape backup. Consequently, it may take longer to recreate the data base.

[ii] Rules for Choosing a Backup System. The following are some simple rules of thumb for developing a backup procedure for your computer system:

- Assign an operator the primary responsiblity of monitoring and conducting all backup procedures and filing responsibilities.

- Require that all media be labeled, noting the date, type of backup, person completing the backup and the data base backed up.

- Store the media off the premises on a daily basis.

- Backup media should be filed by maintaining three previous full-system backups at all times (grandfather, father, son provision).

- Maintain backup media in a stable environment, protecting it against adverse environmental conditions, such as high heat and humidity.

Typically, the more precautions used or developed by the end user, the more assurance the data base will be secure. You should consult the computer vendor about safeguarding your data base.

[3] Selecting the Hardware:

The third step in evaluating a computer system for your practice is to examine the hardware to be used in conjunction with the software package.

Once the software and computer company have been identified, the selection of the hardware is simple. If you assume that the hardware is the focus of the selection process, you risk purchasing a computer system that does not live up to what is promised during the sales presentation. The software design and implementation maximizes the computer processing capability of the hardware. An analogy can be made to purchasing an automobile with an undersized engine: ultimately, the car's performance is reduced.

[a] Operating System

As part of the selection process for the hardware, first determine if the operating system software can be used by the computer hardware. The operating system is the software that instructs the hardware to perform. The combination of the software, operating system and hardware maximizes the overall performance of the computer system. The operating system of a computer system may be purchased directly from the software developer or purchased in combination with the computer hardware.

There are many different operating systems available from computer manufacturers and independent software developers. The operating system employed by the computer manufacturer may be a derivative of an operating system develped by a third party, modified to maximize the performance of the computer hardware. Generally speaking, the three industry standard operating systems in the micro-computer industry are:

- MS-DDS
- CP/M

- UNIX

[b] Operator Vocabulary

It is helpful to know several several key terms and computer concepts when making a hardware selection:

Single User: This concept typically applies to the personal computer market. A "single user" computer system is a computer system that operates only as a stand-alone computer system, to which one operator has access. This is typically a feature of the MS-DDS operating system environment. The need for more than one computer operator to use the system at the same time rules out the feasibility of many such systems. This is one of the primary reasons why personal computer systems have not been very successful as true "business" systems. In most medical practices more than one operator needs access to the computer system at the same time, such as a receptionist who must enter new patient demographic data and the office bookkeeper who needs to enter charges or run statements.

Multiuser: This is a concept used widely by computer manufacturers, but in many cases it is misinterpreted. A multiuser system allows more than one operator to access the computer system via multiple work stations (i.e., terminal or computer). Multiuser capability is not directly related to the computer hardware, but involves the computer software and the operating system. A computer system with more than one work station may be defined as a multiuser system, but the software (application and operating system software) may not be able to operate in a multiuser environment. For example, software applications utilizing the MS-DDS operating system environment may not allow simultaneous system access to different operators.

Local area networking, discussed below, is a software package that allows single user software applications to operate in a multiuser environment. In other words, it allows two separate and distinct software applications to be used simultaneously through a local area network, but it does not allow two operators to utilize the same software package simultaneously.

Multiuser/Multiprocessing: This concept applies to computer systems that allow more than one operator to simultaneously access the same software application without "corrupting" and/or "crash-

(Pub.372)

ing" the system. Most computer systems which operate in a multiuser/multiprocessing mode employ what is called a "file" and/or "record locking" capability. This feature, usually part of the software design, is usually incorporated into the operating system and/or data base manager employed by the software application.

If any of the following needs/conditions are identified, you should select a computer system that operates in a multiuser/multiprocessing mode:

- Need for more than one work station.
- Need for multiple access to the same application (i.e., accounts receivable).
- Need to have accessibility to the same data base file or record.

If these conditions pertain to your practice, many computer hardware systems can be eliminated from the selection process. Similarly, if the software application utilized in conjunction with the computer hardware cannot meet these requirements, it too can be eliminated from the selection process. It is important that you identify your needs in relation to these terms prior to your investigations. Once your needs are determined, they should be specifically included in the request for proposal and stated clearly in the hardware and software sections of the RFP.

Likewise, during the selection process you should require the vendor to demonstrate that the computer system meets the conditions in the proposal to determine whether or not it is capable of performing in the desired environment.

8-Bit versus 16-Bit/32-Bit: During the selection process, references are made as to whether the hardware is an 8-bit, 16-bit or 32-bit machine. Because these terms can often be misleading and therefore misinterpreted, they should not be used as key criteria for selecting your computer system. The term 8-bit or 16-bit refers to the capacity to access and/or retrieve bytes (refer to Glossary) of information at one time. Typically, it is assumed that a 16-bit base machine is faster and/or more powerful than an 8-bit machine.

There are many other factors that influence the computer processing capability of computer hardware. These include, but are not limited to:

(Pub.372)

- The operating system employed by the computer system.
- Design of the software applications.
- Speed of the hard disk drive to access information from the data base.
- The transfer rate of information from the hard disk to the task being performed.
- The general architecture of the computer hardware.

Many excellent computer hardware systems that employ 8-bit technology can be used in a medical practice. Even though the 8-bit technology is older, it is typically very reliable and many software applications have been written to accommodate it. These computer systems should not be ruled out, but they are being overtaken rapidly by computer systems that employ 16- or 32-bit technology.

Expandability: All computer equipment has finite limits, and these limits vary with the manufacturer. It is essential these limits be identified, especially in the following areas:

- Upper limit to CPU memory capacity.
- Total hard disk storage capability.
- Maximum number of terminals the system can handle.
- Total number of printers that can be attached to the system.

You should also consider the operating system's capacity for growth. Some operating systems can be used on larger equipment lines where they can be transferred to other equipment without high conversion costs.

If the computer hardware has been installed at its upper expansion limits, it may not be able to handle the growth of the practice. Buyers have a strong tendency to underestimate growth in terms of volume of business and the need for additional software applications. Typically, once an end user is successful with a specific application, he or she tends to automate another area of the practice. Consequently, adding other applications usually demands that the computer hardware be able to expand with the related software application.

(Pub.372)

[c] Common Mistakes

Practices often make one or several common mistakes when selecting the hardware component for their system.

First, and most common, is the so-called "slick demo." Even though most computer consultants recommend the first demonstration of the system take place at the vendor's office, these demonstrations are often misleading if the following questions are not asked prior to the actual demonstration:

- What is the current size of the files being demonstrated as they relate to transaction history and patient demographic history?
- Is this the same computer system being recommended for our practice?
- How many terminals are currently being utilized in conjunction with the demonstration? If more than one, is this a realistic response time?
- Will the response time be similar to the computer system being recommended, given comparable size of the system?
- Is the software being demonstrated similar to the software that will be recommended for our practice?

Once you have received a demonstration at the vendor's facility, it is also recommended you witness a live demonstration at a current customer's site. You should ask the same questions during this on-site demonstration.

Another pitfall to avoid is the so-called "special deal." Often these special deals end up costing the practice more money in the long-run because the deal can only be given if certain financial considerations have not been compromised with the vendor. As an example, if a huge discount is being given on a line of computer hardware it can indicate that the computer manufacturer is in the process of reducing or terminating the product. Some discounts are valid, but one should be cautious when a special deal surfaces during a computer purchase decision.

As stated earlier, it is also important to avoid the mistake of selecting hardware before the software package has been chosen. The computer itself is not the primary factor in achieving a data processing solution for the practice, and you should place more emphasis on the software application. Psychologically, it is easier for buyers to evaluate and select hardware because it tends to be an objective, not a subjective decision. In other words, it is easier for people to evaluate technical documentation than it is for them to evaluate software features.

Furthermore, it is misleading to assume that hardware can easily be compared based on a product specification sheet. As an example, two similar computer systems may have similar hard disk storage capacity on an "unformatted" basis, but once the system is formatted for the operating system and its software application, the systems could differ significantly in the remaining disk space available for your data base. It is important to keep in mind that computer hardware should not be the sole basis on which to make a purchase decision.

Finally, the people associated with the selection process should also know their technical limitations. The assumption that the person who owns a personal computer is a computer expert is the worst assumption. It is easy to fall into the trap of discussing hardware and its capabilities instead of focusing on the selection process as a complete and total system. Knowing technical limitations also applies to the involvement of family, friends and business associates who become involved in the computer selection process based on their use of a personal computer or their employment by a computer company. Often, the opinions rendered by these individuals are biased and potentially confusing to individuals involved in the selection process.

[4] Service, Support and Maintenance

It is often said that the computer vendor should support the system while the system supports the practice. A key factor for purchasing a system—and one that is frequently overlooked—is the vendor's dedication to supporting the product.

An important question to ask the vendor when purchasing a computer system is "What happens after the system is installed and you or someone in the practice has questions?" Another question to ask is "What happens if something goes wrong or doesn't work right?" The support of a computer system involves many variables

(Pub.372)

including, but not limited to, assisting your personnel, keeping your system up and running properly and modifying or updating the system to deal with changes in the health care industry. A vendor's support staff should be accessible, knowledgeable and, above all, communicative. In the selection process, you should request references from clients as to their knowledge of not only their computer system, but the industry in general.

Support for your computer system can be provided in two ways: either the company from which you purchase the system assumes the responsibility for supporting it, or the support is provided by a third party. It is important to determine where support will come from for both hardware and software. For example, if a major insurance carrier changes its claims reporting format, who will modify the program to accommodate the change? Typically, customer service support is provided by maintenance contracts offered by the computer vendor. Since it is safe to assume that hardware will break down and software will need to be updated, it is desirable to have a maintenance contract for each.

[a] **Hardware Maintenance.**

The hardware maintenance contract can be closely associated with an insurance policy. If the computer hardware components break, the hardware maintenance agreement should provide for the repair and/or replacement of the components and, in most cases, the labor associated with the repairs.

The primary advantage of using the vendor's maintenance organization is that it is familiar with the hardware. The advantage of a third party maintenance organization is its dedication solely to providing this type of service. The primary disadvantage of a third party organization is the trouble associated with "finger pointing," which can happen when each maintenance organization blames the other for the system's problems.

Key items to be addressed in a hardware maintenance contract include:

Description of the Type of Service Provided: Is the maintenance provided on-site or off-site? What is the method of figuring the charges (e.g. fixed rate, time and materials, etc.).

Response Time: Response time is the time it takes the vendor to get to the facility to rectify the problem. This is an important consideration in determining the cost of maintaining the hardware. The rule of thumb is that the quicker response time you desire, the higher the maintenance service. Generally speaking, most maintenance contracts provide for a response time in the range of four to eight business hours.

Access Requirements: This provision specifies that the maintenance organization is able to access the system during normal business operations of the practice. It is helpful to the maintenance organization if you can identify the best times for a vendor to have access to the computer hardware.

Spare Parts/Replacement Parts: The maintenance contract should specify that spare parts are provided for each component and/or guarantee that replacement parts are of comparable or equal value.

Preventive Maintenance: Typically, most hardware maintenance agreements do not provide for preventive maintenance services. This is usually the responsibility of the practice. However, if you desire preventive maintenance services, the hardware maintenance vendor will usually offer them for an additional fee.

Replacement Equipment: This provision requires the maintenance organization to provide temporary hardware components at little or no charge while the problem component is being repaired.

Enforcement: This provision describes the circumstances which would constitute a breach of contract on the part of the maintenance organization.

Renewal Rights: This is typically difficult to negotiate, since most medical practices want the option to continue the maintenance agreement for an indefinite period of time. Typically, hardware maintenance organizations reserve the right to terminate maintenance on computer equipment they deem unrepairable due to neglect and/or general use. However, if you desire this option, it usually involves giving up provisions related to cost protection.

Price Increases: This provision requires the maintenance organization to give written notice on any price increase.

Assignment and Subcontract Rights: Many maintenance organizations unilaterally assign or subcontract their obligations to another maintenance organization. If this is part of the maintenance contract, the medical practice should insist on a provision that allows for assignment to occur only if both the practice and the maintenance organization agree to it in writing.

[b] Software Maintenance

Software maintenance contracts vary from vendor to vendor. Generally speaking, software maintenance contracts provide the following services:

- Software updates or enhancements to the software applications under contract.
- Software diagnosis and program "fixes" or modifications.
- Access to the vendor's customer support service department.
- Revisions/enhancements to software documentation.

A recent trend in the software maintenance area requires end users to install a communications modem. This enables the vendor to provide software and hardware diagnostics. When the vendor is able to conduct on-line diagnostics, it ultimately assists the user by reducing costs related to maintenance services, because it makes an on-site visit unnecessary.

[c] Maintenance Contracts

The rule of thumb in the computer industry is that maintenance contracts should cost approximately one percent to 1.5 percent of the original system cost per month. For example, if the total system cost was $50,000, the associated costs to provide hardware and software maintenance contracts would be $500 to $750. Most vendors provide an initial 90-day warranty for the hardware and software components. The hardware and software maintenance agreements would, subsequently, become effective on the 91st day and either have a remaining term of nine months or twelve months. Again, the terms of maintenance agreements vary from vendor to vendor.

[d] Ongoing Educational Training

In addition to the items identified above, you should inquire about ongoing educational training services provided by the vendor. Ideally, the vendor should provide ongoing educational classes related to the use of the software and computer hardware. Such classes are usually conducted in group sessions and are sometimes referred to as "end-user training classes."

A recent trend is for vendors to provide instructional media to assist in training current and new employees. The use of demonstration and training software can facilitate the training of new employees and reinforce skills learned by existing operators. Training and/or demonstration diskettes are usually made available at no charge to the end user because they reduce the vendor's costs.

[e] Software Documentation

There are, generally, three types of program documentation:

- Operator manuals that serve as reference documents for the use of the software.

- Manager manuals developed to assist the data processing manager or administrator in the use of the software (e.g., references related to maintaining the system security are usually documented in a manager's manual).

- Technical manuals generally provided by the software and hardware vendors. These manuals usually provide information related to the general maintenance of the hardware and software and standard protocols as it relates to system diagnosis.

[f] Installation, Conversion and Training

Another significant factor in the success of a computer system is the quality of training the staff receives. Generally speaking, computer system failure is often linked to the lack of end user training. Poor training also results in underutilization of the computer system and, ultimately, poor end user satisfaction.

To alleviate this problem, it is important to evaluate the vendor's knowledge as it relates to the health care industry. If the vendor does not take time to learn the industry, the vendor will ultimately be unable to support the system. Even with good software, a computer vendor who is inexperienced in health care and/or who does not take the time to thoroughly learn the industry will be unable to properly train your staff. This is a good reason for selecting a vendor dedicated to the health care industry.

(Pub.372)

§ 5.06   MANAGING YOUR MEDICAL PRACTICE

Review of a potential vendor should consider:
- The completeness and practicality of the implementation/conversion plan.
- The ability to obtain references regarding the vendor's prior history in installing a computer system.
- The availablility and responsiveness of the vendor's customer support staff.
- The training tools and/or conversion aids to assist in the installation and training process.

In addition to the installation and training requirements, the medical group may also have to consider the conversion of its existing data to a new system. The conversion process is often ignored in the system evaluation and, if not addressed early, can cause undue pressure and increase costs associated with the conversion.

Items to consider in evaluating the conversion process include:
- Automated file or record conversion capability.
- Vendor's prior history in conducting automated record conversions.
- Whether the vendor provides a conversion plan.
- Identification of the costs associated with doing an automated record conversion.

§ 5.06 Legal Considerations

It is to your benefit to have the practice's legal advisor review all documents pertaining to the acquisition of a computer system. Documents regarding the purchase and maintenance of software and hardware are usually contracts. They should be worded in such a way that you and the vendor are in agreement regarding liability and warranties for the breakdown or updating of computer equipment.

A practice's legal advisor should be involved in the purchase of a computer system and, at the very least, review all of the documents involved with the computer acquisition so that pitfalls typically found in standard or "preprinted" purchase agreements are avoided. Generally speaking, the two types of legal documents associated with a computer acquisition are (1) separate contracts for the computer hardware and software components, and (2) combined purchase agreements encompassing software and hardware.

A computer hardware contract should address the following areas:

Integration or Merger Clause: In most cases, the computer vendor will insist on a clause stating that there are no prior understandings or agreements between parties, except as specified in the written agreement. In this way, the vendor indicates no obligations to the office, except as expressly stated in the written contract. This type of clause eliminates all previous written and oral understandings from the actual agreement. It is recommended that the vendor's proposal and your request for proposal be made part of the contract, which would eliminate the potential impact of the integration clause. By incorporating the RFP and vendor proposal as part of the contract the merger clause, in effect, would not apply to these documents. The vendor should not object to the inclusion of the RFP and the vendor's proposal, since they represent the promises and obligations that originally closed the deal.

Limitation of Action: The Uniform Commercial Code requires that contract actions be instituted within four years after the cause of action arises. However, the limitation of action provision allows the parties to contractually reduce the period of limitation to not less than one year. Most vendors perceive that the end user will not commence litigation until long after the contract is breached. Consequently, they try to reduce the period of limitation to one year.

Disclaimer from Implied Warranties: This type of provision indicates the vendor disclaims all implied warranties. It is recommended that, in exchange for this type of disclaimer, the end user incorporate strong language as it relates to user-oriented acceptance and acceptance testing as part of the contract.

Limitation of Liability: In most circumstances a vendor will try to include a provision that excludes and/or limits vendor liability for consequential and other kinds of damages. Usually, a limit on the vendor's liability equals the amount the user paid under the contract or some other method of liquidated damages, and/or exclusion of consequential and other damages, and a limited remedy of repair or replacement. In exchange for these concessions, a

(Pub.372)

practice should be allowed to recover its conversion and acquisition expenses if the computer vendor's system does not prove to be adequate.

Hardware Specification: This provision describes, in detail, the specifications of each hardware component. It should be in every contract.

Up-Time Warranty: This protects the end user by guaranteeing a percentage (95 to 99 percent) of time that the system is "up" over a one-month period.

Response-Time Warranty: This clause is difficult to draft because of the varied transactions that a system is capable of performing. If this type of provision is included, the vendor and the end user should identify those applications or functions that have the highest frequency of use and, subsequently, establish a response time for those functions. This is a very difficult clause to include and it is often misinterpreted.

Compatibility/Interface Guarantees: If the vendor represents the product as being compatible or able to interface with certain equipment or software, then it would be wise to put this in writing.

Acceptance Testing: Generally speaking, acceptance testing provisions should meet one of the following requirements:

- Provide that the hardware and software meet the specifications as defined in the contract.
- Provide that the system's performance matches the performance guarantees indicated in the contract.
- Provide any compatibility guarantees or interface guarantees are met.

§ 5.07 Computer Systems Checklist

A comprehensive list of points covered in the chapter is provided.

— Management information system services
　— Accounts receivable
　— Accounts payable
　— Billing
　— General ledger

- Payroll
- Insurance files
- Medical records
- Patient demographics
- Special management reports
- Files by exception
- Doctor/patient referrals
- Custom diagnostic coding
- Medication profiles
- Appointment schedules
- Employee vacation/sick day schedules
- Patient recall

- Data Processing Systems
  - Automated pegboard
  - Batch/mail-in service bureau
  - On-line/real-time service bureau
  - In-house system

- Selection Process
  - Assess needs
  - Request for Proposal
    - Determine long- and short-range practice goals
    - Identify vendors
    - Choose vendor(s) servicing hardware and/or software
    - Office and on-site demonstrations
    - Narrow down and reevaluate vendors
    - Purchase negotiations
    - Consultant

- Type of System

- Software
  - Accessibility
  - Security/backup
  - Confidentiality
  - Hardware
  - Compatible with software choice
  - Operating system
  - Single user/multiuser
  - Multiuser/multiprocessing
  - 8-, 16-, 32-Bit
  - Expandable

- Service and Maintenance Contracts
  - Vendor maintenance vs. third-party maintenance organization
  - Preventive maintenance
  - Response time
  - Access requirements
  - Spare parts
  - Replacement/interim equipment
  - Enforcement rights
  - Renewal rights
  - Price increases
  - Subcontracting
  - System conversion
  - Training
  - Ongoing education
  - Warranty/guarantee considerations
    - Integration clause/implied warranty disclaimer
    - Limitation of action/liability
    - Hardware specification

(Pub.372)

- Up-time warranty
- Response-time warranty
- Compatibility guarantee
- Acceptance testing

§ 5.100 Bibliography

Brandefs, J. F. and Pace, G. C.: Physician's Primer on Computers: Private Practice. Lexington, MA: Lexington Books, 1979.

McClug, C. J., et al.: Microcomputers for Medical Professionals. New York: Wiley, 1984.

Appendix 5-A

SAMPLE MANAGEMENT REPORTS

Accounts Receivable Report   Date 06/27/8-   Page   1
                                                  Last Update 06/26/8

	Daily		Month-to-Date		Year-to-Date	
	Current	Charge-off	Current	Charge-off	Current	Charge-off
Beginning A/R Balance:	635,653.95	139,090.07	589,814.55	139,968.01	616,333.91	103,838.50
Gross Charges(+):	.00	.00	249,793.00	.00	2,339,039.00	108.00-
Total Discounts(-):	.00	.00	19,597.33	.00	200,667.77	246.57
Total Receipts(-):	8,099.49	.00	189,499.13	2,877.43	2,091,397.21	31,628.71
Total Refunds/Ret.Checks(+):	.00	.00	772.83	.00	41,079.49	336.99
Total Misc. Debits(+):	.00	.00	576.41	.00	11,671.11	3,707.09-
Total Misc. Credits(-):	.00	.00	304.05	2.33	11,252.42	4,971.72
Total Balance to Charge-off	.00	.00	3,001.82-	3,001.82	68,836.47-	68,836.47
Net A/R Change:	8,099.49-	.00	38,739.91	122.06	18,634.73	27,837.39

A/R Balance Date - 06/26/84   Current A/R   Charge-off A/R   Total A/R
                               $ 627,554.46 $ 139,090.07 $ 766,644.53

FIG. 5-4

(Pub.372)

App. 5-A MANAGING YOUR MEDICAL PRACTICE 5-58

A/R Management Summary Report Date 06/27/8 Page 1
June Fiscal Year: 09/01/8 to 08/31/8

	Total Beginning A/R $	Net(+) Charges	Net(-) Receipts	Net(+/-) Adjustments	Total Ending A/R $	E-O-M Current A/R $	E-O-M Charge-off A/R $	Monthly Coll%	YTD Coll%	A/R Ratio
Last Fiscal Yr's Avg.	683,025.46	200,715.09	188,247.70	1,507.09	696,999.93	610,505.32	86,494.61	94%	94%	3.04
September 198	720,172.41	223,725.59	233,254.27	1,182.25	709,461.48	608,480.27	100,981.21	104%	104%	2.72
October 198	709,461.48	213,685.49	184,169.34	343.65	739,321.48	631,710.12	107,611.36	86%	95%	2.89
November 198	739,321.48	197,356.16	160,331.67	261.23-	776,084.74	661,691.63	114,393.11	81%	91%	3.13
December 198	776,084.74	187,228.66	220,313.09	2,231.91-	740,769.60	618,998.01	121,770.59	118%	97%	3.01
January 198	740,769.60	202,792.25	231,436.92	1,297.41-	710,836.52	587,138.08	123,698.44	114%	100%	2.86
February 198	710,836.52	208,973.85	208,894.65	2,313.05-	709,600.67	584,023.41	124,577.26	100%	100%	2.94
March 198	709,600.67	224,835.51	219,044.98	938.35	723,227.65	588,019.34	135,208.31	94%	99%	2.82
April 198	723,227.65	196,248.21	224,428.48	1,554.94-	693,492.44	560,505.66	132,986.78	114%	101%	2.71
May 198	693,492.44	249,974.07	214,802.39	881.56-	727,782.56	588,814.05	138,968.01	86%	99%	2.78
June 198	727,782.56	230,195.67	191,603.73	270.03	766,644.53	627,554.46	139,090.07	83%	97%	2.94
July 198	.00	.00	.00	.00	.00	.00	.00	0%	0%	.00
August 198	.00	.00	.00	.00	.00	.00	.00	0%	0%	.00
YTD Totals	727,782.56	2,137,015.66	2,082,283.42	9,260.12-	766,644.53	627,554.46	139,090.07			
Avg.-Monthly Totals	724,974.64	213,701.57	208,228.34	826.01-	729,622.07	605,693.55	123,928.61		97%	2.83

FIG. 5-5

(Pub.372)

COMPUTERS IN HEALTH CARE

Physician Management Summary Report
Date 06/27/8   Page 1
Fiscal Year: 09/01/8 to 08/31/8

June

Physician # 1 __   Physician Name: _____

	Gross Charges(+)	Discount(-)	Net Charges(+)	Misc. Debits(+)	Misc. Credits(-)	Total Receipts(-)
Last Fiscal Year's Avg.	25,379.33	.00	25,379.33	.00	.00	.00
September 198	3,150.00	.00	3,150.00	.00	.00	.00
October 198	2,470.00	.00	2,470.00	.00	.00	.00
November 198	3,055.00	.00	3,055.00	.00	.00	.00
December 198	2,247.00	.00	2,247.00	.00	.00	.00
January 198	288.00	.00	288.00	.00	.00	.00
February 198	.00	.00	.00	.00	.00	.00
March 198	.00	.00	.00	.00	.00	.00
April 198	.00	.00	.00	.00	.00	.00
May 198	81.00	.00	81.00	.00	.00	.00
June 198	126.00	.00	126.00	.00	.00	.00
July 198	.00	.00	.00	.00	.00	.00
August 1984	.00	.00	.00	.00	.00	.00
YTD Totals	11,417.00	.00	11,417.00	.00	.00	.00
Avg. Monthly Totals	1,631.00	.00	1,631.00	.00	.00	.00

FIG. 5-6

(Pub.372)

App. 5-A MANAGING YOUR MEDICAL PRACTICE 5-60

Physicians Production Report   Date 06/27/8   Page 1   Last Update 06/26/8

Dr#	Dr. Name	Period	Beginning Date	Gross Charges(+)	Discounts(-)	Net Charges(+)	Debits(+)	Credits(-)	Total Receipts(-)
1	,ARNOLD	Daily MTD YTD	06/27/84 06/01/84 09/01/83	.00 124.00 11,417.00	.00 .00 .00	.00 126.00 11,417.00	.00 .00 .00	.00 .00 .00	.00 .00 .00
2	MD, GEORGE B	Daily MTD YTD	06/27/84 06/01/84 09/01/83	10,782.00 164,494.00	.00 158.40	10,782.00 164,335.60	.00 .00	.00 .00	.00 .00
3	MD, SAM	Daily MTD YTD	06/27/84 06/01/84 09/01/83	21,994.00 199,499.00	.00 .00	21,994.00 199,499.00	.00 .00	.00 .00	.00 .00
4	MD, JAMES A	Daily MTD YTD	06/27/84 06/01/84 09/01/83	18,243.00 161,597.00	.00 27.00	18,243.00 161,570.00	.00 .00	.00 .00	.00 .00
5	MD, BILL	Daily MTD YTD	06/27/84 06/01/84 09/01/83	26,442.00 193,851.00	.00 .00	26,442.00 193,851.00	.00 .00	.00 .00	.00 .00
6	MD, ROBERT	Daily MTD YTD	06/27/84 06/01/84 09/01/83	29,277.00 202,873.00	.00 .00	29,277.00 202,873.00	.00 .00	.00 .00	.00 .00
7	MD, THOMAS	Daily MTD YTD	06/27/84 06/01/84 09/01/83	13,572.00 219,427.00	.00 .00	13,572.00 219,427.00	.00 .00	.00 .00	.00 .00
8	MD, WALLACE	Daily MTD YTD	06/27/84 06/01/84 09/01/83	.00 81.00	.00 .00	.00 81.00	.00 .00	.00 .00	.00 .00
9	MD, HARVEY	Daily MTD YTD	06/27/84 06/01/84 09/01/83	22,815.00 211,932.00	.00 .00	22,815.00 211,932.00	.00 .00	.00 .00	.00 .00
10	MD, ALLAN	Daily MTD YTD	06/27/84 06/01/84 09/01/83	15,912.00 168,445.00	14.40 365.40	15,897.60 168,079.60	.00 .00	.00 .00	.00 .00
11	MD, NORMAN	Daily MTD YTD	06/27/84 06/01/84 09/01/83	.00 621.00	.00 .00	.00 621.00	.00 .00	.00 .00	.00 .00
12	MD, NICK	Daily MTD YTD	06/27/84 06/01/84 09/01/83	1,845.00 46,584.00	.00 .00	1,845.00 46,584.00	.00 .00	.00 .00	.00 .00
13	MD, MARK	Daily MTD YTD	06/27/84 06/01/84 09/01/83	8,046.00 41,760.00	.00 .00	8,046.00 41,760.00	.00 .00	.00 .00	.00 .00

FIG. 5-7

(Pub.372)

COMPUTERS IN HEALTH CARE App. 5-A

Income & Production Summary Report   Date 06/15/84   Page 2

May 1984   Physician #   Name   TOTAL   Fiscal Year: 11/01/83 - 10/31/84

		Month-to-Date			Year-to-Date		
Service Code	Total Code	Description	Amount	%	Volume	Amount	%	Volume
800		ANESTH. FOR LOWER ANTERIOR ABDOM. WALL	.00		0	176.00		2
840		ANESTH FOR INTRAPER-ITONEAL PROC LOW AB.	.00		0	352.00		8
860		ANESTHESIA FOR LOWERABDOMEN/URINARY PROC	.00		0	110.00		2
1200		ANESTHESIA FOR KNEE CLOSED HIP JOINT	.00		0	220.00		4
1250		ANESTHESIA FOR ALL PROC. OF UPPER LEG	.00		0	60.00		3
1382		ANESTHESIA FOR ARTHROSCOPIC PROC.-KNEE	.00		0	176.00		
1800		ANESTHESIA FOR HAND,WRIST, FOREARM	.00		0	1,254.00		
1810		ANES FOR PROCEDURES OF FOREARM,WRIST,HAN	.00		0	264.00		2
1830		ANESTHESIA FOR OPEN SHOC..FRACTURE HAND	.00		0	550.00		4
10140		DEBRIDEMENT;SKIN, PUNCTURE ASPIRATION	.00		0	.00		
11041		TISSUE,MUSCLE,BONE	.00		0	264.00		
11200		ANES EXCISION, SKIN TAGS	.00		0	.00		
11400		ANES EXCISION, BENIGN	.00		0	154.00		
11401		ANES EXCISION BENIGN	.00		0	110.00		
11732		ANES EXCISION OTHER	.00		0	286.00		
11750		ANES AVULSION OR NAIL	.00		0	132.00		
11770		ANES EXCISE FINGER NAIL	.00		0	264.00		
12004		ANES EXCISION OF	.00		0	132.00		
12031		ANES REPAIR WOUND SCALP, LAYER CLOSURE OF	.00		0	264.00		
12051		ANES REPAIR COMPLEX,	.00		0	198.00		
15000		EXCISIONAL PREPARA- TION OR CREATION OF	.00		0	528.00		4
15100		SPLIT GRAFT, TRUNK,SCALP, ARMS, LEGS.	.00		0	242.00		
15200		FULL THICKNESS GRAFTFREE, INCLUDING	.00		0	198.00		
15220		FULL THICKNESS,GRAFTFREE, INCLUDING	.00		0	132.00		
17110		DESTRUCTION BY ANY METHOD OF FLAT WARTS	.00		0	132.00		
19100		BIOPSY OF BREAST (SEP PROCEED)	.00		0	.00		
19101		BIOPSY OF BREAST INCISIONAL	550.00	1.85	2	1,540.00	.73	9
19140		MASTECTOMY FOR GYNE-COMASTIA THROUGH	.00		0	.00		3
19180		MASTECTOMY, SIMPLE COMPLETE; UNILATERAL	418.00	1.41	3	418.00	.20	3
19240		MASTECTOMY, MODIFIEDRADICAL-MOD AXILLARY	308.00	1.04	1	1,870.00	.98	7
		TOTAL INTEGUMENTARY SYSTEM SERVICES	1,276.00	4.30	6	10,158.00	4.79	63
20251		BIOP- INCIS-DEEP-VER-TEBRAL-LUMBAR/CERVIC	.00		0	.00		2
20550		INJECT-TENDON SHEATHLIGAMENT-TRIG. POINT	.00		0	80.00		
20670		INSERT WIRE-PIN SKELTRACTION W/ REMOVAL	.00		0	132.00		6
20680		REMOVAL BURIED WIRE,PIN,SCREW SUPRFCL-	264.00	.89	2	770.00		3
21203		REMOVAL BURIED WIRE,PIN,SCRN,PLATE-DEEP	.00		0	504.00		
21320		OSTEOPLASTY,MANDIBU-LAR RAMUSOSTEOTOMY)	.00		0	440.00		
21450		MANIPULATIVE TREAT- MENT, NASAL BONE FX,	.00		0	132.00		2
21451		TREATMENT OF CLOSED OR OPEN MANDIBULAR	396.00	1.33	1	264.00		2
23140		OPEN TREATMENT OF CLOSED OR OPEN	.00		0	836.00	.39	7
23330		EXCIS-BONE CYST-TUMCLAVIC.,1,2 OR SCAPULA	.00		0	198.00		
23420		REMOVAL FOREIGN BODYSUBCUTANEOUS	.00		0	1,672.00		
23450		REPAIR-COMP SHOULDERCUFF AVULSION-CHRON	.00		0	286.00		
23480		CAPSULOGRAPHY-ANT. MAGNUSEN TYPE PROCED	.00		0	198.00		
23500		OSTEOTOMY-CLAVICLE W/H/OUT INT FIXATION	110.00	.37	1	110.00	.05	1
23515		CLAVIC- FRAC-OPEN REDUCT W/W/OUT FIXAT	.00		0	154.00		
23660		SHOULDER DISLOCATIONOPEN REDUCTION	.00		0	220.00		
23665		SHOULDER DISLOC-WITHFRAC-TUBEROSITY-CLSD	132.00	.44	1	352.00	.06	2
24105		OLECRANON BURS EXCIS				132.00		1

FIG. 5-8

(Pub.372)

App. 5-A MANAGING YOUR MEDICAL PRACTICE 5-62

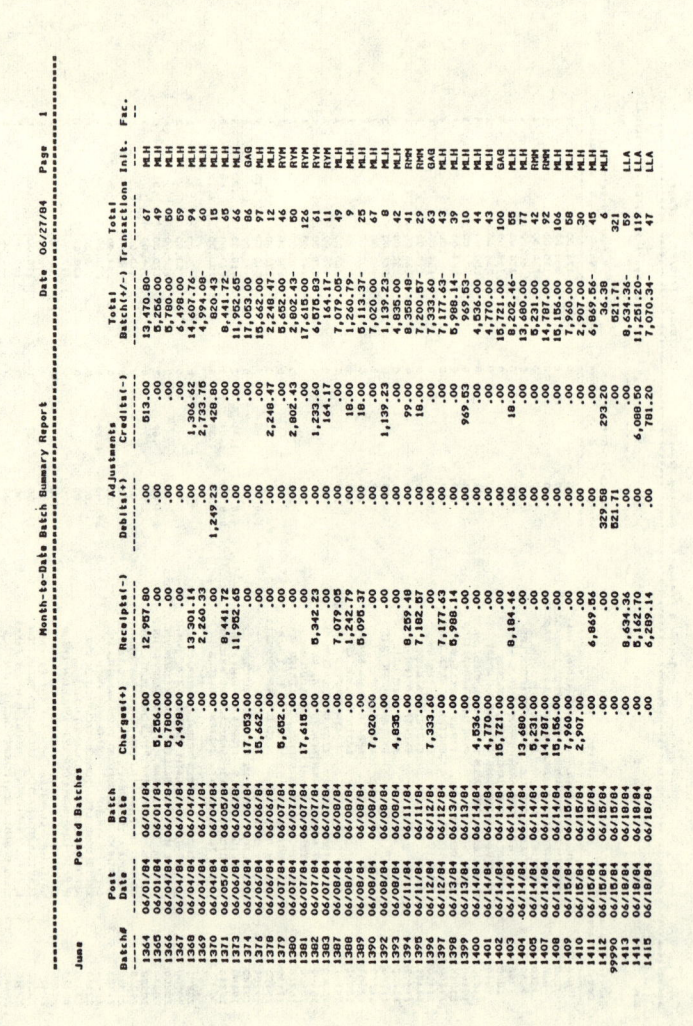

Month-to-Date Batch Summary Report   Date 06/27/84   Page 1

Posted Batches

Batch#	Post Date	Batch Date	Charges(+)	Receipts(-)	Adjustments Debits(+)	Adjustments Credits(-)	Total Batch(+/-)	Total Transactions	Init.	Fac.
1364	06/01/84	06/01/84	5,256.00	12,957.60	.00	513.00	13,470.60	67	MLH	
1365	06/01/84	06/01/84	5,256.00	.00	.00	.00	5,256.00	49	MLH	
1366	06/04/84	06/04/84	5,780.00	.00	.00	.00	5,780.00	60	MLH	
1367	06/04/84	06/04/84	4,499.00	.00	.00	.00	4,499.00	59	MLH	
1368	06/04/84	06/04/84	.00	13,301.14	.00	1,306.42	14,607.56	94	MLH	
1369	06/04/84	06/04/84	.00	2,260.33	.00	2,733.75	4,994.08	60	MLH	
1370	06/04/84	06/04/84	.00	.00	1,249.23	428.80	820.43	15	MLH	
1371	06/05/84	06/05/84	17,053.00	8,441.72	.00	.00	8,441.72	65	MLH	
1373	06/05/84	06/05/84	.00	11,952.65	.00	.00	11,952.65	66	GAG	
1376	06/06/84	06/06/84	15,662.00	.00	.00	.00	15,662.00	97	MLH	
1378	06/06/84	06/06/84	5,652.00	.00	.00	2,248.47	2,248.47	12	RYM	
1379	06/07/84	06/07/84	17,615.00	.00	.00	2,602.43	2,602.43	46	MLH	
1380	06/07/84	06/07/84	.00	5,342.23	.00	1,233.60	6,575.83	60	MLH	
1381	06/07/84	06/07/84	.00	.00	.00	164.17	164.17	126	RYM	
1382	06/07/84	06/07/84	.00	7,079.05	.00	.00	7,079.05	61	RYM	
1387	06/08/84	06/08/84	.00	1,242.79	.00	18.00	1,260.79	9	MLH	
1388	06/08/84	06/08/84	7,020.00	5,095.37	.00	18.00	5,113.37	25	MLH	
1389	06/08/84	06/08/84	.00	.00	.00	.00	7,020.00	67	MLH	
1390	06/09/84	06/09/84	.00	.00	.00	1,139.23	1,139.23	8	MLH	
1392	06/09/84	06/09/84	4,835.00	.00	.00	.00	4,835.00	42	MLH	
1393	06/11/84	06/11/84	.00	8,259.48	.00	99.00	8,358.48	41	MLH	
1394	06/11/84	06/11/84	.00	7,182.07	.00	18.00	7,200.07	29	RMM	
1395	06/11/84	06/11/84	7,333.60	.00	.00	.00	7,333.60	43	GAG	
1397	06/12/84	06/12/84	.00	7,177.43	.00	.00	7,177.43	39	MLH	
1398	06/13/84	06/13/84	.00	5,988.14	.00	.00	5,988.14	10	MLH	
1399	06/13/84	06/13/84	.00	.00	.00	969.53	969.53	42	MLH	
1400	06/14/84	06/14/84	4,536.00	.00	.00	.00	4,536.00	44	MLH	
1401	06/14/84	06/14/84	4,770.00	.00	.00	18.00	15,721.00	43	MLH	
1402	06/14/84	06/14/84	15,721.00	.00	.00	.00	15,721.00	100	GAG	
1403	06/14/84	06/14/84	.00	8,184.46	.00	18.00	8,202.46	55	GAG	
1404	06/14/84	06/14/84	13,680.00	.00	.00	.00	13,680.00	77	MLH	
1405	06/14/84	06/14/84	5,231.00	.00	.00	.00	5,231.00	42	RMM	
1407	06/14/84	06/14/84	14,787.00	.00	.00	.00	14,787.00	92	MLH	
1409	06/15/84	06/15/84	7,940.00	.00	.00	.00	15,156.00	106	MLH	
1410	06/15/84	06/15/84	2,907.00	.00	.00	.00	7,940.00	58	MLH	
1411	06/15/84	06/15/84	.00	4,869.56	.00	.00	2,907.00	30	MLH	
1412	06/15/84	06/15/84	.00	.00	329.58	293.20	4,869.56	45	MLH	
99363	06/15/84	06/15/84	.00	.00	521.71	.00	36.38	6	GAG	
1413	06/18/84	06/18/84	.00	8,634.36	.00	.00	521.31	321	LLA	
1414	06/18/84	06/18/84	.00	5,162.70	.00	4,088.50	8,634.36	59	LLA	
1415	06/18/84	06/18/84	.00	6,289.14	.00	781.20	11,251.20	119	MLH	
							7,070.34	47	LLA	

FIG. 5-9

(Pub.372)

Income & Production Summary Report Date 06/15/84 Page 1

May 1984 Physician # Name TOTAL Fiscal Year: 11/01/83 - 10/31/84

Service Code	Total Code	Description	Month-to-Date Amount	%	Volume	Year-to-Date Amount	%	Volume
2		PATIENT PYMT – CHECK	11,384.25-	.00	124	80,254.17-	.00	788
16		INSURANCE PAYMENT	11,366.80-	.00	66	73,982.54-	.00	422
17		BLUE SHIELD PAYMENT	2,902.94-	.00	19	21,685.70-	.00	164
18		HMO PAYMENT	2,215.00-	.00	12	8,504.20-	.00	50
19		MAPP-HMO PAYMENT				756.00-	.00	4
20		PHP PAYMENT	418.00-	.00	3	1,012.00-	.00	5
23		SHARE PAYMENT	352.00-	.00	1	660.00-	.00	4
24		MEDICARE PAYMENT	238.40-	.00	4	4,577.60-	.00	40
25		MN M/A PAYMENT	1,622.52-	.00	22	4,920.84-	.00	74
26		OUT-STATE M/A PYMT	110.00-	.00	1	1,415.32-	.00	13
27		WORKER'S COMP PYMT	634.00-	.00	4	1,938.00-	.00	3
28		COMPANY PAYMENT				412.00-	.00	3
31		MED/LEGAL PAYMENT	109.76-	.00	1	697.76-	.00	29
32		COLLECTION AGENCY PAYMENT	645.00-	.00	7	1,772.98-	.00	29
51		REFUND PAYMENT	1,108.88	3.64	11	4,963.67	2.54	41
52		REFUND INSURANCE CO	96.00	.32	2	96.00	.05	2
53		REFUND BLUE SHIELD	353.00	1.16	5	619.60	.32	7
54		REFUND MAPP/HMO				144.00		1
56		REFUND MN M/A	.00		0	35.20		
	2	TOTAL RETURNED CHECKS	30,430.79-	100.00	282	195,721.46-	100.00	1653
	3	TOTAL RETURNED CHECKS AND REFUNDS	30,430.79-	100.00	282	195,721.46-	100.00	1653
	4	NET RECEIPTS	30,430.79-		282	195,721.46-		1653

FIG. 5-10

App. 5-A MANAGING YOUR MEDICAL PRACTICE

Detail Processing Report - Credit Balances Date 08/16/84 Page 2

RP Account	RP Name/Address	Date	Patient Name	Transaction Description	Trans. Amount	New Balance	Dr	Svc	CODES Mod Pl Diag	BC	FC	NC	Ref. Batch
152239	BERNICE, M E MAGNOLIA, W ST PAUL	070284 070284 MN 072484	BERNICE	PREVIOUS BALANCE PREVIOUS STATEMENT WRITE-OFF PER MGMT CURRENT ACTIVITY	115.44-* 38.64 38.64 *	76.80-	98	99970 99980 99943		54			753
152477	IRENE, RT 3 BOX, WEBSTER	070284 070284 MI 072084 WI 072584	IRENE	PREVIOUS BALANCE PREVIOUS STATEMENT PATIENT PYMT - CHECK BLUE SHIELD PAYMENT CURRENT ACTIVITY	206.48 * 206.48- 28.70- 235.18-*	28.70-	98 98	99970 99980 17		12	20		741 743
152571	PHILIP, APACHE LANE, MENDOTA HEIGHTS	070284 070284 MN 071384 080284	CHARLES	PREVIOUS BALANCE PREVIOUS STATEMENT PATIENT PYMT - CHECK CURRENT ACTIVITY	15.20 * 15.20- 15.20- 30.40-*	15.20-	98	99970 99980 2		10	20		733 757
152676	DARYLE D, MALVERN ST, ST PAUL	070284 070284 MN 073184 080284	CONNIE	PREVIOUS BALANCE PREVIOUS STATEMENT SMALL BALANCE W/O PATIENT PYMT - CHECK CURRENT ACTIVITY	43.00 * 43.00- 43.00- 86.00-*	43.00-	98 98	99970 99980 99952 2		10	20		754 757
152761	GARY L, OTTAWA AVE, ST PAUL	070284 070284 MN 071384	GARY	PREVIOUS BALANCE PREVIOUS STATEMENT INSURANCE PAYMENT FED EMP GOV DEN PLAN CURRENT ACTIVITY	1,195.00 * 1,225.00- 1,225.00-*	30.00-	98	99970 99980 16		15	20		733
152778	KAREN L, CAMBODIA AVE, FARMINGTON	060484 MN 073084	KAREN	PREVIOUS BALANCE INSURANCE PAYMENT LONE STAR LIFE INS CURRENT ACTIVITY	.00 * 75.00- 75.00-*	75.00-	98	99970 16		10	20		748
152819	EILEEN M, BEAUMONT ST, ST PAUL	070284 070284	EILEEN	PREVIOUS BALANCE PREVIOUS STATEMENT	126.80-*	126.80-		99970 99980		12			
153004	RICHARD, SUMMIT AVE, ST PAUL	070284 070284	RICHARD	PREVIOUS BALANCE PREVIOUS STATEMENT	70.00-*	70.00-		99970 99980		12			
153017	JAMES, ADRIAN ST, ST PAUL	070284 070284 MN 072784 072784	MARY	PREVIOUS BALANCE PREVIOUS STATEMENT DISCOUNT, BLUE SHIELD U/C REFUND BLUE SHIELD CURRENT ACTIVITY	300.00-* 50.00 225.00 275.00 *	25.00-	93 98	99970 99980 99904 53		12			753
153044	CATHERINE, JUNO, ST PAUL	070284 070284		PREVIOUS BALANCE PREVIOUS STATEMENT	65.50-*	65.50-		99970 99980		12			753
153046	REBA B, S SARATOGA, ST PAUL	070284 070284 MN 070984 080284	REBA	PREVIOUS BALANCE PREVIOUS STATEMENT PATIENT PYMT - CHECK CURRENT ACTIVITY	220.00 * 220.00- 100.00- 320.00-*	100.00-	98 98	99970 99980 2		12	20		727 757

FIG. 5-11

(Pub.372)

FIG. 5-12

Detail Ageing Report - Net Production   Date 08/16/84   Page 4

Resp. Party Name Resp. Party J Phone-1 Phone-2	Address	Balance	Current	31-60	61-90	91-120	121-150	151-OVER	C	LP-Date Amount Type	BC FC MC
,VERNON 153771	SOMERSET RD WOODBURY MN 55125	300.00	300.00	.00	.00	.00	.00	.00	1		10
738- ,DAVID 932- 179	1ST WESTMORELAND #A COLORADO SP CO 80907	288.00 *	.00	.00	.00	.00	.00	288.00	1		19 16
644 ,DONNA M 12645	8TH ST E #7 INVERGROVE HTS, MN 55075	8.00 *	.00	.00	.00	.00	.00	8.00	1	11/11/83 35.00 32	19 26
450- ,DEBBIE J 153696	BEECH ST PAUL MN 55106	180.00	.00	180.00	.00	.00	.00	.00	1	08/15/84 144.00 16	10 11
774- ,JACK MD 153827	KENILWORTH DR WOODBURY MN 55125	504.00	504.00	.00	.00	.00	.00	.00	1		15
738- ,CONNIE M 150024	BOX WEBSTER WI 54893	50.00 *	.00	.00	.00	.00	.00	50.00	1	07/26/84 25.00 32	19 21
,ROBERT J 153073	JAMES AVE ST PAUL MN 55105	98.00	.00	.00	.00	.00	98.00	.00	1	05/21/84 73.68 17	12 90 21
699- ,JESSIE 11455	ERIE CROSBY, MN 56441	126.00 *	.00	.00	.00	.00	.00	126.00	1		19 16
546 ,RAYMOND MD 153359	DAYTON AVE ST PAUL MN 55104	12.15-	12.15-	.00	.00	.00	.00	.00	1	08/02/84 35.33 17	15 20
644- ,MARY 152272	STRYKER AVE ST PAUL MN 55107	246.24	.00	.00	.00	.00	.00	246.24	1	01/13/84 209.76 24	54 90 26
222- ,MICHAEL 153867	BLAIR AVE ST PAUL MN 55103	504.00	504.00	.00	.00	.00	.00	.00	1		10
488- ,SHER A 153313	VAN BUREN ST PAUL MN 55104	300.00	300.00	.00	.00	300.00	.00	.00	1		19 13
488- ,SANDRA K 13744	5 AVE NO SO ST PAUL MN 55075	40.00 *	.00	.00	.00	.00	.00	40.00	1	04/13/84 140.00 52	19 23
426- ,ARNE 2478	MAPLE ST CLEAR LAKE WI 54005	98.00 *	.00	.00	.00	.00	.00	98.00	1		19 16
,TERRY 153842	OAKDALE #116 W ST PAUDALE MN 55118	340.00	340.00	.00	.00	.00	.00	.00	1		12
450- ,DIANA 153874	CONROY TR INVER GROVE HGT MN 55075	100.00	100.00	.00	.00	.00	.00	.00	1		54
457- ,ROBERT 153824	MATILDA ST ROSEVILLE MN 55113	160.00	160.00	.00	.00	.00	.00	.00	1		60
483- ,THOMAS 153890	W SHRYER ROSEVILLE MN 55113	160.00	160.00	.00	.00	.00	.00	.00	1		60
644- ,DENISE A 153128 771-	7TH ST SO #2 SOUTH ST PAUL MN 55075	300.00	.00	.00	.00	.00	300.00	.00	1		10 90 14
455-											

(Pub.372)

App. 5-A MANAGING YOUR MEDICAL PRACTICE 5-66

TTD Ageing Summary Report Date 06/03/85 Page 6

Category - CHARGE OFF

Date	Active Accts	Total	Current	%	31-60	%	61-90	%	91-120	%	121-150	%	150-over	%
01/08/85	317	53,264.13	.00	0	.00	0	.00	0	.00	0	.00	0	53,264.13	100
02/04/85	318	55,171.88	.00	0	.00	0	160.00	0	716.00	1	196.00	0	54,099.38	98
03/04/85	315	54,155.13	.00	0	.00	0	.00	0	160.00	0	716.00	1	53,279.13	98
04/01/85	314	54,030.13	.00	0	.00	0	.00	0	.00	0	160.00	0	53,870.13	100
05/07/85	322	55,732.97	.00	0	.00	0	.00	0	.00	0	62.40	0	55,670.57	100
06/03/85	321	55,652.22	.00	0	.00	0	.00	0	.00	0	.00	0	55,652.22	100
Average	318	54,667.74	.00	0	.00	0	26.67	0	146.00	0	189.07	0	54,306.01	99

FIG. 5-13

(Pub.372)

COMPUTERS IN HEALTH CARE

TTD Ageing Summary Report
Date 06/03/85 Page 4
Category - Welfare-No Medicare

Date	Active Accts	Total	Current	%	31-60	%	61-90	%	91-120	%	121-150	%	150-over	%
01/08/85	56	11,932.25	2,105.00	18	2,108.00	18	1,232.00	10	868.00	7	2,168.00	18	3,451.25	29
02/04/85	56	10,975.25	1,712.00	16	2,108.00	19	1,576.00	14	1,072.00	10	448.00	4	4,059.25	37
03/04/85	55	10,251.05	1,212.00	12	2,260.00	22	1,388.00	14	1,588.00	15	1,340.00	13	2,463.05	24
04/01/85	55	10,748.05	1,978.25	18	1,772.00	16	2,080.00	19	1,212.00	11	1,068.00	10	2,637.80	25
05/07/85	67	12,104.30	4,486.30	37	2,642.00	22	1,448.00	12	1,052.00	9	824.00	5	1,852.00	15
06/03/85	59	10,104.00	2,860.00	28	3,800.00	38	374.00	4	936.00	9	632.00	6	1,502.00	15
Average	58	11,019.15	2,392.26	22	2,448.33	22	1,349.67	12	1,121.33	10	1,046.67	9	2,650.89	24

FIG. 5-14

(Pub.372)

App. 5-A MANAGING YOUR MEDICAL PRACTICE 5-68

TTD Ageing Summary Report   Date 06/03/85   Page 1

Category - Net Production

Date	Active Accts	Total	Current	%	31-60	%	61-90	%	91-120	%	121-150	%	150-over	%
01/08/85	1036	168,295.76	62,935.49	37	36,520.69	22	28,140.92	17	10,734.96	6	10,191.88	6	19,768.82	12
02/04/85	1001	166,624.77	60,158.70	36	47,699.61	29	17,992.98	11	16,492.79	10	5,880.20	4	18,400.49	11
03/04/85	941	154,208.89	49,868.82	31	44,518.90	28	27,011.67	17	11,640.18	7	10,268.57	6	15,900.75	10
04/01/85	962	166,946.57	53,299.78	32	42,387.22	25	24,793.21	15	16,178.94	10	8,755.26	5	21,532.16	13
05/07/85	1060	182,072.26	83,172.80	46	36,616.92	20	21,281.72	12	11,998.93	7	10,713.80	6	17,983.09	10
06/03/85	1019	205,551.89	60,358.10	29	70,772.16	34	25,361.09	12	15,160.84	7	9,834.25	5	24,065.45	12
Average	1003	174,783.36	61,682.28	35	46,419.25	27	24,096.93	14	13,701.11	8	9,274.49	5	19,607.29	11

FIG. 5-15

(Pub.372)

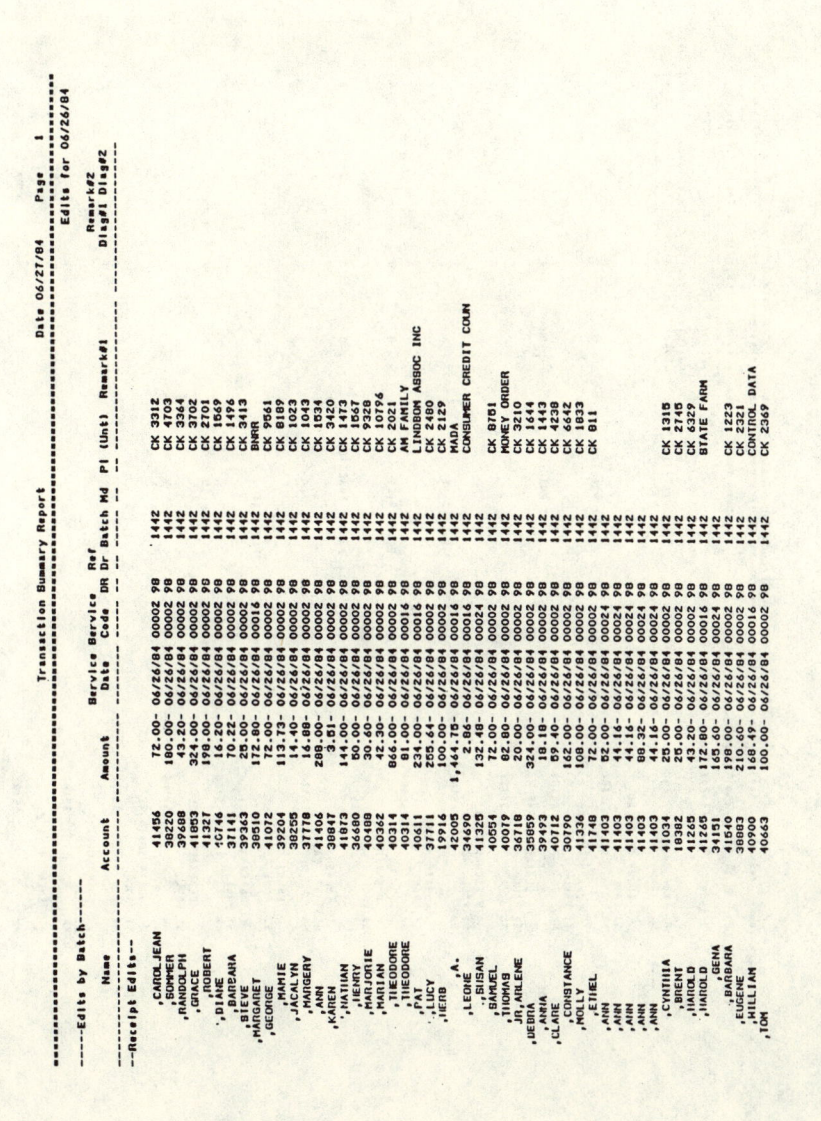

FIG. 5-16

App. 5-A MANAGING YOUR MEDICAL PRACTICE 5-70

Referring Doctor/Location Summary Report   Date 08/17/84 Page 1

Location Code: 1   Name: ST PAUL,
July   1984   Fiscal Year: 04/01/84 - 03/31/85   Monthly Total   Yearly Total   Last Years Total   Total
                                                         0   28   188   216

Ref Dr Cd	Ref Dr Name / Address	Phone	Specialty	Monthly Total	Yearly Total	Last Years Total	Grand Total
ZH	LOWRY BUILDING ST PAUL, MN 55102	222-	OB/GYN	0	0	0	1
59	PAYNE AVENUE ST PAUL, MN 55101	771-	FAMILY PRACTICE	0	0	1	1
02	LEXINGTON AVE N ST PAUL, MN 55112	483-	FAMILY PRACTICE	0	1	0	1
02	W EXCHANGE, # ST PAUL, MN 55102	227-	OB/GYN	0	0	1	1
05	SMITH AVENUE ST PAUL, MN 55102	227-	PEDIATRICS	0	2	5	7
06	N SMITH AV ST PAUL, MN 55102	227-	PEDIATRICS	0	0	6	6
85	EMERSON AVE. WEST ST. PAUL, MN 55118	457-	FAMILY PRACTICE	0	0	2	2
T4	FRONT ST. ST. PAUL	488-	PEDIATRICS	0	1	1	2
IX	MANDAMA BLVD. ST PAUL, MN 55108	641-	PEDIATRICS	0	0	0	2
17	CENTRAL MED BLDG ST PAUL, MN 55104	645-	PEDIATRICS	0	0	2	2
20	NORTH SMITH AV ST PAUL, MN 55102	227-	PEDIATRICS	0	1	4	5
09	SHERMAN ST # ST PAUL, MN 55102	224-	OB/GYN	0	0	1	1
22	SHERMAN ST # ST PAUL, MN 55102	224-	FAMILY PRACTICE	0	0	1	1

FIG. 5-17

(Pub.372)

July

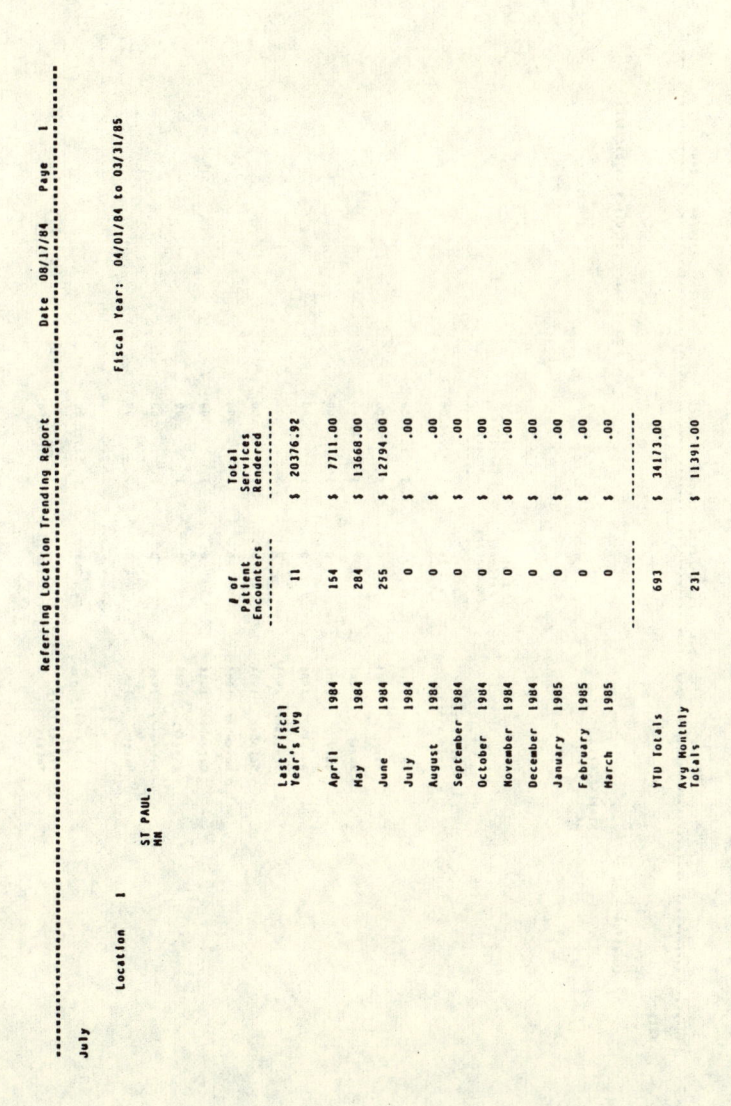

Referring Location Trending Report   Date 08/17/84   Page 1

Fiscal Year: 04/01/84 to 03/31/85

Location 1   ST PAUL,
             MN

	# of Patient Encounters	Total Services Rendered
Last Fiscal Year's Avg	11	$ 20376.92
April 1984	154	$ 7711.00
May 1984	284	$ 13668.00
June 1984	255	$ 12794.00
July 1984	0	.00
August 1984	0	.00
September 1984	0	.00
October 1984	0	.00
November 1984	0	.00
December 1984	0	.00
January 1985	0	.00
February 1985	0	.00
March 1985	0	.00
YTD Totals	693	$ 34173.00
Avg Monthly Totals	231	$ 11391.00

FIG. 5-18

App. 5-A MANAGING YOUR MEDICAL PRACTICE 5-72

Referring Location Trending Report   Date 08/17/84   Page 2

Fiscal Year: 04/01/84 to 03/31/85

Location 2 MINNEAPOLIS, MN

	# of Patient Encounters	Total Services Rendered
Last Fiscal Year's Avg	25	$ 1226.00
April 1984	26	$ 1092.00
May 1984	0	$ .00
June 1984	232	$ 12429.00
July 1984	0	$ .00
August 1984	0	$ .00
September 1984	0	$ .00
October 1984	0	$ .00
November 1984	0	$ .00
December 1984	0	$ .00
January 1985	0	$ .00
February 1985	0	$ .00
March 1985	0	$ .00
YTD Totals	258	$ 13521.00
Avg Monthly Totals	129	$ 6760.50

FIG. 5-19

(Pub.372)

5-73 COMPUTERS IN HEALTH CARE App. 5-A

Referring Doctors Trending Report Date 08/17/84 Page 5
Fiscal Year: 04/01/84 to 03/31/85

July

Doctor   TOTAL

Specialty: Location:

	# of Patient Encounters	Total Services Rendered
Last Fiscal Year's Avg	82	$ 3968.83
April 1984	13	$ 628.00
May 1984	10	$ 526.00
June 1984	42	$ 2321.00
July 1984	0	.00
August 1984	0	.00
September 1984	0	.00
October 1984	0	.00
November 1984	0	.00
December 1984	0	.00
January 1985	0	.00
February 1985	0	.00
March 1985	0	.00
YTD Totals	65	$ 3475.00
Avg Monthly Totals	22	$ 1158.33

FIG. 5-20

(Pub.372)

Appendix 5-B

SAMPLE APPOINTMENT SCHEDULING REPORTS

App. 5-B   **MANAGING YOUR MEDICAL PRACTICE**   5-76

```
Big Clinic, P.A.        Appointment Recap   8/12/84 to 8/13/84         Report Date 08/13/84  Page   3  ASRI
==================================================================================================
Big Clinic, P.A.                                                                    Client Totals

                              ---- Appointment Slot Utilization ----

                    Count    Prct.
                   --------  ------
Appointment Slots    172

Work In / Call In Slots   28   16.27 %

Appointment Slots Taken    2    1.16 %

Work In / Call In Taken              %

Slots Blocked Out                    %   Actual Block Out Time      Hours 00 Minutes


                                ---- Appointment Information ----

                    Count    Prct.
                   --------  ------
Appointments Made      1

Appointments in Limbo          %   Average Length  45 Minutes    Patients with A/R Accounts

Reschedules by Resource        %   Minimum Length  45 Minutes    Patients Marked New

Reschedules by Patient         %   Maximum Length  45 Minutes

Cancellations by Resource      %

Cancellations by Patient       %   Average Age   8

Walk Outs                      %   Minimum Age   8

No Shows                       %   Maximum Age   8

Patients Seen          1  100.00 %


                        ---- Appointments Distributed by Visit Type ----
                          Avg                    Avg                    Avg                    Avg
     Visit Type   Count   Len     Visit Type  Count Len    Visit Type  Count Len    Visit Type  Count Len
     ----------  ------   ---    ----------- ------ ---   ----------- ------ ---   ----------- ------ ---
    ALLERGY SHOT                 BIOPSY                   CONSULT                  Code - D
    Code - E                     Code - F                 Code - G                 HISTORY
    INJECTION                    Code - J                 Code - K                 Code - L
    Code - M                     NEW BACK                 OB CHECKUP               PAP
    Code - Q                     RE-CHECK                 Code - S                 Code - T
    Code - U                     VISIT          1   45    WELL BABY                Code - X
    Code - Y                     NOT SPECIFIED
```

FIG. 5-21

(Pub.372)

COMPUTERS IN HEALTH CARE App. 5-B

```
Big Clinic, P.A.          Daily Appointment Schedule for Tuesday   Apr 17 1984      Report Date 04/17/84  Page   6
=================================================================================================================

Department   1 Family Practice                                      Resource   4 Brandt MD,John C            Page

         Length                                      Birth    Schd  Reschd          New
   Time   (Min)    Patient Name       Phone Number    Date    Init   R P    Account (X)  Visit Type    Remarks
   ----   ------   ------------       ------------    -----   ----   ---    ------- ---  ----------    -------

   8:00A    30    WEBER,HEATHER D.    389-6517      7/24/75    JBK          14081519      VISIT        MEASLES
   8:30A    30    RICHTER,LYNN M      715-468-2601  5/09/64    JBK          13897196      PAP
   9:00A    30    PAUL,JASON STEPHEN  698-5350      9/05/73    JBK    1     14633525      INJECTION
   9:30A    30    URMAN,MARK          444-4793      1/17/70    JBK          14458915      VISIT         UNKNOWN ILLNESS
  10:00A    30    NORD,BORG           332-323-3333  1/22/22    JBK                    X   INJECTION     CHEMO
  10:30A
  11:00A    30    ROTHLISBERGER,RANDALYN 326-2719 12/25/76     JBK    1     14209276      VISIT         COLD
  11:30A
  12:00P
  12:30P
   1:00P          << Break >>
   2:00P   120    JUMPKEY,JIMMY       123-4324      1/24/56    JBK    1                X  VISIT         SORE THROAT
   2:30P
   3:00P
   3:30P
   4:00P
   4:30P
   5:00P
   5:30P
   6:00P          << Break >>
```

FIG. 5-22

(Pub.372)

App. 5-B MANAGING YOUR MEDICAL PRACTICE 5-78

```
Big Clinic, P.M.            Manual Backup Schedule for Tuesday  Apr 17 1984       Report Date 04/17/84 Page  1

Department  1 Family Practice                              Resource  1 Kline MD,James B.      Page   1
           ----------------- Slot 1 -----------------   ----------------- Slot 2 -----------------   ----------------- Slot 3 -----------------
Time   Patient Name / Remarks 1 Visit / Phone        Patient Name / Remarks 1 Visit / Phone        Patient Name / Remarks 1 Visit / Phone

8:00A  << Unavailable >>                             << Unavailable >>                              << Unavailable >>
8:15A  << Unavailable >>                             << Unavailable >>
8:30A  << Unavailable >>                             << Unavailable >>                              << Unavailable >>
8:45A  << Unavailable >>                             << Unavailable >>
9:00A  KIBLER,NICOLE            VISIT               HANSON,VANESSA           VISIT
        3 WK RET, FBS CBC       737-4315             1 WK RET                 483-1292
9:15A  RICHMOND,LUCINDA RAE    CONSULT
        TUBAL CONSULT           218-829-0282
9:30A       "   "   "
9:45A
10:00A
10:15A
10:30A
10:45A
11:00A LANNERS,MARK M           Code - Q
        CAMP PI                 1-679-4892
11:15A      "   "   "
11:30A      "   "   "
11:45A      "   "   "
1:00P
1:15P
1:30P
1:45P
2:00P
2:15P
2:30P
2:45P
3:00P
3:15P
```

FIG. 5-23

(Pub.372)

Big Clinic, P.A.   Credit Problem List for Tuesday Apr 17 1984   Report Date 4/17/84   Page 1 ASRF

                         New   Rsrc R.P.
Patient
Account   Patient Name   (X) Time Num. Account   Responsible Party Name   Phone #1   Phone #2   BC FC NE Balance

11898493 SAX,GREGORY J   9:20A 2 80005277 FOLSTROM,HARVEY M   434-6254   10 90 14 1,165.00
14551917 RICHMOND,LUCINDA RAE   9:15A 1 80004692 RICHMOND,LUCINDA R   218-829-0282   19 16   610.00
14645057 FILBIN,THOMAS MICHAEL 8:00A 4 80005231 FILBIN,EDWIN J   473-6999   10 90 23   375.00
14645172 HANSON,VANESSA   9:00A 1 80005157 HANSON,VANESSA   483-1292   54 90 20   587.50

       Total Patients

FIG. 5-24

App. 5–B MANAGING YOUR MEDICAL PRACTICE 5–80

Big Clinic, P.A.　　　　　　New Patients Added on 4/17/84　　　　　　Date 04/17/84　Page 1　ASRD

Patient Name / Account	Appointment Date	Time	Lgth	Visit Type Cd.	Description	Ph. Number Birth Date	Remarks	Num.	Resource Name
BENNETT,BILLIE M.	4/20/84	8:00A	15	V	VISIT	999-9546 12/28/28	SPOT ON LIP	1	Kline MD,James B.
TWEEDY,CARL LEON JR	4/18/84	1:30P	120	N	NEW BACK	987-2536 2/09/54	FITTING FOR BRACE REF: DR. LANGDON	3	Brandt MD,Carl W
LEFORGE,DAWN C	4/18/84	1:00P	30	O	OB CHECKUP	687-3241 2/07/58	6 MONTH	3	Brandt MD,Carl W
WINTERS,CARSON C	5/01/84	8:00A	15	V	VISIT	568-1093 7/13/72	FLU	1	Kline MD,James B.
JANSCO,JODI	4/17/84	12:00P	30	V	VISIT	983-8611 2/17/62	TUMOR REF: DR. GLEASON	6	CT SCAN ROOM 413A
KINLEY,SHERRIE	4/18/84	8:00A	15	V	VISIT	983-8495 10/15/48	SORE THROAT	1	Kline MD,James B.
WEST,LINDA	4/17/84	8:30A	15	V	VISIT	684-2658 3/09/50	RASH ON HANDS	1	Kline MD,James B.

Total Patients   7

FIG. 5-25

(Pub.372)

Big Clinic, P.A.   Chart Pull List for Tuesday   Apr 17 1984   Report Date 4/17/84   Page 1 ASRE

	Patient Name	Account	New (1)	Time	Length	Phone Number	Birth Date	Visit Type	Num.	Resource Name
*	JANSCO,JODI	11898493	X	12:00P	30	983-8611	2/17/62	VISIT	6	CT SCAN ROOM 413A
*	SAL,GREGORY J	13257086		9:20A	20	434-6254	8/20/70	VISIT	2	Traynor MD,Michael S
*	KIBLER,NICOLE	13897196		9:00A	15	757-4315	3/30/71	VISIT	1	Kline MD,James B.
*	RICHTER,LYNN M	14081519		7:00A	30	715-468-2601	5/09/64	VISIT	5	CT SCAN ROOM 413A
*	WEBER,HEATHER D.	14406609		8:30A	45	389-6517	7/24/75	RE-CHECK	4	Brandt MD,John C
*	LANNERS,MARK M	14551917		11:00A	60	1-679-4892	11/26/71	Code - Q	1	Kline MD,James B.
*	RICHMOND,LUCINDA RAE	14645057		9:15A	30	218-829-0282	10/04/76	CONSULT	1	Kline MD,James B.
*	FILBIN,THOMAS MICHAEL	14645172		8:00A	30	473-6999	1/04/77	VISIT	4	Brandt MD,John C
*	HANSON,VANESSA A.			9:00A	15	483-1292	8/30/72	VISIT	1	Kline MD,James B.

Total Appointments   9

FIG. 5-26

(Pub.372)

App. 5-B   MANAGING YOUR MEDICAL PRACTICE

```
Big Clinic, P.A.              Appointments Cancelled by Resource              Date 4/17/84  Page  1  ASRA
===========================================================================================================
                       --- Appointment ----   -- Visit Type --  Ph. Number                     Resource
Patient Name / Account Date    Time    Lgth   Cd. Description   Birth Date   Remarks     Num.  Name
-----------------------------------------------------------------------------------------------------------
<< Unavailable >>      4/23/84 9:00A   180                                   SURGERY - O.R. 110A
                                                                             TONSILECTOMY       1 Kline MD,James B.

<< Unavailable >>      4/23/84 11:30A  120                                   SITE VISIT AT DISC 1 Kline MD,James B.

DORSCHNER,SCOTT        4/17/84 10:40A  20     R  RE-CHECK       829-3607 ARM                    2 Traynor MD,Michael S
14142105                                                        12/16/76

<< Unavailable >>      4/19/84 8:00A   240                                   SURGERY - COLOSTOMY 4 Brandt MD,John C
                                                                             ROOM 912 C UNITED

JONES,JEREMIAH J.      4/17/84 12:00A  60     V  VISIT          123-456-7890                    6 CT SCAN ROOM 413A
                                                                1/01/33

TEST,TEST              4/18/84 12:00P  60     A  ALLERGY SHOT   213-443-4443 AAAAAAAAAAAAAAAAAA 6 CT SCAN ROOM 413A
                                                                1/01/01      BBBBBBBBBBBBBBBBBB

Total Appointments  6
```

FIG. 5-27

(Pub.372)

Big Clinic, P.A.   Appointments Requiring Rescheduling   Date 4/17/84 Page 1 ASRA

		Appointment		Visit Type	Ph. Number		Resource
Patient Name / Account	Date	Time	Lgth	Cd. Description	Birth Date	Remarks	Num. Name
RICCI,NINA DELTREAN 14529251	4/17/84	1:00P	240	A ALLERGY SHOT	774-1810 6/05/81	ALLERGY SKIN TESTS	1 Kline MD,James B.
ROTHLISBERGER,RANDALYN 14209276	5/28/84	8:15A	15	C CONSULT	326-2719 12/25/76		1 Kline MD,James B.
SAHR,MICHAEL 14518510	4/20/84	3:40P	20	V VISIT	632-2201 1/05/79		2 Traynor MD,Michael S
WEBER,HEATHER D. 14081519	5/28/84	10:00A	0	O OB CHECKUP	389-6517 7/24/75		2 Traynor MD,Michael S
KANE,OUY CHANG	6/14/84	8:00A	180	H HISTORY	322-1323 12/30/48	SEVERE ALLERGIES REF: DR. WILSON	2 Traynor MD,Michael S

Total Appointments   5

FIG. 5-28

(Pub.372)

Appendix 5-C

COMPARISON OF SERVICE BUREAUS AND IN-HOUSE COMPUTER SYSTEMS

Facts to Consider

Fact: Service bureau costs are based on the number of active accounts, number of statements produced, number of insurance claims generated and the cost of communication devices/telephone lines.

Result:

- Rising service bureau costs due to the significant increase in prepaid/capitated reimbursement for outpatient physician services. Direct loss of revenue on part of service bureau.

- Loss of revenue means fewer dollars appropriated for research and development and new product development. Loss of revenue = increase in service bureau costs = less service.

Fact: Nationwide, service bureaus have a shrinking base. A recent study conducted by the Minnesota Academy of Family Practitioners Computer Committee indicates a strong shift from service bureaus to "in-house" practice-owned systems. Over 98 percent of new systems planned by current users and 90 percent of those planned by current nonusers will be with their own computers. Only 58 percent of those using service bureaus are satisfied. Most of the dissatisfaction expressed by those using service bureaus is related to cost.

Result:

- Shrinking client base = shrinking revenues.

- Loss of income = increase in service bureau costs.

- Loss of income = less dollars for research and development projects.

- Less research and development = inability to keep pace with ongoing changes in the health care industry.

(Pub.372)

Fact: A major trend in health plan development is in the area of Health Maintenance Organizations (HMOs and PPOs). In the state of Minnesota, over 35 percent of eligible enrollees are covered by an HMO, PPO or IPA health insurance plan. This creates a demand for practices to identify, analyze and monitor the cost of services and emphasizes management information, such as length of stay by procedure/diagnosis, cost of services by diagnosis/doctor, etc.

Result:

- The design of service bureau software is not a true data base. Inability to generate reports given multiple file parameters.
- Inability to produce management reports to monitor cost of services of prepaid health plans.
- Special or custom management report's = cost to clinic to produce with significant time delays.

Fact: Major service bureaus are experiencing a loss of ciients to in-house systems because their existing products cannot meet the data processing needs of today's practicing physician.

Result:

- Service bureaus are seeking or have purchased the marketing rights to sell in-house systems.
- Service bureaus sell products which they have not developed and experience higher costs to the market because of demands on staff to learn, install and train end users.
- Continued loss of revenue because of the one-time infusion of income of in-house sales and continued loss of "bread and butter" income from loss of service bureau clients.

Fact: A service bureau's on-line products experience significant periods of "down time."

Result:

- Loss of productivity and efficiency in the clinic setting = higher operating costs.
- Need to upgrade communications equipment = increased costs to clients or higher internal expenses.

(Pub.372)

- Cost of service bureau products is approximately 30 to 40 percent higher than in-house system.

Fact: A service bureau cannot provide solutions for other data processing applications for the clinic (payroll general ledger, accounts receivable, word processing, etc.).

Result:
- Loss of clients to in-house computer systems.
- Clinic's inability to control cost in areas which can easily be automated with an in-house system.
- Clinic must purchase dedicated in-house systems to meet this need, which results in lack of consistency in data processing area and increase in operating costs.

Fact: As practice productivity increases (new business, HMO contracts, mergers) cost of service bureau proportionately increases.

Result:
- Larger practices are forced to underwrite costs of smaller practices because of fixed cost of service bureau.
- The practice is unable to control costs of data processing.

Fact: Service bureaus approach marketing by promoting elimination of tasks associated with in-house system.

Result:
- Any expenses involved are built into their cost.
- Most in-house systems offer mail room services.
- Cost to produce insurance claims statements is higher than in-house systems.
- In-house system's ability to "hold" statements, produce special orders by account type, generate reports for credit balance statements, etc. = reduced forms and handling costs.

(Pub.372)

Appendix 5-D

GLOSSARY OF BASIC COMPUTER TERMINOLOGY

(Pub.372)

GLOSSARY OF COMPUTER TERMS

ACCESS TIME

The amount of time it takes for the system to retrieve requested data. It is measured from the time data is requested to the time the data is displayed.

APPLICATION

The procedure or problem to which a computer is applied. Common applications include payroll, general ledger, accounts receivable, and budgeting.

APPLICATION SOFTWARE

A computer program or set of programs that tells a computer how to perform a function or manipulate the data into the desired configuration.

AUXILIARY STORAGE

A storage device is an addition to the "core" or main storage of the computer. Auxiliary storage is the permanent storage for information. It includes magnetic tapes, cassette tapes, cartridge tapes, hard disks, diskettes. Auxiliary storage can't be accessed as fast as main storage.

BACKUP

Duplicate data files, equipment, or procedures used in the event of failure of a component or storage media.

BASIC

Beginner's All-purpose Symbolic Instruction Code. An easy-to-learn high level language used most frequently with mini-computers. Originally it was developed as an algebraic time-sharing language. More recently a number of mini-computer manufacturers have extended the limits of BASIC so that it can be used for mini-computer business applications.

BATCH PROCESSING

An approach to computer processing in which groups of like transactions or programs are accumulated (batched) to be processed at the same time.

FIG. 5-29

(Pub.372)

BIT

The common abbreviation for binary digit (0 or 1). A number of bits together are used to represent a character to the computer.

BOOT

Start-up of computer operation by loading the initial computer programs. This is typically done by pressing a particular key.

BRIDGING

The process whereby an operator can go from function to function withou having to go back to the various individual program menus. Bridging can be accomplished by:

(1) Using the assigned Programmable Function keys.

(2) Using the "ESC" escape key and typing the desired function code.

BUG

A mistake in the design or makeup of a computer system or program.

BYTE

A group of bits or binary digits processed as a unit. In most computers a byte equals eight bits and can represent one alphabetic character or two digits.

CENTRAL PROCESSOR

The hardware component that combines the operating system instructions, program instructions, and required data in one central location so that the computer can manipulate the data into the desired configurations.

CHARACTER

One of a set of symbols which express information. Letters, numbers, or other symbols commonly found on a keyboard.

FIG. 5-30

CHARACTER PRINTER

A device attached to the computer that prints much like a typewriter. It prints one character at a time. Its speed is measured in characters per second (CPS).

CHIP

A chip is commonly used to mean an integrated circuit (IC) on a silicon chip A computer is usually made up of several ICs or chips.

COBOL

Common Business Oriented Language. A high-level procedural computer language used for business programming.

CODE or CODING

Common terms used to mean writing a computer program. These may also refer to the program itself.

COMPILER

A program that translates a high level computer language into codes understood by the machine.

COMPUTER

A device which rapidly handles data for future retrieval and manipulation.

CONFIGURATION

A term used by computer people in referring to the equipment that will be assembled to work as a unit for a business. It includes the options chosen a well as peripheral devices.

CONSOLE

A CRT or teletypewriter used to control and monitor computer operations.

CONTROLLER

A device used to manage peripheral devices such as CRTs, printers, disk drives, or tape drives.

FIG. 5-31

CONTROLLER CABLE

A Multicolor ribbon cable connecting the disk drive to the computer.

COPY

To duplicate a diskette.

CORE

A particular type of main computer memory. Another kind is MOS.

CPU

Central Processing Unit. This usually refers to the computer's main memory and the part of the computer that runs a program, called the processor.

CRT

Cathode Ray Tube. A television-like screen used to display data from the computer. With a typewriter keyboard, it is sometimes called a terminal. Often CRT and terminal are used as interchangeable terms.

CURSOR

The blinking position indicator on the CRT.

DASD

Direct Access Storage Device. Examples are: diskette, cartridge disk, and fixed disk drives.

DATA

Information—numeric or other.

DATA BASE

A set of data records that are organized in a logical manner so they can be easily accessed and used.

FIG. 5-32

(Pub.372)

DATA SET

A Data Set refers to either a modem or a file.

DBMS

Data Base Management System. A DBMS is a set of programs for manipulating and using a data base.

DEBUG

The process of finding and correcting errors in computer programs.

DEDICATED LINE

A communication line (the link between a terminal and a computer) that is dedicated from a single point to a single point (point-to-point) as opposed to a dial-up, or switched, line.

DEGRADATION

This slows the response of a computer system in the operator's eyes. This phenomenon is seen when the number of terminals trying to use the system increases beyond the ability of the CPU to respond.

DIAL-UP LINE

A line that is given to a terminal that dials into the computer, as opposed to a dedicated line.

DISK DRIVE

The mechanism within which the disk, storing information used by the computer system, rotates. It is connected to the CPU and contains electronic circuitry that feeds signals from the disk to the computer and back.

DISKETTE

A circular piece of flexible mylar, about the size of a 45 rpm record, coated with magnetic film and encased in a square protective jacket. It is used to store information, such as an Accounts Receivable file, to be used with a computer. Standard sizes are 8" and 5-1/4".

FIG. 5-33

(Pub.372)

DISPLAY SCREEN

Same as CRT. A television-like screen used to display data from the computer.

DP

Data Processing. Use of a computer to process data.

DISTRIBUTED PROCESSING

The use of computers at various locations, each of which is tied to a central computer. This allows preliminary processing to be handled by the "distributed" computers and eases the load on the central computer.

DUMP

Mass copying of memory from a storage device such as a disk to another storage device, or a printer, so that it can be used as a backup or analyzed for errors.

ERROR MESSAGE

A message from the computer telling the operator that the entered information is inaccurate or inappropriate for the field.

EXECUTE

The act of running a computer program.

FIELD

A data item in a record or file. Examples would be a customer number or a telephone number.

FILE

A group of related data records usually arranged in some sequence according to a key in each record. For instance, a Payroll file would contain one record for each employee. It would probably be arranged by the employee number contained in each record.

FILE MAINTENANCE

Updating the file to reflect changes in information. Data might be added, altered, or deleted. File maintenance also refers to reorganizing files, or deleting records in mass storage that are no longer in use, etc.

FIG. 5-34

FIXED DISK

A device in which the disk pack is sealed and cannot be removed. Being sealed, it cannot be exposed to dust and dirt. It can therefore be operated at higher speeds, with greater reliability, than removable units.

FLEXIBLE DISK

Same as diskette.

FLOPPY DISK

Same as diskette.

FLOWCHART

A diagram representing the logical flow of a program or system.

FORMAT

To prepare a new diskette for use by the system. Formatting destroys all data on the diskette. All new diskettes must be formatted before they can be used by the computer.

FORTRAN

FORmula TRANslation. Fortran is a high level language used primarily for coding mathematical or engineering problems for the computer.

HARD COPY

Printing data on a printer instead of displaying it on a CRT.

HARD DISK

A term used to refer to a disk to differentiate it from a diskette. The reference may be to either a cartridge disk or a fixed disk.

HARDWARE

The physical components of the computer system. Examples include the display device or video tube, printer, and data storage unit.

FIG. 5-35

HEAD

A device within a disk drive which picks up electronic information from the diskette, or records information on it.

HEX

Short for hexadecimal. A numbering system based on 16 rather than 10. Most computers operate using hexadecimal numbers.

HIGH LEVEL LANGUAGE

A computer programming language that approaches English in its syntax. Usually easier to learn than a low level language such as assembly language. BASIC, COBOL, and RPG are examples of high level languages.

INITIALIZE

To title, arrange, and prepare a diskette for use or reuse.

INPUT

To write to a computer's memory, or when the computer writes to one of its peripheral devices.

INTERACTIVE

A software program that provides give-and-take between the operator and the machine. The program may ask a question to elicit a response from the operator or present a series of choices from which the operator can select. May also be referred to as "conversational" mode.

KB

Kilobyte. One thousand twenty-four (1024) bytes of information. Commonly used to refer to the memory size of the CPU. A 64KB computer would contain 64 x 1024, or 65,536 bytes of memory in the CPU.

KEYBOARD

An input device usually attached to a CRT or teleprinter. It looks like a typewriter keyboard. The data typed into it using its keys goes into the computer.

FIG. 5-36

KEYSTROKE

A keystroke is a single press of a key on a keyboard. A count or estimate of keystrokes is often used to determine how long a function will take or to price data entry services.

LEASED LINE

Usually synonymous with dedicated line.

LETTER QUALITY PRINTER

A printer which forms whole characters and provides output much like a standard office typewriter in quality. Also known as a correspondence quality printer (CQP).

LINE PRINTER

A printer that composes and prints a whole line at a time. Its speed is measured in lines per minute (LPM).

MACHINE LANGUAGE

The hexadecimal code which the machine has built to be able to interpret programs directly. Compilers and assemblers translate program code into machine language.

MAG TAPE OR MAGNETIC TAPE

A mass storage device which uses reels of magnetic tape similar to the tape used in home tape recorders. Mag tape usually refers to a specific 3/4" reel tape, as opposed to cassette tape.

MAIN FRAME

The computer itself, not including peripherals.

MASS STORAGE DEVICE

A disk, cassette, or mag tape that has the capacity to store a number of records.

FIG. 5-37

(Pub.372)

MASTER FILE

A file that contains the main, permanent information used in a system. Other files are transaction files or files used as temporary work areas.

MATRIX PRINTER

A matrix printer uses a grid of dots, usually 5 by 7. Characters are formed by striking certain dots in the grid.

MB

Megabyte. One million bytes or characters. Commonly used to refer to the amount of information that can be stored on a mass storage device such as a disk or tape. A 10MB disk would hold ten million characters of information.

MEMORY

The capacity to record and maintain units of data in a specific computer system.

MENU

A list of functions within a program.

MICROPROCESSOR

A single miniaturized circuit that contains the complete computer processing logic. The circuit is typically 1/2-inch by 1 inch, or smaller, in several layers.

MINI-FLOPPY

A 5-1/4" diskette.

MODEM

A device attached between a computer and a phone line that translates data into sound, or sound into data, depending on the direction of transmission. MODEM stands for MOdulate-DEModulate.

MODULE

A component which may be added to the computer system, either hardware or software.

FIG. 5-38

MOS

There are currently two kinds of computer memory in use, core and MOS. MOS stands for Metal Oxide Semiconductor. MOS is found in hand calculators. It is cleared when power is turned off. Core retains data even after power is turned off.

MTBF

Mean Time Between Failures. A way of gauging the general reliability of a piece of equipment.

MULTIPROCESSING

A system with two or more computer units that can work together.

MULTIPROGRAMMING

A computer operating system that can handle two or more computer programs at the same time. Actually no two programs are executed at the same time. Their execution is interlaced. Because the computer is so fast, it appears to the user as though more than one program is executing.

OBJECT LANGUAGE

The machine language put out by a program translating system, such as a compiler or assembler.

OBJECT PROGRAM OR OBJECT CODE

A program that has been compiled, or assembled, and is ready to be run. Source language is what you start with before translation.

OEM

Original Equipment Manufacturer. A term commonly used to refer to a computer sales organization that has an arrangement to sell a manufacturer's product. In other industries they would be referred to as dealers or distributors.

OFFLINE

A device that isn't currently attached to the computer is said to be offline. Offline storage is data on disks or tapes where the disk or tape isn't currently mounted on a drive.

FIG. 5-39

ONLINE

The opposite of offline. A device that is currently attached to the computer.

OPERATING SYSTEM

The part of the software which internally manages the computer's activities. It is a set of very complex computer programs, normally supplied by the vendor, that controls, monitors, and executes programs. It can schedule and load programs, produce the computer log, control multi-programming, and route and schedule terminal communications.

OUTPUT

Reading data from a computer's memory or one of its peripheral devices.

PASCAL

A high level programming language, gaining popularity on micro-computer systems and some mini-computers.

PASSWORD

A code word or group of characters which a computer system would require to allow an operator to perform certain functions. An operator's password might allow him to update payroll hours, but not run checks.

PERIPHERAL

A device other than the computer itself used in computer processing. Disk drives, tape drives, CRT's, and printers are peripheral devices.

PINS

Sprockets which control advance of paper through the print cycle within the printer.

POS

Point Of Sale. Capturing data at the time of the original transaction rather than at some later time. Most common uses are in the retail environment.

FIG. 5-40

(Pub.372)

PRINTER

An instrument which produces permanent copy (output) on paper.

PRINTOUT

The product of printer (output).

PROGRAM

A set of computer routines used to solve a problem. The instructions are executed in the order they're written.

PROGRAM BLOCK

A group of programs controlled by the same menu.

PROGRAMMING LANGUAGE

A set of rules and conventions used to prepare the source program for translation by the computer. Each language has its own rules. Examples of programming languages are BASIC, COBOL, and RPG.

RAM

Random Access Memory. The portion of computer memory generally available to execute programs and store data. Memory locations can be both read from, and written to, at high speeds.

RECORD

A set of related data items, such as an employee's name, employee number, marital status, pay rate, date of employment, etc. This record is then one element of a file containing records on each of a company's employees.

RECOVERY

Restoring an error or condition to a previously correct state.

REPORT GENERATOR

A computer program designed to be used with very little training. It is designed to allow the user to retrieve information from files in various report formats.

FIG. 5-41

(Pub.372)

ROM

Read Only Memory. A portion of computer memory where information is permanently stored. This information can be read at high speed, but can never be altered. It is not available to execute programs or to store data.

RPG

Report Program Generator. A programming language used on some small business computers. It is usually considered a high level language.

RUN

To execute a program.

SCREEN

Same as CRT. A television-like screen used to display data from the computer.

SLOT

A groove in the main board, for insertion of program chips.

SOFTWARE

Computer programs including application programs, generators, operating systems, compilers, assemblers, and interpreters.

SORT

Arrange records in order by a key.

SOURCE LANGUAGE

The code a programmer produces in either a high or low level language, before it is translated into object or machine language.

SOURCE PROGRAM OR SOURCE CODE

A program written in source language.

SUB-MENU

A menu within, or called from, another menu.

FIG. 5-42

(Pub.372)

SYMBOLICS

Same as source code. A program written in source language.

SYSTEM

A set of programs, a set of hardware, or a set of programs and hardware, that work together for some specific purpose.

SYSTEM PROMPT

A symbol indicating computer is ready to communicate with you. For example (ENTER).

TELECOMMUNICATIONS

Transmission of data over long distances using phone lines, microwave, etc.

TERMINAL

A device used to enter information into the computer system and/or retrieve information from it. With many systems this would refer to a CRT, but it may also be a printing terminal.

TEXT ENTRY

To type information into the computer keyboard.

TIMESHARING

A method whereby several users can use the same computer at the same time.

TUBE

Same as CRT. A television-like screen used to display data from the computer.

TURNKEY VENDOR

One who provides a complete system including the computer, software, training, and installation.

UPGRADE

Advance, modify, accelerate, or improve hardware, firmware, or software.

FIG. 5-43

VDT

Visual display tube. Same as CRT. A television-like screen used to display data from the computer.

WORK FILE

A temporary computer file used to manipulate data for processing or to assemble data for output. Under normal circumstances, records can be processed more efficiently in a work file than in master data files.

FIG. 5-44

Appendix 5-E

REQUEST FOR PROPOSAL

The documents contained herein have been developed to assist your practice in submitting requests for proposal to purchase a computer system. These documents provide you with a plan to review, evaluate and select a computer system that is most appropriate for your practice. Please note that these documents should be modified at your discretion, given any unique characteristics or circumstances appropriate to note in your request for proposal.

TABLE OF CONTENTS

Section	Page Number
Directions on How to Use This Document	5–104
Questions to Ask Vendor's Existing Clients	5–107
Vendor Evaluation	5–109
Request for Proposal Format	
Cover Letter	5–110
Vendor Proposal Requirements	5–111
Practice Profile	5–113
Vendor Background/Information Questionnaire	5–115
Proposal System Configuration Format	5–117
Software Design Evaluation	5–119
Evaluating the Vendor	5–124
Software Features Evaluation	5–129

DIRECTIONS ON HOW TO USE THIS DOCUMENT

(1) Make a complete copy of the document.

(2) Using the copy, spend the necessary time to fill in the blanks for the following items:

(a) Sample RFP letter

(b) Vendor proposal requirements

(c) Practice profile

(d) Practice objectives

The remaining documents contained herein are for the computer vendors to complete.

(3) After completing the copy of the document, have your secretarial staff type in the answers on the original document.

(4) Compose a list of five to ten computer vendors who specialize in medical computer systems. Please note that your best source of which vendors to select is the recommendations and/or input you receive from your peers in practice and other physicians currently utilizing an in-house computer system. Magazine advertisements, direct mail, yellow pages, and your state and local medical societies are also good sources in helping to make up your computer vendor list.

(5) Mail a copy of the request for proposal, which begins with the sample RFP letter you have completed, to each of the computer vendors on your list. Deter "sales techniques" at this point by suggesting vendors spend more time preparing their RFP.

(6) Based on your original vendor mailing list, you should anticipate receiving no more than three to eight completed RFPs. Vendors who do not respond properly will probably be eliminated at a subsequent date. Once you have received the completed RFPs, documents that would contain the point values assigned to each of the vendors and any additional costs for the categories within each vendor should be collated by your staff. These collated points should then be transferred to the evaluation summary sheet and submitted to your evaluation committee.

(7) Select the three vendors whose RFPs best satisfy your practice, business, software and hardware objectives. The simplest way to choose is to select the three vendors with

(Pub.372)

the highest point accumulations. However, strong consideration should be given to unique circumstances that prevail for each vendor. It is sometimes difficult to assess a point in an evaluation criteria which is subjective and not objective.

(8) Contact the three selected vendors directly by telephone. Inform the other vendors by letter that they have not been selected and provide them with three consolation items:

- Thank them for the time they spent generating the proposal.
- If appropriate, tell them why they were not selected.
- Provide them with the names of the three vendors selected for final evaluation.

(9) Request a reference list of satisfied users from the three vendors selected. Call each vendor's references and let them educate you about what to ask the vendor and what to look for in the demonstration. A sample reference list document that itemizes such questions is provided. It is important that the recommendations you collect be consistent with each of the references.

(10) Set up half-day demonstrations. You will get more out of a demonstration at the vendor's office than at the office of a satisfied user. It is difficult, at times, to visit an existing user's site owing to the time commitment involved in a demonstration and the activities the user needs to complete for a normal workday. Before the demonstration, review the practice requirement statements contained in the RFP to prepare yourself properly for the demonstration. Your basic philosophy should be to have the vendors prove their capabilities and explain how those capabilities can benefit your practice. If necessary, you may want to tour a practice similar to your own, but do so only after the vendor's private demonstration.

(11) Choose the final vendor. The selection should be based upon the point value system, price, demonstration and subjective feelings you have developed for the vendor. Consult the professionals, but follow your instincts. We

(Pub.372)

suggest you involve your accountant, if appropriate, when it comes to the financial considerations of your purchase. In addition, you may want to have your attorney review the vendor's purchase agreement/contract.

(12) Finally, commit the practice to make a decision. Execute the necessary documents and get on with implementing your decision. Do not procrastinate. Give the vendor you choose all your support and the enthusiastic backing the vendor needs to be successful with your conversion and installation. We suggest that once the contract is executed you schedule a meeting with the vendor to begin developing a timetable for implementing your decision. It is in your best interests to begin working with your vendor as soon as possible.

We wish you the best of success.

QUESTIONS TO ASK VENDOR'S CLIENTS

(1) How long has the system been installed in your practice?

(2) What was/were the key factor(s) that lead you to purchase the system you have, instead of another vendor's system?

(3) What was your previous accounts receivable system?

(4) Was the conversion to computer handled efficiently and accurately?

(5) What was the timetable for installation/conversion?

(6) Was installation/conversion on schedule?

(7) Was the training of your staff thorough?

(8) Is additional/ongoing training/assistance readily available?

(9) How often has your system been "down" and is service/repair handled on a timely basis?

(10) What is the service response time?

(11) Do you feel the system recommended for your practice was sized adequately or is it too small/too large to meet your present/future needs?

(Pub.372)

(12) Does the software have all the capabilities to meet your needs?

(13) Is there good documentation?

(14) If you had it to do over again, would you purchase the same system? If not, why not?

COMPUTERS IN HEALTH CARE App. 5–E

VENDOR EVALUATION

EVALUATION CRITERIA	MAXIMUM POINTS	VENDOR #1 POINTS	VENDOR #1 CAPITAL EXPENSE	VENDOR #1 ADDITIONAL EXPENSE	VENDOR #2 POINTS	VENDOR #2 CAPITAL EXPENSE	VENDOR #2 ADDITIONAL EXPENSE	VENDOR #3 POINTS	VENDOR #3 CAPITAL EXPENSE	VENDOR #3 ADDITIONAL EXPENSE
Software Design Yes = 1 point No = -1 point	26		N/A	N/A		N/A	N/A		N/A	N/A
Evaluating the Vendor Yes = 1 point No = -1 point	25		N/A	N/A		N/A	N/A		N/A	N/A
Software Features Evaluation:										
• Clinic Master Files	70		N/A						N/A	
• Billing	145		N/A			N/A			N/A	
• Patient/Guarantor Maintenance	95		N/A			N/A			N/A	
• Insurance	110		N/A			N/A				
• Management Reports	75		N/A			N/A			N/A	
• Referring Doctor	55		N/A			N/A				
• Collection Management	105		N/A			N/A			N/A	
• System Utilities	100		N/A			N/A			N/A	
• System Print	65		N/A			N/A			N/A	
• Telecommunications	35		N/A			N/A				
Proposed System Configuration										
• Total Hardware Cost				N/A			N/A			N/A
• Total Software Cost				N/A			N/A			N/A
• Total Training Cost				N/A			N/A			N/A
• Total Monthly Software Maintenance				N/A			N/A			N/A
• Total Monthly Hardware Maintenance				N/A			N/A			N/A
TOTALS										
VENDOR RANKING										

FIG. 5-45

(Pub.372)

NOTE: Mail everything from here to the back of this document to the vendors.

CLINIC LETTERHEAD

Date

Vendor Name

Vendor Address

Subject: Request for Proposal

Enclosed you will find a Request for Proposal (RFP) which our organization has developed to begin the selection process of purchasing a computer system for our practice. We would appreciate it if your firm would review and submit a completed proposal to our organization for the selection committee to review. All proposals must be postmarked or received by _____.

It is our intention to select a computer system which meets not only our current needs as specified in the RFP, but which also meets the growth and applications software that we feel might be appropriate to add in the future. We would like to begin implementation of our computer system as soon as good business judgment permits. We will be pleased to answer any of your questions concerning the applications requirements, statistical volumes as it relates to our practice, hardware capabilities and other issues related to the purchase of an in-house computer system which may not be covered in this RFP. Please note that we would appreciate you not attempt to preempt the selection process outlined in this RFP. It is our goal to avoid formal sales presentations until our selection committee has had the opportunity to review each RFP and subsequently select vendors whose computer systems we would like to see demonstrated. If you have any questions, please address them to _____, our Evaluation Director.

We anticipate three vendors will be chosen for closer examination based on the information obtained in the RFPs. Each of the vendors will have an opportunity to demonstrate the system capabilities and open negotiations to install their computer system in our practice. Final vendor selection will be made between _____ and _____.
Again, we anticipate an immediate implementation after the selection has occurred.

(Pub.372)

Respectfullly submitted,

(Signature)
Name
Title

VENDOR PROPOSAL REQUIREMENTS

All proposals must be received or postmarked no later than _____.

Please mail or deliver the proposal, along with any supporting documentation, to the attention of _____ at the following address:

(Signature)
Name
Title
Name of Evaluation Director
Clinic/Practice Name
Address
City, State, Zip Code

Your proposal should contain the following:

(1) The completed Vendor Background/Information Questionnaire, which provides an opportunity to describe your company and any unique characteristics that should be considered in our evaluation process. Please attach any supporting documentation or literature which you feel is appropriate by referencing an exhibit number.

(a) Discuss years of service and types of experiences within the ambulatory/clinical health care field.

(b) Provide the actual number of existing installations and a breakdown of the specialty type of those users.

(c) Project your growth for the next twelve-month period.

(Pub.372)

(d) Describe unique or significant ambulatory health care relationships or experiences of your organization.

(2) The enclosed System Proposal. Detail the following components of your recommended hardware and software configuration, pricing each item separately whenever possible. In addition, please identify the hardware and software maintenance costs (monthly and/or annual) for each component.

(3) Answers to all questions detailed in the sections of this RFP.

   (a) Evaluating the Software Design

   (b) Evaluating the Vendor

   (c) Software Features Matrix

(4) A list of users, with telephone numbers and initial contact persons who might serve as a reference or provide a demonstration site. Please identify users who have had the system installed for at least 24 months and three to five users for less than six months.

(5) A copy of your standard contract and related maintenance agreements for the system you are recommending.

We acknowledge the effort and time required to prepare the information outlined above is not insignificant. Please note that strong consideration will be given to the quality of your work in completing this RFP.

Dates pertinent to this RFP are as follows:

   RFP release date: _____

   RFP submission date: _____

   Selection of final vendors: _____

   Vendor presentations scheduled _____ to _____

   Site visits: To be scheduled

   Final selection: _____

   Estimate of start date: _____

Again, we appreciate your time and energy and look forward to reviewing your completed RFP.

(Pub.372)

PRACTICE PROFILE

Practice Profile:

Current Method of Managing Accounts Receivable:

General Statistical Information:
    (1) Number of F.T.E. doctors _____
    (2) Number of office locations _____
    (3) Average number work days per month _____
    (4) Average number patients seen per day _____
    (5) Average number new patients per day _____
    (6) Average number services rendered per patient encounter _____
    (7) Average number active accounts per month _____
    (8) Average number statements sent per month _____
    (9) Average number insurance claims processed per month _____
    (10) Estimate of current patient population _____
    (11) Number months on-line patient transaction history desired _____
    (12) Total number nonmedical personnel:
        (a) Office managers/department heads _____
        (b) Receptionists _____
        (c) Bookkeepers _____
        (d) Insurance clerks _____
        (e) Collection clerks _____
        (f) Medical transcriptionists _____
        (g) Miscellaneous: _____
    (13) Estimated number terminals/work stations _____

Data Processing Objectives:

  To properly address our data processing needs, we have given priority to some of our objectives in purchasing an in-house system for our practice.

(Pub.372)

App. 5-E MANAGING YOUR MEDICAL PRACTICE

(1) Improve credit/collection capability _____

(2) Reduce outstanding accounts receivable and increase cash flow _____

(3) Improve overall office efficiency _____

(4) Stabilize or reduce overhead expenses _____

(5) Immediate access to management information _____

(6) Increase office productivity _____

(7) Facilitate decision making with comprehensive management reporting _____

(8) Prepare and initiate marketing activities _____

(9) Conduct research _____

(10) Provide tighter monetary and management controls _____

(11) Others: _____

Software Objectives:

We would like each vendor's proposal to contain quotations on the following software programs. In addition, we have given priority to our software objectives as they relate to current versus future implementation.

Current Future
- (1) Medical Management System Matrix (per Software Features)
- (2) General Ledger
- (3) Accounts Payable
- (4) Payroll
- (5) Patient Recall
- (6) Appointment Scheduling
- (7) Continuing Medical Education Reporting
- (8) Inventory

(Pub.372)

(9) Fixed Asset Accounting

(10) Amortization Schedules

(11) Word Processing (Multiuser)

(12) AMA NET

(13) Financial Modeling/Budgeting

VENDOR BACKGROUND/INFORMATION QUESTIONNAIRE

Directions:

Please respond to the following items. If appropriate, attach supplemental documentation/literature.

(1) Provide a brief overview of your company (date company founded, philosophy, etc.).

(2) Describe any unique characteristics that should be considered in the evaluation process, especially significant ambulatory health care experiences or relationships that contribute to your company.

(3) Briefly describe your twelve-month marketing objectives.

(4) With regard to your company's research and development activities, provide a list of development projects currently in process and future research and development activities. What is your company's organizational/philosophical approach to research and development? Estimated research and development budget?

(5) Describe your organizational approach to the following company products and services:

  (a) Customer Service.

  (b) Education and Training:

    (i) Initial training:

    (ii) Ongoing training:

  (c) Hardware Maintenance.

  (d) Software Maintenance.

(6) Complete the following items as they relate to your company's organization/human resources:

(Pub.372)

(a) Total number of employees _____

(b) Total number customer service representatives _____

(c) Total number software programmers _____

   (i) Research and development programmers _____

   (ii) Maintenance programmers _____

(d) Total number conversion/installation staff _____

(e) Total number management/administrative staff _____

(f) Total number hardware technicians _____

(g) Total number marketing/sales _____

(h) Total number current installations _____

(i) Total number of medical specialties represented _____

REQUESTED FORMAT FOR PRESENTING SYSTEM CONFIGURATION

Component	Quantity Recommended	Unit Price	Extended Pricing	Maintenance Per Month	Availability
A. Hardware:					
CPU					
Modem					
Work Stations					
Printers					
SUBTOTAL HARDWARE					
B. Software:					
List individually					
SUBTOTAL SOFTWARE					
C. Conversion and Training:					
D. TOTAL SYSTEM COSTS:					

FIG. 5-46

(Pub.372)

App. 5–E MANAGING YOUR MEDICAL PRACTICE 5–118

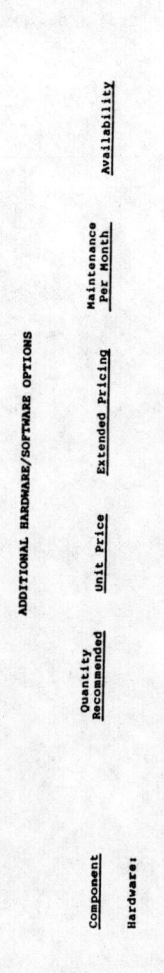

ADDITIONAL HARDWARE/SOFTWARE OPTIONS

Component	Quantity Recommended	Unit Price	Extended Pricing	Maintenance Per Month	Availability
Hardware:					
Software:					

FIG. 5-47

SOFTWARE DESIGN EVALUATION

Directions:

This section contains evaluation criteria as it relates to the generic software design and system capabilities that we feel are important in selecting a software application for our practice. For each item listed, place an "X" in the appropriate "Yes" or "No" column. If you would like to clarify or further describe your response, space is provided on the right hand portion of the document. Space is also provided on the back of each page.

This document will be used during the vendor interview and demonstration portion of the selection process. The design of the software should maximize operator efficiency, reduce labor intensive data processing functions, and optimize the capability of the computer hardware.

(Pub.372)

SOFTWARE DESIGN MATRIX

Page Number: 1

Software Design	Availability Yes / No	Rating Code (Clinic Use Only)	Comments (Continue on reverse if needed)
1. The software is menu and/or function driven versus "prompt/answer" (scrolling).			
2. The software is designed to operate in a "multiuser" and multitasking environment.			
3. The operating system utilized by the computer hardware is recognized by the computer industry as a "mainstream" software product. Please specify name of operating system.			
4. The programming language utilized by the vendor is recognized by the computer industry as a standard and can be easily interpreted and maintained by a third party programming support group. Please specify programming language.			
5. Software applications offered by the vendor can be installed as separate stand alone and/or integrated applications.			
6. Operator "commands" (instructions) are consistent for all software applications.			
7. Software applications proposed by the vendor can be accessed without requiring the operator to understand and access the operating system.			
8. Screen formats (design/layout) are consistent and standardized for all software applications.			

FIG. 5-48

(Pub.372)

COMPUTERS IN HEALTH CARE

SOFTWARE DESIGN MATRIX

Page Number: 2

Software Design	Availability Yes	Availability No	Rating Code (Clinic Use Only)	Comments (Continue on reverse if needed)
9. The software incorporates/utilizes a "full" screen handler to maximize operator efficiency, validation of data entered by field and/or for the entire screen.				
10. Error or required data entry field messages are user friendly and easily identified (i.e., reverse video screen attributes).				
11. A "forms handler" is utilized to manage system output, assign a forms type to facilitate printing, and enable the user to customize system output.				
12. The operator is able to "bridge" or "transfer" between programs and applications without accessing a menu or the operating system.				
13. Software supports video attributes (i.e., color).				
14. Word processing is integrated with the software applications.				
15. Operator is able to access software application menus and functions through a maintenance program or listing.				
16. Software is capable of supporting remote terminals and printers.				

FIG. 5-49

(Pub.372)

SOFTWARE DESIGN MATRIX

Page Number: 3

Software Design	Availability Yes / No	Rating Code (Clinic Use Only)	Comments (Continue on reverse if needed)
17. Personal computers can be integrated as a system work station and/or a stand alone computer.			
18. The software supports "record locking" and "unlocking" during computer processing.			

19. A user definable, multilevel security maintenance program is provided by:
  Operator
  Terminal
  Application program
  Function			

20. The application programs have comprehensive utility programs to enable the user to maintain the system (i.e., backup utilities, purge programs).			
21. User definable master maintenance programs are provided to enable the user to customize program and system files (i.e., service code master file).			
22. All system masters can be changed, added, and deleted.			
23. The software applications can support multiple billing entities on one computer system.			
24. The software applications utilize a reverse "B" tree data base to facilitate I/O transfer of data elements.			

FIG. 5-50

(Pub.372)

COMPUTERS IN HEALTH CARE   App. 5–E

SOFTWARE DESIGN MATRIX

Page Number: 4

Software Design	Availability Yes / No	Rating Code (Clinic Use Only)	Comments (Continue on reverse if needed)
25. The data base file structures are not limited to a maximum size (i.e., patient name/demographic information).			
26. The software should be capable of moving to substantially larger computer equipment without significant reprogramming and costs.			

FIG. 5-51

(Pub.372)

EVALUATING THE VENDOR

Directions:

This section contains the vendor evaluation techniques that will be used to assess the organizational strengths and weaknesses of each vendor. We have prepared a list of specific vendor qualities we feel are important in selecting a company. For each item listed, place an "X" in the appropriate "Yes" or "No" column. If you would like to clarify or further describe your response, space is provided on the right hand portion of the document. Space is also provided on the back of each page.

This document will be utilized during the vendor interview and demonstration portion of the selection process. It is our goal to become familiar with your organization, given the long-term relationship which we hope to enter into with a company.

EVALUATING THE VENDOR MATRIX

Page Number: 1

	Availability		Rating Code (Clinic Use Only)	Comments (Continue on reverse if needed)
	Yes	No		

1. The vendor is dedicated to developing and marketing software applications to the health care community.

2. All of the software applications are designed, developed, and supported by the vendor.

3. The vendor employs experienced medical professionals involved in the installation and training of the computer system.

4. A "turnkey" service is provided by the vendor:
   a. Software applications
   b. Computer hardware
   c. Direct software maintenance and support services
   d. Direct hardware maintenance and support services
   e. Ongoing customer service programs (i.e., telephone support, training programs)

5. Vendor employs full-time in-house programmers for software maintenance and research/development activities.

6. Vendor is actively involved in research and development programming activities.

7. Direct vendor software maintenance and support maintenance agreements are available to the end user providing:
   a. Telephone support services
   b. Ongoing training programs
   c. Guaranteed access and implementation of all software updates and enhancements

FIG. 5-52

(Pub. 372)

App. 5-E   MANAGING YOUR MEDICAL PRACTICE   5-126

EVALUATING THE VENDOR MATRIX

Page Number: 2

	Availability		Rating Code (Clinic Use Only)	Comments (Continue on reverse if needed)
	Yes	No		
8. The vendor offers on-line diagnostic services via a communications modem.				
9. Professionals in clinic management are involved in the development and design of the system.				
10. Personnel involved in the installation, conversion, and training process are experienced professionals in clinic management and data processing.				
11. The vendor has actively been involved in providing computer systems for the health care industry for a minimum of two years.				
12. Software application source is available via the software license agreement.				
13. Comprehensive initial and ongoing education and training services are provided by the vendor.				
14. End user has a vehicle to submit direct feedback regarding software changes and enhancements and new software applications.				
15. 24 hour or next day service guaranteed.				

FIG. 5-53

(Pub.372)

EVALUATING THE VENDOR MATRIX

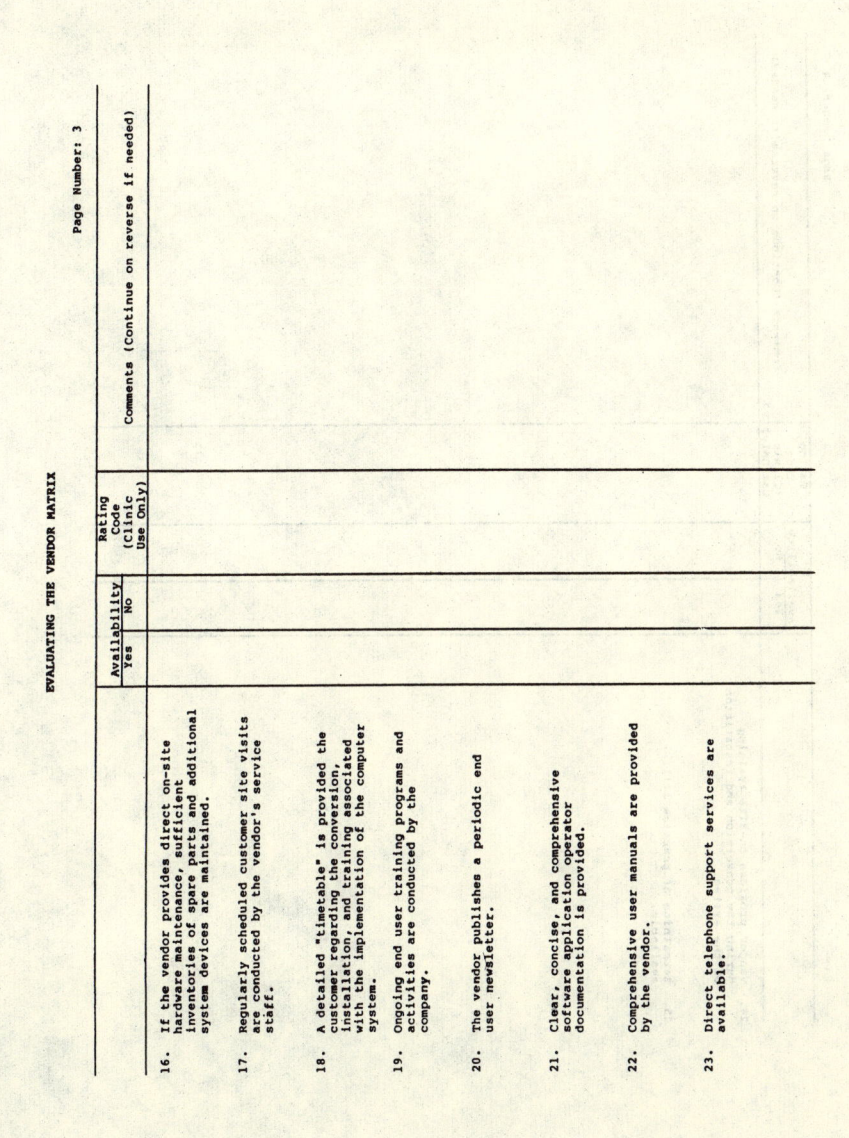

Page Number: 3

	Availability Yes / No	Rating Code (Clinic Use Only)	Comments (Continue on reverse if needed)
16. If the vendor provides direct on-site hardware maintenance, sufficient inventories of spare parts and additional system devices are maintained.			
17. Regularly scheduled customer site visits are conducted by the vendor's service staff.			
18. A detailed "timetable" is provided the customer regarding the conversion, installation, and training associated with the implementation of the computer system.			
19. Ongoing end user training programs and activities are conducted by the company.			
20. The vendor publishes a periodic end user newsletter.			
21. Clear, concise, and comprehensive software application operator documentation is provided.			
22. Comprehensive user manuals are provided by the vendor.			
23. Direct telephone support services are available.			

FIG. 5-54

(Pub.372)

App. 5-E MANAGING YOUR MEDICAL PRACTICE 5-128

EVALUATING THE VENDOR MATRIX

Page Number: 4

	Availability		Rating Code (Clinic Use Only)	Comments (Continue on reverse if needed)
	Yes	No		
24. Vendor provides on-site training during the conversion and installation of the system.				
25. Retraining of practice still available.				

FIG. 5-55

(Pub.372)

SOFTWARE FEATURE EVALUATION

Directions:

This section contains the software evaluation techniques to be used in determining whether the projected software will meet our practice needs. There are three major components: (1) Code Values, (2) Additional Costs and (3) Documentation Reference.

We have prepared a list of requirements and we ask each vendor to evaluate their system capabilities for each item. Vendor evaluations should be entered in each of the three columns (Code Value, Additional Cost and Documentation Reference) for each requirement.

Vendor proposals submitted without a completed vendor evaluation section will be disqualified.

Code Value:

Vendors should read each specific requirement and assign a code value according to their software product capability. We fully anticipate no vendor will be capable of achieving a perfect score (5 points for every requirement). We will be using your point value response not only for our initial evaluation purposes (selection of three vendors), but also in our demonstration and final selection phase. It is in our mutual best interests for you your code value to reflect an accurate accounting of your software capabilities:

- 5 = This feature is currently available and is part of the system outlined in your proposal.
- 4 = This feature is currently available as an option (at an additional cost to the system outlined in your proposal).
- 3 = This capability is not presently available but is currently under development and will be offered as part of our standard system within one year (see Additional Cost).
- 2 = This capability is unavailable today but is under study and will be offered as part of our standard system later (see Additional Cost).
- 1 = This feature is unavailable and we have no plans to offer it in the future. However, we will custom program this for you (see Additional Cost).

(Pub.372)

0 = This feature is unavailable, and we will NOT offer it or custom program it (see Additional Cost).

Additional Cost:

Additional cost may represent the price of optional software, optional hardware, custom programming and all other expense items not specifically covered in your proposal. We fully anticipate optional software and other additional expenses will be incurred. We simply want all items of additional expense (outside the system proposed) identified clearly for "intelligent" evaluation.

If two or more specific requirements can be accommodated with one optional software package, one custom programming task, etc., be sure to enter the additional cost on one requirement line only and bracket or identify those requirement lines that will be satisfied by this single additional expense. Additional cost should represent your "best guess" based on the limited information provided in this Request for Proposal. You may prefer to enter a low-high range of cost estimate. For mutual protection, further discussions will be conducted with the vendor(s) selected so Additional Costs can be precisely identified prior to contract signing.

Documentation Reference Column:

Most medical computer systems are complex, with numerous reports, system capabilities, and features. We strongly suggest you correlate each one of our requirement lines to your appropriate documentation reference and support your capabilities with written or illustrative proof. For instance, reference a page number in your brochure illustrating a completed insurance form. Provide the reader with specific proof that the capabilities exist. We have a special interest in reviewing how your company plans to accomplish or print certain information. Your documentation reference column will greatly assist us in quickly finding and appreciating your abilities and strengths.

You may also use this column to reference any additional notes or comments you care to make on your requirement or your answer. Basically, we request you use this column extensively to guide the reader through your system.

(Pub.372)

SOFTWARE FEATURES MATRIX
MEDICAL MANAGEMENT SYSTEM

Page Number: 1

Clinic Custom Master Files	Code	Additional Cost	Documen-tation Reference	Feature Description (Continue on reverse if needed)
1. Ability to set up the following clinic information: a. Clinic name b. Address, city, state, zip code c. Federal ID number d. Fiscal year e. Business telephone number f. Appointment telephone number				
2. Option to select finance or rebilling charges. In addition, provide user defined parameters to "hold" finance or rebilling charges on specific account types (i.e., insurance only).				
3. Ability to design automatic dunning messages.				
4. Ability to have user define all purge parameters for the following: a. Patient/guarantor demographic files b. Patient transaction files				
5. Allow up to 99 different doctors with the following information for each doctor: a. Doctor name b. Department c. Provider numbers assigned by insurance carriers d. Social Security number e. Board certification number f. Board specialty name g. Miscellaneous information (i.e., date doctor joined practice)				
6. Provide a user defined facility master file to facility-reporting of services by doctor by facility or location where service rendered (i.e., satellite clinics).				

FIG. 5-56

(Pub.372)

App. 5-E MANAGING YOUR MEDICAL PRACTICE 5-132

SOFTWARE FEATURES MATRIX
MEDICAL MANAGEMENT SYSTEM

Page Number: 2

Clinic Custom Master Files	Code	Additional Cost	Documentation Reference	Feature Description (Continue on reverse if needed)
7. User defined service code master file to accommodate up to 99,999 procedures and transaction codes that includes: a. Custom description capability b. Cross-reference capability c. Repricing by service code by location				
8. Ability to establish up to 999 different insurance companies to include the following information: a. Insurance name b. Clinic provider number c. Insurance form type (i.e., HCFA 1500) d. Insurance submitter number for electronic claims submission e. Accept assignment status by insurance carrier f. Cross-reference codes (i.e., service codes, place of service) g. Totals of claims by page or individual claim h. Multiple doctor versus single doctor claim submission requirements				
9. Ability to establish CPT modifier master codes within user defined descriptions.				
10. Provide place of service file which includes the capability to assign multiple cross-reference codes to unique insurance filing requirements.				
11. Enable the practice to define financial classifications for each patient account (i.e., poor credit, bankruptcy).				

FIG. 5-57

(Pub.372)

SOFTWARE FEATURES MATRIX
MEDICAL MANAGEMENT SYSTEM

Page Number: 3

	Code	Additional Cost	Documentation Reference	Feature Description (Continue on reverse if needed)
Clinic Custom Master Files				
12. Provide chart location master file to facilitate chart retrieval (i.e., satellite locations, microfiche). This chart location code can be assigned by operator for each patient.				
13. Ability to establish up to 99,999 ICD-9-CM diagnosis codes with custom descriptions.				
14. Enable the practice to assign up to 100 different adjustment transaction codes.				

FIG. 5-58

(Pub.372)

App. 5–E MANAGING YOUR MEDICAL PRACTICE 5–134

SOFTWARE FEATURES MATRIX
MEDICAL MANAGEMENT SYSTEM

Page Number: 1

Billing	Code	Additional Cost	Documentation Reference	Feature Description (Continue on reverse if needed)
1. Allow the practice to determine the frequency of billing (i.e., daily, monthly, cycles).				

2. Provide automated data entry controls of:
  a. Batch totals
  b. Account/patient edits (i.e., name, address, etc.)
  c. Detailed transaction edits of batch (i.e., date of service procedure code, diagnosis code)				

3. Provide prepricing at the following levels:
  a. Procedure code
  b. Insurance type (i.e., Medicare)
  c. Modifier code
  d. Place of service				

4. Allow practice to change pricing/fee schedule automatically by:
  a. Procedure code
  b. Range of procedures
  c. Percentage rate increase
  d. Fixed amount rate increase
  e. Round prices to nearest dollar				

5. Ability to manually override prepricing at time of charge entry.				
6. Ability to further define charge description on an exception basis.				

FIG. 5-59

(Pub.372)

5-135 COMPUTERS IN HEALTH CARE App. 5-E

SOFTWARE FEATURES MATRIX
MEDICAL MANAGEMENT SYSTEM

Page Number: 2

Billing	Code	Additional Cost	Documen- tation Reference	Feature Description (Continue on reverse if needed)
7. Ability to correct erroneous charge/ payment/adjustment entries nonreflective on patient billing documents and financial reporting.				
8. Provide daily audit trail reports of all financial data entry activity.				
9. Ability to utilize either a superbill, standard statement, or mailer format.				
10. The billing statement format should include the option to print the following items: a. Summarized ageing of the account b. Allow all account transactions, rather than only the detail since the last billing, to be printed each time a statement is produced c. Miscellaneous remarks entered to patient's demographic file d. Secondary insurance company name on superbill format e. Finance/rebilling message f. Number of service description lines				
11. All billing statement formats should include a perforated return tab to facilitate the ease of proper payment and account identification.				
12. Printing of "demand" patient bills and duplication of a previous bill.				

FIG. 5-60

(Pub.372)

SOFTWARE FEATURES MATRIX
MEDICAL MANAGEMENT SYSTEM

Page Number: 3

Billing	Code	Additional Cost	Documentation Reference	Feature Description (Continue on reverse if needed)
13. Ability to issue general messages to patient base on billing statements.				
14. In the statement production process, provide the ability to "hold" and/or batch billing statements based on the following parameters: a. Balances under a user defined amount b. Credit balances c. Zero balances with current charges d. Account number ranges e. Insurance type f. Multiple page billing statements g. Physician h. Financial status/class (i.e., credit holds)				
15. Ability to generate billing statements in alphabetical, account number, or zip code sequence.				
16. Produce a credit balance detail transaction report to facilitate the processing of patient refunds.				
17. Generate patient mailing labels based on clinic designed criteria.				
18. Provide the option to select one of the following billing arrangements: a. Family billing: Ability to link/assign multiple patients to one guarantor b. Nonfamily billing: Ability to assign only one guarantor to one patient				

FIG. 5-61

SOFTWARE FEATURES MATRIX
MEDICAL MANAGEMENT SYSTEM

Page Number: 4

		Code	Additional Cost	Documentation Reference	Feature Description (Continue on reverse if needed)
	Billing				
19.	Any and all accounts should be immediately accessible on-line/real time through any terminal (unless "security" protected).				
20.	Ability to "view" transaction detail by the following parameters: a. Operator defined date of service b. Patient encounter (multiple services per visit)				
21.	Viewing of transaction detail should include the following: a. Charges b. Payments c. Adjustments d. Insurance filing e. Dates of service f. Place of service g. Doctor rendering service h. Service codes i. Diagnosis codes j. Modifier codes k. Batch date/batch number l. Remarks/miscellaneous description m. Patient name				
22.	Provide clear identification of the guarantor and each patient with the accounts receivable display or view function.				
23.	Provide written procedures for maintaining control logs and balancing procedures. The clinic must be able to prove easily that the total system is in balance with itself.				

FIG. 5-62

(Pub.372)

App. 5-E MANAGING YOUR MEDICAL PRACTICE 5-138

SOFTWARE FEATURES MATRIX
MEDICAL MANAGEMENT SYSTEM

Page Number: 5

	Code	Additional Cost	Documentation Reference	Feature Description (Continue on reverse if needed)

Billing

24. Procedures to correct errors in daily transactions.

25. Clear identification of data fields on each audit trail report.

26. Provide a charge ticket/route slip audit trail.

27. Cash drawer balancing routine for payments requested at the time of service.

28. Ability to request/demand print a charge ticket/route slip before the appointment or when the patient arrives.

29. In regard to data entry (i.e., charges, payments) functions provide the following:
   a. Full screen entry and validation of data
   b. Consistency in data entry methods to process transactions
   c. Batch entry method to ensure proper audit trails and maximize operator efficiency
   d. Operator manually assign or allow the system to assign batch numbers
   e. Verification of all batch totals prior to posting (does not allow unbalanced batches to be posted).
   f. Option to select automatic bank deposit slips

FIG. 5-63

(Pub.372)

SOFTWARE FEATURES MATRIX
MEDICAL MANAGEMENT SYSTEM

Page Number: 6

Billing	Code	Additional Cost	Documentation Reference	Feature Description (Continue on reverse if needed)
g. Charge entry procedure should allow operator to enter transactions via a one screen format for each patient or multiple patients per screen				
h. Unlimited number of diagnosis codes assigned to one procedure				
i. Default transactions to the attending or assigned physician				
j. Ability to post transactions immediately or as part of an "end of day" processing function				
k. Ability to enter receipts and adjustments at the same time				
l. Patient name and date of birth verification during data entry				

FIG. 5-64

(Pub.372)

App. 5-E   MANAGING YOUR MEDICAL PRACTICE   5-140

SOFTWARE FEATURES MATRIX
MEDICAL MANAGEMENT SYSTEM

Page Number: 1

Patient/Responsible Party (Guarantor) Registration and Maintenance	Code	Additional Cost	Documentation Reference	Feature Description (Continue on reverse if needed)

1. Ability to allow the following user defined fields in the patient/guarantor files:
   a. Patient name
   b. Patient registration date
   c. Patient birth date
   d. Calculate age of patient
   e. Patient's sex
   f. Social Security number
   g. Patient employer
   h. Patient address
   i. Patient insurance information
      i. Primary insurance
      ii. Secondary insurance
      iii. Subscriber's name
      iv. Relationship to subscriber
      v. Group/contract numbers
      vi. Accept assignment option
   j. Billing type code (i.e., no finance charges
   k. Financial class (credit status)
   l. Responsible party/guarantor name
   m. Responsible party/guarantor address
   n. Telephone numbers (home/work)
   o. Chart location
   p. Miscellaneous information lines
   q. Referring physician code/identification

2. Ability to allow the following supplemental user defined fields in the patient/guarantor files:
   a. Guarantor employer name
   b. Guarantor employer address
   c. Patient next of kin
   d. Next of kin relationship
   e. Next of kin telephone number
   f. Next of kin address
   g. Miscellaneous informtaion (i.e., health history)

FIG. 5-65

(Pub.372)

SOFTWARE FEATURES MATRIX
MEDICAL MANAGEMENT SYSTEM

Page Number: 2

Patient/Responsible Party (Guarantor) Registration and Maintenance	Code	Additional Cost	Documentation Reference	Feature Description (Continue on reverse if needed)
3. Provide a function to allow an operator to locate a patient and/or guarantor name, alphabetically or by account number. This function must provide the following: a. "Scroll" or page forward or backward through the data base b. Ability to bridge or transfer data to other demographic file programs				
4. Patient and guarantor files must be able to be manually or automatically flagged for credit reasons.				
5. On-line/real time access to demographic files. Ability to add new records or update existing records utilizing one function, one screen. a. Identification of duplicate patient names during new patient entry				
6. Ability to generate a registration form/ face sheet for the patient's medical record based on user defined fields selected from the demographic files.				
7. Provide the ability to view all patients associated with a guarantor. This should display the guarantor's billing information.				
8. Describe the method of how patients and guarantors are linked or associated for family billing.				

FIG. 5-66

(Pub.372)

App. 5-E MANAGING YOUR MEDICAL PRACTICE

SOFTWARE FEATURES MATRIX
MEDICAL MANAGEMENT SYSTEM

Page Number: 3

Patient/Responsible Party (Guarantor) Registration and Maintenance	Code	Additional Cost	Documentation Reference	Feature Description (Continue on reverse if needed)
9. Ability to review billing information (i.e., balance due, services) on-line for a specified time period or default to most current transactions. This billing information should include: a. Ageing status b. Current balance c. Key billing information d. Last payment e. Last payment date f. Amount of last payment g. Payment type h. Detailed itemization of all transactions posted to the account i. Ability to scroll or page forward/backward through the patient's transaction file				
10. Allow the production of chart labels at the time of new patient registration.				
11. Provide automatic or manual assignment of account numbers.				
12. Produce a custom charge ticket on a demand or batch basis independent of an appointment scheduling system.				
13. Should the practice elect to establish/set up an additional billing entity, provide the ability to transfer patient/guarantor files to the other billing entity without reentering the information.				

FIG. 5-67

(Pub.372)

5-143 COMPUTERS IN HEALTH CARE App. 5-E

SOFTWARE FEATURES MATRIX
MEDICAL MANAGEMENT SYSTEM

Page Number: 4

Patient/Responsible Party (Guarantor) Registration and Maintenance	Code	Additional Cost	Documen- tation Reference	Feature Description (Continue on reverse if needed)
14. Provide a user defined program to purge demographic information with a zero balance and no activity from the system or be designated as an inactive file (compacted file) which is available to be reactivated.				
15. Provide system security by function to prevent designated personnel from adding/changing demographic information.				
16. Ability to utilize a program or report writer/generator to develop and analyze demographic file information separately or in conjunction with the transaction files.				
17. Provide verification messages to the operator regarding "required fields," "updated accounts," etc.				
18. Produce "rolodex" cross-reference cards for new patients.				
19. Generate a chart pulling list by doctor.				

FIG. 5-68

(Pub.372)

App. 5–E MANAGING YOUR MEDICAL PRACTICE 5–144

SOFTWARE FEATURES MATRIX
MEDICAL MANAGEMENT SYSTEM

Page Number: 1

Code	Additional Cost	Documen- tation Reference	Feature Description (Continue on reverse if needed)

Insurance

1. Allow the assignment of all insurance information to the patient record or file versus the responsible party.

2. Enable the clinic to assign a minimum of two (2) insurance carriers per patient record.

3. Ability to automatically generate more than one claim per patient in order to coordinate the benefits between major third party carriers.

4. Assign a priority status to automatic insurance in order to identify primary versus secondary carrier.

5. Provide user definable frequency of processing for automatic insurance (i.e., daily, weekly, monthly).

6. Ability to assign up to 999 insurance carriers for automatic claims processing.

7. Ability to print demand insurance claim forms.

8. Ability to print demand itemized bills.

FIG. 5-69

(Pub.372)

FIG. 5-70

SOFTWARE FEATURES MATRIX
MEDICAL MANAGEMENT SYSTEM

Page Number: 2

Insurance	Code	Additional Cost	Documentation Reference	Feature Description (Continue on reverse if needed)
9. Enable the operator to enter insurance and bill requests via a batch mode to facilitate data entry and efficiency.				
10. Resubmit any insurance claim previously generated.				
11. Provide automatic and request insurance audit trail reports.				

12. Provide a custom insurance master program to include the following:
  a. Selection of cross-referenced service, diagnosis, modifier, and place of service codes to print on an insurance carrier's forms unique to that insurance carrier
  b. Generate claims by individual doctor or multiple doctors on a per claim basis
  c. Insurance claim totals by page or total claim (multiple pages)
  d. Ability to selectively accept assignment by insurance carrier (i.e., Medicare) for all patients				

13. Provide an "insurance forms generator" software package to eliminate "costly" revisions to insurance claim processing requirements set by the insurance carrier.				

14. Generate an "insurance transaction" which can be viewed to the patient's file documenting:
  a. Date claim was processed
  b. Insurance carrier
  c. Inclusive service dates
  d. Total amount of claim				

(Pub.372)

App. 5-E MANAGING YOUR MEDICAL PRACTICE 5-146

SOFTWARE FEATURES MATRIX
MEDICAL MANAGEMENT SYSTEM

Page Number: 3

		Code	Additional Cost	Documentation Reference	Feature Description (Continue on reverse if needed)
	Insurance				
15.	Ability to demand an insurance claim or itemized bill at the time of service.				
16.	Ability to enter "prior authorization" numbers received from the insurance carrier to allow it to print on the claim form.				
17.	Provide the ability to enter the following items to enable it to print on the insurance claim form by patient encounter: a. Date of illness b. Date of injury c. Admit/discharge dates d. LMP date e. Accept assignment by encounter f. Facility where services were rendered				
18.	Provide the option to utilize a "units" field in charge entry to process multiple visits (i.e., hospital visits, injections) for insurance carriers. System calculates beginning and ending date of service.				
19.	Ability to transmit insurance claims via magnetic media or telecommunications to major third party carriers. a. Nine track tape option b. Eight inch diskette option c. Telecommunications (1200 Baud modem)				
20.	Provide detailed aged accounts receivable figures by insurance carrier (horizontal presentation of ageing categories).				

FIG. 5-71

(Pub.372)

SOFTWARE FEATURES MATRIX
MEDICAL MANAGEMENT SYSTEM

Page Number: 4

Insurance	Code	Additional Cost	Documen-tation Reference	Feature Description (Continue on reverse if needed)
21. Provide accounts receivable summary by insurance carrier on a daily, month to date, and year to date basis: 　a. Total gross charges (+) 　b. Discounts (-) 　c. Net charges (+) 　d. Adjustments (+, -) 　e. Net receipts (-)				
22. Insurance field messages automatically generated on a patient's statement.				

FIG. 5-72

(Pub.372)

SOFTWARE FEATURES MATRIX
MEDICAL MANAGEMENT SYSTEM

Page Number: 1

Management Reports	Code	Additional Cost	Documentation Reference	Feature Description (Continue on reverse if needed)

1. Provide production reports with monthly, year to date and prior year to date figures for the following:
   a. Clinic/practice
   b. Physician
   c. Procedure
   d. Facility (location of services rendered)

2. Provide daily, month to date, and year to date accounts receivable figures for the clinic and payor type to include:
   a. Beginning A/R balance
   b. Gross charges
   c. Total discounts
   d. Total receipts
   e. Total refunds/returned checks
   f. Total miscellaneous debits
   g. Total miscellaneous credits
   h. Actual net change in A/R

3. Generate a "trended" monthly accounts receivable summary report based on the practice's fiscal year to include:
   a. Beginning of the month A/R balance
   b. Net charges (+)
   c. Net receipts (−)
   d. Net adjustments (+, −)
   e. End of month A/R balance
   f. Monthly collection percentage
   g. Year to date collection percentage
   h. Accounts receivable ratio

4. Provide a "trended" monthly physician production report based on the practice's fiscal year to include:
   a. Gross charges
   b. Discounts (−)
   c. Net charges (+)
   d. Miscellaneous debits (+)
   e. Miscellaneous credits (−)
   f. Total receipts (−)

FIG. 5-73

(Pub.372)

SOFTWARE FEATURES MATRIX
MEDICAL MANAGEMENT SYSTEM

Page Number: 2

Management Reports	Code	Additional Cost	Documentation Reference	Feature Description (Continue on reverse if needed)
5. Provide statistical reports for patient office visits, hospital services, procedures, etc., to include monthly, year to date, and prior year to date figures.				
6. Provide diagnosis (ICD-9-CM) and/or CPT frequency report for a user requested period of time by the following: a. Clinic b. Attending physician c. Facility d. Insurance type e. Billing type				
7. Provide report writer/generator capabilities for all data files and integrate with word processing. This feature should also be able to produce the following: a. Listing by patient b. Mailing labels c. Generate a MailMerge file				
8. Produce collection statistics monthly, year to date, prior year to date, and collection ratio.				
9. Generate a daily transaction audit report of all transactions posted to the system. This report should list the day's transactions by either type (i.e., total charges) or batch number.				
10. Provide a monthly batch summary to list all posted and open batches that have been entered into the system for the previous month.				
11. Produce a credit balance report to facilitate researching patient refunds and eliminate unnecessary production of patient bills.				

FIG. 5-74

(Pub. 372)

SOFTWARE FEATURES MATRIX
MEDICAL MANAGEMENT SYSTEM

Page Number: 3

	Code	Additional Cost	Documentation Reference	Feature Description (Continue on reverse if needed)
Management Reports				
12.				Generate user defined A/R ageing reports to enable the practice to analyze the A/R by insurance type, billing type, etc. The presentation of these reports should be horizontal for the following ageing categories: Current, 31-60 days, 61-90 days, 91-120 days, 121-150 days, 151+ days.
13.				Ability to "view" management reports via the terminal rather than printing the report.
14.				Provide the capability to monitor patient accounts which have been referred to a professional collection agency.
15.				Ability to analyze payments, discounts, miscellaneous credits and debits by type (i.e., cash versus insurance payments) for each month and on a year to date basis.

FIG. 5-75

COMPUTERS IN HEALTH CARE

SOFTWARE FEATURES MATRIX
MEDICAL MANAGEMENT SYSTEM

Page Number: 1

Referring Doctor	Code	Additional Cost	Documentation Reference	Feature Description (Continue on reverse if needed)

1. Ability to establish a data base of referring physicians to include the following:
  a. Referring physician name
  b. Practice name
  c. Address
  d. Telephone number
  e. Specialty type
  f. Location assignment (i.e., ABC Clinic, professional building)				

2. Allow each referring physician to be assigned to a "location code/identifier" which is user defined.
  a. Name and location
  b. Address
  c. Miscellaneous information				

3. Provide the operator the ability to search the referring physician data base alphabetically to obtain specific information (i.e., telephone number).				
4. Generate a management report showing comparative data on each referring physician's referrals for the month, preceding year's average, year to date, and monthly average totals.				
5. Generate a management report based on the parameters listed in item 4 above, except by location code/identifier.				
6. Generate a management report to analyze referring physicians grouped by location.				

FIG. 5-76

(Pub.372)

App. 5-E   MANAGING YOUR MEDICAL PRACTICE   5–152

SOFTWARE FEATURES MATRIX
MEDICAL MANAGEMENT SYSTEM

Page Number: 2

Referring Doctor	Code	Additional Cost	Documentation Reference	Feature Description (Continue on reverse if needed)
7. Ability to "view" the referring physician and location summary data via the terminal rather than printing the report.				
8. Ability to integrate the referring physician data base with word processing (i.e., MailMerge list).				
9. Generate referring physician mailing labels and/or custom letters.				
10. Ability to analyze patient referrals by the following: a. ICD-9-CM diagnosis codes b. CPT codes c. Insurance type d. Location e. Patient's sex f. Attending physician g. Service date h. Place of service				
11. Ability to analyze patient referrals by referring physician specialty.				

FIG. 5-77

(Pub.372)

SOFTWARE FEATURES MATRIX
MEDICAL MANAGEMENT SYSTEM

Page Number: 1

Collection Management	Code	Additional Cost	Documen- tation Reference	Feature Description (Continue on reverse if needed)
1. Calculate month to date and year to date collection percentage utilizing net receipts and net charges				
2. Calculate accounts receivable ratio.				
3. Automatic and manual user defined notes and dunning messages on statements.				
4. Automatic and manual collection letters integrated with word processing.				
5. Ability to alter automatic collection dunning message and letters on an individual-account basis.				
6. Ability to record and view on-line patient account representative collection notes.				

FIG. 5-78

App. 5–E MANAGING YOUR MEDICAL PRACTICE 5–154

SOFTWARE FEATURES MATRIX
MEDICAL MANAGEMENT SYSTEM

Page Number: 2

Collection Management	Code	Additional Cost	Documentation Reference	Feature Description (Continue on reverse if needed)

7. Capability to generate a custom collection letter for a specific group of patients by one or more of the following parameters:
   a. Patient account numbers
   b. Account balance (i.e., all balances over $100.00)
   c. Insurance type
   d. Ageing category
   e. Bill type (i.e., accept insurance only)
   f. Dunning message type
   g. Terms				

8. Capability to generate mailing labels as defined above.				
9. Capability to generate a patient listing as defined above.				

10. Ability to generate a collection letter transaction to the patient's file which can be viewed indicating the following:
   a. Collection letter type
   b. Date letter was generated
   c. Current balance				

11. Ability to monitor "terms" arrangements made with the clinic for:
   a. Amount of payment meets conditions
   b. Payment date
   c. Ability to suppress automatic collection letter if terms and conditions are met
   d. Generate collection terms detail report listing the account number, terms, current balance, and terms status
   e. Generate collection terms summary report listing statistics related to number of accounts meeting or failing to meet the terms conditions				

FIG. 5-79

(Pub.372)

SOFTWARE FEATURES MATRIX
MEDICAL MANAGEMENT SYSTEM

Page Number: 3

Collection Management	Code	Additional Cost	Documen-tation Reference	Feature Description (Continue on reverse if needed)
12. Report generation of patient account representative's monthly activity and results.				
13. Ability to track collection agency performance.				
14. Monitor payments made on accounts placed with a professional collection agency.				
15. Provide capability to suppress automatic collection letters on specific types of patient accounts (i.e., medical assistance).				
16. Ability to assess a rebilling or finance charge based on ageing criteria (user defined).				
17. Ability to suppress rebilling or finance charges on specific types of patient accounts (i.e., insurance only, HMO accounts).				
18. Ability to initiate an automatic or manual "credit flag" on patient accounts which can be displayed and viewed on patient demographic files.				
19. Ability to generate a hard copy detailed report by patient summarizing all collection activity.				

FIG. 5-80

(Pub.372)

App. 5–E　　MANAGING YOUR MEDICAL PRACTICE　　5–156

SOFTWARE FEATURES MATRIX
MEDICAL MANAGEMENT SYSTEM

Page Number: 4

Collection Management	Code	Additional Cost	Documentation Reference	Feature Description (Continue on reverse if needed)
20. Provide a "collection document" (i.e., card) which can be produced and utilized in addition to or in lieu of real time/on-line collector's notes.				
21. Generate ageing reports by billing type, insurance, etc. in a horizontal format utilizing the following ageing categories: 0-30 days, 31-60 days, 61-90 days, 91-120 days, 121-150 days, and 151+ days. This report should display the following information: a. Patient name b. Responsible party/guarantor name c. Address d. Telephone number e. Age analysis f. Last payment date g. Last payment amount h. Insurance type i. Billing classification				

FIG. 5-81

(Pub.372)

SOFTWARE FEATURES MATRIX
MEDICAL MANAGEMENT SYSTEM

Page Number: 1

System Utilities and Maintenance Programs	Code	Additional Cost	Documentation Reference	Feature Description (Continue on reverse if needed)
1. Ability to "partition" the hard disk drive to allow segregation of application program files (i.e., word processing files).				
2. User definable program to allow the operator to dedicate terminal function keys to a specific application and/or functions to increase operator efficiency by reducing keystrokes.				
3. Ability to analyze mass storage (hard disk) availability in order to monitor system files.				
4. User definable system security program by operator, terminal, application program, and functions.				
5. Provide the user the ability to define the parameters to remove data systematically with the application programs. These programs should provide comprehensive hard copy audit trail reports.				
6. Provide system utility programs that are an integral part of the application programs to backup data in order to protect, preserve, and recreate data base files.				
7. Ability to "backup" files incrementally (i.e., new or changed data) or on a complete basis.				

FIG. 5-82

(Pub.372)

SOFTWARE FEATURES MATRIX
MEDICAL MANAGEMENT SYSTEM

Page Number: 2

System Utilities and Maintenance Programs	Code	Additional Cost	Documentation Reference	Feature Description (Continue on reverse if needed)
8. Provide a user definable program to perform daily, weekly, monthly, and annual (i.e., fiscal year-end) processing functions to ensure proper maintenance of the system.				
9. Ability to utilize "job streams" to perform routine daily processing tasks versus a function-by-function set of commands.				
10. Automatic data increment.				
11. Automatic diskette formatting procedure as part of the backup utility program.				
12. Automatic diskette load procedure as part of the backup utility program.				
13. Ability to utilize a streaming tape cassette for tape backup purposes.				
14. Automatic tape cassette formatting procedure as part of the backup utility program.				
15. Provide a program to integrate a personal computer (i.e. IBM PC, IBM XT, IBM AT, Apple) as system work station.				

FIG. 5-83

SOFTWARE FEATURES MATRIX
MEDICAL MANAGEMENT SYSTEM

Page Number: 3

System Utilities and Maintenance Programs	Code	Additional Cost	Documentation Reference	Feature Description (Continue on reverse if needed)
16. Ability to transfer system data files to a personal computer utilizing industry standard "diff files."				
17. Provide remote terminal capability and support remote terminal printing via standard telephone line and communications modem (300, 1200 or 2400 Baud) async.				
18. Software should include daily transaction audit program which can be performed in case of hard disk errors or system failure.				
19. Provide the capability to restore backup data and recreate "key" files.				
20. Provide communication programs to support standard async communication protocol.				

FIG. 5-84

App. 5–E MANAGING YOUR MEDICAL PRACTICE 5–160

SOFTWARE FEATURES MATRIX
MEDICAL MANAGEMENT SYSTEM

Page Number: 1

System Print Utilities	Code	Additional Cost	Documentation Reference	Feature Description (Continue on reverse if needed)
1. Capability to "spool" all output.				
2. Provide the operator the capability to designate/select the system printer for the designated system output.				
3. Provide the operator the capability to change the current terminal printer (i.e., letter quality to dot matrix printer) depending on the system output.				
4. If printer failure occurs, provide the operator the ability to advance the output to a specific page number.				
5. Ability to transfer system output to a diskette or tape medium.				
6. Provide the ability to print data from remote data bases (i.e., AMA NET).				
7. Support the ability to have remote printer capability (i.e., satellite office).				
8. Capability to view system output prior to printing (80 and 132 column format).				

FIG. 5-85

(Pub.372)

SOFTWARE FEATURES MATRIX
MEDICAL MANAGEMENT SYSTEM

Page Number: 2

System Print Utilities	Code	Additional Cost	Documentation Reference	Feature Description (Continue on reverse if needed)
9. Assign a "forms type" to all system output (i.e., superbills versus insurance) to eliminate printing information on the wrong forms.				
10. Compressed printing capability to allow system output to be printed on 9-1/2" x 11" pinfed paper.				
11. Provide forms alignment capability to enable the operator to "set" printer prior to printing the actual output.				
12. Provide a forms/printing management system to view the status of system output.				
13. Enable all terminals to have printing capability via a local or system printer.				

FIG. 5-86

App. 5–E MANAGING YOUR MEDICAL PRACTICE 5–162

SOFTWARE FEATURES MATRIX
MEDICAL MANAGEMENT SYSTEM

Page Number: 1

Telecommunications	Code	Additional Cost	Documentation Reference	Feature Description (Continue on reverse if needed)
1. Provide a user oriented modem set-up procedure.				
2. Provide capability to interface personal computer (i.e., IBM PC or Apple) within the system utilizing modem.				
3. Capability to utilize the following Baud rates to asynchronous modems: a. 300 Baud b. 1200 Baud c. 2400 Baud				
4. Converse through modem with save of data.				
5. Transmit files through the modem.				
6. Receive a file through the modem.				
7. Ability to access the following remote data bases: a. AMA NET b. Dow Jones c. Electronic mail				

FIG. 5-87

(Pub.372)

CHAPTER 6

Financial Management

> **SCOPE**
>
> Good financial management of a medical practice entails working within a budget. By forecasting realistic revenues and expenses based on business averages and physician needs, and seeing how closely actual business income approximates them, a physician can pinpoint the strengths and weaknesses of the practice. Budgeting necessitates keeping a detailed general ledger of all expenses and income, each subdivided into specific accounts with running balances that can be easily examined and compared to figures for previous years. Records for accounts payable and employee payroll are of particular importance. You must establish a system whereby purchases and payments for office needs are centralized so that the chance for discrepancies in billing is minimized. Likewise, you must keep permanent payroll records to show how much has been withheld from employee paychecks for tax purposes and how much you are liable for in taxes, if penalties for disorganized finances are to be avoided. The system of financial management you choose must ultimately do two things: (1) provide accurate financial information that will facilitate the management of the practice and allow you to exploit potentially lucrative concepts such as cash flow; and (2) provide information required by the government for determining tax liabilities. For this reason many physicians find it practical to enlist the services of a professional consultant or accountant in managing their financial affairs.

SYNOPSIS

§ 6.01 Budgeting and Financial Forecasting
    [1] Forecasting Expenses
    [2] Forecasting Revenue
    [3] Cash Flow
    [4] The Budget Forecast

§ 6.02 Financial Reports
    [1] Income Statement
        [a] Cash Receipts
        [b] Business Expenses
        [c] Income Statement Breakdowns
        [d] Supplemental Accounts Receivable Report
        [e] Trend Analysis Report
    [2] Practice Comparisons
    [3] Cash Flow Reports

§ 6.03 Accounts Payable
    [1] Centralized Purchasing
    [2] Receipt Controls
        [a] Purchase Orders
        [b] Packing Invoices
        [c] Supplier Statements
    [3] Paying Bills
    [4] Accounts Payable Filing System
    [5] Accounts Payable Check Writing System
    [6] Petty Cash Expenditures

§ 6.04 Payroll
    [1] Time Cards
    [2] Individual Earnings Record
    [3] Vacation Records
    [4] Sick Pay Records
    [5] Individual Earnings Reports to Employees
    [6] Check Writing System
    [7] Payroll Taxes
        [a] Standard Withholdings
        [b] Penalties
    [8] Payroll Tax Reports
    [9] Non-Employee Compensation

§ 6.05 General Ledger
    [1] Bank Deposits
    [2] Checkbook Disbursements
        [a] General Disbursements
        [b] Payroll Check Disbursements
    [3] Reconciling Records

§ 6.06 Choosing an Accountant
    [1] Criteria for Selection
    [2] Professional Credentials

§ 6.07 Cash Flow Management
  [1] Money Market vs. Checking Account
  [2] Early Contributions to Pension and Profit Sharing
  [3] Periodic Bonuses
  [4] Early Pay Discounts
§ 6.08 Financial Management Checklist
§ 6.09–§ 6.99 Reserved
§ 6.100 Bibliography

§ 6.01 Budgeting and Financial Forecasting

> Working within a budget allows you to determine the strong and weak spots of the practice. To create a budget, you must keep a record of both fixed and variable expenses. This record can help you forecast a reasonable patient volume and the type and number of procedures you will need to perform to break even, as well as show the difference between actual practice income and available cash flow. Established practitioners, who can look back on figures from earlier years, generally find making expense and revenue forecasts easier than do new practitioners who must rely largely on projected values.

Working within a budget need not be a burden or restraint. Rather, budgeting can be an excellent tool that assists you in keeping control of your practice. When used properly, a budget can provide the information needed to decide whether or not something is affordable and where the money for it will come from. It can also serve as a guide for measuring the strengths and weaknesses of the practice.

A budget can be extremely helpful in a group practice, where important financial decisions need to be reviewed, studied, discussed and decided on in an orderly fashion. The budget can also be used to make financial forecasts by helping to set goals in terms of overhead control and, when combined with projected revenue forecasts, to estimate the amount available for salaries, fringe benefits, pension and profit sharing, etc. Each month, the financial forecast or budget can be compared with the actual operation revenues to help spot the areas of a practice that stand out, for good or for bad reasons. It can generally provide information on trouble areas early enough to allow preventive or corrective action to be taken.

(Pub.372)

[1] Forecasting Expenses

Before you can put together a budget, various financial data must be collected. The first step is to assemble all the known expenses of the practice. This will be easier for an established practitioner, since figures from previous years are available. A physician starting a new practice will have to combine existing figures with projected averages.

The initial figures to be entered into the budget include rent, utilities, other occupancy costs, telephone, staff salary, payroll taxes, employee fringe benefits, dues and journals, cleaning expenses, business insurance, professional fees and debt service. Each of these expenses should be placed in a separate category for each month in which the expense is to be paid.

A new practice will also have certain "start-up" costs, including initial equipment acquisitions, leasehold improvements, office supplies and medical supplies. These should be incorporated into the first month of the budget.

The next category of expenses would be variable expenses, or expenses that vary with the volume of work done in the office each month. Variable expenses should be calculated as a percentage of income, rather than in fixed dollar amounts.

The percentage of income that should be devoted to specific expenses will vary with the specialty. For example, according to statistics calculated by the Society of Medical/Dental Management Consultants, a family practitioner should budget 3.8 percent for professional supplies, 1.9 percent for office supplies and 2.8 percent for laboratory fees. According to the same statistics, though, a dermatologist should budget seven percent for professional supplies, while a cardiovascular surgeon should budget less than 0.2 percent. Medical business consultants or other physicians in the field can help a starting practitioner determine appropriate percentages for his or her specialty. Once these areas of expense are identified, they should be listed on a columnar pad for each month and projected for at least six months.

The total of fixed expenses (i.e., rent, utilities, telephone equipment lease and loan payments, as opposed to variable expenses like professional, office and laboratory supplies) equals the amount necessary to maintain the practice whether or not a patient is seen. Fixed expenses should also be logged and projected in their own category.

[2] Forecasting Revenue

To determine a practice's potential for profit, it is necessary to project revenue forceasts consistent with expense forecasts. Established practices, particulary those with good computer management, have good criteria for predicting revenues: not only do they have data from the previous six months, they also have information on growth rates, and how fee increases affect revenues over an interval of months. However, for a physician starting a practice, the revenue forecast is the most difficult part of the budget.

A new physician must generate revenue to hit a "break even" point as soon as possible, which means regularly generating enough revenue to pay all of the office and living expenses. The new physician should endeavor to break even within six months of opening a practice. (In this sense, "break even in six months" means being able to pay the current monthly expenses, not including the first six months' operating losses, from the current monthly revenues.) This initial goal should be the criteria used to established minimum projected revenues for the first six months.

To determine how realistic these minimum goals are, you should calculate how many patients you will need to see to meet these goals, and how many procedures will have to be performed. A surgeon, for example, may not need to see as many patients and may meet the break even level by performing a few surgeries. A primary care physician, however, may need to see a number of patients to generate adequate charges. He or she should figure out the average daily charges needed to meet established minimum goals and divide this figure by the expected charge per patient to determine the necessary patient volume. This hypothetical patient volume can then be compared with actual volume to determine whether the physician has sufficient volume or needs to increase it.

[3] Cash Flow

The cash flow of a practice depends on the volume of charges generated. Since a substantial portion of medical charges are disbursed on a credit basis, there is usually a time lag between billing and collection that must be considered in the financial model. Cash revenues may be anticipated by reviewing previous collection experience. A new practitioner should realize that the figures for accounts receivable in a medical practice typically represent between two and three months of charges.

[4] The Budget Forecast

Once the initial information is assembled, the entire forecast can be put together:

- The first section of the forecast should show the expected patient flow and charge volume.
- The second section should show the accounts receivable and collections.
- The third section should show the practice's expenses.
- The fourth section should calculate profit (the expected cash receipts less expenses).
- The fifth section should show the physician's draws and fringe benefits. For a physician starting a practice, the draw amount should equal the minimum needed to pay personal living expenses. For incorporated medical practices, the amount of physicians' salaries and fringe benefits should be listed in this area.

(See Figure 6–1 for a sample spreadsheet of a medical practice's projected revenues, expenses and profits for one year.)

The financial forecast and budget can be used to enhance practice profitability. By reviewing the forecast, you can anticipate profits and look for areas of improvement if anticipated profits are not realized. For example, you can determine whether you will need to work more hours or see more patients to increase income. You can also look at how additional revenue will affect expenses and net profit and how to cut overhead or extract money out of the budget for equipment, property or business trips.

As the practice begins its fiscal year, your forecast helps you to keep on target by comparing actual monthly financial reports to those forecast. Doing so reveals whether or not the practice is ahead

FINANCIAL MANAGEMENT § 6.01[4]

WILLIAM S. JOHNSON, M.D.
FINANCIAL FORECAST
1985

	1	2	3	4	5	6	7	8	9	10	11	12	12 MTH TOTAL
PRODUCTION:													
DOCTOR JOHNSON	10000.00	12000.00	13000.00	14000.00	15000.00	17000.00	19000.00	20000.00	20000.00	20000.00	20000.00	20000.00	200000.00
-LESS WRITE-OFFS & ADJ	-500.00	-600.00	-650.00	-700.00	-750.00	-850.00	-950.00	-1000.00	-1000.00	-1000.00	-1000.00	-1000.00	-10000.00
NET PRODUCTION	9500.00	11400.00	12350.00	13300.00	14250.00	16150.00	18050.00	19000.00	19000.00	19000.00	19000.00	19000.00	190000.00
COLLECTIONS:													
PATIENTS	3000.00	6000.00	9500.00	11400.00	12350.00	13300.00	14250.00	16150.00	18050.00	19000.00	19000.00	19000.00	161000.00
TOTAL COLLECTIONS	3000.00	6000.00	9500.00	11400.00	12350.00	13300.00	14250.00	16150.00	18050.00	19000.00	19000.00	19000.00	161000.00
BUSINESS EXPENSES:													
STAFF SALARIES	1600.00	1600.00	1600.00	1600.00	1600.00	1600.00	1600.00	1600.00	1600.00	1600.00	1600.00	1600.00	19200.00
RENT,UTIL,& OCC	500.00	500.00	500.00	500.00	500.00	500.00	500.00	500.00	500.00	500.00	500.00	500.00	6000.00
PROFESSIONAL SUPPLIES	114.00	342.00	541.50	649.80	703.95	758.10	812.25	920.55	1028.85	1083.00	1083.00	1083.00	9120.00
OFFICE SUPPLIES	57.00	126.00	199.50	239.40	259.35	279.30	299.25	339.15	379.05	399.00	399.00	399.00	3375.00
CONV., DUES & JOURNALS	25.00	25.00	25.00	1000.00	25.00							25.00	1125.00
TELEPHONE	300.00	300.00	300.00	300.00	300.00	300.00	300.00	300.00	300.00	300.00	300.00	300.00	3600.00
MISCELLANEOUS	300.00	300.00	300.00	300.00	300.00	300.00	300.00	300.00	300.00	300.00	300.00	300.00	3600.00
PROFESSIONAL FEES	250.00	250.00	250.00	250.00	250.00	250.00	250.00	250.00	250.00	250.00	250.00	250.00	3000.00
LABORATORY FEES	84.00	615.00	973.75	1168.50	1285.88	1383.25	1464.63	1655.37	1850.12	1947.50	1947.50	1947.50	16279.00
TAXES	160.00	160.00	160.00	160.00	160.00	160.00	160.00	160.00	160.00	160.00	160.00	160.00	1920.00
BUSINESS INSURANCE	300.00						1000.00						1300.00
MARKETING	500.00	50.00	50.00	50.00	50.00	50.00	50.00	50.00	50.00	50.00	50.00	50.00	1050.00
HOSPITAL PAYMENT	210.00	210.00	210.00	210.00	210.00	210.00	531.00	531.00	531.00	531.00	531.00	531.00	4966.28
INTEREST	58.50	108.32	124.54	107.40	83.24	38.28							
TOTAL BUSINESS EXPENSE	4458.50	4586.32	5334.29	6535.10	5707.41	5808.93	7263.12	6606.08	6949.03	7120.50	7120.50	7145.50	74535.28
NET PROFIT FROM PRACTICE	-1458.50	1413.68	4265.71	4864.90	6642.59	7491.07	6986.88	9543.92	11100.97	11879.50	11879.50	11854.50	86464.72
PERSONAL DRAW	-2800.00	-2800.00	-2800.00	-2800.00	-2800.00	-2800.00	-2800.00	-2800.00	-2800.00	-2800.00	-2800.00	-2800.00	-33600.00
LOAN PYMT (DRAW)	-4258.50	-1386.32	1465.71	2064.90	3842.59	4691.07	4186.88	6743.92	8300.97	9079.50	9079.50	9054.50	52864.72
LOAN BALANCE	5000.00	9258.50	10644.82	9179.12	7114.21	3271.63							

FIG. 6–1. A 12-month financial forecast for a starting practice.

(Rel.1–2/87 Pub.372)

of or behind goals and whether or not corrective action is necessary. If a questionable item comes up, such as whether or not an expenditure should be made for a certain item, you can use the forecast to determine how such an expenditure will affect profits. (See Figure 6–2.)

A group practice can use the initial budget to calculate the amount available for individual physician salaries. The individual physicians could use these figures to estimate taxes, determine the amount of spendable cash for the year or calculate the size of bonuses.

The financial forecast is an excellent tool for securing bank financing, as bankers appreciate a well-organized customer with a plan for how loans will be used and repaid. Moreover, if the financial forecast is put together properly and shows effective results, you will know whether the bank's terms for financing are sensible and whether monies will be available to repay the loan.

§ 6.02 Financial Reports

> All practices should keep a record that divides income and expenses into specific subaccounts and carries running balances for each. The record allows you to see which expenses absorb the largest amount of practice income and whether something should be done about it. A separate record should be established for accounts receivable. The practitioner who keeps accurate, itemized records in these areas will have the information necessary to control cash flow, determine which areas of the practice are profitable and unprofitable, and compare his or her practice's current performance against its past performance and the performance of the average practice in the same specialty.

A number of financial reports are important in helping you monitor your practice. It is crucial that you prepare these reports properly if you are to determine the strengths and weaknesses of your practice.

[1] Income Statement

The income statement is a detailed chart that records all types of income, expenses and profit. A properly prepared income statement details all sources and disbursements of income.

[a] Cash Receipts

Separate accounts should be kept for:

Patient Income: All patient payments.

Capitation Income: Income paid whether or not services are rendered, particularly reimbursement from HMO third parties.

Interest: All interest from savings accounts, money markets, certificates of deposit and any other investments.

Other: All miscellaneous income, including income from miscellaneous insurance reports, depositions, expert witness testimony, speaking engagements, etc.

[b] Business Expenses

Separate accounts should be kept for:

Staff Salaries: The gross amount paid for staff salaries. Larger practices may wish to break this account into subaccounts for nurse, medical assistant and business office salaries.

Payroll Taxes: All payroll tax expenses for employees, i.e., the employer's share of FICA, state unemployment and federal unemployment liability.

Staff Fringe Benefits: This account would include all the fringe benefits paid for the staff, such as health insurance, life insurance, disability insurance and medical reimbursement.

Staff Pension and Profit Sharing: Employer contributions to the pension and profit sharing plan for the staff.

Rent, Utilities and Occupancy: All expenses for occupancy costs, including rent and utilities (although telephone would be listed under a separate account).

Medical Supplies: All medical supplies, including drugs, gowns, specimen cups, needles, etc. Subaccounts may be made for important supplies bought consistently, such as chemotherapy drugs for an oncologist. An ophthalmologist dispensing contact lenses or eyeglasses should have a separate account showing the sales of those products and the cost of goods sold.

Office Supplies: All of the office business supplies, including letterhead stationery and postage.

Conventions and Meetings: All of the expenses for continuing education and business meetings, including travel expenses, registration fees and lodging.

THE ALPHA BETA CLINIC, PA
FINANCIAL BUDGET
1987–88

	6-30-88 ACTUAL	6-30-88 PROJECTED	DIFFERENCE
CHARGES:			
Dr. Alpha	$121,303	$126,950	($5,647)
Dr. Beta	$72,505	$73,540	($1,035)
			$0
			$0
TOTAL CHARGES	$193,808	$200,490	($6,682)
less w/o & adj	($15,212)	($14,025)	($1,187)
NET CHARGES	$178,596	$186,465	($7,869)
CASH RECEIPTS:			
Patient	$176,385	$186,455	($10,070)
Interest	$0	$0	$0
Other	$3,885	$4,575	($690)
TOTAL RECEIPTS	$180,270	$191,030	($10,760)
BUSINESS EXPENSES:			
Staff Salaries	$28,594	$30,000	($1,406)
Rent, Util, & Occ	$5,813	$5,815	($2)
Professional Supplies	$7,217	$6,495	$722
Office Supplies	$4,276	$6,112	($1,836)
Convs, Dues, & Journals	$7,506	$6,275	$1,231
Telephone	$4,160	$4,440	($280)
Miscellaneous	$253	$200	$53
Repairs	$1,000	$500	$500
Laundry	$717	$550	$167
Car Expense	$5,000	$5,190	($190)
Professional Fees	$4,304	$4,210	$94
Laboratory Expense	$1,627	$4,210	($2,583)
Taxes	$5,210	$6,000	($790)
Business Insurance	$4,514	$2,400	$2,114
Equipment Lease	$11,719	$26,686	($14,967)
Promotion	$2,360	$3,000	($640)
Staff Fringe Benefits	$5,253	$6,250	($997)
Depreciation Expense	$1,350	$1,350	$0
Interest	$0	$150	($150)
All Other			$0
TOTAL BUSINESS EXPENSE	$100,873	$119,833	($18,960)
PROFIT	$79,397	$71,197	$8,200

FIG. 6–2. A comparison report for a new practice contrasting forecast revenue and expenses to actual income and expenses of the first five months.

Dues and Journals: Professional dues and journal fees, including memberships in state medical societies, local societies, subspecialty societies, etc. The cost for subscriptions to professional journals should also be placed in this account.

Telephone: Basic telephone charges, the telephone lease and long distance charges. Most offices include Yellow Pages advertising in this account, since it is generally part of the regular monthly telephone bill, but it might be better for accounting purposes to place the Yellow Pages advertisement costs in a separate marketing account.

Miscellaneous Expenses: Subaccounts for small expenses that cannot be categorized separately, including subscriptions for magazines in the reception room, bank service charges, etc.

Car Expense: The expenses pertaining to business use of the car. Group practices may wish to have subaccounts in this category for each car used by the practice.

Professional Fees: Outside professional fees, such as consulting fees, legal fees, collection fees and pension management fees. Casual labor may also be listed in this area if it is a small expense. If casual labor becomes a larger item, a separate account should be set up.

Physician Fees: Payment to physicians from outside the practice, e.g., for consultant or coverage fees.

Laboratory Fees: Outside laboratory fees, including tests performed at the pathology laboratory.

Business Insurance: Business insurance would include professional liability, property and casualty, worker's compensation, etc. It would not include fringe benefit types of insurance, such as life, disability or medical insurance.

Promotion: All marketing and promotion expenses for the practice.

Equipment Lease: Lease payments on business and office equipment.

Depreciation Expense: The amount of depreciation charged against capital assets. Although this is not a cash expense, it is an actual practice expense.

Interest: The actual amount of interest charged to the practice and paid by the practice. Principal payments should not be included as an expense.

Physician Salaries: Gross physician salaries. A group practice may wish to have subcategories of each physician's salary listed in order of status.

Physician Pension and Profit Sharing Contributions: The actual amount contributed for the physician's staff. If these plans are distinct from one another, each should be set up as a subaccount.

Physician Fringe Benefits: Fringe benefits paid to the physician(s), such as life, health and disability insurance and medical reimbursement.

[c] Income Statement Breakdowns

The income statement report should detail:

- The balance in each of the income accounts.
- Business operating expenses.
- Profit before physician salaries and fringe benefits are substracted.
- Physician salary and fringe benefit expenses.
- Taxable profit (if practice is a corporation; unincorporated practices would not pay income tax, as profit is added to physician's personal income tax return).

(For a sample income statement, see Figure 6-3.)

Each expense should be shown as a dollar amount, and also as a percentage of receipts that can be used in statistical comparisons for the preceding and following years.

Larger practices may wish to break down income statements into subincome statements by department so that rates of profitability can be determined for each part of the practice. The sum of departmental income statements would equal the totals on the practice income statement.

[d] Supplemental Accounts Receivable Report

Physician income statements are generally based on income declared at the time it is collected, rather than at the time it is charged or billed. This is different from public corporations that

SUNSHINE CLINIC, P.A.

STATEMENT OF INCOME

3/1/85 TO 3/31/85

	CURRENT PERIOD	% OF RECEIPTS	7/1/84 TO DATE	% OF RECEIPTS
CASH RECEIPTS				
PATIENTS	$ 50,799.	100.0	$ 481,753.	99.7
INTEREST			1,047.	0.2
OTHER			180.	0.0
TOTAL CASH RECEIPTS	$ 50,799.	100.0	$ 482,981.	100.0
BUSINESS EXPENSES				
STAFF SALARIES	9,445.	18.6	93,619.	19.4
RENT, UTILITIES & OCCUPANCY	1,179.	2.3	9,964.	2.1
PROFESSIONAL SUPPLIES	2,246.	4.4	30,973.	6.4
OFFICE SUPPLIES	828.	1.6	7,272.	1.5
CONV., DUES AND JOURNALS	46.	0.1	4,383.	0.9
TELEPHONE	341.	0.7	3,157.	0.7
MISCELLANEOUS	28.	0.1	697.	0.1
REPAIRS	1,619.	3.2	2,422.	0.5
LAUNDRY	14.	0.0	140.	0.0
CAR EXPENSE	400.	0.8	5,224.	1.1
PROFESSIONAL FEES	806.	1.6	7,583.	1.6
LABORATORY FEES	1,671.	3.3	15,104.	3.1
TAXES	956.	1.9	14,637.	3.0
BUSINESS INSURANCE			26,928.	5.6
EQUIPMENT LEASE	901.	1.8	8,109.	1.7
PROFESSIONAL EXPENSE	44.	0.1	850.	0.2
STAFF FRINGE BENEFITS			1.	
TOTAL BUSINESS EXPENSE	$ 20,524.	40.4	$ 231,064.	47.8
NET PROFIT FROM PRACTICE	$ 30,275.	59.6	$ 251,917.	52.2
DOCTOR JONES	5,000.	9.8	76,200.	15.8
DOCTOR SMITH	5,000.	9.8	48,100.	10.0
DOCTOR DOE	5,000.	9.8	63,270.	13.1
PENSION PLAN			16,100.	3.3
PROFIT SHARING PLAN			19,300.	4.0
FRINGE BENEFITS			977.	0.2
TAXABLE INCOME	$ 15,275.	30.1	$ 27,970.	5.8

UNAUDITED REPORT PREPARED BY PROFESSIONAL CONSULTING GROUP, INC.

FIG. 6-3. An illustrated income statement and balance sheet for a small to mid-size practice. Note how physician benefits are separated from total business expenses and how subaccounts are given as both a dollar figure and a percentage of receipts. This gives the physicians an idea of which expenses use the bulk of income.

(Rel.1-2/87 Pub.372)

§ 6.02 [1]   MANAGING YOUR MEDICAL PRACTICE   6–14

SUNSHINE CLINIC, P.A.

BALANCE SHEET

AS OF 3/31/85

ASSETS

CURRENT ASSETS
CHECKING ACCOUNT #1 $ (22,117.)
SAVINGS ACCOUNT   49,328.
COLLECTIONS SAVINGS ACCOUNT   8,232.

TOTAL CURRENT ASSETS $ 35,444.

FIXED ASSETS
ORGANIZATION EXPENSE $ 975.
    ALLOWANCE FOR AMORTIZATION   (975.)

TOTAL ASSETS $ 35,444.
                                                                ============

LIABILITIES

PAYROLL PAYABLES

STOCKHOLDER'S EQUITY
CAPITAL STOCK $ 1,500.
RETAINED EARNINGS   5,974.
CURRENT PROFIT   27,970.

TOTAL STOCKHOLDER'S EQUITY $ 35,444.

TOTAL LIABILITIES & STOCKHOLDER'S EQUITY $ 35,444.
                                                                ============

UNAUDITED REPORT PREPARED BY PROFESSIONAL CONSULTING GROUP, INC.

FIG. 6–3 (cont.)

declare income at the time it is charged, rather than at the time it is collected. Although this kind of accounting is appropriate for both management and tax purposes, it tends to overlook production and accounts receivable volumes. To keep track of the charges, adjustments and accounts receivable, it is recommended that you design a supplemental report to be presented with the income statement.

The supplemental accounts receivable report should track the accounts receivable on a month-by-month basis. The report is divided into six columns: the first column for the date; the second column for the charge amount; the third column for payments; the fourth column for debt or credit adjustments; the fifth column for the accounts receivable balance; and the sixth column for the accounts receivable balance. The first row across supplies information for the first month of the fiscal year, the second row across the second month, etc. The report should be carried for the entire fiscal year. (See Figure 6–4.)

By reviewing the accounts receivable report, you can keep track of production, along with the dollar amounts of accounts receivable and the size of the accounts receivable relative to the monthly charges. Since the average accounts receivable for physician's offices represents two to three months of charges, you may be alarmed if your accounts receivable goes unpaid for more than three months. Because write-offs and adjustments are also shown on this report, you may be alarmed by growth in this area as well.

[e] **Trend Analysis Report**

To obtain a quick review of the overall management of the practice, it is recommended that you develop a trend analysis report. A trend analysis report outlines key areas of the practice on a month-by-month basis. Year-to-date figures, year-to-date averages and previous year averages should also be included to permit comparison. These figures will enable you to determine any strengths or weaknesses of the practice. The key areas of the trend analysis are:

- Charges (broken down by doctor, location, etc.).
- Write-offs and adjustments.
- Net charges (total charges less write-offs and adjustments).
- Collection percentage (cash receipts from patients divided by net charges).

ACCOUNTS RECEIVABLE CONTROL

MONTH	CHARGES	PAYMENTS	W/O & ADJ	OTHER	A/R BAL
JUNE 30, 1984					275417.00
JULY	62210.00	-55867.00	-3113.00		278647.00
AUGUST	57139.00	-56824.00	-1930.00		277032.00
SEPTEMBER	53964.00	-56344.00	-1549.00		273103.00
OCTOBER	60388.00	-52014.00	-2538.00		278939.00
NOVEMBER	54819.00	-51349.00	-7712.00		274697.00
DECEMBER	51835.00	-56817.00	-8417.00		261298.00
JANUARY	60146.00	-56623.00	-4900.00	-1507.00	258414.00
FEBRUARY	51023.00	-45116.00	-3525.00	-7000.00	253796.00
MARCH	56674.00	-50799.00	-4616.00		255055.00

MANAGEMENT REPORT PREPARED BY PROFESSIONAL CONSULTING GROUP

FIG. 6–4. An accounts receivable control record for nine months of a practice's fiscal year. The previous accounts receivable balance, plus charges, minus payments, plus or minus adjustments should equal the current accounts receivable balance. This figure is confirmed by totaling ledger cards.

- Dollar amount of accounts receivable (write-off percentage).
- Size of accounts receivable as measured by average monthly charges (computed by dividing the accounts receivable by the average net charges).
- Patient receipts.
- Interest income.
- Other income.
- Total income.
- Operating expenses.
- Operating overhead percentage.
- Practice profit.
- New patients.
- Patients seen.

(For a sample month-by-month trend analysis, see Figure 6–5.)

[2] Practice Comparisons

In addition to comparing actual financial records with those initially forecast, each quarter you should compare financial reports with the same fiscal period from the previous year. Differences should be calculated to determine areas in which the practice has improved or fallen behind. By doing this you can quickly spot unexpected changes in the practice. This data also helps in various decision-making processes, such as determining necessary fee increases. Unusual increases in supplies, for example, can alert you to problems such as inefficient purchasing. (See Figure 6–6.)

Year-to-year practice comparisons can also help you in personal planning. An increase in profits, for example, may alert you to the need for additional tax planning. Decreases in profit, on the other hand, may alert you to the need to cut back personal spending or reduce pension and profit sharing benefits. When detailed practice comparisons are not made, you might overlook a decrease in profit as a result of an unexpected change (such as an increase in write-offs and adjustments) because you first see only positive changes (such as an increase in patient volume).

You should also undertake a statistical comparison of your practice's figures with the statistical averages for your specialty on

§ 6.02 [2] MANAGING YOUR MEDICAL PRACTICE 6–18

U. S. A. FAMILY PRACTICE, P.A.
MONTH-AT-A-GLANCE
1985

	FEBRUARY	MARCH	APRIL	MAY	Y-T-D	YTD AVG	PREV YR
CHARGES:							
HOSPITAL	42719.00	40225.00	12900.00	35795.00	131639.00	32909.75	37988.50
OFFICE	93742.00	98865.00	76319.00	130986.00	399912.00	99978.00	97512.42
TOTAL	136461.00	139090.00	89219.00	166781.00	531551.00	132887.75	135500.92
DR. HANSON	27129.00	24533.00	8126.00	19410.00	79198.00	19799.50	20523.00
DR. ANDERSON	19513.00	25255.00	6579.00	31279.00	82626.00	20656.50	24769.33
DR. NELSON	29457.00	28384.00	21639.00	32589.00	112069.00	28017.25	28297.08
DR. HARRISON	23268.00	21973.00	18236.00	27298.00	90775.00	22693.75	21899.08
DR. WITT	21855.00	21747.00	18087.00	33312.00	95001.00	23750.25	24901.08
DR. ANLOW	8422.00	10526.00	10126.00	13371.00	42445.00	10611.25	11832.50
DR. HUBBERT	6817.00	6672.00	6426.00	9522.00	29437.00	7359.25	3289.00
TOTAL	136461.00	139090.00	89219.00	166781.00	531551.00	132887.75	135510.08
WRITE-OFFS & ADJ.	-12258.00	-18089.00	-14736.00	-14441.00	-59524.00	-14881.00	-13466.42
NET CHARGES	124203.00	121001.00	74483.00	152340.00	472027.00	118006.75	122043.66
COLLECTION %	87.90	89.97	123.77	86.38	93.60	93.60	100.90
WRITE-OFF %	8.98	13.01	16.52	8.66	11.20	11.20	9.94
ACCOUNTS RECEIVABLE	392557.00	405147.00	387438.00	408191.00		398333.25	
# OF MOS. IN A/R	3.25	3.26	3.54	3.49		3.39	
CASH RECEIPTS:							
PATIENTS	109178.00	108866.00	92191.00	131587.00	441822.00	110455.50	123140.08
CAPITATION INCOME	9994.00	8262.00	7364.00	7469.00	33089.00	8272.25	5688.00
INTEREST							25.58
OTHER	351.00	-26.00		8509.00	8834.00	2208.50	905.92
TOTAL	119523.00	117102.00	99555.00	147565.00	483745.00	120936.25	129759.58
BUSINESS EXPENSES	64798.00	69583.00	65826.00	70120.00	270327.00	67581.75	79338.33
OVERHEAD %	54.21	59.42	66.12	47.52	55.88	55.88	61.14
PROFIT	54725.00	47519.00	33729.00	77445.00	213418.00	53354.50	50421.25

4.00

MANAGEMENT REPORT PREPARED BY PROFESSIONAL CONSULTING GROUP

FIG. 6–5. A four-month trend analysis report. The physician can use this report to spot strengths and weaknesses of the practice.

an annual basis. Although no two practices are exactly alike, this type of comparison can be used as a measuring stick for key areas of the practice, such as production, overhead and profit. In addition, it allows you to create specific budgetary goals that are within reason. Assume, for example, that an internist doing a comparison finds that the average internist spends 2.5 percent of receipts on medical supplies. If he or she is spending five percent of receipts on supplies,

(Pub.372)

U. S. A. FAMILY PRACTICE CLINIC P. A.
PRACTICE COMPARISON
MAY, 1985

	1985	1984	DOLLAR CHANGE	PERCENTAGE CHANGE
CHARGES:				
TOTAL CHARGES	$ 629438.00	$ 598382.00	$ 31056.00	5.19
WRITE-OFFS & ADJ.	-59524.00	-49928.00	-9596.00	19.22
NET CHARGES	$ 569914.00	$ 548454.00	$ 21460.00	3.91
HOSPITAL CHARGES	$ 131639.00	$ 173466.00	$ -41827.00	-24.11
OFFICE CHARGES	399912.00	404328.00	-4416.00	-1.09
TOTAL CHARGES	$ 531551.00	$ 577794.00	$ -46243.00	-8.00
CASH RECEIPTS:				
PATIENTS	$ 441822.00	$ 530565.00	$ -88743.00	-16.73
CAPITATION INCOME	33089.00	10251.00	22838.00	222.79
OTHER	8833.00	4334.00	4499.00	103.81
TOTAL RECEIPTS	$ 483744.00	$ 545150.00	$ -61406.00	-11.26
EXPENSES:				
STAFF SALARIES	$ 92229.00	$ 91819.00	$ 410.00	.45
RENT, UTILITIES	32061.00	31116.00	945.00	3.04
PROFESSIONAL SUPPLIES	21470.00	23201.00	-1731.00	-7.46
OFFICE SUPPLIES	5473.00	14749.00	-9276.00	-62.89
CONV., DUES, JOURNALS, & PR	2637.00	800.00	1837.00	229.63
TELEPHONE	10947.00	7752.00	3195.00	41.22
MISCELLANEOUS	216.00	309.00	-93.00	-30.10
REPAIRS	562.00	204.00	358.00	175.49
LAUNDRY	1300.00	1377.00	-77.00	-5.59
CAR EXPENSE	103.00	-1577.00	1680.00	-106.53
HMO REFERRALS	15.00	1923.00	-1908.00	-99.22
PROFESSIONAL FEES	16657.00	9387.00	7270.00	77.45
X-RAY FEE		5874.00	-5874.00	-100.00
LABORATORY FEES	24445.00	30725.00	-6280.00	-20.44
TAXES	19269.00	21547.00	-2278.00	-10.57
BUSINESS INSURANCE		-1978.00	1978.00	-100.00
EQUIPMENT LEASE	13875.00	15500.00	-1625.00	-10.48
PROFESSIONAL EXPENSE	114.00	84.00	30.00	35.71
STAFF FRINGE BENEFITS	5735.00	6704.00	-969.00	-14.45
DEPRECIATION	8207.00	9200.00	-993.00	-10.79
INTEREST	5003.00	4479.00	524.00	11.70
TOTAL BUSINESS EXPENSE	$ 260318.00	$ 273195.00	$ -12877.00	-4.71
PROFIT	$ 223426.00	$ 271955.00	$ -48529.00	-17.84
ACCOUNTS RECEIVABLE	$ 427435.00	$ 388048.00	$ 39387.00	10.15
# OF MONTHS	3.00	2.90	.10	3.45
COLLECTION %	77.52	96.74	-19.21	
WRITE-OFF %	9.46	8.34	1.11	
OVERHEAD %	53.81	50.11	3.70	

FIG. 6–6. A comparison report for an established practice contrasting 1985 receipts to 1984 receipts.

(Rel.1–2/87 Pub.372)

it should prompt immediate review of purchasing and supply consumption. Using outside statistics can help you to avoid repeating financial mistakes that might not be evident from your practice's statistics when they are considered by themselves.

Although some statistical information is available through publications such as *Medical Economics,* a proper and accurate statistical comparison requires the services of a specialized medical business consultant. Top consultants have a broad base of statistics derived from their own experience, and through national organizations such as the Society of Medical/Dental Management Consultants they have access to statistics from many different practices across the country.

[3] Cash Flow Reports

Many business people ask their accountants the same question: "If I show a profit, how come there's no cash in the bank?" Accountants are often unable to give a satisfactory answer because their clients do not understand the principles of cash flow. To understand cash flow, and the difference between income and cash, a brief review of accounting methods is necessary.

The two basic methods of accounting are accrual accounting and cash basis accounting. Accrual accounting considers items income at the time they are charged, rather than when they are collected. Under the accrual method of accounting you can have thousands of dollars of gross income yet have no cash collections. Likewise, expenses under the accrual method are determined when they occur, rather than when they are paid. Thus, you can have substantial expenses under the accrual method of accounting even though you have not paid any bills. Income under the accrual method of accounting is determined by taking accrued income (physician charges) and subtracting accrued expenses (bills, paid or unpaid). You can see how a business can show substantial profits under the accrual method of accounting, yet have little or no cash.

For most physicians, cash basis accounting is more advantageous. Under the cash basis of accounting, income is considered income when it is collected, and expenses are considered expenses when paid, with certain exceptions:

Loans: Loan proceeds are not considered income.

Capital Expenditures: Equipment, office furniture and leasehold improvements are common examples of capital expenditures that are not deductible when purchased. For taxes and financial purposes, these items are considered assets or investment.

Depreciation: Since capital acquisitions are not considered deductible when acquired, a depreciation deduction is allowed. Depreciation deduction allows a portion of the asset to be written off or deducted each year until the entire asset is deducted.

Salaries: The gross amount of salaries is deductible. Since employers are required to withhold payroll tax, the net amount actually paid to the employees is less than the gross salary. Gross salaries are deductible whether or not the payroll taxes have been paid.

Payroll Taxes: Since gross salaries are deductible, payroll taxes are not deductible when paid. (The exception is the employer's share of of FICA taxes and unemployment taxes, which are paid out of the profits rather than out of the employees' salaries.)

Principal Payments: Principal payments are not deductible. (Good cash flow management requires a loan to be repaid at approximately the same rate it is depreciated. The lack of a deduction for principal payments is offset by the depreciation deduction.)

A mature practice that has not made any recent capital expenditures, has depreciated most of its assets, has no debt, pays most of its bills on time and employs the cash basis of accounting will note little difference between cash flow and income. Other practices will need to be aware of how their cash flow is affected and in many cases will need cash flow reports in addition to the normal profit and loss statement.

The normal cash flow statement prepared by an accountant is called a statement of changes in financial position; it is generally difficult for the nonaccountant to understand. When a cash flow report is needed, the physician should request that the accountant prepare a special report showing the actual income and expenses, defining income as all sources of cash and defining expenses as all expenditures of cash, or have the accountant take the income from the income statement and illustrate adjustments affecting cash flow. (See Figure 6–7.)

Cash Flow Statement
June 30, 1983

Total Cash Receipts		$ 9,223.45
Less:		
Total Business Expense		− 6,604.65
Personal Draw		− 3,935.40
Federal Income Tax		− 400.00
Payroll Taxes		+ 95.60
Payment to 1st National		− 400.00
		$ − 2,021.00
Available Cash	5-31-83	$ 3,333.80
Minus June Decrease		− 2,021.00
Available Cash	6-30-83	$ 1,312.80

FIG. 6–7. A simplified cash flow statement

§ 6.03 Accounts Payable

Without an organized system for accounts payable, a practice can end up paying for goods never ordered, goods never received or goods of shoddy and defective quality. Where possible, purchasing duties should be delegated to one person. This person creates a file in which purchasing orders, packing invoices and company billing statements can be compared for discrepancies before any payments are issued.

(Pub.372)

> Accounts payable should be paid out of a checkbook or computer system designed specifically for that purpose, and either one or two specific dates each month should be set as deadlines for bill payment. Subaccounts in accounts payable, such as petty cash and change-making funds, should be kept distinct from one another.

Accounts payable—keeping track of the purchases and bills of the practice other than payroll—is an important part of bookkeeping. However, since most physicians' overhead is small, compared to business overhead in general, physicians have generally paid little attention to this area. As a result, some common errors are committed:

- Checks are issued to solicitors of business because the accounts payable clerk thinks they are presenting a legitimate bill, rather a solicitation. A recent scam that affected many physicians involved a company billing for "Yellow Pages" ads. Many physicians, apparently unaware that the bill for Yellow Pages advertising is incorporated into the general telephone bill, paid for what turned out to be publication of their names in a obscure "yellow pages" book.
- Payment is made for supplies never ordered. Large vendors occasionally send supplies to the wrong office and bill that office. Without a proper accounting system, the accounts payable person will pay the bill, thinking it is legitimate.
- Payment is made for supplies ordered but never received. A supplier may fill a portion of the order and mistakenly bill for the entire amount.
- Credit is not given for damaged or returned items.
- Interest or service charges are billed because payment was not made on goods received late or never received at all.
- A negotiated or promised discount is not received. Occasionally, after a discount from a vendor has been agreed upon, the vendor fails to give that discount.
- Credit for early payment is not received. Many creditors give a one or two percent discount if a bill is paid within ten days. When a timely check is issued, the bookkeeper must be sure that full credit is given on the account.

- An extra charge is added for shipping and handling. When shipping and handling has been promised as included in the supplier's price, it is important to make sure you are not billed for an additional charge.
- Inferior supplies or supplies at excessive cost are delivered. In today's competitive office supply market a number of unscrupulous suppliers call offices and promise quality supplies at lower prices. Thanks to a quick sales pitch, these supplies, which are not wanted, needed or economical, are ordered, shipped and billed.

[1] Centralized Purchasing

The first step in organizing accounts payable is to establish a centralized system of ordering. You should delegate responsibility for ordering supplies to one person. (In a large practice, the supply ordering responsibility may be divided. For example, one person might be put in charge of medical supplies and another person put in charge of office supplies.) Putting one person in charge of supplies eliminates redundant orders, adds objectivity to the purchasing process since the purchaser is generally not buying supplies directly for his or her own use and eliminates the need for salespeople to talk to many different people in the office. Centralized purchasing permits the employee in charge of purchasing to become familiar with prices of various supplies, the various suppliers of products used in the office and the best prices and services offered by the suppliers so that he or she can shop around to get the best bargain on an item. An across the board discount is frequently granted to practices that give a certain amount of business to a supplier.

[2] Receipt Controls

Purchasing and billing for an item generates many notices and statements. To avoid any discrepancy between the initial order and final billing, you must establish an orderly system whereby all notices and statements pertaining to an order can be filed.

[a] Purchase Orders

A purchase order should be used to keep track of supply purchases. The purchase order documents supplies ordered and prevents suppliers from alleging requests for supplies never ordered. Purchase orders may also be used to authorize employees to makes purchases if orders are signed by the person in charge of purchasing. (See Figure 6–8.)

[b] Packing Invoices

When supplies are received they are accompanied by a packing invoice. The user of the supplies (i.e., the person most familiar with them) should check the packing invoice so that any damaged or missing supplies are noted before the invoice is placed in inventory. The person reviewing the delivered supplies should sign the packing invoice after it has been reviewed for discrepancies and forward the invoice to the person in charge of purchasing. That person should then pull the outstanding purchase order to note that the supplies have arrived. (See Figure 6–9.)

[c] Supplier Statements

Although some suppliers request that bills be paid directly from the packing invoice, most do not even put the price on the packing invoice. Instead, periodic (usually monthly) statements are sent to the physician for supplies delivered. This is where the person issuing the accounts payable checks may pay for an incorrect statement, which is why it is extremely important that tight control be maintained on purchase orders and supply invoices. These documents should be compared with the itemized statement to confirm the accuracy of the statement and challenge any discrepancy. Before any checks are issued, these supply statements must be carefully reviewed and matched with the packing invoices. (See Figure 6–10.)

Any discrepancies on the bills should be immediately noted and the supplier should be contacted. Suppliers are usually cooperative about correcting their errors and making proper adjustments. Occasionally, though, complete documentation is necessary before the supplier will properly adjust the account.

When reviewing statements, the following steps should be taken in addition to an item-by-item comparison of details on the statement to the packing invoices:

- The beginning balance should be checked and compared to the end balance of the previous statement.

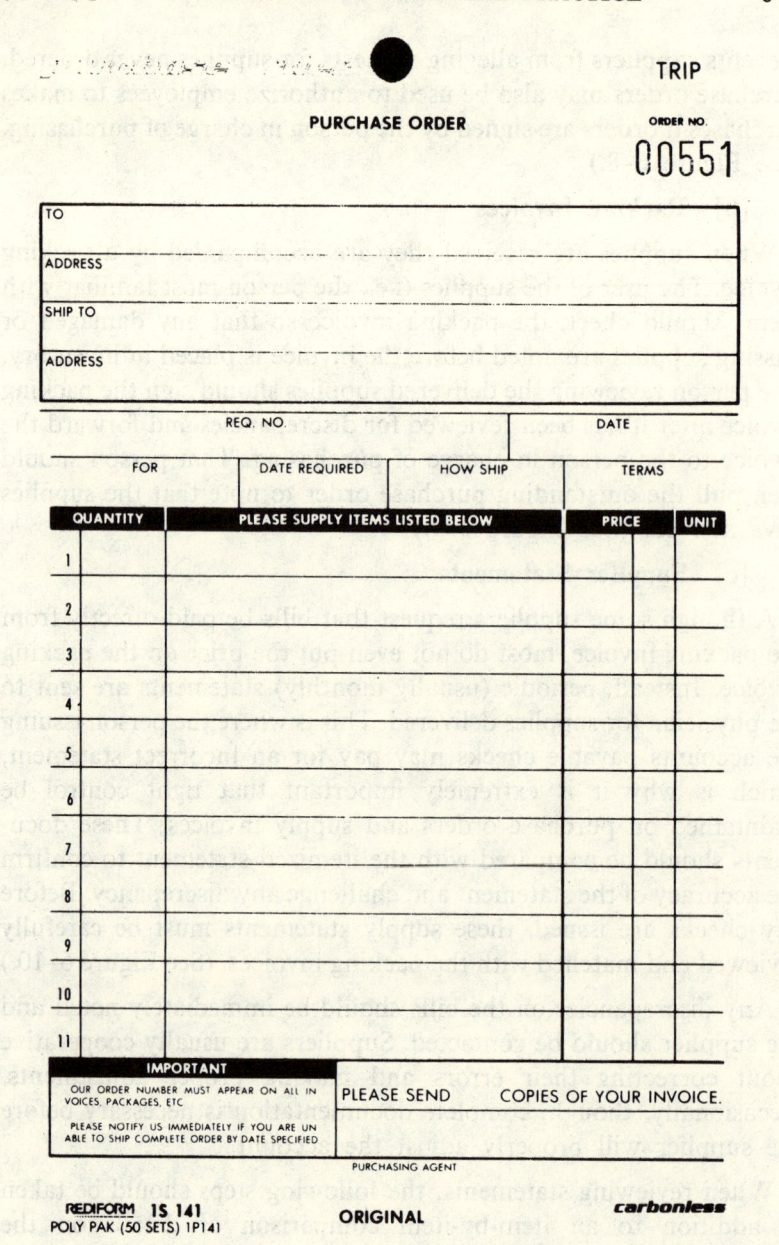

FIG. 6–8. A purchase order can be used to keep track of supplies ordered and compared to the shipping invoice.

FINANCIAL MANAGEMENT § 6.03 [2]

FIG. 6–9. A typical supplier statement. Before a bill is paid it should be compared to the shipping invoice and original purchase order.

§ 6.03 [2]   MANAGING YOUR MEDICAL PRACTICE   6–28

FIG. 6–10. A typical shipping invoice. When the invoice arrives it should be compared with the purchase order.

- The statement should be reviewed to make sure proper credit has been given for any payments made since the last statement.
- Any interest charge should be checked against the terms arranged with the supplier.

(Matthew Bender & Co., Inc.) (Rel.5–1/91 Pub.372)

- The mathematical computation on the statement should be checked.
- The statement should be checked to make sure proper credit has been given for an across the board discount or a discount given for early payment.

Some items billed monthly do not carry packing invoices that confirm amounts due. Common examples are the monthly charges for rent, telephone, Yellow Pages, utilities and lease. Items due quarterly, semi-annually or annually include business insurance (including malpractice), dues, subscription fees, third party contracts and various fringe benefit payments. A list of these items should be prepared according to the frequency of payment of the item. The list should detail:

- To whom the check is being issued.
- The purpose of the check.
- The frequency of the check.
- The dollar amount of the check.

The origin of the information listed on these sheets should be the documents that spell out the terms of the various agreements. For example, the amount of rent and frequency of payment should come directly from the lease arrangement. The amount of the telephone bill should be based on the basic charge from the telephone company and the amount for Yellow Pages ads should be based on the agreement made at the time the Yellow Pages ads were contracted for; additional charges, such as long distance telephone calls, should be backed up and documented with a telephone log. Items such as the electric and gas bills should use an estimated cost based on the range of monthly bills. Using these lists as a guide to bills to be paid you avoid missing payments and can spot erroneous bills. Statements from these sources should otherwise receive the same scrutiny as statements from suppliers.

[3] Paying Bills

Some offices pay bills only once a month. If this is the case, bills should be paid at the end of the month to assure that all expenses for the month are paid and included on the financial report for that

(Pub.372)

month. Bills immediately due on the first of the month, such as rent, should be paid at the end of the preceding month with the rest of the bills due for that month. However, it is recommended that two specific days, one at the middle and one at the end of the month, be established for paying bills to spread out the work flow and cash flow and take advantage of early payment discounts.

When bills are paid, the checkbook should be balanced. If there is an excess of cash in the account after payment of bills, it should be moved into an interest bearing account (such as a money market fund). If there is a deficit in the checking account, funds should be withdrawn from the interest bearing account and deposited in the checking account to avoid a service charge. Business checking account minimum balances are generally based on the activity in the account. Your banker should be able to tell you the minimum balance you must maintain to avoid service charges.

[4] Accounts Payable Filing System

A good system for keeping track of accounts payable need not be complicated. You should first establish a file for unfilled purchase orders. This file should contain all of the orders placed with a vendor but not yet filled. Most small offices will find a simple manila file folder labeled "Unfilled Orders" sufficient for this file, although a larger practice may need to alphabetize the purchase orders by supplier for quick retrieval.

Another file should be established for unpaid invoices. As invoices are received from the recipient of supplies, the purchase order should be pulled, attached to the invoice and filed with the invoice in an unpaid invoice file.

Finally, statements received from the various suppliers can be placed in a file labeled "Bills to Pay." When it is time to pay bills, unpaid invoices should be pulled from the unpaid invoice file and attached to the applicable supplier statement before any checks are written. As bills are then paid, the statement should be marked "paid," and the date and check number should be recorded on the statement.

Paid-up statements should be filed alphabetically in a file for the practice's fiscal year. Generally, an expandable, alphabetical file is the best way to file paid-up invoices. (See Figure 6–11.)

(Pub.372)

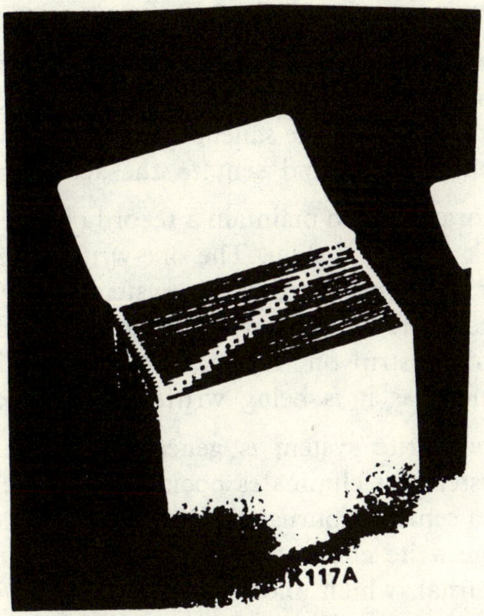

FIG. 6-11. An expandable alphabetized file. All paid-up statements, except for capital expenditures, would be filed in this file. At the end of the fiscal year, this file should be closed, labeled as a paid-up statement file for that fiscal year and a new file started. The old file should be kept for three years from the filing date of the IRS tax return.

A separate paid-up file should be established for capital assets. This should be a permanent file and assets should remain in this file until disposed of. The capital assets file should include all capital expenditures, such as for equipment, office furniture, expensive leasehold improvements, etc. Not only will this file serve as a backup to the depreciation schedule in the event of an IRS audit, it will also serve as an excellent inventory of equipment for valuation purposes.

[5] Accounts Payable Check Writing System

The most common checks found in the medical offices are standard business checks with check stubs attached in a three-ring binder. Physicians using outside accountants can send these stubs to the accountant. Offices wishing to maintain possession of the check stubs generally order check stubs with carbon backing or make

(Pub.372)

photocopies of the check stubs and send the copies to the accountants.

Another common system of check writing is a standard business check with a separate check register. The separate check register, which is used to record all the salient information about the check, can then be photocopied and sent to the accountant.

A more elaborate way to maintain a record of checks is to have a one-write check writing system. The one-write system works in a manner similar to the pegboard billing system. The checks come in "shingles" attached to a pegboard designed for check writing, and each has a carbon strip on the back. A journal sheet is placed beneath the check as it is being written for a separate record.

While the one-write system is generally more expensive than other check systems, it eliminates bookkeeping time for recording each check on a separate journal sheet or check stub. Furthermore, most of the one-write check systems are designed to serve as an expenditure journal, which allows for the filing of various check records into subaccounts. The problem with this system is that the check is recorded in only one place (in other words, it is not recorded both in a check register or on a check stub and in a separate general ledger). This sometimes creates problems when the accountant and bookkeeper need to review check listings at the same time. A good checkwriting system can be efficiently used if it is employed mainly as a record of checks and a photocopy of the check record can be sent to the accountant for entry into the general ledger.

With the automation of medical offices, and with the availability of numerous accounts payable programs, a number of offices are computerizing disbursement systems (see Chapter 5, Computers in Health Care). With an automated accounts payable system, checks are issued directly from the computer: special checks designed to go on the computer are printed out and their salient information is automatically recorded in a log or journal. Because some checks will still need to be written by hand (for example, when an immediate need for a check comes up and the computer is not available to print one), a system to enter checks written by hand so that they may be included in the journal manually is also available.

A good accounts payable system on a computer (see § 5.02[7]) is complicated and generally not found in the medical community, except in larger practices. Accounts payable management done by hand is reasonably simple unless there is a tremendous volume. An automated system does not obviate the responsibility for checking to insure proper receipt of goods and proper payment of bills.

[6] Petty Cash Expenditures

You should have a small petty cash fund on hand for small, unpredictable expenses (e.g., postage due, a small office supply item needed in a hurry, coffee for the office staff). Accounting for petty cash can be done in a small spiral notebook with the following columns sketched in:

- Date
- Description
- Deposit
- Disbursement
- Balance

The amount kept in the petty cash fund is determined by the size of the office. Typically, fifty dollars is sufficient for a small office.

The original funding of the petty cash fund comes from the main checkbook. A check for cash is disbursed and the cash is placed in a petty cash box. The first entry in the notebook is this deposit entry, showing a balance, in this case, fifty dollars. Each time a disbursement is made out of petty cash, a receipt is obtained and the amount is recorded in the disbursement column. The date of each transaction is recorded and the new balance of the petty cash fund is determined by subtracting the disbursement from the previous balance. An envelope should be kept in the back of the notebook for petty cash receipts. (See Figure 6–12.)

At any given time, the amount in petty cash, when totaled, should equal the balance shown in the notebook. Any discrepancies should immediately be recorded in the notebook and the new balance reflecting the actual petty cash should be shown. When the balance in the petty cash fund reaches a certain level, perhaps fifteen dollars, a check should be issued from the general checking

Dr. Paul Jones
Petty Cash Record

Date	Description	Deposit	Disbursement	Balance
1-1-85	Office Check #3845	10000		10000
1-29-85	Postman		2000	8000
2-15-85	Office Coffee		1498	6502
2-20-85	Note Pads		468	6034
3-12-85	To Dr Jones – Lunch Meeting		2000	4034
3-31-85	Office CK #4132	5966		10000

FIG. 6–12. A standard petty cash record.

account to bring the balance back up to maximum (in this case, fifty dollars).

At the end of the fiscal year, the receipts from the petty cash fund should be filed with the other receipts. The individual receipts can stay in the petty cash receipt envelope and then be filed in the record of expenses under "petty cash disbursement."

Many people confuse a petty cash fund with a change fund used for making change when a patient pays in currency. Petty cash money should not be used for making change, as it may complicate the balancing of the petty cash. The size of a change fund should be based on the volume of currency in the office, with fifty dollars usually satisfactory for a small office. The change fund balance should always equal the amount put into it in the beginning. Every day it should be confirmed that there are (in this case) fifty dollars in the fund comprised of the lowest denomination bills (or coins) received. Higher denomination bills should be deposited with the bank and should balance with the cash receipts postings for the day when combined with noncurrency deposits.

§ 6.04 Payroll

Although payroll is a form of disbursement, it should be kept distinct from payments made for accounts payable and its records should be kept permanently. Employees should keep some type of time card for the hours worked each week, and be informed of vacation time, sick days and the value of all personal benefits in accordance with the practice's personnel policy. For the sake of convenience, it is recommended that employees be paid twice a month rather than every two weeks. Each check should contain gross and net pay figures and detailed explanation of all withholdings. The physician should also keep a copy of these figures to determine employer liability for unemployment, social security, and state and federal taxes, and in addition, records on any payments to non-employees above the established limit for taxation. Failure to have the necessary employee and taxation forms on record or to keep accurate records can result in late or improper tax deposits made to the government and a severe penalty for which the physician will be entirely responsible.

It is important that a medical practice establish payroll records from the beginning. Many experts recommend that the records be kept permanently. Payroll records are used to determine many financial arrangements including pension benefits and other matters that may not be payable for many years. When an employer fails to keep proper payroll records, the IRS and department of labor tend to favor the employee in disputes brought to their attention.

Most physicians fall under federal jurisdiction and must comply with the Fair Labor Standards Act. All physicians must comply with the employment regulations of their state. Failure to document proper payment for overtime hours employees have worked can result in problems with the Department of Labor, which may respond to the complaint of a disgruntled employee or even initiate its own review of an employer's records. To avoid such problems, the bottom line is: keep good payroll records.

[1] Time Cards

A time card should be made to keep track of hours worked by each employee. The use of time cards does not mandate a time clock. Many employers only request that employees record the times they arrive and leave and compile their total working hours each day. Each pay period, the time cards should be added up by the employee and turned in to the person in charge of payroll, who should review the time cards for accuracy, overtime, tardiness or leaving early. It is recommended that the employee sign a statement at the bottom of each time card that certifies the hours marked are accurate and also acknowledges that any cheating or lying is considered grounds for immediate dismissal and loss of benefits. (See Figure 6–13.)

[2] Individual Earnings Record

Individual earnings records should be kept for each employee. Employee earnings records are based on the calendar year, regardless of whether it coincides with the fiscal year of the practice, and they should include the amount of each payroll check issued, the employee's gross salary and any monies withheld. Earnings records should be broken down into two sections: demographic information and the actual earning information. (See Figure 6–14.)

The demographic data on the individual earning record should include the employee's:

- Complete name.
- Complete address.
- Social security number.

Date	Hours & Fraction		Time	Date	Hours & Fraction		Time
		In				In	
		Out				Out	
		In				In	
		Out				Out	
		In				In	
		Out				Out	
		In				In	
		Out				Out	
		In				In	
		Out				Out	
		In				In	
		Out				Out	
		In				In	
		Out				Out	
		In				In	
		Out				Out	
	Sick Pay Hours				Sick Pay Hours		
	Vacation Pay Hours				Vacation Pay Hours		
	Balance from Other side				Balance from Other side		
	Total Hours				Total Hours		

Time Record of: _____ For period: _____ To: _____

Time Record of: _____ For period: _____ To: _____

I certify the hours shown have been completed by me and are correct to my best knowledge.

I certify the hours shown have been completed by me and are correct to my best knowledge.

FIG. 6–13. A time card need only be a sheet that records and totals the employee's hours and carries an employee acknowledgement of honesty.

- Number of exemptions claimed for tax purposes.
- Date of original employment.
- Birth date.
- Status as regards coverage under the company pension plan.
- Marital status.

(Rel.2–2/88 Pub.372)

§ 6.04 [2]   MANAGING YOUR MEDICAL PRACTICE   6–38

FIG. 6–14. An individual earnings record breaks down each employee's salary by paycheck and into quarterly totals.

(Rel.2–2/88 Pub.372)

FINANCIAL MANAGEMENT

The earnings section of the individual earnings record should include:

- Subdivisions detailing monthly, quarterly and annual earnings.

- Date.

- Check number.

(Text continued on page 6-39)

- Hours worked.
- Overtime hours.
- Regular hours.
- Pay rate.
- Salary for pay period.
- Gross regular salary for pay period.
- Gross overtime.
- FICA tax withheld.
- Federal withholding.
- State withholding.
- Local withholding.
- Other withholding (employee savings plan, insurance, expense reimbursement, etc.).
- Net check amount.

Each pay period the totals from the individual earnings record should be computed to make certain they balance with aggregate payroll figures. Each month, individual totals should be computed and balanced with the aggregate for the month. Each quarter, the individual record should be computed and balanced. These figures can be used to prepare federal and local tax deposits, along with quarterly payroll tax reports. At the end of the year, the individual earnings records can be used to prepare employee W-2 forms. Individual payroll records can also be used to calculate pension benefits accrued by employees.

[3] Vacation Records

To avoid having key people take vacations at the same time, it is important to set up a vacation calendar each year and record when people will be away. When a conflict occurs, you should give priority to employees based on procedures outlined in the personnel policy.

An individual vacation record should be kept for each employee. Each record should contain the employee's:

(Pub.372)

- Name.
- Social security number.
- Date of employment.
- Rate at which vacation time accrues (based on the applicable personnel policy).
- Chosen vacation dates.
- Explanation for vacation.
- Vacation time accrued.
- Vacation time used.
- Remaining balance of vacation time.

This simple record can help prevent vacation liabilities and misunderstandings between employee and employer over the amount of vacation due.

[4] Sick Pay Records

Individual sick pay records should contain the same basic information found on the employee's vacation record adjusted to reflect the amount of sick pay allowed under the personnel policy. Keeping an accurate sick pay record for each employee eliminates uncertainty as to whether or not an employee should be docked pay when he or she is absent from work as a result of illness. (See Figure 6–15.)

[5] Individual Earnings Reports to Employees

Since employees "see" only their net check, and not the various amounts withheld from their gross pay, they may undervalue their actual salary and benefits. Many employers prepare an annual record for each employee to outline the true remuneration he or she receives. (See Figure 6–16.)

- Name.
- Gross salary.
- Overtime salary.
- Bonuses, if paid.

Monetary values would also be given for:

FINANCIAL MANDATORY § 6.04 [5]

VACATION PAY RECORD

Date	Explanation	Unpaid Hours Used	Hours Earned	Hours Used	Balance Due (hours)

SICK PAY RECORD

Date	Explanation	Unpaid Hours Used	Hours Earned	Hours Used	Balance Due (hours)

FIG. 6–15. A combined sick pay and vacation pay record.

- Accrued vacation time.
- Accrued sick time.
- Employer contributions to the pension plan.
- Employer contributions to the profit sharing plan.

(Pub.372)

Approximate Benefit Analysis

Employee _____

Position _____

Benefit	Estimated Cost
Salary Base (with 40 hour week)	
FICA paid by employer	
State Unemployment Insurance	
Federal Unemployment Insurance	
Worker's Compensation Insurance	
Life/Health Insurance	
Pension & Profit Sharing Plans	
Vacation (weeks)	
Sick Pay (days)	
Paid Holidays (days)	
Uniforms	
Extra Bonuses	
Total	

FIG. 6–16. An individual earnings report that assigns a monetary value to all employee fringe benefits in addition to salary. A summary of benefits would typically include the employee's:

- Employer-paid health insurance.
- Employer-paid life insurance.
- Employer-paid disability insurance.
- Accrued medical reimbursement.
- Uniform allowances.

(Pub.372)

- Car allowances.
- Paid holidays.
- Fringe benefits (such as free coffee or food supplied by the physician).
- Total remuneration received.
- Worker's compensation insurance premiums.
- State unemployment insurance.
- Federal unemployment insurance.
- Employer share of FICA taxes.

This special report may shock the employee, as the total package of benefits paid by the employer typically comes to a far greater amount than the employee realizes. Normally, the individual report is prepared and discussed at the employee's individual performance and salary review.

[6] Check Writing System

Unless your practice is very small, you may find using the same checkbook for accounts payable and payroll cumbersome. If you employ more than a few people, the office should have special checks for payroll. It is not necessary to have a separate checking account or payroll, but it is advantageous to have separate checks and check records for each type of account.

When a payroll check is written, the employer's check stub and the employee's check stub should both show:

- Hours worked, including regular hours and overtime hours.
- Gross amount of check.
- Gross amount of regular check.
- Gross amount of overtime.
- Gross amount of bonus.
- FICA taxes withheld.
- Federal taxes withheld.
- State taxes withheld.

(Pub.372)

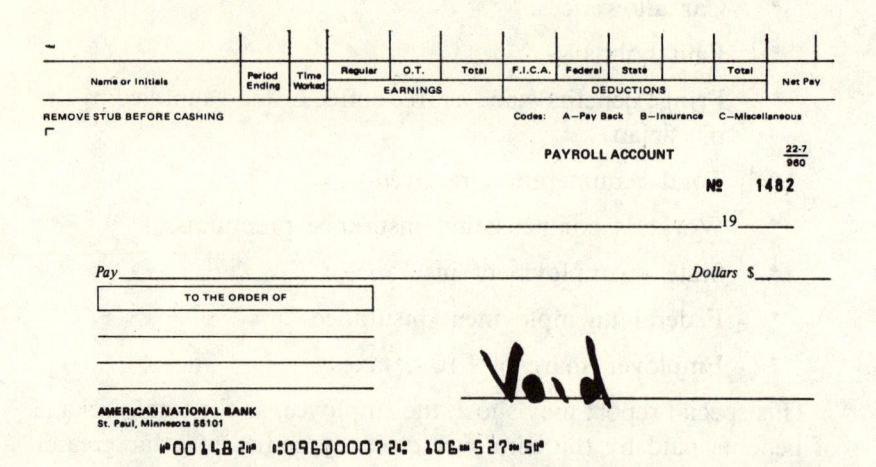

FIG. 6–17. A one-write payroll check. With the help of carbons, the detailed information is entered on the employee's check stub and in the employer's check register journal. The journal sheet can be added and cross-footed to assure mathematical accuracy before the check is disbursed.

- Local taxes withheld.
- Other withholdings (savings, insurance, dues, expense withholdings, etc.).
- Net check.

(See Figure 6–17 for a sample payroll check.)

Since all of these items need to be recorded in different places, a pegboard payroll system is very feasible if you have five or more employees and your system is not automated.

The pegboard accounts payable system is advantageous because it creates an employee check stub, carbon copies for an individual employee record and carbon copies for a journal sheet that can be used to quickly balance all of the payroll before the checks are disbursed. For larger practices an automated system is the most streamlined. Once the original program is set up, each pay period's time records are entered into the computer and the computer automatically computes proper withholdings, employee records, employee stubs, check registers, etc. Information stored in the computer can also generate quarterly summaries for payroll tax reports and annual W–2 statements.

(Pub.372)

To avoid months with excessive payroll and minimize the number of payroll checks issued, it is recommended that payroll be done twice monthly, rather than every two weeks. Doing payroll twice monthly requires 24 pay periods annually, contrasted to 26 biweekly periods and two months of the year that have three pay periods. It is common for employers paying twice a month to pay employees on the 15th and the last day of the month. If the 15th or last day of the month falls on a Saturday, checks are issued the Friday before; if the 15th or last day of the month falls on Sunday, the checks are issued on the following Monday.

[7] Payroll Taxes

Employers are required by law to withhold payroll taxes from employees. The IRS requires that employees file with their employer a W–4 form providing their complete name, address and social security number, the number of exemptions they claim, and certification that the information they supply is accurate. Employers are required to withhold as though the employee had filed for single status with no exemptions if an employee fails to file a W–4. If an employee claims more than 12 exemptions on the W–4, the employer is required to send a copy of the W–4 to the IRS. An employer may become responsible for an employee's income taxes (up to a minimum of what withholdings would have been with a single, no exemption election) if a properly completed W–4 is not filed and the employee fails to pay income taxes. (See Figures 6–18 and 6–19.)

[a] Standard Withholdings

Mandatory withholdings from an employee's pay are as follows:

FICA: The Federal Insurance Contribution Act, commonly known as social security. The tax collected under FICA is used to fund old age and survivor annuities and the Medicare program. Currently, the rate of withholding for this tax is 7.05 percent on the first $39,600.

Federal Withholding: The employer is required to withhold an amount from the employee's check based on earnings, marital status and the number of exemptions the employee claims. The federal government prepares an employer's tax guide that supplies figures

FIG. 6–18. A W–4 form, to be completed and filed by the employee.

FINANCIAL MANAGEMENT § 6.04 [7]

Line 5 of Form W-4

Additional amount, if any, you want deducted from each pay.—If you are not having enough tax withheld from your pay, you may ask your employer to withhold more by filling in an additional amount on line 5. Often, married couples, both of whom are working, and persons with two or more jobs need to have additional tax withheld. You may also need to have additional tax withheld because you have income other than wages, such as interest and dividends, capital gains, rents, alimony received, taxable social security benefits, etc. Estimate the amount you will be underwithheld and divide that amount by the number of pay periods in the year. Enter the additional amount you want withheld each pay period on line 5.

Line 6 of Form W-4

Exemption from withholding.—You can claim exemption from withholding only if last year you did not owe any Federal income tax and had a right to a refund of all income tax withheld, **and** this year you do not expect to owe any Federal income tax and expect to have a right to a refund of all income tax withheld. If you qualify, check Boxes 6a and b, write the year exempt status is effective and "EXEMPT" on line 6b, and answer Yes or No to the question on line 6c.

If you want to claim exemption from withholding next year, you must file a new W-4 with your employer on or before February 15 of next year. If you are not having Federal income tax withheld this year, but expect to have a tax liability next year, the law requires you to give your employer a new W-4 by December 1 of this year. If you are covered by social security, your employer must withhold social security tax.

Your employer must send to IRS any W-4 claiming more than 14 withholding allowances or claiming exemption from withholding if the wages are expected to usually exceed $200 a week. The employer is to complete Boxes 7, 8, and 9 only on copies of the W-4 sent to IRS.

Table 1—For Figuring Your Withholding Allowances For Estimated Tax Credits and Income Averaging (Line E)

Estimated Salaries and Wages from All sources	Single Employees (A)	Single Employees (B)	Head of Household Employees (A)	Head of Household Employees (B)	Married Employees (When Spouse not Employed) (A)	Married Employees (When Spouse not Employed) (B)	Married Employees (When Both Spouses are Employed) (A)	Married Employees (When Both Spouses are Employed) (B)
Under $15,000	$ 90	$150	$ 30	$150	$ 50	$120	$ 0	$120
15,000-25,000	120	250	0	250	70	170	310	170
25,001-35,000	190	300	0	300	130	250	800	220
35,001-45,000	250	370	0	370	170	320	1,500	250
45,001-55,000	690	370	0	370	230	340	2,210	330
55,001-65,000	1,470	370	220	370	310	370	3,020	330
Over 65,000	2,460	370	920	370	680	370	3,400	370

Worksheet to Figure Your Withholding Allowances to be Entered on Line 4 of Form W-4

A Personal allowances ▶ **A**
B Special withholding allowance (not to exceed 1 allowance—see instructions on page 1) ▶ **B**
C Allowances for dependents ▶ **C**

If you are not claiming any deductions or credits, skip lines D and E.

D Allowances for estimated deductions:

1 Enter the total amount of your estimated itemized deductions, alimony payments, qualified retirement contributions including IRA and Keogh (H.R. 10) plans, deduction for a married couple when both work, business losses including net operating loss carryovers, moving expenses, employee business expenses, penalty on early withdrawal of savings, and charitable contributions for nonitemizers for the year ▶ **1** $

2 If you do not plan to itemize deductions, enter $500 on line D2. If you plan to itemize, find your total estimated salaries and wages amount in the left column of the table below. (Include salaries and wages of both spouses.) Read across to the right and find the amount from the column that applies to you. Enter that amount on line D2. ▶ **2** $

Estimated salaries and wages from all sources:	Single and Head of Household Employees (only one job)	Married Employees (one spouse working and one job only)	Employees with more than one job or Married Employees with both spouses working [1]	
Under $15,000	$2,800	$3,900		40%
15,000-35,000	2,800	3,900	of estimated salaries and wages	23% of estimated salaries and wages
35,001-50,000	8% of estimated salaries and wages	3,900		20%
Over $50,000	10%		7% of estimated salaries and wages	18%

3 Subtract line D2 from line D1 (But not less than zero) ▶ **3** $
4 Divide the amount on line D3 by $1,000 (increase any fraction to the next whole number). Enter here ▶ **D**

E Allowances for tax credits and income averaging: use Table 1 above for figuring withholding allowances

1 Enter tax credits, excess social security tax withheld, and tax reduction from income averaging $
2 Enter the column (A) amount from Table 1 for your salary range and filing status (single, etc.). However, enter 0 if you claim 1 or more allowances on line D4 $
3 Subtract line 2 from line 1 (If zero or less, do not complete lines 4 and 5) $
4 Find the column (B) amount from Table 1 for your salary range and filing status
5 Divide line 3 by line 4. Increase any fraction to the next whole number. This is the maximum number of withholding allowances for tax credits and income averaging. Enter here ▶ **E**

Example: A taxpayer who expects to file a Federal income tax return as a single person estimates annual wages of $12,000 and tax credits of $650. The $12,000 falls in the wage bracket of under $15,000. The value in column (A) is 90. Subtracting this from the estimated credits of 650 leaves 560. The value in column (B) is 150. Dividing 560 by 150 gives 3.7. Since any fraction is increased to the next whole number, show 4 on line E.

F Total (add lines A through E). Enter total here and on line 4 of Form W-4 ▶ **F**

[1] If you earn 10% or less of your total wages from other jobs or one spouse earns 10% or less of the couple's combined total wages, you can use the "Single and Head of Household Employees (only one job)" or "Married Employees (one spouse working and one job only)" table, whichever is appropriate

(Rel.1–2/87 Pub.372)

§ 6.04 [7]   MANAGING YOUR MEDICAL PRACTICE   6-48

Control number	OMB No. 1545-0008			
2 Employer's name, address, and ZIP code		3 Employer's identification number		4 Employer's State number
		5 Stat employee ☐ Deceased ☐ Legal rep ☐	942 emp ☐ Subtotal ☐ Void ☐	
		6 Allocated tips	7 Advance EIC payment	
8 Employee's social security number	9 Federal income tax withheld	10 Wages, tips, other compensation	11 Social security tax withheld	
12 Employee's name, address, and ZIP code		13 Social security wages	14 Social security tips	
		16		
		17 State income tax	18 State wages, tips, etc.	19 Name of State
		20 Local income tax	21 Local wages, tips, etc.	22 Name of locality

Form W-2 Wage and Tax Statement 1984   Copy 1 For State, City, or Local Tax Department
Employee's and employer's copy compared ☐

FIG. 6–19. A W–2 form, to be filled in by the employer and sent to the employee at the end of the year for taxation records.

for the amount of withholding, for which the employee will receive credit on his or her income taxes.

State and Local Taxes: Like federal withholding taxes, state and local withholding taxes are withheld by the employer and credit is given to the employee on income taxes. Generally, the states and localities supply booklets to help determine the amount of withholding based on the employee's marital status, claimed exemptions and earnings.

In addition to the amounts of taxes withheld from an employee, an employer is required to pay certain payroll taxes out of revenue:

FICA: The government requires that the employer match each dollar of tax withheld from the employee. Mismatching dollars count as 100 percent employer expense.

Federal Unemployment Taxes: The federal government requires that a tax be paid based on the gross payroll for unemployment. Although unemployment programs are administered by the various states and localities, the federal tax is used to subsidize state and local revenue when they fall short. The rate of the federal tax may change since a credit is applied against the federal rate, depending on the state a physician practices in. A local IRS office must be

(Rel.1–2/87 Pub.372)

contacted to determine the rate of withholding. The current maximum base per employee is $7,000.

State Unemployment Taxes: An unemployment tax is assessed by and directly paid to the state. This tax is used to finance the bulk of unemployment benefits. The rate generally varies from state to state, and typically is based on an experience rating. An employer with a small employee turnover generally has a lower rate than an employer with high employee turnover. Local authorities must be contacted to determine the correct rate and base charges for the state. Normally, a rate is assigned to employers on an individual basis, rather than in blanket fashion.

[b] Penalties

The government requires employers to make periodic payments of payroll taxes. Since the government considers withholding taxes employee money, the employer is considered a fiduciary. In general, the government severely penalizes employers delinquent in paying these taxes. An immediate five percent penalty is the standard assessment if payroll taxes are only a day late.

The first step toward avoiding payroll tax penalties is to determine the amount for which you, as an employer, are liable. For state withholding taxes, the amount of liability is computed by adding the total state withholdings of employees. The federal tax deposit is slightly more complicated. It currently requires that the total FICA taxes withheld be multiplied by two and added to the federal withholding of employees.

The second step toward avoiding payroll tax penalties is to know when the tax is due. The earliest any payroll tax is due is three days after the time it is withheld. A physician who wishes to simplify tax deposits and avoid learning all of the rules may wish to simply calculate taxes each time a payroll is done and make the proper deposits within this three day period, whether or not they are due. A physician willing to become slightly more involved in stretching out the tax deposits can follow these basic rules:

- If the total liability, i.e. FICA tax times 2, plus federal withholding, cumulative, is less than $500, the amount should be paid by the 15th of the month following the calendar quarter in which the taxes are withheld.

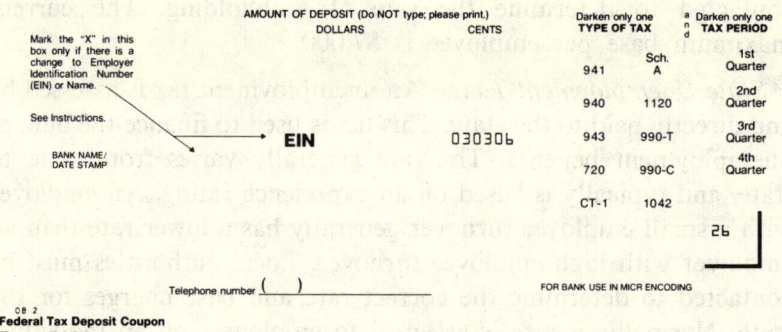

§ 6.04 [7]   MANAGING YOUR MEDICAL PRACTICE   6–50

Federal Tax Deposit Coupon
Form 8109 (Rev. 9-85)

FIG. 6–20. A federal tax deposit form. Generally, an employer uses this form for payroll tax deposits. When federal and state taxes are to be withheld the "941" box should be checked off and the proper calendar quarter should be checked. This form should be sent with a check to the bank, which then deposits this money with the IRS so that the taxpayer receives credit.

- If the cumulative tax liability is over $500, but less than $3,000, the amount must be deposited by the 15th of the month following the withholding.

- If the amount of cumulative withholding is $3,000 or more, the deposit must be made within three days.

(These three rules are simplifications of standard IRS rules.)

The advantage of not paying taxes until the due date is that the employer enjoys the extra cash flow and can theoretically earn interest on the money. Most physicians do not have large enough payrolls to consider doing this and some who do forget to pay the tax on time and incur a penalty far in excess of the interest they earn. However, large practices with large payrolls generally take advantage of the possibilities.

The IRS requires payroll tax deposits to be made directly to a bank acting as a federal depository. To ensure that proper credit is given to the employer's account, a special coupon issued by the IRS is used to make the payroll tax deposit. (See Figure 6–20.)

The government sends coupon books directly to the employers when they apply for the federal identification number. If coupons become lost or otherwise unavailable, the local IRS office should be immediately contacted and generic forms obtained so that payroll tax deposits may be made. The IRS does not consider not having the coupon book an adequate reason for making a late deposit.

[8] Payroll Tax Reports

The federal government, and many states, require quarterly tax reports that summarize the withholding information and reconcile the withholding from employees and employer fair share of FICA

(Text continued on page 6-51)

with payroll tax deposits. These tax reports are used to determine employer liability and penalties. The quarterly tax reports are due the last day of the month following the calendar quarter. (See Figure 6–21.)

An annual unemployment report is used to calculate the exact amount of unemployment taxes due. Although this report is due annually, a deposit for unemployment taxes must be made by the 30th of the month following a calendar quarter if the total employer liability exceeds $100.

Most physicians rely on assistance from outside accounting professionals in preparation of quarterly and annual tax reports.

[9] Non-Employee Compensation

A physician makes payment to individuals besides employees, such as outside consultants or maintenance workers. Federal law requires that a business paying an unincorporated business or individual an amount more than $600 in a calendar year keep track of the amount paid and report that amount to the government and employee at the end of the year for tax purposes (many states require the same information). Furthermore, current law requires that proper identification numbers be filed on these forms. If an unincorporated business refuses to give the identification number, the "employer" must withhold 10 percent of the gross amount and deposit that money with payroll taxes. Since many physicians are unaware of this, they end up without proper records for these disbursements and without proper identification numbers. Failure to comply with this law may result in a 10 percent penalty.

To keep track of these disbursements throughout the year, you must keep a record similar to an individual employee record for all unincorporated businesses that provide you with more than $600 worth of services. You must also request the recipient's proper identification number and maintain that on file.

§ 6.05 General Ledger

> The general ledger is a record of all accounts kept by a practice for both income and expenses. It includes bank deposits, which are generally equal to the sum of all sources of income, and checkbook disbursements for items such as payroll checks and general practice

§ 6.05 MANAGING YOUR MEDICAL PRACTICE 6-52

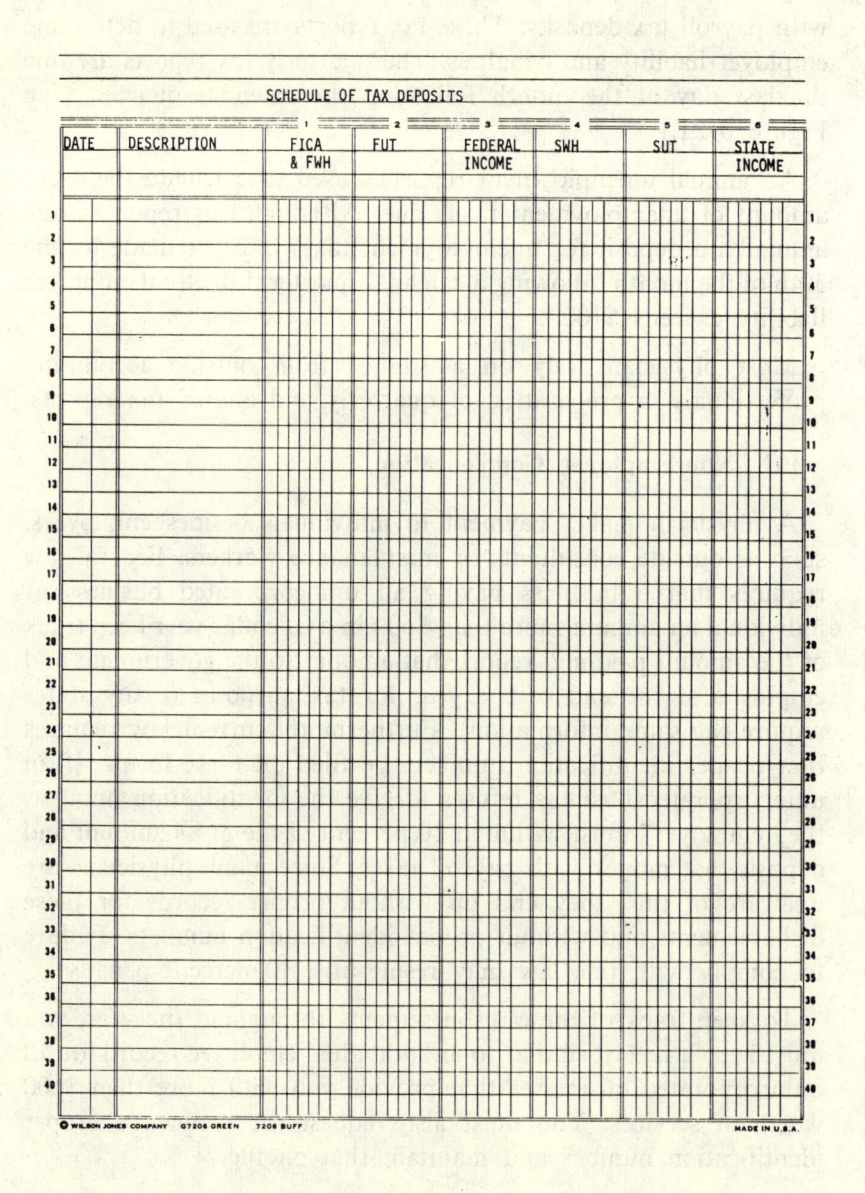

FIG. 6–21. A schedule of tax deposits.

expenses. When properly detailed, the general ledger allows an employer to account for every credit and debit and to regularly reconcile total balances and individual running balances. Although outside accountants are usually retained to compile the majority of

(Pub.372)

information in the general ledger, it behooves an employer to understand the basic principles behind it.

The general ledger is defined as the various groups of accounts kept by a business and the balancing of those accounts. A practice must keep a general ledger to show adequate accounting for income, expenses, assets, liabilities and equity.

Normally, an outside accounting firm is used to provide a substantial portion of services relating to the general ledger. Small practices may do a portion of the general ledger processing themselves and leave final balancing of quarterly or year-end adjustments to an accountant. Larger practices may employ an in-house accountant, although outside accountants are generally retained at the end of the year to compile a financial report.

The medical office's general ledger can be broken down into a few major sections. The source of most information for the general ledger is the business checking account. Accounts receivable and accounts payable are generally not salient for a medical office general ledger, since most physicians are on a cash basis of accounting (i.e., they count income as cash collected and expenses as bills paid). Only under an accrual method of accounting, in which income is considered income when charges are made and expenses are considered expenses at the time they are are incurred, is it necessary to bring both the accounts payable and accounts receivable into the general ledger.

[1] Bank Deposits

Deposits add to the balance of an asset account (the bank account). In the dual-entry method of accounting, a credit entry must be made for each debit entry and vice versa. That is, with each bank deposit, the checking account is debited and an offsetting credit entry is made into another account, usually the patient receipt account. Normal credit entries in the medical office include:

- Income from patient services.
- Interest income.
- Miscellaneous income (EKG reading fees, court deposition, expert witness fees, etc.).

- Liability account (bank loan proceeds, a stockholder loan, etc.).

- Equity contribution (proprietorship capital payments from the doctor, initial capitalization of corporation, additional capitalization of corporation, etc.).

Since the practice's bank deposit is usually equal to the sum of all its various incomes, the cash journal generally breaks down income items and carries a running balance for each. Unusual items, such as bank loans or capitalization, would be posted to the liability and equity accounts.

[2] Checkbook Disbursements

Since disbursements from the checkbook are charged against an asset account (i.e., the checking account), the checking account is credited for each disbursement. Since each credit must have an offsetting debit entry to balance the general ledger, each disbursement must also have a debit entry. Normal debits for a medical office include:

- Expenses (charged against the proper expense account).
- Patient refunds (charged against patient receipts).
- Capital acquisitions (on equipment, office furniture or leasehold improvements).
- Principle payments on debt.
- Dividends paid.
- Draws by the proprietor (e.g., physician draws for unincorporated practices).
- Loans (typically stockholder loans to the physician).

[a] General Disbursements

For the practice that keeps a general ledger manually, the bulk of financial transactions will be disbursements. The best way to handle them is by setting up a spreadsheet divided into columns. The first column contains the date of the disbursement, the second column describes whom the check was written to, the third column indicates the check number and the fourth column shows the amount of the check. To the right of the check amount column

(Pub.372)

(column four), numerous columns should be set up for categorizing the various expenses. Each column would be considered the expense account for that type of item. The final column should be reserved as a general column for unusual disbursements (loan payments, capital expenditures, etc.). Each month the check amount column is totaled and balanced against the sum total of the other columns. The year-to-date totals in the expense columns may be used as account balances; each of the figures listed in the general column (the last column), however, must be posted to their relevant account so that a running balance is maintained.

[b] Payroll Check Disbursements

The most difficult expense to handle in the general ledger is the payroll expense. Each payroll check generally has at least four credit entries—net payroll check, FICA tax withheld, federal withholding and state and local withholding—and one debit entry, the salary expense. For simplicity, it is recommended that payroll checks be listed separately from general accounts payable checks. The listing sheets or journal sheets for payroll checks should include columns for:

- Date
- Employee
- Check number
- Gross amount of payroll (the debit amount)
- FICA withholding
- Federal withholding
- Other withholding
- Net check

The totals of each payroll journal should be balanced; in other words, the sum of the net check and withholding should equal the gross. The following could then be entered into the expense journal:

- Debit: salary expense
- Credit: disbursements from checkbook
  FICA withholding liability
  federal withholding liability

(Pub.372)

state withholding liability
any other withholding liability

When a payroll tax deposit is made, the bulk of the check is generally applied against the liability of payroll taxes withheld. The portion of the deposit representing the employer's share of FICA is charged to business expenses.

[3] Reconciling Records

A reconciliation of the checkbook with the general ledger, using total deposits from the cash journal and total disbursements from the disbursement journal, should confirm totals through one of two equations.

(1) Beginning balance
 + Deposits from cash journal
 = Disbursements from the disbursement journal
 = New balance

or

(2) Balance per bank statement
 − Outstanding checks issued for the month that have not yet cleared the bank
 + Outstanding deposits made for the month that have not yet cleared the bank
 = Bank balance

After the bank reconciliation is completed, all of the deposits and checks have been listed, spread and cross-footed and the general items have been posted, all of the accounts should be totaled. The sum of the balances in the asset and expense accounts should equal the sum of the balances in the income, liability and equity accounts. This is what accountants refer to as the trial balance. (See Figure 6–22.)

Although this section cannot give a complete lesson in accounting, it should familiarize the physician with some of the basic accounting terminology and general accounting problems faced by the medical office. A complete understanding of bookkeeping systems would require formal training and schooling, which is why

Checking Account Reconciliation Report

As of _____

Beginning Balance — — —	$ _____
Plus Deposits & Bank Credits	_____
Less: Total Checks Issued & Bank Debits	_____
Ending Balance — — —	$ _____
Balance Per Bank Statement	$ _____
Less Outstanding Checks	_____
Subtotal	$ _____
Outstanding Deposits	_____
Ending Balance — — —	$ _____

Comments & Notes

_____

_____

_____

_____

_____

_____

_____

_____

_____

FIG. 6–22. A form to be used when reconciling checkbook balance to general ledger balance. Reconciliation should be done on at least a monthly basis.

most offices use the services of an accountant. In fact, unless the office has an experienced bookkeeper, it is desirable to have the general ledger prepared in its entirety by an outside accounting group.

(Pub.372)

§ 6.06 Choosing an Accountant

> Many physicians retain professional accountants to oversee their financial records. Criteria for selecting an accountant include good references and membership in an accredited professional organization. A good accountant should be able to communicate with the physician and make basic money management concepts understandable.

You should not be embarrassed or intimidated by the prospect of hiring an accountant, especially when you consider the importance of having the practice's finances organized and the penalties that can result from their mismanagement.

The financial report in the medical office should serve two purposes: it should be adequate for preparation of necessary income tax returns and it should provide useful, understandable information. The first rule for hiring an accountant, therefore, is to select one with whom you can communicate. By going over the income and expense categories mentioned in this chapter and spending time together at the outset, you and your accountant can produce a useful management report.

[1] Criteria for Selection

You should select an accountant in much the same way you would select a staff employee. First, you should create a pool of prospective accountants. Begin with referrals from other physicians and ask if the accountant:

- Provides reports that contain useful management information.
- Makes reports understandable.
- Takes time to explain reports and answer questions.
- Provides timely service.
- Produces quick financial reports.
- Has ever been late filing tax returns.
- Always files extensions.
- Represents you in the event of an IRS audit.
- Discusses the consequences of financial decisions (i.e., does he or she recommend alternative strategies to minimize taxation?).

(Pub.372)

If you don't get a positive response to these questions, keep looking for referrals. If you are considering an accountant who has not been referred to you, ask the accountant for three or four references and ask the same questions of those references.

[2] Professional Credentials

The following list gives the meaning of some accounting credentials:

American Institute of Certified Public Accountants (AICPA): AICPA is a national organization of certified public accountants. Although its main certification and purpose centers around public auditing (mainly large and major publicly held corporations), many members have sought to accommodate small businesses. Some specialize in the medical area and some firms have divisions or accountants on staff who specialize in servicing physicians. A licensed CPA has passed a rigorous examination and has a minimum of three years experience. Continued membership in the AICPA requires adherence to basic ethical requirements.

National Society of Public Accountants (NSPA): This society is comprised of accounting firms throughout the nation serving small businesses. Most members of the NSPA are not CPAs. Membership in the NSPA requires adherence to a different code of ethics.

Accreditation Council of Accountancy: This organization provides accreditation in accounting and taxation. Accountants who have been accredited have passed rigorous examinations, must maintain the council's code of ethics and must keep up to date through minimum continuing education.

Enrollment to Practice Before the IRS (Enrolled Agents): Accountants passing a rigorous tax examination conducted by the Internal Revenue Service are granted privilege to practice before the IRS. Enrolled agents may practice before the IRS in the same capacity as CPAs and attorneys.

Society of Medical/Dental Management Consultants (SMD): This national organization of consultants specializes in the medical/dental area. Many members of the SMD provide accounting services to physicians. Since members of SMD have limited their practice to physicians and dentists, you are assured that you are receiving service from experienced specialists.

(Pub.372)

Society of Professional Business Consultants: This national organization of consultants also provides services exclusively to professionals, including physicians.

Once you have three or four accountants in mind, make appointments to see them. Ask the prospective accountant for a resume of his or her accounting degree, certifications and memberships. During the interview, ask the following questions:

- If I select your organization, will I be working directly with you? If not, whom will I be working with?
- How long have you been in public accounting?
- How many (name your specialty) have you worked with?
- In what ways will your reports help me manage my practice? How quickly will I receive my financial report at the end of the month?
- Can you provide me with comparative statistical data on other specialists in my field for the key areas of my practice? How often do you recommend we sit down and do tax planning?
- What kind of advice could you give me to help minimize my taxes?
- Are you familiar with professional associations? Corporate pension plans?
- What would be the cost for monthly service? What services would that fee include? What services would cost additionally? What would be my annual fees?

Have the accountant show you sample reports and see if you can understand them. If you can't, see if the accountant can explain them to you so that you can get a clear picture of their meaning.

Changing accountants is difficult. Nevertheless, if you feel you are not getting the proper service from your accountant or that you are getting reports that have no meaning for you, do not hesitate to change after talking with the accountant and giving him or her a chance to correct the problem.

§ 6.07 Cash Flow Management

By taking advantage of money market funds, pension plans, bonuses and early pay discounts a physician can use cash flow to increase profits and minimize expenses.

It is not unusual for a great deal of money to move through a medical practice, particularly a group practice. By managing cash flow wisely—i.e., taking advantage of cash balances to earn money and avoid service charges—a practice can increase this income and reduce expenses.

[1] Money Market vs. Checking Account

As a minimum requisite of cash flow management, you should set up a money market account (which has a higher yield than most checking accounts that pay interest) in addition to a checking account for the practice. The bank will tell you the minimum balance needed for the checking account so that you will not incur service charges. The bookkeeper should constantly be aware of this minimum balance and, as the checking account balance exceeds that minimum, the excess should be transferred to the money market account. The money should remain there unless checks drawn on the account make it necessary to transfer money back from the money market fund to avoid slipping below the minimum balance.

[2] Early Contributions to Pension and Profit Sharing

Many physicians make good use of their money by making early contributions to their pension and profit sharing plans. Some even go without a salary for a few months to "prefund" their fiscal year retirement plan contributions. Placing money into the pension account early offers several advantages:

- The money in the pension account is available for higher yielding investments than money in the money market.
- The money is in the account for a longer period of time and thus earns more interest.
- Earnings in the pension profit sharing plan escape initial taxation. The tax savings generated are used to compound the investments and earnings.

(Pub.372)

[3] Periodic Bonuses

Rather than allow money to accumulate in the practice, physicians typically distribute profits on a periodic basis. This permits them to put their income to best use immediately.

[4] Early Pay Discounts

A typical supplier statement might note the following terms: "2/10, net/30." This means that a two percent discount may be taken if the bill is paid in ten days, otherwise the balance is due in 30. A two percent discount, acquired by paying the bill 30 days early, is equivalent to an annual yield of 24 percent. Alert your bookkeeper to take advantage of early payment discounts whenever possible.

§ 6.08 Financial Management Checklist

A review of steps for managing practice finances is given.

— Prepare a financial report

— Incorporate financial forecast of revenues and expenses into budget and monthly operating statement

— Design and implement financial reports
  — Income statement
  — Monthly trend analysis
  — Practice comparison
  — Cash flow reports

— Implement complete accounts payable system to monitor and keep control of accounts receivable
  — Centralize purchasing
  — Keep purchase orders
  — Check packing invoices
  — Review supplier statements
  — Select time(s) at which bills will be paid
  — Establish filing system for control and tax purposes

(Pub.372)

- Establish petty cash account for minor expenditures
- Include proper documentation and receipt file

— Establish accurate payroll system and records
- Time cards
- Individual earnings records
- Sick pay records
- Individual earnings and compensation report to employees
- Check writing system with base stub
- Payroll tax withholdings and deposits
- Employee W-4 forms
- Non-employee compensation records

— General ledger
- Chart of accounts
- Manual
- Computerized

— Bank deposits
- Duplicate records
- Identify revenue source

— Checkbook disbursement system
— Cash flow management
- Savings accounts
- Money market accounts
- Minimum balance
- Advanced pension and profit sharing contributions
- Bonuses to physicians
- Early pay discount

(Pub.372)

§ 6.100 Bibliography

Lusk, E. J. and Lusk, J.G.: Financial and Managerial Control: A Health Care Perspective. Germantown, MD: Aspen Systems Corp., 1979.

Silvers, J. B. and Pralhalad, C.K.: Financial Management of Health Institutions. Flushing, NY: Spectrum Publications, distributed by Halstad Press, 1974.

CHAPTER 7

Credit and Collections

SCOPE

While physicians recognize the need to be compensated for services, they may also feel guilty if the cost of services that maintain or enhance a patient's quality of life place that patient under economic stress. Nevertheless, the medical office must have an effective credit and collection policy if it is to continue serving patients fairly. A credit and collection policy must be consistent with the physician's professional philosophy, consider all possibilities in the physician-patient-third-party insurer relationship and be reasonable enough to satisfy all parties involved. Over the years, third parties have complicated the collection process in the medical office. In many cases, special forms for billing, coding of every medical procedure and diagnosis and contractual relationships with third parties have become necessary. As a result, the medical office suddenly needs to have different credit and collection policies for patients and groups of patients, as well as billing methods to accommodate the third party. In circumstances where it is necessary to enter a participation agreement, the physician should know what the insuror considers relative values for services performed and the physician's own personal and community profile. If a patient does not pay at the time services are rendered, the physician should have a follow-up system for sending out statements and collection letter reminders and for making phone calls. Accounts of patients who ignore paying must often be turned over to collection agencies, credit bureaus and occasionally to a conciliation court. A physician should always keep meticulous records of any collection transactions as both a reminder to the office staff and proof of an outstanding account. Regularly monitoring accounts receivable can inform the physician in advance of any problem accounts and possibly forestall the need to resort to drastic collection activities.

(Pub.372)

MANAGING YOUR MEDICAL PRACTICE

SYNOPSIS

§ 7.01 Guidelines for Establishing a Credit Policy
    [1] Credit Philosophy
    [2] Marketing
    [3] Physician-Patient Legal Relationship

§ 7.02 Written Collection Policy

§ 7.03 Collecting from Third Parties
    [1] CPT Codes
    [2] Diagnostic Codes
    [3] HCPCS
    [4] Relative Values
    [5] Profiles
    [6] Participation Agreements
        [a] Pros and Cons of Participation in Third-Party Agreements
        [b] Evaluating Contracts
    [7] Assignment of Benefits

§ 7.04 Collecting from Patients
    [1] Time-of-Service Payments
    [2] The Statement Process
        [a] Sequence
        [b] Computerized and Manual Collection Statements
    [3] Collection Letters
        [a] Collection Letter Procedure
        [b] Credit Arrangements
        [c] Special Circumstances
    [4] Collection Letter Services
    [5] Collection Telephone Calls
        [a] Sample Telephone Calls
        [b] Obtaining a Commitment from the Patient
    [6] Collection Agencies
        [a] Finding an Agency
        [b] Trying Out Agencies
        [c] Monitoring Agencies
    [7] Credit Bureaus
    [8] Conciliation Court
        [a] Advantages and Disadvantages
        [b] Conciliation Court Procedures

§ 7.05 Monitoring Collections

(Pub.372)

        [1]   Areas to Review
        [2]   Manual vs. Computerized Monitoring
§ 7.06   Collections Checklist
§ 7.07–§ 7.99   Reserved
§ 7.100   Bibliography
Appendix 7–A   Credit and Collection Policy
Appendix 7–B   Credit Letters

§ 7.01 Guidelines for Establishing a Credit Policy

> A physician must have a credit and collection policy compatible with his or her professional philosophy. That policy, however, must also be agreeable to the patient and consistent with credit and collection policies to which the patient is accustomed. A good policy will (1) consider the right of the physician to compensation for services rendered; (2) consider the right of the patient to well-rendered services; (3) take into account the likelihood of involvement with third-party insurers; and (4) stay within the boundaries of laws established to define the creditor-debtor relationship.

A credit and collection policy is as essential for the life of a medical practice as it is for any business that provides consumer services. However, before a physician can establish a credit policy, he or she must consider a number of important factors.

[1] Credit Philosophy

Physicians are healers, frequently involved in life and death crises. What is important to the physician professionally is the care of patients, not the collection of money. Many physicians despise the business side of medicine and entrust it to an assistant. This works well if the credit and collection procedures implemented by the medical assistant are consistent with the physician's philosophy. If they are not, disgruntled patients will find they can avoid payment of their bills simply by complaining to the doctor and undermining the assistant's policy.

In developing a philosophy toward collections, you should consider the following points:

- Medical services are generally a necessity, not a luxury.
- Most patients are generally honest and make every effort to pay their bill.

(Pub.372)

- People do not "plan" on becoming ill, so their budgets often cannot accommodate unexpected medical bills.

- Patients who need medical services, but who have not had medical care recently, may find the cost extremely high, not unlike the "sticker shock" people experience when they look at new cars.

- Many physicians have paid a great deal of tuition and are in debt when they complete their residencies.

- Because schooling and residency programs go on for an extensive period of time, physicians lose some earning power while they are in school.

- Most physicians assume grave responsibilities and work long hours under stress.

- To provide competent medical services, a physician must maintain a competent staff and facilities. Funding of the physician's staff and facilities must come from patient collections.

- When a patient refuses to pay, the revenues lost must be subsidized by patients who do pay.

- A substantial portion of medical costs are paid by insurance. When patients fail to pay, it may be because they have illegally retained the insurance payments.

[2] Marketing

The next consideration in developing credit lines and credit policies is marketing. Having 100 percent collections does not mean much if you are only seeing two patients. Some physicians adopt a strict "cash only" policy, and as might be predicted, these physicians do not have the largest practices. They can't stand to lose any of their charges to patients who are unable or unwilling to pay their bills and adopt a credit policy that is convenient and efficient for them but unreasonable for patients.

A physician who is uncertain of how to establish a credit policy might want to ponder some marketing considerations:

- In today's credit-oriented society many people are used to doing business on a credit basis. The physician who demands cash may lose patients who feel that the physician is more interested in money than in health.

- Since a good many medical costs are covered by insurance it may be unreasonable to expect a patient to pay for covered services before they are reimbursed.

- By having insurance benefits assigned directly to the physician, the actual cost to and financial burden upon the patient is less. This may create an image of affordability of the medical services.

- While many patients are credit-oriented, others prefer to pay at the time of service, especially for procedures not covered by insurance. A billing system should be designed to accommodate both groups of patients. Patients want to know what is expected of them financially. The medical office that is uncomfortable with, confused about or unable to discuss its credit policy creates confusion and apprehension in the patient.

- Patients with outstanding balances who, for financial reasons, are unable to pay the entire bill, yet are satisfied with the physician's services, usually prefer to get the bill paid off. Talking with patients and working with them on payment arrangements often makes them feel better.

- Patients with large bills, who are uncertain about how they are going to pay them, may delay or avoid seeking necessary medical services because of guilt.

- The value of services performed diminishes in the mind of the patient with time. The quicker the patient knows the fee and charge for services, the better the chances that the charges will seem reasonable.

If billing and collections are the business side of a medical practice, a physician must appreciate marketing considerations when establishing a credit policy. Few physicians are in a position to ignore the consequences of a poor collection tactics. Fortunately, most items that are positive from a marketing aspect are congruent with good credit policies.

(Pub.372)

[3] Physician-Patient Legal Relationship

A credit and collection policy must demonstrate a basic awareness of both patient and physician rights. The policy must recognize the physician's right to be paid for services performed, and the patient's right to refuse or defer payment under certain circumstances. For example, it may be difficult for the physician to collect from a patient for a broken appointment when no services have been performed.

The policy should also demonstrate an awareness of the responsiblities involved in a relationship with third parties. If the physician does not have a contractual relationship with the third party, whatever reimbursement the patient receives or does not receive is between the patient and the third party and the physician must rely on the patient to pay him or her the amount billed for. On the other hand, if the physician has a contractual relationship with the third party—for example, a Blue Cross participation agreement—the policy must direct collection efforts and responsibilities to the proper party.

All physicians must be aware of a number of federal laws that must be complied with when establishing a credit and collection system:

Truth in Lending: Congress passed the Truth in Lending Act in 1968 and amended it in 1975 (Fair Credit Billing Act) and 1980. The purpose of this law was to protect consumers from excessive finance charges or service charges. When a business falls under the truth in lending laws, it places a substantial burden on the business to continually provide information to credit customers on their legal rights and total amount of finance charges. Detailed credit card billings, for example, are a result of the truth in lending law. A physician can avoid the truth in lending law if his or her collection policy keeps within specific boundaries:

- No interest is charged.

- No finance charges or any other charges for the extension of credit are made.

- No formal written agreements for installment payments where there are more than four installments (including the down payment) are made.

- If there are any collection charges, past due charges or late charges they are not related to the size of the bill.

Because of these exclusions, many physicians are able to avoid the regulations of truth in lending legislation.

Equal Credit Opportunity Act: This law, passed in 1974, was designed to eliminate discrimination in credit practices. The creditor falling under this act cannot consider an applicant's sex, color, race, religion or national origin. The creditor may not inquire about birth control methods, an applicant's plans to have children or the applicant's marital status. The creditor may not elect to exclude income items such as part-time employment or retirement benefits, alimony, child support or separate maintenance payments when considering whether or not to extend the applicant credit. Physicians affected by this act are subject to additional paperwork and potentially large fines for any violations.

Fortunately the law allows an exclusion for businesses that grant only incidental credit, and most physicians avoid the law under this exclusion. The physician who avoids truth in lending regulations may also avoid the equal credit opportunity act.

Fair Debt Collection Act: This act became effective in 1978. It was designed to regulate the activities of the professional debt collector. Any creditor, however, who uses a name other than that of the business falls under this act. The physician avoids falling under the Fair Debt Collection Act simply by collecting debts in the name of the business.

These laws are covered in greater detail in Chapter 12, "Law for the Medical Office." Physicians who do not take steps to avoid being affected by these laws must comply with them. You should obtain a copy of the regulations of these laws to find out if your practice falls within their purview. These regulations, published by the federal government, outline the various rules the physician must follow to comply with the Truth in Lending Law.

§ 7.02 Written Collection Policy

Once a collection policy is agreed upon it should be written out for the benefit of office workers who will do the collecting and for the benefit of the patient. The policy should detail (1) the various types of charges collected; (2) the party responsible for paying them; (3) when charges are due; and (4) when and where any exceptions to the policy are allowed.

Once a physician has considered and discussed the philosophical, marketing and legal considerations of a satisfactory collection policy, he or she should write it out. A written collection policy makes the physician's position on credit and collections clear to both employees responsible for collecting the accounts receivable and to patients who owe money.

If you do not take time to develop and express a solid position on collections, you can confuse all parties involved. A sure way to render collection procedures ineffective is to make office workers uncomfortable with a credit policy based on inconsistent decisions that allow patients to get around the personnel who normally do the collecting by going directly to you.

A written collection policy should include the following provisions:

Definition of Different Types of Charges: Normally in a physician's office different types of charges are handled in different ways. For example, a physician may require a cash payment for a new patient's first visit to the office. That same physician, however, is unlikely to require a cash payment for a new patient if the first charge is at the hospital as a result of a consultation ordered by another physician. If the patient has insurance coverage, and the physician allows assignment of benefits, services covered by the insurance company and those not covered may be treated differently. The physician may be willing to extend patient payments for the uncovered portion for several months, but expect immediate and full payment from the insurance company for the insured portion.

Definition of the Responsible Party: In most cases the patient is responsible for payments, regardless of whether he or she has assigned benefits to the physician. Minors and incapacitated adults are the exceptions. Another exception is the patient whose third-party insurer has contractual arrangements with the physician. For example, in the event of Blue Cross/Blue Shield coverage, a participating physician may not bill the patient for monies due from Blue Cross/Blue Shield. The physician may only bill the patient for that portion of the bill for which the patient is responsible.

When the Bill Is Due: Once the type of payment and the

responsible party are defined, the timing allowed for payment must be defined. Is the payment for services due at the time rendered, upon receipt of the first statement, within thirty days of the first statement, within sixty days, etc?

Terms: If the policy allows any exceptions with regard to when payment is due or how and from whom it is accepted, these should be outlined in the credit policy.

Appendix 7-A provides an illustrated sample of a written office collection policy.

Each physician or group of physicians must design their own policy. Considering the rapidly changing contracts and physician participation in third party contracts, the collection policy may need to be reviewed and revised periodically. It is important from both a marketing and collection standpoint to have a key person in the office familiar with third party reimbursement. Although it is not necessary for your office to be familiar with every third party, if your office is not familiar with a particular carrier it should be able to direct the patient to a source from which he or she can get more information. The collection policy should be very firm, yet still be able to accommodate patients who are unable to make full payment in a timely fashion (it is unrealistic to think this will not occur). Patients should be encouraged to communicate with the physician's credit department, and the burden of communication should initially be placed on the patient.

§ 7.03 Collecting from Third Parties

Owing to the great number of third party insurers a physician may encounter, it is a good idea to have an office credit manager who is experienced in dealing with private insurers, government regulated medical aid programs, major national carriers such as Blue Cross/Blue Shield and physician organizations. Among the many things that must be known before the physician can receive proper compensation for services from third parties are the proper procedure and diagnostic codes on standardized forms; the relative value of services performed and the physician and community profiles that some insurers use to determine reimbursement; and the intricacies of physician-third party relationships as regards participation agreements or the assignment of benefits directly to the physician. The physician and/or credit manager should do a comparative study of participation agreements and assignation of benefits to determine

(Pub.372)

which are the easiest and the most likely to guarantee satisfactory compensation.

It is no longer good business for a physician to ignore third parties. Indeed, it is almost impossible, since a majority of health care payments are funded through insurance and governmental programs. The physician who ignores third parties and places the full burden for services on the patients does them a disservice and hurts his or her collections and public image.

You and your staff should be familiar with how third party reimbursement works and what can be done to obtain the most from third parties. If you have a direct contract with the third party, billing errors can result in a direct loss to the practice. In cases where you do not have a relationship with the third party, you may receive an indirect loss if improper billing procedures are employed: you may simply never be paid for the bill or payment may be delayed if the patient was counting on insurance reimbursement and did not receive it. A good credit manager in a medical office will be more familiar with the various third parties than the average patient, and will help address any contingency as it arises.

[1] CPT Codes

Many procedures share the same name but differ in definition (for example, what takes place during a five-minute office visit is usually different than what occurs during a forty-five minute office visit). Procedures that have more than one name can cause further confusion. For the third parties to gain any type of control or understanding of these procedures, it became necessary for them to develop and assign codes to all of the procedures performed by physicians.

The American Medical Association publishes a text called "Current Procedure Terminology–5." It provides the "CPT" codes generally used by insurance companies to identify medical procedures. Nearly all major insurance companies require that bills sent to them be coded in accordance with the definitions of "Current Procedure Terminology–5." Most physicians use CPT coding for all billing.

[2] Diagnostic Codes

Most insurance companies do not pay for medical services performed for well patients; i.e., they generally do not cover examinations and minor office calls. Thus, a diagnosis and its meaning determine whether or not an insurance company will cover a claim. As it is difficult for the insurance companies to keep track of the meaning and importance of various diagnoses, many have adopted diagnostic coding.

The standard codes used in medicine today are taken from the International Classification of Diseases, Ninth Revision, Clinical Modification. This text, copyrighted by the Commission on Professional and Hospital Activities and published by Edward Brothers, Inc., Ann Arbor, MI. is commonly referred to as the "ICD-9" or the "ICD-9-CM." It lists the majority of possible diagnoses and assigns each a code number. The insurance companies are thus able to determine whether or not a procedure is covered by looking up its diagnostic code.

In an effort to handle those carriers who use ICD-9 coding and to maintain standardization, many physicians automatically use ICD-9 coding themselves. All of the quality computer medical programs provide for coding in this area. The physician must remember that ignoring the diagnosis code on the patient's billing statement or on the third party billing form, or using less specific diagnoses, may result in a lower reimbursement or no reimbursement at all.

[3] HCPCS

To further complicate coding, the Health Care Financing Administration (HCFA) developed an HCFA Common Procedure Coding System (HCPCS) in 1984. The HCPCS was designed to be more specific than CPT codes. For example, while CPT has one code for office supplies, the HCPCS codes break down the supplies into specific items. Other common areas where the HCPCS codes are necessary include oncology chemotherapy, injections and laboratory procedures. HCPCS codes are now required by Medicare providers when applicable.

It is unfortunate that the additional detail in billing provided in

HCPCS was not done by expanding standard CPT codes. In addition to creating the need for another coding book for HCPCS procedures, the codes themselves are alpha-numerical codes, in contrast to CPT codes which are simply numerical. Many of the medical software programs cannot be adapted to this alpha-numerical change without substantial software costs.

[4] Relative Values

In an effort to provide a rational and equitable method for determining fees, a system of relative values for physician procedures was begun in the early 1950's in California. The relative values developed did not determine fees; rather, they weighed the value of various procedures in relation to one another. Over the years, state medical associations began to adapt, publish and provide relative value indexes for their members.

During the 1970's, however, the U.S. government became concerned that the production and distribution of relative values by the medical associations was too closely linked to minimum or maximum prices in a geographic area and could result in price fixing. As a consequence, the production of relative value indexes ceased and physicians were asked by some associations to return indexes to be destroyed. Nevertheless, insurance companies continued to produce relative value studies as internal documents virtually unavailable to physicians and the public. These studies enabled insurance companies to monitor reimbursements and determine the value of fees for minimum/maximum reimbursement levels—the idea being that, as insurance companies are run by business people who have never performed medical procedures, only through the relative value system can they gain some perception of the value of procedures performed.

Today the relative value index is available from McGraw-Hill Book Company, Heightstown, NJ for physicians in private practice. This index can be a helpful tool to the physician developing a fee schedule and monitoring profiles and reimbursement levels.

[5] Profiles

All insurance companies need to maintain some sort of control over the amount they pay health care providers to prevent themselves from overpaying. Most insurance companies base reimbursement on profiles. Profiles are created from information available to the insurance companies on the physician's specialty, geographic location, etc. All fees charged for various procedures are calculated so that highs, lows, means, medians and modes may be determined.

Medicare establishes a profile for each physician and for the community at large. The profile for the physician is based on the fees for various procedures submitted by the physician directly or by the physician's patients. The community profile is based on the average fee profiles for all of the physicians in a particular area as defined by Medicare.

For claims submitted by the physician, Medicare will pay 80 percent of whichever is lower, the physician's profile or the community profile. The patient is responsible for the remaining 20 percent. Blue Cross and other third-party carriers provide similar coverage.

Many physicians, who ask why they should bill Medicare, Medicaid, Blue Cross, etc. for their full fee when they know they will only be paid a portion, submit a lower bill to take advantage of the higher community profile. Unfortunately, this ultimately hurts both the physician and patient, since it creates an artificially low profile for the physician and for the community at large. As a result, both the physician and the patient are penalized in the long run.

Generally you can obtain a copy of your profile from the third party upon request. You should keep a copy of your profile on record for monitoring. To monitor the profile for various third parties, you can convert fees allowed by third parties back to their original amount with the conversion factor derived from the relative value index (see Figure 7–1).

Profile information is also important to your collection staff. With the profile information, they will know whether the payments they receive from patients are proper. If, for example, the third party pays less for a procedure than is allowed by the physician's profile (this in fact does happen as a result of computer and human error), your staff can note this immediately and contact the insurance company.

PROFILE RECORD

Conversion Factors Allowed

	1985		1986		1987	
	Effec. Date	Conver. Factor	Effec. Date	Conver. Factor	Effec. Date	Conver. Factor
1) Workers' Compensation						
Medicine	____	____	____	____	____	____
Anesthesia	____	____	____	____	____	____
Surgery	____	____	____	____	____	____
Pathology	____	____	____	____	____	____
Radiology	____	____	____	____	____	____
2) Blue Cross/Blue Shield						
Medicine	____	____	____	____	____	____
Anesthesia	____	____	____	____	____	____
Surgery	____	____	____	____	____	____
Pathology	____	____	____	____	____	____
Radiology	____	____	____	____	____	____
3) Medicare						
Medicine	____	____	____	____	____	____
Anesthesia	____	____	____	____	____	____
Surgery	____	____	____	____	____	____
Pathology	____	____	____	____	____	____
Radiology	____	____	____	____	____	____
4) Medicaid						
Medicine	____	____	____	____	____	____
Anesthesia	____	____	____	____	____	____
Surgery	____	____	____	____	____	____
Pathology	____	____	____	____	____	____
Radiology	____	____	____	____	____	____

FIG. 7–1. This profile record can be used to keep track of the conversion factor allowed by various third parties and to determine which third-party agreements are more economically feasible.

(Pub.372)

PROFILE RECORD (Cont.)

Conversion Factors Allowed

	1985		1986		1987	
	Effec. Date	Conver. Factor	Effec. Date	Conver. Factor	Effec. Date	Conver. Factor
5) Insusror #1 __(name)__						
Medicine	____	____	____	____	____	____
Anesthesia	____	____	____	____	____	____
Surgery	____	____	____	____	____	____
Pathology	____	____	____	____	____	____
Radiology	____	____	____	____	____	____
6) Insuror #2 __(name)__						
Medicine	____	____	____	____	____	____
Anesthesia	____	____	____	____	____	____
Surgery	____	____	____	____	____	____
Pathology	____	____	____	____	____	____
Radiology	____	____	____	____	____	____
7) Insuror #3 __(name)__						
Medicine	____	____	____	____	____	____
Anesthesia	____	____	____	____	____	____
Surgery	____	____	____	____	____	____
Pathology	____	____	____	____	____	____
Radiology	____	____	____	____	____	____

Effec. = Effective   Conver. = Conversion

In this way you can monitor fees yearly and get the most for services without damaging the practice or community profile.

(Pub.372)

[6] Participation Agreements

Many third parties such as Blue Cross/Blue Shield, Medicaid and Medicare offer physicians a variety of participation contracts. In some instances, even if the the physician does not sign a provider agreement, patients will be reimbursed for the services he or she performs. For example, a physician may decide not to enter into a provider agreement with Blue Cross but may see Blue Cross patients. Under these circumstances the physician will not be able to collect directly from Blue Cross, but he or she may submit forms on behalf of the patient. The patient will then be reimbursed for services for which he or she has paid the physician. (See Chapter 10, "Accounts Receivable Management.")

Medicaid, on the other hand, requires that the physician bill Medicaid directly and accept payment from Medicaid as payment in full. The physician does not have the option of non-participation for seeing Medicaid patients. In the event a non-participating physician sees a Medicaid patient, neither the patient nor the physician are reimbursed for services.

[a] Pros and Cons of Participation in Third-Party Agreements

The common reasons physicians give for participating with a particular third party are:

- The physician may fear he or she will lose patients because the insurer does not reimburse the patient who sees a nonparticipating physician (as in Medicaid) or because it becomes less convenient for the patient to obtain reimbursement (as would be the case with Blue Cross).

- A contractual arrangement with a third party that provides direct payment to the physician prevents the patient from absconding with the reimbursements. Probably every physician's office has experienced a situation where the patient receives reimbursement from an insurance company and uses it for something other than paying the physician's bill. The patient may then stretch out payments to the physician over a long period of time or neglect to pay altogether.

- By participating with the third party the physician receives direct reimbursement. This eliminates the potential delay between the time the patient receives the payment, deposits the payment and issues a new check to the physician.
- By dealing directly with the third party the physician can process the claim as quickly as possible and receive reimbursement sooner. The non-participating physician must leave claims processing up to the patient, which can result in an additional thirty to sixty days before collection.

Physicians who do not enter into provider agreements give the following reasons:

- They do not wish to comply with specific billing requirements of the third party.
- The physician prefers to deal directly with the patient in collection of payments. Quite simply, this shifts the burden of collection from the third party to the patient.
- By placing the burden of payment directly on the patient, the physician may request immediate or quick payment.
- The physician does not wish to get into a position in which the third party dictates or controls the fee. By entering the third party agreement, the physician generally has to comply with the profiles and not bill the patient for charges in excess of what the profiles allow.

[b] Evaluating Contracts

The decision whether or not to participate with third party carriers should be made on a situation-by-situation basis. Each contract with a third party should be evaluated separately and from a business, rather than emotional, standpoint. There are several points to consider when evaluating third party contracts:

- The contract may call for you to do things which you find professionally objectionable. An example is a third party contract that prohibits you from prescribing certain drugs. Another example is a provider contract that requires you to make referrals to specific physicians or other health care facilities which you do not currently use for professional reasons. You must try to be objective about this.

- Check the type of additional administrative burdens placed on you when you sign the participation agreement. For example, will you need to have certain procedures approved before you can perform them? Some third parties require a participating physician to prepare a referral slip for patients being referred to another participating physician. Maybe the third party has an unusual billing form which your current system would be unable to handle. The cost of handling additional forms might exceed the benefit of participation.

- Determine what your profile is and what percentage of your fees will be paid. If the third party requires that you reduce or write off a portion of your fees, this cost must be considered. You should also determine how the level of fees and the profiles will be developed by the third party.

- How much coverage does the third party guarantee the patient? If the coverage to the patient is minimal, there may be little benefit to your participation. If, on the other hand, the insurance carrier covers most of the services you will be asked to provide, it may be more beneficial to join.

- Determine how the program will affect your patient volume. If the program is popular and a number of new patients come into the practice as a result of your participation, some minimal costs or write-offs may be made up for in volume. If a number of your current patients will be signing up for the program or wish to sign up for the program, you may benefit by being a provider.

- Find out if participation will lessen competition for medical services. If the contract enables you to provide an alternative to competitive or alternative care such as an HMO, it might be to your advantage to participate. You must have foresight when analyzing this type of program and understand that failure to offer services on a competitive and economic basis with other providers may result in the loss of patients.

- If you encourage patients to sign up for coverage under a particular program as a result of your participation in that program, and the program controls where the patients go—as an HMO program or an IPA program does—you may be benefitting the third party more than yourself. If you decide later to terminate the arrangement, or if the third party terminates the arrangement, patients you brought in to the arrangement may be prohibited from going to you under the terms of their contractual arrangement with the third party. (One advantage of a PPO is that the patients may stay in the PPO network or they may leave the PPO network and still receive reimbursement. This is in contrast to the IPA, in which the patient must continue to see a participating physician.)

- Review the termination provisions of the contract to determine if you can terminate the contract in an acceptable manner. Determine your rights in the event the third party terminates the contract or decides not to renew it.

From a credit and collection standpoint, you generally do well to participate in a third party program if the profile is within five percent of your fees, and the third party accepts the standard AMA insurance form or a very similar form. In the event the paperwork is excessive or the profiles are unacceptably low, do not sign the contract if at all possible. From a credit/collection standpoint, signing up as a Medicare provider in October of 1984 proved devastating to many physicians. Because the Medicare profile was so low for the physicians, their write-offs increased substantially and their cash collections decreased.

[7] Assignment of Benefits

Most insurance companies allow a patient to assign benefits directly to a health care provider. To do so, there does not have to be any type of arrangement between the physician and the insurance company. Physicians generally encourage patients to do this, as it enhances their collection program without taking risks. Because assigning benefits directly to the physician does not relieve the patient of the responsibility for his or her bill, in a way it guarantees the physician the best of both worlds.

Assignment of benefits speeds up the collection process, since patients can sign forms at your office. From there, the forms can be

§ 7.04 Collecting from Patients

processed and sent directly to the insurance company. Often, when this is done, payment from the insurance company is received prior to the patient getting his or her first bill. In this case the patient will be relieved of a substantial portion of the bill.

§ 7.04 Collecting from Patients

> A physician should be flexible about the amount of time needed for payment of medical bills, but not to the point where patients never settle a bill.

There are a number of in-house systems a physician can use to collect from patients with accounts due, including (1) time-of-service payments, (2) a series of itemized statements, (3) collection letters, and (4) collection telephone calls. Whoever the physician puts in charge of in-house collection systems should be experienced in handling a range of patient personalities, from those who are simply forgetful to those who purposely avoid paying the bill. Some patients do not realize the seriousness of delinquency and force the physician to go to outside services such as (1) collection letter agencies, (2) collection agencies, (3) credit bureaus, and ultimately (4) small claims court. Since an outside agency generally charges the physician a percentage of the outstanding bills it collects on, the physician should do comparative shopping to choose an agency, taking into account how long an agency will keep an account open, accountability and frequency of reporting. Whether done in-house or through an agency, the practice should keep strict records of all transactions and any promises made by the patient. These can be used to remind the patient and staff and, if need be, as proof in court.

If approximately 60 percent of physician's fees are now covered by insurance, then approximately 40 percent come directly out of the patient's pocket. If patients and their insurers could be counted on to pay their share of the bill on time all of the time, there would be no need for thorough credit policies. However, as the proliferation of payment plans and collection agencies indicates, this expectation is impractical.

[1] Time-of-Service Payments

It is generally recommended that your office encourage the

patient to pay at the end of a visit. Whether the collection policy you decide upon requires payment at time of service or not, your office should always be able to accommodate patients who wish to pay this way. Many people prefer to pay at the time of service if it can be handled quickly and orderly, and the office should never be "too busy" to oblige them.

The first step in receiving payment at the time of service is to use an orderly routing slip or charge slip for all office procedures (see Chapter 4, "Office Systems"). If you use a properly designed routing slip, the receptionist will have charge information for the day available when the patient is leaving the office. Depending on the office's credit policy, the receptionist can begin in one of the following ways:

- "Your charges for the day are $25.00, Mr. Brown. Would you like to make a payment today?"
- "Your charges were $25.00 today, Mr. Brown. Will that be cash or a check?"
- "Your charges were $25.00 today, Mr. Jones. Since you are a new patient, our office requires that payment today. In the future you will have the option of paying at time of service or at the time you receive your first statement."

All of these examples are polite, tactful ways for a receptionist to carry out the office policy. If the patient fails to make payment at the time of service for whatever reason, the receptionist can follow up by saying something like this:

- "Here's a statement of your charges for today, Mr. Jones. This statement is detailed, showing all of the procedures and your diagnosis. For your convenience I am going to give you an envelope along with your statement so that you may make payment the next time you pay bills. It's nice to see you again. We look forward to seeing you on the _____" (give next appointment date).

[2] The Statement Process

If the patient fails to make payment at the time of service, it is necessary for you to have another method to collect the amount due.

(Pub.372)

It is recommended that patients who do not pay at the time of service be given an itemized copy of their charges along with an envelope. This encourages them to pay the next time they pay their bills. If this fails, however, you should send the patient a bill within thirty days of the service date. To ensure this, your policy should be designed to bill all accounts at least monthly. Cycle billing is popular and very feasible with computer systems. If you send out all statements once a month, it is recommended that you send them on approximately the twelfth of the month. This has proved effective since most people have major bills due at either the end of the month or the beginning of the month that could preempt payment of what they consider less urgent bills.

[a] Sequence

The sequence of statements should be followed in a systematic fashion:

First Statement: The first statement should be a "normal" statement showing all of the procedures performed, the diagnostic codes, the previous balance, the charges for current services, the credits for any payments or credit adjustments and the current balance.

Second Statement: The second statement should show all of the items outlined on the first statement and include aging information if possible. Computer systems can easily illustrate the age of the patient's bill. In addition, the second statement should carry a mild reminder to the patient that the bill is tardy. Perhaps the most subtle way to get the point across is to begin with a "Please."

Third Statement: The third statement should contain all of the elements of the first statement along with a firmer message. Some examples of effective messages are:

- "Good credit is a privilege. Don't abuse it by neglect or oversight of this overdue balance."
- "Don't jeopardize your credit standing by neglecting payment on this past-due account."
- "If you have overlooked this past due balance, there's no time like now for prompt payment."

Fourth Statement: The patient's account is now seriously overdue. Depending on the mailing date of the first statement, the patient's account is anywhere from four to five months old. A firm message should be placed on the account at this time, such as:

- "This account is now past due. Immediate payment is now necessary."
- "This account is delinquent. Payment in full is expected."

Fifth Statement: The fifth statement should be the last statement before final notice is given that the account will be turned over to collections or that the patient will be brought to conciliation court. The patient should receive a statement with a firm message:

- "This account is seriously delinquent. Full payment must be made to maintain credit with this office."
- "This account is seriously overdue. Payment in full is now necessary to protect your credit rating."

Sixth Statement: This should be the patient's final statement. It may be similar in format to the first statement, with a collection notice, or totally different. However, it should contain a message to the following effect:

- FINAL NOTICE. IF THIS ACCOUNT IS NOT PAID IN FULL WITHIN ___ DAYS, IT WILL BE REFERRED TO THE ABC CREDIT AGENCY FOR ACTION.

Additional methods to improve the collections of accounts receivable should be employed. Telephone calls and collection letters are extremely effective, but sometimes get temporarily put off by the office personnel. The office with a letter system has a "safety net" to make sure all patients get eight opportunities to pay their bill before serious collection action is taken (i.e., the request for payment at the time of service, the early pay statement and six mailed statements).

(Sample credit letters are provided in Appendix 7–B.)

[b] Computerized and Manual Collection Statements

Computer systems can be programmed to automatically carry out the statement process. Most systems can determine the status of an account by age of charges, or by computing all credits and debits to the account since the date of last payment. Generally speaking, physicians employ relatively liberal collection policies and they often allow a payment to bring an account current.

If you use a manual aging system, your staff will have to visually inspect each ledger at the time of billing. On a manual system a record is usually kept of what collection message is being sent to the patient. Messages are usually standardized and the bookkeeper keeps track of them by simply recording on the ledger the number of the message going out to the patient (see Figure 7-2).

[3] Collection Letters

Collection letters are an effective way to encourage patient payment. Form letters approved by the physician can be set up to avoid any confusion about the type of messages going out to the patients. Like the messages on the patient statements, the collection letters can be numbered and the type of letter sent out to the patient can be kept track of simply by recording the number of the collection letter on the billing card. Physicians who have a computer and/or word processor can produce standardized collection letters easily enough. Physicians who do not own such equipment may wish to have the collection letters preprinted and then type in the patient's name and other salient information as the occasion arises. Collection letters should generally be sent within 60 to 90 days of billing.

[a] Collection Letter Procedure

The sequence of collection letters should proceed as follows:

Collection Letter 1:

Dear Mr. Jones,

It has been 90 days since you received services from our physicians. You have neglected to pay your bill. As stated in our patient information brochure, it is our policy to require payments within 30 days of receipt of the first statement. As of this time, you have neglected to make payment on your account. If you are unable to make a payment on your account, we will make arrangements. We will do so only if you contact our credit department.

If you unable to pay this account, please contact our credit department today. We will appreciate your attention to this matter.

Very truly yours,

Harvey Hanson
Credit Manager

CREDIT & COLLECTIONS § 7.04 [3]

Front side of collection work card

Back side of collection work card

FIG. 7–2. This collection work card is used to keep track of the collection letters and dunning notices sent to patients. Use of a collection card keeps everyone involved with the patient's account informed of what collection procedures have been taken and prevents the credit clerk "forgetting" what was sent to the patient. It also gives the physician or office supervisor control over what followup work is being done on delinquent accounts. Gummed labels that emphasize the number of the message are available from suppliers (see Figure 7–3).

(Pub.372)

§ 7.04 [3]   MANAGING YOUR MEDICAL PRACTICE   7–26

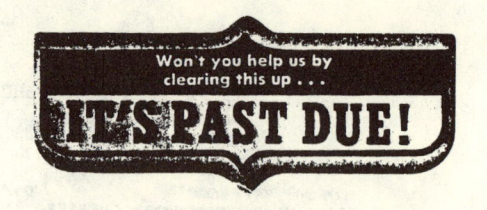

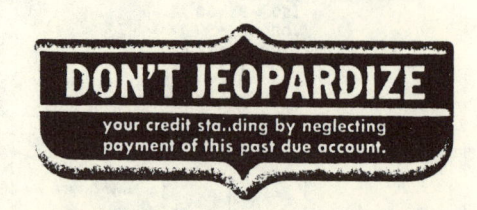

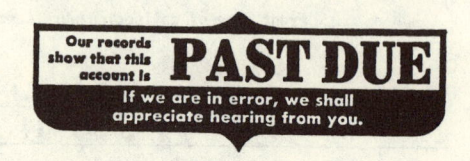

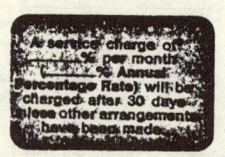

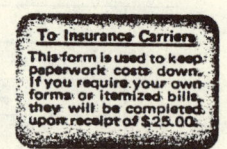

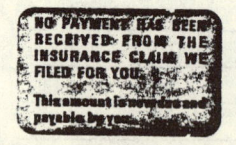

FIG. 7–3. Collection stickers can be attached directly to a copy of the patient's statement as a form of reminder.

If after thirty days there is no response to that letter, a second collection letter should be sent. (At this time the account is approximately 120 days old.) The second credit letter should say something to this effect:

Collection Letter 2:

Dear Mr. Jones,

Last month we wrote to you calling your attention to the fact that

(Pub.372)

your account was unpaid. As stated in our previous letter, it is a credit policy of this office to accept payment within thirty days of the receipt of our first statement. To date your bill remains unpaid although it is seriously delinquent.

As stated in our previous letter, we will make arrangements with you if you are faced with a problem paying this bill. We will do so, however, only if you contact our office.

Please contact our office today so that this problem may be solved.

Very truly yours,

Harvey Hanson
Credit Manager

If after thirty days from sending the second letter (180 days delinquent) the patient has not contacted the office to make credit arrangements, the final notice letter should go out. The final notice letter should be brief and to the point.

Collection Letter 3:

Dear Mr. Jones,

We have made numerous attempts to contact you regarding the payment of your bill. To date you have neither paid the bill nor contacted our office to make arrangements to pay the bill. As a result we are forced to notify you that **IF PAYMENT ON THIS ACCOUNT IS NOT MADE WITHIN THIRTY DAYS, THIS ACCOUNT WILL BE REFERRED TO THE AGGRESSIVE CREDIT AGENCY FOR FURTHER ACTION.**

Please make payment in full immediately to avoid collection agency problems and further damage to your credit rating.

Very truly yours,

Harvey Hanson
Credit Manager

[b] Credit Arrangements

If in the course of sending out the first two letters the patient contacts the office to make credit arrangements, you should set up suitable terms. The terms the patient and credit manager agree

(Pub.372)

upon should be recorded, and a letter should be sent to the patient confirming the terms so that there is no confusion.

Confirmation of Terms Letter:

Dear Mr. Jones,

Thank you for contacting our office to discuss your unpaid balance in the amount of $325.00.

As we have agreed upon on the telephone, we will expect monthly payments on the 15th of each month, in the amount of $75.00, until the bill is paid in full. We are happy to be able to help you in this matter and appreciate your contacting our office to make credit arrangements.

> Very truly yours,
>
> Harvey Hanson
> Credit Manager

If the patient breaks the terms of this agreement, without calling and changing the terms, new letters should be sent out. For example the credit letter would be as follows:

Broken Terms of Agreement Collection Letter:

Dear Mr. Jones,

On June 15, 1985, you agreed to make monthly payments on the 15th of each month, in the amount of $75.00, until the balance of your account was paid in full. To date we have not received your payment for September 15, 1985. In order to bring your account up to date we are requesting you to send in a payment of $150.00 to cover your September 15 payment and your October 15 payment. Your next payment will then be due November 15.

Please send in the payment today. If you are unable to do so, please contact our office immediately so that we can discuss your situation.

In order to eliminate further problems with this account, please handle this situation at once.

> Very truly yours,
>
> Harvey Hanson
> Credit Manager

If the patient breaks his or her terms and does not reconcile the situation by making up the delinquent payments, a final notice should be sent to the following effect:

Final Notice:

Dear Mr. Jones,

We have previously discussed your bill and have agreed upon a payment schedule satisfactory to both of us. In spite of this, you have neglected to make payments on your account in accordance with those terms.

As a result of your action, WE FIND IT NECESSARY TO TURN YOUR ACCOUNT OVER TO THE AGGRESSIVE COLLECTION AGENCY IN THIRTY DAYS IF FULL PAYMENT OF YOUR ACCOUNT IS NOT MADE.

In order to avoid to having your account turned over to our collection agency and in order to protect your credit rating, please pay your account today.

Very truly yours,

Harvey Hanson
Credit Manager

[c] Special Circumstances

The series of collection letters described above can be adapted to cover unusual circumstances. The following sample collection letters are routinely used in a medical office:

Form Collection Letter 1:

Dear Mr. Smith,

We recently received payment from your insurance carrier, Blue Cross/Blue Shield, in the amount of $810.00. The balance of $302.00 represents the balance you owe. (A $100.00 deductible and $202.00 co-payment.)

Our office policy requires payment to be made thirty days from receipt of statement. Because you have Blue Cross coverage, the amount due was unclear until we received payment. We now ask that you pay this balance.

If you are unable to pay the balance at this time, please call our office so that we may make credit arrangements.

Very truly yours,

Harvey Hanson
Credit Manager

Form Collection Letter 2:

Dear Mr. Smith,

When you registered as a patient at our office, you indicated that you preferred to pay your bill upon receipt of your first statement. Thirty days have elapsed since we have sent your first statement, yet we have not received payment. We would appreciate a prompt payment of your bill at this time.

If you are unable to make payment at this time, we will make other arrangements, but we will do so only if you contact our office. If you have any questions about the bill, please contact us so that we may discuss them.

We appreciate your attention to this matter.

Very truly yours,

Harvey Hanson
Credit Manager

Form Collection Letter 3:

Dear Mr. Smith,

As you are aware, your account is currently ninety days delinquent. It is our normal process to send delinquent accounts through our routine collection process. We prefer not to do that with you, however, and request that you check the appropriate box, sign this letter, and return it within fifteen days.

[ ] I prefer to handle this account by making a full payment at this time. Payment in full is enclosed.

[ ] I am unable to pay the entire amount of this bill at this time. I will make monthly payments of ____. My first payment of ____ is enclosed.

[ ] I do not feel I should pay this bill for the following reason:

[ ] I do not intend to pay this bill. You may turn the account over to your collection agency. (Failure to respond to this letter may result in such action.)

―――――――――

Patient's Signature

Thank you for your attention to this matter.

Very truly yours,

Harvey Hanson
Credit Manager

There are advantages to using collection letters instead of statements. A patient with a delinquent account who has received a few statements comes to recognize what they look like and in many cases will not even open them if he or she does not intend to pay the bill. Letters are generally opened, and if they are brief and to the point, the patient will read them in their entirety.

To expedite the processing of letters, form manufacturers have developed standard message slips. These message slips, like a personal letter, can be sent independent of statement. Some message slips are printed on paper approximately the same size as a business check, on the theory that the patient will at least open the letter in anticipation of a possible check.

Use of routine statements and collection letters generally results in better payments on accounts receivable. In addition, it supplies proof that the physician who ultimately resorts to firmer action (i.e., collection agency referrals or conciliation court), has given the patient numerous opportunities to pay his or her bill. For example, an office going through a routine collection system with a six-month rule for turning the account over to a collection agency or to conciliation court would give the patient an opportunity to pay the bill at the time services were performed, six statements, and the three letters detailed above. This is a total of ten notices to the patient. No physician should hesitate about taking firm action against patients who neglect ten notifications. (Remember this system gives the patient numerous opportunities to make full or partial payments.)

(Pub.372)

[4] Collection Letter Services

A number of collection agencies have collection letter services whose purpose is to insure that letters are sent to the patient. The agencies rationale is that, in many cases, the patient will pay the third party immediately, even after refusing to respond to the numerous attempts by the physician's office to collect the bill.

A quality letter collection service generally offers several advantages:

- Once the account is turned over to the collection letter service, the physician is assured that the letters are going out. Many times, the medical office is "too busy" to do all of the collection follow-up.

- The collection letter is sent by a third party and in many cases patients notified by a third party immediately pay their bill.

- A letter service is generally cost effective, particularly when compared to using an agency. Many collection letter services guarantee the charge for the letter service will represent only X percentage of the resulting collection.

The main disadvantage of using the collection letter service is that there is generally little or no flexibility in the type of letters sent

(Text continued on page 7-33)

to the patient. Because letter services deal with all types of clients (even though the firm may specialize in physicians, it may deal with all specialties) they must have a relatively generalized format. The need to use specific terms is generally not conducive to using a collection letter service.

A collection letter service should be employed if your office is unable to send out its own collection letters. Many physicians also find it cost effective to use a collection service as an interim step between the final notice sent out by the physician's office and the collection agency or conciliation court.

[5] Collection Telephone Calls

The telephone can be an excellent tool in the collection process. Used properly, it can be the most effective method of bringing payments into the doctor's office. The telephone brings the physician's business assistant right into the home or office of the patient. Most people give the telephone priority when it rings. In addition, when the telephone call is from the physician's bookkeeping department, the patient can no longer set the problem aside in a pile on his or her desk or temporarily eliminate the problem by throwing it in the trash. He or she must confront the problem.

Unfortunately the telephone is generally not used as effectively as it could be in the medical office. This is usually the result of inadequate training of office personnel and the general feeling among staff that working on collections is a disagreeable task.

Medical assistants should be taught not to think of themselves as adversaries of the patient. Rather they should take the position that they are there to help the patient solve the problem of paying the bill. The assistant must help the patient realize that if he or she does not pay the bill, it places an unjust burden on those who do pay.

Those collecting for the physician should also be made to realize that the majority of people are honest and that, typically, when the physician is not paid, it is out of neglect. A patient may feel he or she should wait until "next month," so the bill can be paid in full (although they come to the same conclusion the next month, and so on.) Or they may want to get other credit accounts settled first, since most physicians don't charge interest or, if they do, it is generally a lower rate than department stores or credit cards

(Pub.372)

charge. Furthermore, patients are generally aware that failure to pay the department store results in swift credit action: generally department stores contact the customer after a delinquent statement has been sent and no payment has been received.

In many cases utilization of routine collection letters will result in the patient contacting the office to discuss the bill or make credit arrangements. However, if the patient does not contact the office the assistant must take steps to contact the patient.

[a] Sample Telephone Calls

You should establish a rule on the number of times the office should attempt to contact the patient. If, for example, the number chosen is four, an assistant will make four attempts to reach a patient by telephone. Each attempt should be made at a different time of the day and be recorded on the patient's ledger card or collection card.

Once contact has been made with the patient, the assistant should introduce himself or herself and explain the problem, as in the following example:

"Hello, Mr. Smith. This is Jane Johnson from the USA Clinic. Our auditor was in earlier this week to review our accounts receivable and pulled your account. He pointed out that your account was 120 days old. I pulled out your records and noted that we had sent you four statements. A letter asking you to call us was also sent. To date we have not heard from you. Is there any problem that you are having that you would like to discuss with us?"

The assistant should then wait for a reply from the patient. The assistant should realize that the patient may be experienced in avoiding direct answers and making up excuses as to why the bill was not paid and why the office had not been contacted. "Deadbeat" patients will have developed methods of dealing with collection calls, since they are generally delinquent to more than one creditor and have already received several severe collection calls from stores and agencies. Here are some common excuses with appropriate comments by the assistant:

<u>Call 1</u>

Patient: "That's awfully strange, Mrs. Johnson. I haven't received any bills from you."

Assistant: "Well, that is indeed strange, Mr. Smith. We haven't received any of your statements back. In any event the amount owed by you at this point is $100.00. Is that something you can afford to pay today?"

If the patient answers in the affirmative, the assistant should get a specific date when the payment will be made and confirm it again with the patient before hanging up. If the patient says he or she is unable to pay the entire amount at this time, the assistant should suggest partial payments spread over time. The assistant should try to obtain promises from the patient, including specific payment amounts and dates. All items promised by the patient should be recorded on the patient's ledger card or collection for follow-up (see Figure 7–4).

Call 2

Patient: "Well, I sure did get that bill, Mrs. Johnson. I was just waiting for my insurance to pay it. They should be paying it any day now."

Assistant: "Most insurance companies will pay in thirty days, Mr. Jones. We would recommend that you follow up on that right away. Since you didn't assign your benefits to us, however, we will need to get payment directly from you. Could you pay the amount due today?"

Call 3

Patient: "Well, I did get your statement, but I didn't really understand it. I was going to call up to get some sort of clarification, but I've just been too busy to do so."

Assistant: "Well, let me go over your bill right now with you, Mr. Smith. Here's a detailed listing of the procedures Dr. Nelson performed and the price for those procedures. (List the procedures and the costs.) Does that all make sense to you, Mr. Smith, or do you have any questions? (If the patient says it doesn't make sense or if the patient wants further clarification, continue the discussion.) Can you make a payment on your account today?"

Call 4

Patient: "I sure did get that statement. I'm outraged. It's obvious Dr. Nelson cares more about his charges than he does about his patients. My neighbor had the same thing done last week and his

MANAGING YOUR MEDICAL PRACTICE 7-36

STATEMENT
USA Clinic

- Jane Johnson
  2186 Thompson Street
  New Richmond, VA 34210

-

NUMBER	DATE	DESCRIPTION	CHARGE	PAYMENT	CURRENT BALANCE
	1-31-84	Office Call	25 00		25 00
	2-15-84	Brief Office Call	15 00		40 00
	6-2-84	Spoke to patient; will pay $15 on the 15th each month until paid			
	6-17-84			15 00	25 00
	8-1-84	Spoke to patient. Promised to pay balance on 8-15-84			
	8-17-84			25 00	—

PLEASE PAY THE LAST FIGURE IN THIS COLUMN

FIG. 7-5. With a manual collection system, the credit clerk can write credit messages directly on the patient's card. Using a photocopy of this ledger as the patient's statement keeps the credit clerk informed and automatically shows the patient that the credit clerk is informed and will know of any payment promises made.

doctor only charged him half as much. Surely you don't expect me to pay that entire bill?"

(Rel.1-2/87 Pub.372)

Assistant: "I wish you would have contacted us earlier if you felt that way, Mr. Smith. In any event you should be assured that Dr. Nelson's fees are in line with the prevailing charges in the community. Dr. Nelson is considered one of the leading physicians in the community and his fees are in no way out of line with others.

Dr. Nelson's fees are annually reviewed by the various third parties in the community and have always been approved. I'm sorry that you feel that the fees are excessive, but I'm afraid I'm unable to authorize any type of discount. May we expect payment on your account today?"

Call 5

Patient: "Who did you say you were? You sound awfully young to be calling me about my bill. I go back a long way with Dr. Nelson and he's never had any young whippersnapper call me before. Who do you think you are, calling me up about my bill?"

Assistant: "My age is not at issue here, Mr. Smith. Dr. Nelson has assigned me this responsibility to follow up on your account. If we are to avoid further collection action on this account, you will need to deal directly with me. I'd like to help you get this matter solved. Is there any reason this account hasn't been paid that you'd like to discuss or can we expect payment of this account?"

Call 6

Patient: "I have received your statement. I'm sorry, but I was laid off from work a month ago and have been unable to secure other employment. I've got some more interviews next week and I'm sure something will happen. Your account is going to receive payment when I gain employment."

Assistant: "Mr. Smith, I'm so sorry to hear that you have been laid off. You should have let us know so that we could have marked your account. As you might expect, our policy here is to help patients in financial difficulty and we certainly want to help you. I wonder if you could make a minimum payment of $25.00 so that I can put this account on hold until next month at which time things will undoubtedly be getting better for you?"

Call 7

Patient: "You are darn right I got your statements. You're lucky I haven't sued you! Dr. Nelson really screwed me up and I have to go to that new doctor. He got me back on track, but I sure don't intend to pay your bill."

Assistant: "I'm sorry to hear you feel that there was a problem, Mr. Smith. I'm making note of that and will report it to Dr. Nelson. I'll have Dr. Nelson give you a call to discuss the problem."

Call 8

Patient: "I don't intend to pay that bill. I've turned the whole matter over to my attorney. You'll have to deal with him."

Assistant: "We'll be happy to deal with him, Mr. Smith. Can you give me his complete name and phone number?"

Call 9

Patient: "Yes, I received your statement. Quite frankly we're in very tough financial shape right now and are not going to be able to pay that bill."

Assistant: "That presents quite a problem, Mr. Smith. If you are unwilling to work with us at all, I'm afraid your account may need to be referred for further collection action. If we can set up a payment schedule, however, we can avoid that altogether . Would it be possible for you to make monthly payments of $25.00?"

[b] Obtaining a Commitment from the Patient

The person making the collection call should attempt to get the patient to promise to pay the entire bill within a few days. If the patient says that is not possible, the person making the call should suggest a payment schedule that would allow the bill to be paid in four or less installments. As a last resort, the assistant should attempt to get the patient to make specific payments that would extend the entire payment period for more than four periods. However, the assistant should record the patient's promise and tell the patient he or she is unauthorized to accept such low payments under normal circumstances, but will discuss the situation with the supervisor and try to get approval.

The assistant must always try to get a specific promise or specific refusal to pay the bill. In the event the patient refuses to pay the bill, the account should be pulled from the normal collection system. If the patient has turned the account over to an attorney, threatens a malpractice suit or expresses dissatisfaction with the services performed by the physician, these details should be recorded and the entire matter should immediately be turned over to the physician. The physician should then contact his or her attorney or malpractice insurance carrier, as the case may be, to seek out proper counsel. In the event the patient is not refusing to pay the bill, the assistant should attempt to get the following promises:

- A specific payment amount.
- A specific date the payment will be made, or dates the payments will be made.

Once obtained, these details should be recorded on the patient's ledger collection card. If possible, the patient should be called within a few days after the promise date if the check does not arrive. Under no circumstances should the account go beyond thirty days without followup. If the patient makes a promise twice, or if the assistant is unable to reach the patient who has broken a promise, then the account should be pulled and referred to a collection agency or conciliation court.

When making collection calls, the assistant must remember to display a helping attitude, yet be firm with the patient and obtain commitments. The assistant must have a thick skin and be able to disregard any insults or attempts at intimidation.

[6] Collection Agencies

If you follow all of the procedures outlined above, and after six months the patient has failed to make payments or has made inadequate payments on his or her account, you should resort to more severe collection followup. For most physicians the best answer to problem accounts is a good collection agency. Although some physicians simply write off an account after six months, this course of action should be avoided. Only in situations where the patients have contacted the physician and the physician is aware of unusual circumstances should the account be written off.

It is common to have trouble finding a good collection agency. An agency may employ harsh or unreasonable tactics in dealing with patients. Another common problem in dealing with collection agencies is that they often devote attention only to the larger bills because the agency is paid on a percentage basis. In the physician's

(Pub.372)

office the accounts receivable is made up of many little bills rather than a few large bills.

[a] Finding an Agency

The following steps are recommended when determining which collection agency to employ:

1. *Obtain Recommendations from the Hospital and from Colleagues:* You should learn what collection agencies are used by the hospital you work with. If you are a specialist, find out what agency referring doctors use. Occasionally, when an agency is working for both the physicians and hospitals, it pools delinquent accounts and exerts more pressure on delinquent patients.

2. *Contact Representatives of the Collection Agency:* Contact the agencies used by the hospital and by other colleagues, and ask a representative to come to your office to discuss the agency's services. Ask the representatives to bring references from other physicians they deal with, particularly physicians in your specialty.

3. *Interview Representatives of Various Agencies:* Ask the following questions:

    - How do you charge for services? Most agencies charge on a percentage of collections so that, in essence, the physician has a guaranteed fee (40 percent is common, although the fee may range as high as 50 percent).

    - What steps will you take when accounts in the $10.00 to $25.00 range are turned over? In the $25.00 to $50.00 range? In the $50.00 to $100.00 range? In the over $100.00 range?

    - If I charge interest on delinquent accounts, who receives that income, the agency or our office?

    - If a patient threatens a malpractice suit, how will the agency handle it?

    - Do you have any other physicians in my specialty with whom you are currently dealing? May I call these doctors for references?

- What percentage does your agency end up collecting based on all of the accounts turned over to it? (While it is obvious that the percentage the agency collects will depend on the condition of accounts turned over to it, the national average tends to be approximately 40 percent.)
- What type of accounting will you give me on a monthly basis so that I can monitor the credit action being taken on those accounts with which you are dealing?
- If I decide to pull an account from the agency, what steps must I take and how will I be charged for this?
- At what point will you turn accounts back to me so I can write them off? (Most agencies tend to retain accounts indefinitely since, if they are ever collected, the agency is due a fee. The authors recommend the physician demand accounts be returned to his or her office automatically if no results are forthcoming after the agency has had the account for six months.)
- How long has your agency been in business?
- Who are the principal owners of your agency?
- Does your agency participate with the credit bureau so that all of the accounts turned over to you and not collected are reported on the patient's credit rating file?

Eliminate any agencies that respond to the above questions in a manner you feel is negative. After you have interviewed three or four different collection agencies, call their references. Contact other physicians using the agency, ask if they are satisfied with the agency and if they have ever had any type of problem with the agency. Ask the reference if the agency gives adequate accounting on a monthly basis so that you know what work is being done with agency accounts and what amounts have been collected. Ask what percentage of accounts turned over to the agency are collected and compare the answer you get with what the agency representative said during the interview.

[b] Trying Out Agencies

Select two collection agencies to work with, based on the information provided through the interview with the agency representative and the references. Call representatives from each of the agencies and give them the following information:

(Pub.372)

- Tell each of the agencies that they are one of two your office will be working with and that the office will monitor both of them. Although initially accounts should be distributed evenly between the two, the agency performing the best will most likely get the larger accounts.

- Tell the agencies you expect to get monthly reports showing the accounts they are working on, the beginning balance, payments received and the ending balance for each of the accounts. (This information can be balanced against the business office records of outstanding accounts at the agencies.)

- Inform the agency that it will be expected to return all accounts deemed uncollectable, and unless special conditions prevail, no account should remain with the collection agency for more than six months. Circumstances that allow the agency to hold accounts for more than six months might include a situation where the agency is collecting payments on the account or in the middle of special collections actions such as taking a patient to court or garnishing wages.

If the agencies agree to these terms, the physician should begin using them.

[c] Monitoring Agencies

Unless your office is extremely large, two agencies should be satisfactory. Split accounts between them and evaluate the collection ratios on an annual basis. Generally, it is unfair to the agencies to evaluate them more frequently. If you find a large discrepancy in performance, or if you wish to try a new agency, drop the agency with the poorer performance and replace it.

To monitor an agency's performance, have your bookkeeper keep track of accounts turned over, accounts returned and payments made. This can be done by keeping the following information on a worksheet in a columnar notepad:

- Date
- Description
- Amount turned over

(Pub.372)

- Amount of payments received
- Amount returned by the collection agency
- Outstanding balance at the collection agency
- Agency fee

Entries should be made in this log as they occur. To evaluate the agencies, simply subtotal the accounts and divide the payments received by the agency by the total amounts turned over. The resulting percentage is the differential you should use to compare agencies (as mentioned earlier, a 40 percent ratio is average).

[7] Credit Bureaus

A credit bureau maintains credit records on consumers and gives consumers credit ratings based on that information. That information is generally provided to the credit bureaus by their members, i.e. the businesses with whom consumers deal (like medical practices).

Generally the cost of being a member in the credit bureau is minimal. For this fee a physician receives the following benefits:

- When the patient's account becomes delinquent, the physician has the option to report it to the credit bureau. This is generally a strike against the patient's rating and by itself may give the patient incentive to pay the physician.

- Once the physician's bill has been recorded on the credit bureau records, it stays there until it is paid. In some cases the patient finds it necessary to pay off a medical bill to obtain much wanted credit, such as a mortgage.

- If the physician's credit clerks begin to suspect a problem with collections on the patient's account or feel the patient is giving them the "run-around," they may contact the credit bureau to find out the patient's credit history. This information can be valuable in determining how swiftly an account should be referred to a collection agency or conciliation court. It also permits the credit clerk to be firmer in dealings with the patient over the telephone or through collection letters.

- If a patient does not leave forwarding addresses, this information may be available through the credit bureau. This information helps the credit clerk locate a delinquent account. Sometimes an honest patient moves without giving a proper forwarding address to the physician. Getting this information from the credit bureau may result in payment on the account that otherwise would have been written off or transferred to a collection agency.

- In the event that the physician's office seeks and obtains a judgment against a patient, the credit bureau may help locate the patient's place of employment for the purpose of garnishing wages.

- When the physician is a member of the credit bureau, this may be noted on the credit and collection letters so that the patient will be aware that not paying the bill may have adverse effects on his or her credit rating.

It is generally advisable for the physician to become a member and participate with the local credit bureau. Even if the physician never gets paid for an account, he or she will have the satisfaction of knowing that the patient's credit rating has been affected by his or her refusal to pay the physician.

[8] Conciliation Court

Generally, the maximum claim that can be filed with the conciliation (small claims) court is approximately $1,200.00, although this depends upon the state and county in which suit is brought. Claims in excess of the maximum should be filed through the regular court system, for which it is usually prudent to engage an attorney.

Many physicians don't use a conciliation court because they are confused as to how it works or think that they themselves need to file the claim. It is important for a physician to have an understanding of how conciliation court works. In many situations, the large fee charged by a collection agency can be avoided by taking the patient to conciliation court.

[a] Advantages and Disadvantages

The advantages of using conciliation court include:

- The physician need not be present or personally take the matter to court. The situation may be handled by the physician's bookkeeper or credit clerk.
- In many cases the patient does not show up for a court appearance and an automatic judgment is awarded to the physician.
- In the event the patient does show up, it is unlikely he or she will win. If the procedures being billed for were, in fact, performed under normal circumstances for regular fees, there is little chance the physician will lose.
- Once judgment is obtained, the physician may garnish the patient's wages and obtain a lien on bank accounts or personal property.
- In many cases, the patient pays the bill when served with notice that the matter is being brought before the conciliation court, or at least pays at the time the judgment is granted against the patient.

Disadvantages of the conciliation court system include:

- A representative of the office must take time away from other matters to attend conciliation court. (This generally can be minimized by taking the bulk of accounts to the court all at once.)
- When a judgment is obtained against the patient, the collection clerk must locate the patient's assets or place of employment for garnishing purposes. In the event the patient is transient and does not have a stable home or employment, a judgment against the patient will do the physician little good.
- Using conciliation "costs" the physician in terms of the assistant's time and effort. If, in the final analysis, no revenues are brought into the office, this is a loss. (The collection agency by contrast, will not "cost" the physician anything unless revenues are brought into the office.)

[b] Conciliation Court Procedures

Although the actual procedures vary from county to county across the country, the conciliation court procedure generally involves the following steps:

1. Obtain Statement of Claim and Summons and Affidavit of Identification forms from the district court of the county in which the delinquent patient resides. Generally, there is a small fee for these forms.
2. Complete and file the Statement of Claim and Summons form and filing fee with the district court of the county in which the defendant resides.
3. Your office will be notified when to appear at the court. A representative of the office will need to appear. If the defendant does not appear, you win by default. If the defendant appears, your representative should be prepared to present the case with proof of claim. The proof of claim consists of copies of statements, medical charts and other records documenting services performed.
4. Within a few days, your office will be notified by mail of the judgment decision. After that, there is a ten-day waiting period for either party to file an appeal in municipal or county court. If a patient does not show up for a court appearance, and can show good reason for not appearing, the case may be reopened.

If the patient is found at fault and pays, a letter should be sent to the clerk of conciliation court stating that the case has been satisfied. In the event the defendant does not pay, the physician's collection clerk must send an Affidavit of Identification to the District Court along with a filing fee. A wage lien may be obtained by sending a filing fee to the county where the defendant is employed to receive a Writ of Execution, sending a garnishment exemption notice to the defendant (there must be a ten-day wait at this point) and sending a notice to the county sheriff with the original copy of the Writ of Execution and a check to cover the sheriff's fee.

A bank lien may be obtained by getting a Writ of Execution from the county where the bank is located and sending to the bank a letter along with the Writ of Execution, Execution Levy Disclosure forms and copies of the garnishment exemption notice.

Before a practice becomes involved in conciliation court proceedings, the collection clerk should review the process several times to determine the exact procedures and time involvement to see the case through from beginning to end. Collection clerks who have used the conciliation court a number of times are in a good position to evaluate the best course of action: writing the account off, turning it over to a collection agency or taking the patient to court.

§ 7.05 Monitoring Collections

By keeping track of the write-off percentage, collection percentage, dollar amount of accounts receivable, size of accounts receivable compared to monthly charges, and aging of accounts receivable, a physician can get a fairly good idea of how collection is proceeding and whether too many accounts are going unpaid. Once it becomes a chore for the office to keep track of these figures manually, the physician should consider computerizing the collection system.

If a physician's office is to maintain full control over credit and collections, good monitoring systems must be set up. Monitoring systems should provide information in the aggregate, so that the physician knows whether credit and collections are under control. The system should also permit you to obtain specific account information needed to follow up on delinquent patients and third parties. The physician must know what type of information he or she should receive and review on a monthly basis and how he or she should interpret that data.

[1] Areas to Review

Among the key items you should review on a monthly basis to monitor the overall control of accounts receivable are:

Write-off Percentage: Write-off percentage is the ratio of the total of write-offs, discounts, disallowed charges, etc. divided by the gross charges. It is this percentage that ultimately determines the amount of charges never collected. Having this information available enables you to measure trends in the practice and be alert to any substantial changes.

Collection Percentage: The collection percentage is the ratio of cash receipts divided by charges. Some physicians determine their collection percentage using gross charges; other physicians use net charges (net charges being defined as the total charges minus write-offs and adjustments). Obviously, it is important to establish a consistent method of determining the collection percentage and, when comparing collection percentages with other physicians, make you know how they have determined theirs. The author recommends defining collection percentage as the ratio of cash receipts from patients divided by *net* charges. The value of the collection percentage determined this way is that over the course of a twelve-month period, the collection percentage should equal 100 percent. (Remember the amount of write-offs is measured in the write-off percentage.) The exception is in the case of a growing practice, where charges are constantly growing. In this case, the collection percentage does not reach 100 percent until charges level off.

Dollar Amount of Accounts Receivable: The physician should constantly check the dollar amount in accounts receivable to detect any excess growth in accounts receivable in terms of dollars.

Size of Accounts Receivable Compared to Monthly Charges: This figure relates the size of the accounts receivable in accordance with average monthly charges. If, for example, a physician's average charges are $10,000 and there is $25,000 in accounts receivable, the figure would be determined as 2.5 (i.e. $25,000/$10,000 = 2.5.). This means that the physician has 2.5 months of his or her average charges in accounts receivable. This is a significant figure, as it automatically adjusts for an increase in accounts receivable resulting from an increase in charges. When monitoring the accounts receivable figure by dollar amount, the physician should always check the size of accounts receivable relative to monthly charges if the figures show an increase in the dollar amount.

Aging of Accounts Receivable: Aging of accounts receivable breaks down the book value of accounts receivable according to specific periods of time. It show the dollar amount and the percentage of the total accounts receivable for each aging category, typically 30 days, 60 days, 90 days, 120 days, 150 days and 180 days and older. A computerized system can provide the aging information according to responsible party (see Figure 7–5).

For example, the aging report can be broken down by private patients, Blue Cross/Blue Shield, Medicaid, Medicare, etc. By consulting this information on a consistent basis, the physician can determine if there is a change signaling a collection problem.

You should meet with the person responsible for collections on a monthly basis to discuss any trends in these figures. If there is an unusual occurrence, such as an increase in the delinquencies of Blue Cross accounts, request that the person in charge of collections look

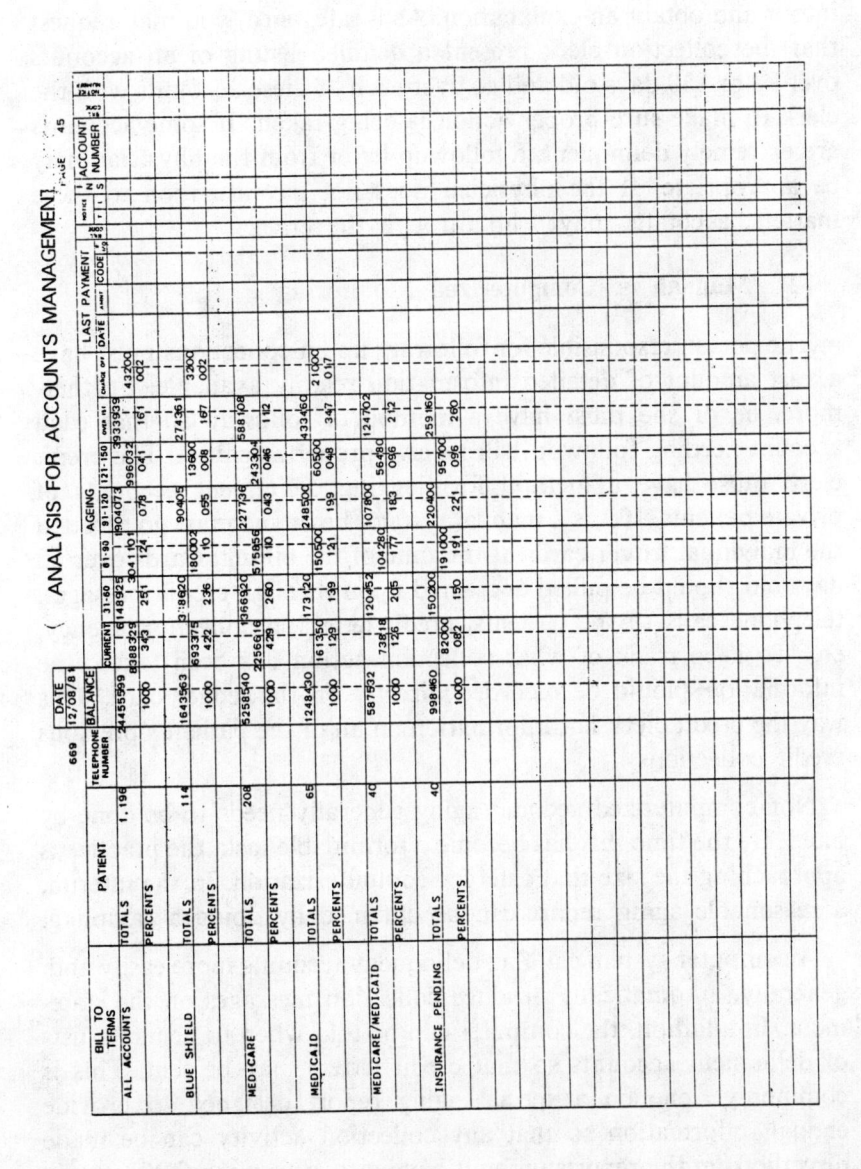

FIG. 7–6 This aging report illustrates an aggregate report for each major category in this physician's office. The physician uses the report to watch for delinquencies in any particular area.

(Rel.1–2/87 Pub.372)

into it and obtain an explanation. As a safeguard, you may request that the collection clerk present a detailed listing of all accounts over 90 or 120 days old and go over each of these accounts with the clerk to make sure proper action is being taken. If some accounts are extremely delinquent, a followup letter from the physician may be appropriate. If the physician does not pay attention to these matters, accounts may "slip through the cracks."

[2] Manual vs. Computerized Monitoring

The person responsible for following up on collections must have a vast amount of detailed information readily available. Furthermore, he or she must have a method of followup so that each account needing followup will receive proper attention. The credit clerk must have a method for flagging delinquent accounts of private patients. If it is a manual system, he or she must go through the individual ledger cards at the time of the billing. Cards over 30 days old should be pulled and acted upon through credit messages, telephone calls to the patients, credit letters, a collection agency, etc. To keep track of what collection action has been taken, the information should be recorded directly on the ledger card. This way the credit clerk has information on all of the patient's previous credit collections.

Non-computerized account aging generally needs to be done by hand. By the time this has become a formidable task, the practice is approaching the size that calls for computerization. In the interim, a reasonable aging report can be obtained by doing a sampling.

A computer system can flag delinquent accounts more easily and, generally, automatically produce collection messages on the statement. In addition, the computer can be told when to generate lists of delinquent accounts so that credit letters may be sent. This is commonly done on a special aging report designed to provide enough information so that any collection activity can be made directly from the reports without having to review the CRT screen. Some systems produce collection work cards that can be used to record what credit activity has been performed on them. Other systems allow this information to be entered directly into the computer.

Third party payments can be more difficult to monitor when they are not on a computer. Computerized systems can generally give an aging analysis by account and responsible party. As outlined in Chapter 10, "Accounts Receivable Management," the claims should be filed in an unpaid file until paid. Each month the unpaid

(Text continued on page 7-51)

file should be reviewed to determine which accounts are older than thirty days. Accounts older than 90 days which are due from third parties should be reported to the physician so that, if possible, he or she can send a personal letter. In many cases this carries more weight than any communication from a credit manager or clinic administrator.

§ 7.06 Collection Checklist

A comprehensive checklist for collecting from both patients and third-parties is provided.

- Collecting from Third Parties
    - Use proper coding procedures
        - CPT codes
        - HCPCS codes
        - ICD-9-CM diagnostic codes
    - Profiles
        - Know the practice profiles for community and specialty
        - Watch the profiles and use them to monitor payments
    - Be aware of relative values for procedures
    - Enter into participation agreements that will benefit the pactice
    - Negotiate for assignment of benefits when possible
    - Keep claims up-to-date and processed weekly
    - Establish follow up procedure for the office
- Collecting from Patients
    - Offer the patient a convenient opportunity to pay for procedures at the time that they are performed
    - If the patient does not wish to pay at the time of service, give the patient a statement of the charges along with an "early-pay" envelope as a first statement
    - Statement process

- Statement 1 should itemize procedures performed and give diagnostic codes, previous balance, charge for services, credits for any payments, credit adjustments and the current balance
- Statements 2–5 should be balance-forwarded typed statements with proper credit messages
- Statement 6 should be the patient's final notice
- Collection letters
- Collection letter services
- Collection telephone calls
- Collection agencies
- Credit bureaus
- Conciliation court
— Monitoring Collections
- Write-off percent
- Collection percent
- Dollar amount of accounts receivable
- Size of accounts receivable
- Size of accounts receivable to monthly charges
- Aging accounts receivable

§ 7.100 Bibliography

Lusk, E. J. and Lusk, J. G.: Financial and Managerial Control: A Health Care Perspective. Germantown, MD: Aspen Systems Corp., 1979.

Silvers, J. B. and Pralhalad, C. K.: Financial Management of Health Institutions. Flushing, NY: Spectrum Publications, distributed by Halstad Press, 1974.

Appendix 7-A

CREDIT AND COLLECTION POLICY

It is the policy of the U.S.A. Clinic to provide the finest quality of medical care available. In an effort to make our services available to as many patients as possible on an affordable basis the U.S.A. Clinic employs firm practice management. This enables us to provide the highest level of care, and at the same time be sensitive to cost containment. In an effort to be fair to all patients, the U.S.A. Clinic has adopted the collection policy outlined below. Please read the policy to learn how the services from the U.S.A. Clinic will be provided to you in an affordable way.

Insurance Coverage and Third Parties.

To help reduce paperwork and relieve patients of financial burdens, the U.S.A. Clinic has entered into a contractual arrangement with the following insurance companies and third parties:

1. Blue Cross and Blue Shield of the U.S.
2. U.S. State Medicaid Program
3. HMO of U.S. City

Patients covered under these programs will be responsible only for the services not covered, deductibles and participations in accordance with their specific contracts. The U.S.A. Clinic will bill the insurance carrier third party directly for that portion of the bill for which they are responsible. If you have coverage under one of these plans and are uncertain as to what items are covered or what you will be responsible for, please discuss this with our credit manager, Mr. Harvey Hanson, before services are commenced. It is our policy to work with patients when confusion arises over these issues to eliminate future problems.

As a service to our patients, we will generally bill other third parties directly when patients assign benefits directly to the U.S.A. Clinic. In those cases, the insurance company will generally pay U.S.A. Clinic directly and the patient need pay only deductibles, co-insurance amounts and noncovered services. If a problem with the third party occurs, we will provide the patient with information on services performed so that the patient may receive all benefits due

(Pub.372)

under his or her plan. In these cases, however, the patient must remember that he or she assumes ultimate responsibility for the bill and that the U.S.A. Clinic has no control or authority over the patient's insurance company.

New Patients

New patients visiting our clinic are expected to pay in full for services when they are performed. Please bring insurance coverage information including the insurance company's name, policy number, group numbers and type of coverage. Since new patients are expected to pay for services when performed, they should be prepared to do so at the completion of the first visit. For the convenience of new patients U.S.A. Clinic will accept payment via Mastercard or Visa credit cards.

Established Patients

Established patients are always welcome to pay for services when performed or to charge services on their Visa or Mastercard. As a convenience to our patients, our business office will accept payments at the time of service to avoid billing costs and future inconvenience to our patients. Patients will always be given a complete itemized statement suitable for reimbursement from insurance companies at they time they visit our office.

Established patients who wish to charge services may do so. For these accounts, it is our policy to bill every thirty days. Patients making charges at our office are expected to pay the bill in full within thirty days of receipt of statement.

Patients who have large bills from U.S.A. Clinic as a result of extended care or hospitalization and who are unable to make full payment of their bill as a result of financial difficulties should contact our credit manager, Mr. Harvey Hanson, as soon as possible. It is the policy of this clinic to help work out payment terms to patients in financial need, but we can do so only if Mr. Hanson is contacted to make arrangements.

Summary

If you have any questions regarding our collection policies, please contact Mr. Hanson to discuss them. Mr. Hanson is familiar with most of the major third party contracts and may be able to answer questions regarding your coverage or direct you to people who can do so. Things don't always go as planned. If a problem comes up that you didn't anticipate, and you are unable to pay your bill, contact Mr. Hanson. This will let us know you are receiving your bill and are not making efforts to avoid payment. Thank you for being cooperative in our collection policy and thank you for selecting U.S.A. Clinic as your provider of health care services.

Appendix 7-B

CREDIT LETTERS

Credit letters like those presented here can be purchased directly from medical publishers. These collection letters can be used if you wish to avoid sending out personalized collection letters on your office letterhead. A medical practice might consider sending out variations on these letters in the following sequence:

CREDIT POLICY

DR. ARTHUR J. PETTERSON, P.C.
7801 WINPARK DRIVE, SUITE 204
MINNEAPOLIS, MINNESOTA 55427
TELEPHONE: (612) 545-3200

DATE_____   BALANCE DUE $_____

The purpose of this reminder is to clarify our credit policy and thus avoid any misunderstanding now and in the future.

Our office policy is to extend 30 days credit to those patients who request it. All accounts are billed monthly and are due and payable upon receipt of statement. **Extension of credit beyond 30 days must be approved by our office.**

As of this date, no payment has been received on the balance shown above, nor have you contacted our office to explain why. An immediate remittance or response is requested.

Sincerely

_____
Office Secretary

FIG. 7-7.

(Pub. 372)

7–57   **CREDIT & COLLECTIONS**   **App. 7–B**

Co-operation is a two-way street

We've done more than our share to call to your attention your past due balance of $ _____.

Your co-operation as noted below will demonstrate that you intend to meet your obligations and protect your credit standing.

☐ Wish I could pay it all, but the enclosed check is the best I can do right now.

☐ I am sending full payment in this envelope.

☐ I'll send you a check not later than _____.

MEDICAL ARTS PRESS OR THE BILL-A-PAK CO., MPLS, MN 55427   ← DETACH ALONG THIS PERFORATION →   USE THE ENVELOPE BELOW FOR YOUR REMITTANCE

FROM _____

PLACE STAMP HERE

DR.   P.A.
WINPARK DRIVE
MINNEAPOLIS, MN 55427

FIG. 7–8.

(Pub.372)

App. 7–B   MANAGING YOUR MEDICAL PRACTICE   7–58

FINAL NOTICE

, M.D., P.C.
MEDICAL ARTS BLDG.
MINNEAPOLIS, MINN. 55402

TELEPHONE: (612) 827-4003

AMT. ENCLOSED $ _____

BALANCE DUE $ _____

Because your account is long past due, we would normally turn it over to a collection agency. We would, however, prefer dealing directly with you. Please read and check one of the three options below and return to us.

☐ 1. I would prefer to settle this account. Please find full payment enclosed.

☐ 2. I would prefer to make monthly payments of $ _____ until this balance is cleared up. I understand that no interest will be charged for this delayed payment schedule.

☐ 3. I would prefer that you assign this account to an agency for collection. (Failure to return this past due reminder will result in this action.)

Signed: _____

If you have any questions, please do not hesitate to call me.

Sincerely,

_____
Office Secretary

FIG. 7–9.

(Pub.372)

STOP SERVICE ORDER

███████████, M.D., P.C.
██████, MEDICAL ARTS BLDG.
MINNEAPOLIS, MINN. 55402

TELEPHONE: (612) 827-4003

DATE_____   BALANCE DUE $_____

Repeated requests by this office for settlement of your balance as shown above have brought no response from you.

Under these circumstances, it becomes necessary to inform you that a **STOP SERVICE ORDER** for any future medical services by members of our staff is now in effect. This includes both you and those for whom you are financially responsible.

Two options are available to you:

(1) Make immediate provision to settle your account, **in which** case this order will be rescinded; or

(2) Designate in writing another medical facility to whom **we** should transfer your records.

Be assured that <u>we stand ready to be of service in any true emergency,</u> but as of this date no further routine medical services will be available to you or your dependents from this office.

FIG. 7-10.

CHAPTER 8

Risk Management and Insurance

by

Earl Cook, Michael E. Mitchell and Joseph Miller

SCOPE

In many areas the practicing physician faces far greater risks—personal, public and professional—than any other business person. The consequences of these risks can range from minor inconvenience to financial ruin. For that reason, the physician should make an effort to eliminate risks wherever possible. Risk management begins with identifying the cost of losing or replacing specific assets and weighing the value against the cost of insuring them. Many common property losses and financial risks can be avoided through commonsense safety precautions and efficient control of personnel and office protocol. For major risks—life insurance, malpractice insurance, loss of practice, etc.—the physician should contact an insurance consultant to draw up a contract that provides adequate coverage. Both the physician-employee and the sole-owner of a practice must consider the benefits of practice coverage—such as auto insurance, fire insurance, fiduciary liability, insurance for other employees—and personal coverage—including life insurance, disability income and buyout insurance—since they are often interrelated. A contract should carry standard provisions for medical practice and practitioner insurance, and be amended with riders for any provisions found lacking.

SYNOPSIS

§ 8.01 Risk Identification
    [1] Property Losses
        [a] Direct Losses
        [b] Consequential Losses
    [2] Liability Losses

[3] Practice Loss
§ 8.02 Risk Prevention
    [1] Internal Control
    [2] Avoiding Malpractice Actions
    [3] General Risk Avoidance
§ 8.03 Insurance Coverage for the Practice
    [1] Property Losses
        [a] Direct Losses
        [b] Consequential Losses
    [2] Liability Losses
        [a] Professional Liability
        [b] Public Liability
        [c] Employer's Liability
        [d] Auto Liability
        [e] Fire Tenant's Legal Liability
        [f] Fiduciary Liability
        [g] Umbrella Liability
§ 8.04 Insurance Coverage for the Physician-Employee
    [1] Life Insurance
    [2] Disability Income
        [a] The Initial Policy
        [b] Sick Pay Plan
        [c] Major Contract Provisions
        [d] Other Contract Provisions
        [e] Riders
        [f] Policy Exclusions
    [3] Group Insurance
        [a] Questions
        [b] Overhead Expense
        [c] Disability Buyout
        [d] Medical Insurance
§ 8.05 Risk Management Checklist
§ 8.06–§ 8.99 Reserved
§ 8.100 Bibliography
Appendix 8-A Malpractice Avoidance Checklist

§ 8.01 Risk Identification

The physician should identify all potential risks in the areas of direct and consequential property loss, loss through liability and loss of practice. By determining, where possible, the cost and replacement value of specific items the physician can obtain an idea of which noncatastrophic losses are worth insuring against.

The first step toward developing a risk management program is to identify and measure potential risks. This ensures that no risk is overlooked and avoids unnecessary worry and the purchase of unnecessary insurance. Once you have measured and listed potential losses, you will be in a position to decide which losses would be catastrophic and unacceptable and which would be acceptable. You will also have enough information to weigh the cost of risk avoidance (insurance) against the potential risk of noncatastrophic losses.

Some risks are common to all businesses, or to medical practices in general. Additional risks or risks special to your practice can be identified with the help of an insurance agent or risk management consultant.

[1] Property Losses

Property losses fall into two categories: direct losses, in which tangible assets or investments are damaged or destroyed; and consequential losses, such as loss of clients, which may be the result of a direct loss.

[a] Direct Losses

Direct losses are the easiest to list. They can often be compiled through inventories.

Furniture: You should take a complete inventory of all office furniture. Every piece should be assigned a cost, and a replacement value which, in most cases, is greater than cost.

Medical and Business Equipment: Another inventory including cost and replacement value should be done for medical and business equipment.

Leasehold Improvements: A physician's leasehold improvements are generally all the changes he or she puts into an office to make it suitable for a medical practice, such as extra plumbing for sinks, carpeting, wallpaper, examination room walls, special lighting, etc. Although a tenant's rights to leasehold improvements are generally limited to the term of the lease, it is not uncommon for a physician to invest a great deal of money in them. Loss of the building or any circumstance that leads to the physician having to move his or her office could entail loss of this investment.

Accounts Receivable: The accounts receivable typically represent one and one-half to three month's worth of charges. Loss of accounts receivable could result in a tremendous financial loss and an immediate obstacle to cash flow.

Patient Records: The cost of setting up and maintaining a patient's chart is a minimum of $1.50 for a new chart and far more for an established patient's chart. The actual dollar amount involved to replace the chart is the direct loss. The value of the information lost may be immeasurable.

Other Valuable Papers: These could include all sorts of business information, ranging from insurance company profiles to corporate minutes to personnel records. The cost to replace these papers in the event of a loss could be substantial in terms of employee manpower.

Embezzlement: The most common types of embezzlement in the medical office are misappropriation of patient receipts and false postings in the accounts receivable file. Other areas where the physician is vulnerable include accounts payable, payroll and the petty cash fund.

Continued Overhead Costs: In the event of a destruction of the office or practice you can incur the cost of continued overhead for such things as employee salaries. In the event a partner becomes disabled, the continued overhead cost could be even greater. Most of the cost would continue for at least a limited amount of time.

Automobiles: An automobile can be an essential tool of the practice if you have to do much traveling between the office and hospitals, nursing homes or other offices. If your practice's automobile is destroyed you will be liable not only for replacing it but also for associated interim expenses, such as car rental.

[b] Consequential Losses

Direct losses are often compounded by a number of consequential losses that have a greater or incalculable monetary value.

Loss of Patients: Almost any of the above losses can result in inconvenience to and the eventual loss of a patient. If your office is temporarily shut down, the patient may be forced to see another physician in the interim. If the patient feels the services obtained through the temporary physician are better than yours, he or she may never return.

Loss of Patient Goodwill: Any inconvenience can result in a loss of goodwill between you and a patient. For example, if a patient's account is embezzled and the situation is not properly handled, it is possible that the patient will be billed a second time when, in fact, he or she has paid the bill. Any time the patient's goodwill is lost or diminished, the chances of losing the patient, losing patient referrals and exposing yourself to a malpractice suit increase.

Loss of Employees: Recruitment and training of an employee often take substantial time and money. A direct loss whose consequential loss is the loss of an employee can damage your practice.

Loss of Income: Any time a practice is closed, its earning power is zero. Since your compensation comes directly from practice earnings, not operating the practice means you earn no income.

[2] Liability Losses

In addition to relatively straightforward property losses, you should review the more complex risk of losses associated with personal and professional liability.

Professional Liability: Professional liability, or the risk of a lawsuit as a result of malpractice or alleged malpractice, is undoubtedly the greatest, most frightening area of potential risk in your risk management program. Owing to inflation and liberal juries and judges, malpractice claims in the last fifteen years have exceeded what insurers consider reasonable maximums.

Public Liability: In comparison to professional liability, a physician's public liability may seem a trivial concern. However, it is important and you must identify it as a potential risk. Public liability is any liability that does not have a professional origin; for example, a patient falling in the office or getting his or her hand caught in a door. In severe cases—for example, a patient who is left permanently disabled as a result of a fall—your public liability risk can be substantial.

Worker's Liability: As an employer you are liable for employee injuries on the job. Although the risk for a person in the medical office is less than that of an iron worker, for example, the potential for harm still exists. Worker's compensation laws are in effect throughout the country, and it is generally not possible for a medical office to cover this risk without worker's compensation insurance.

Automobile Liability: Liability for a business owned automobile is probably one of a medical practice's greatest and best known potential risks. Less well known, though, is the liability for an automobile not owned by the practice. As an employer, you incur liability for any employee who conducts company business in his or her own car. Even though it may not be routine practice for your employees to use their own cars for practice business, you are liable even if the employee is only running out to make a bank deposit or pick up supplies from a store.

Fire Liability: Fire liability is another little-known risk. If a fire that destroys an entire office building originated in your office, it is possible you could be sued for the entire, potentially enormous loss.

[3] Practice Loss

Death or disability of one or more owners of the practice could result in immediate loss of the entire practice. Before you are re-established the value of goodwill, patient records and accounts receivable could diminish and a forced liquidation of the office furniture and medical equipment could result in a selling price far below cost or replacement value. In short, your most valuable assets could disappear overnight if you do not identify and take steps to avert or minimize this potential risk.

§ 8.02 Risk Prevention

Part of being a good businessman is using all available safeguards to prevent avoidable risks. In the medical profession these safeguards include internal control over employees and accounts, general risk prevention against such problems as burglaries and loss of the practice through the death of a partner, and protection against malpractice suits. Most forms of risk prevention involve a combination of common sense and good business sense.

Once you have identified risks, you must find the best, most practical and least expensive way to avoid them. Although each medical office must be considered individually, there are some areas common to all in which loss can be prevented or minimized.

(Pub.372)

[1] Internal Control

Techniques for internal control should derive largely from the personnel and employment policies you establish at your practice's outset.

Quality Personnel: The best way to prevent embezzlement problems is to hire good personnel (see Chapter 2, Staff Recruiting, Development and Management). Be sure to check references personally, and remember that an applicant's past employer will frequently say things on the telephone that he or she would not put in writing.

Divide Bookkeeping Duties: Split up the accounting process as much as possible. For example, have different people open the mail, deposit the checks and post payments to patient accounts.

Use Prenumbered Documents: By using prenumbered receipts, charge slips, checks and deposit slips it is easier to discover when they are missing and if they have been used to conceal embezzled funds.

Endorse All Checks Immediately: Have an endorsement stamp made up that says 'For Deposit Only' and that specifies your business account and account number. Do not endorse insurance checks over to patients: they may never get beyond an employee's desk and could present tax problems in the event of an audit. Deposit insurance checks in the practice checking account and issue patients refund checks.

Keep Duplicate Deposit Slips: Match duplicates against total cash receipts posted for each day to check for discrepancies.

Personally Approve All Adjustments, Discounts and Write-Offs: No adjustment, discount or write-off should be permitted if it does not carry your signature or initials. The total of these items should be balanced monthly.

Balance Ledger Cards: Make sure the sum total of patient accounts equals the control total of accounts receivable.

Send Detailed Charge and Payment Statements to Patients. This way, if a patient's payment is omitted from his or her account, the patient is better able to report it.

Insist Employees Take Vacations: Some devoted employees never take vacations because they are afraid to leave their duties to someone else. However, in some situations temporary assignment of their duties to another person may uncover discrepancies.

Don't Type Checks: Hand write checks. The modern typewriter can easily lift-off what has been written on the check and change names or figures. Don't allow erasable ink pens in your office either.

Invoice and Statement Control: Have your bookkeeper present the invoice and statements with the check when you pay for supplies or services. This way the vendor of services can be clearly identified and verified.

Keep Financial Records in the Office: Do not allow employees to remove financial records from the office. No matter how dedicated the employee, do not let him or her take records to work on at home.

Periodically Add Up Journal Sheets: Every now and then take the time to add up the figures of the bookkeeper. This will let the bookkeeper know you are watching things and would detect any massive errors or cheating.

Periodically Check an Entire Day's Records for Accuracy. For example, check the appointment book against all of the patients which have been in for the day. Check to make sure that all patients who have been in have had charges posted to their accounts. Check the deposit for the day against the daysheet postings and review any discrepancies with your accountant. Let your employees know you are reviewing the records: it may turn up an embezzler or discourage one from starting.

Have the Completed Daysheet Placed on Your Desk for Review: Even if you don't have time to review the sheets each day, the routine delivery of daysheets to your desk each day gives the impression that you review them.

Don't Cheat: Remember that you set rules of the office. If you "occasionally" take a few dollars out of petty cash for lunch and don't put in an IOU or business document that acknowledges it, you give employees the impression that this is acceptable behavior. If you accept cash payments from patients with the intent of omitting receipts from the financial records, you are sanctioning dishonest policies.

(Pub.372)

Be Alert: Watch for warning signals from your employees, such as:

- Casual office procedures or sloppy bookkeeping.
- Resisting change.
- The appearance of living beyond means or a noticeable change in spending habits.
- IOUs in the petty cash.
- Switching vendors for no apparent reason.
- High pressure collection tactics that yield no visible results.
- Staff involved with financial matters who don't allow others to help in the bookkeeping or running of the accounts receivable tape at the end of the month.
- Missing petty cash slips and cash receipts.
- Resentment expressed toward your lifestyle or income.

A detailed internal control checklist is provided in Figure 8-1.

[2] Avoiding Malpractice Actions

Every physician should use malpractice prophylaxis. Most preventive measures are simply good business practice.

Do Not Disclose that You Have Professional Liability Insurance: It is well known that many patients feel malpractice awards don't "hurt" doctors since they are covered by insurance. It is important to have malpractice insurance, but do not discuss it with patients.

Use X-Rays as a Diagnostic or Confirmatory Aid Where They Are Established Practice: Don't try to "save" the patient money. If it turns out that you missed something because an x-ray was not taken when it should been, you could be accused of malpractice.

Do Not Criticize the Work of Other Physicians: Criticizing the work of another physician weakens that physician's defense and may invite retaliation. It is best to handle any professional incompetence you perceive through peer review. Report questionable practices to the medical society and/or appropriate hospital administration.

Secure Legal Counsel when Participating as a Witness at a

INTERNAL CONTROL CHECKLIST

	YES	NO
CASH COLLECTION & RECEIPTS		
1. Is a seperate change fund being maintained?		
2. Are receipts issued for all cash payments?		
3. Are they prenumbered?		
4. Are they preprinted?		
5. Is a carbon copy kept?		
6. Are payments received indicated as check or cash on the receipts and daysheets?		
7. Is cash balanced to agree with daysheets?		
8. If a receipt is spoiled, is it voided and left in the book or attached to daysheet?		
DEPOSITS		
1. Is a deposit prepared daily?		
2. Are receipts deposited daily?		
3. Are deposits held overnight stored safely?		
4. Are total receipts being deposited?		
5. Are payments by check listed on the deposit form?		
6. Are the carbon copy deposit forms attached to the daysheet or kept in book?		
7. Is the bank statement opened only by the Doctor or the accountants?		
8. Do employees cash personal checks with deposit monies?		
PETTY CASH CONTROL		
1. Do you have a petty cash fund?		
2. Do you itemize petty cash expenditures?		
3. Are receipts kept for petty cash expenditures?		
4. Do you keep a running balance of the petty cash fund?		
5. How much is in the fund now? Does the cash balance agree with the records?		
6. Are petty cash monies kept separate from any change funds?		
7. Are employee purses and personal belongings kept in a separate location away from the reception area?		
EMPLOYEE CONTROL		
1. Are employees who handle cash bonded?		
2. Are employees required to rotate duties and responsibilities?		
3. Are refund checks approved by the Doctor?		
4. Are "write-offs" approved by the Doctor?		
5. Is control maintained over accounts in collection?		

FIG. 8-1. An internal control checklist is helpful for assessing the effectiveness of employee-directed monetary transactions and any areas where a backup system may be wanting or necessary.

Coroner's Inquest. It is prudent to consult an attorney who specializes in malpractice cases before participating at a coroner's inquest or autopsy, especially if you are inexperienced. If you make inaccurate statements, they could be construed as negligence on your part.

Keep Office Equipment in Excellent Working Order at All Times: Equipment in poor condition may lead you to misinterpret important information or give the wrong results for tests that are your responsibility.

Furnish Proper Notice of Termination of Services to Avoid Charges of Abandonment: In the event you decide to terminate services to a particular patient, make sure that written notice is given to the patient and recorded in the patient's records. Policies on abandonment vary with the community and availability of other physicians.

Maintain Permanent, Adequate Records: It is important to keep comprehensive records for patient files, since you may not remember all the details of a particular patient's case and since, at some point, another physician may become involved in a case and need to review the patient's files. In the event of a malpractice suit, the medical records may be your only defense. Do not destroy medical records. If space is a problem, consider microfilming.

Be Knowledgeable about a Physician's Legal Duty to a Patient: If this is unclear, speak to your malpractice insurer. Much information is available on the dos and don'ts and in some areas continuing education courses are offered on the subject.

Whenever Possible and Necessary Have a Witness Present when Consulting with a Patient: Especially in the case of women patients treated by a male physician, have a nurse or medical assistant in the examination room. Certain procedures—for example, pelvic examinations for a female patient or artificial insemination—should not be done under any circumstances without a witness present. You should be aware of the standards for your particular medical community.

Review All Bad Debts before Giving Them to a Collection Agency or Conciliation Court: A patient may not pay a bill because he or she has already paid it, or is under the impression that a third-party insurer is taking care of it.

Consult an Attorney about Making Personal Assets Less Vulnerable to Professional Damage Suits: This should be done as part of your financial planning.

Never Guarantee Results: Guarantees are uninsurable and considered unethical. You are in no position to guarantee results and you open yourself up to a malpractice suit by doing so.

Keep Abreast of the Average Standards of Your Specialty: Participate in group study and attend local meetings to keep up to date on current practice. Make it a habit to meet periodically with detail men to find out what new products are coming on the market. Set aside time to read contemporary professional journals.

(Pub.372)

Be Diplomatic and Courteous in Dealing with Patients: Even the most difficult patients must be handled politely. Don't allow the patient's behavior to make you act unprofessionally.

Furnish Proper Instructions for Patient Care and Prescriptions: Take time to discuss with each patient the therapy or care you recommend. In many cases, a medical assistant or nurse can be trained to go over detailed instructions with patients. Whenever possible, it is a good idea to give the patient written instructions. This makes the patient more comfortable with what's going on and is the best deterrent to misunderstanding.

Give the Patient an Idea of the Fee before the Procedure Is Performed: While this seems common sense, many physicians perform services without giving the patient any information regarding cost. The fee is part of the crucial information the patient should have, especially if it is going to be sizable.

Refrain from Giving or Renewing Prescriptions over the Telephone. If the problem the patient is having is important enough to prompt a telephone call, it is probably important enough so that the patient should come to see you. This not only reduces the risk of malpractice, it can help to build your practice.

Keep All Scheduled Appointments: It is not always possible for you to keep on schedule, but if you are off schedule consistently, if you cancel appointments and if you usually make your patients wait, they may feel you are incompetent or hurried and disorganized.

Help Patients Secure Consultants: Do not be afraid or hesitate to refer patients to consultants when appropriate. Failure to do so can lead to a question of malpractice if a problem occurs.

Keep Relations with Patients Strictly Confidential: Violation of this rule by any staff member should be grounds for immediate termination. As in other areas, you are the leader and are expected to treat information professionally and confidentially.

Recommend a Competent Substitute to the Patient when You Will Be Absent from the Practice: Don't leave for vacation without having adequate coverage arrangements for your patients. A contingency plan should be available in the event you become ill or disabled. This is generally more of problem for the single practitioner than for the group practitioner.

Don't Practice Medicine You Are Not Properly Qualified to Perform: No physician is confident in all areas of medicine. You must know know your limits and refer work to others when appropriate.

Secure Proper Written Consent in All Cases: Without documentation of informed consent you can be charged with assault, or worse, especially if a procedure is controversial or a failure.

Avoid Using Any Unapproved or Experimental Procedures or Drugs: In the event your practice is participating in a drug study, the patient must sign informed consent forms prior to the use of drugs. For the most part, it's probably best to leave experimental procedures and drugs to the universities and other research facilities.

Furnish Assistants with Proper Instructions and Monitor Their Follow-through: It is important that medical assistants be properly trained to carry out their responsibilities. Take time to give your staff specific instructions on how you want things done. Lack of communication in this area is extremely dangerous.

Exercise Caution Continuously: Be especially careful in the labeling of containers, observing casts for fractures, etc.

Make Sure the Number of Visits Are Adequate for Patient Care: Inform patients if they are going to need followup and record this on the medical record to avoid accusations that you never discussed it with them. A recall system for contacting patients who fail to follow up is also helpful. Regardless of whether you have a recall system, though, you should place the burden of followup on the patient by informing him or her of its importance.

Avoid Admitting Anything Against Your Own Interests on Services You Have Performed or That Someone Else Has Performed on Your Behalf: It can be used against you. A physician should never criticize staff in front of patients.

Secure Proper Authorization for Any Autopsy in which You Participate. You can perform an autopsy only after you have obtained proper permission. Failure to obtain authorization from the proper party can result in a lawsuit.

A comprehensive checklist of steps the physician should take to avoid a malpractice suit is provided in Appendix 8-A.

[3] General Risk Avoidance

Every medical office should periodically review steps it takes to avoid risks, whether to prevent an office burglary or an employee injury that results from carelessness. Some routine methods for avoiding risks include:

Security Locks: Physician's offices are prime targets for burglars looking for petty cash, checks and narcotics. Make sure your office has high quality dead bolt locks and that they are securely bolted each night.

Fire Resistant Safe: Use a fire resistant safe to store cash, the change fund, office checks and narcotics. If you have a deposit that cannot be taken to the bank until the next day, this too should be placed in the safe. Any unposted patient checks should also be placed in the safe.

Back Up and Remove Computer Files: All computer files should be backed up at least once a week and a copy of the tape or disk removed from the premises. This not only avoids the potential loss of data through computer breakdown, but also allows for data to be recreated in the event of a fire or other catastrophe.

Microfilm Billing: Offices not on computer may backup their accounts receivable with a microfilm billing service. A microfilm billing service usually keeps a copy of the microfilm until the next film is made. An alternative to using a microfilm billing service is to make duplicate copies of ledger cards periodically and remove them from the premises.

Periodically Microfilm Patient Records: Since patient records are so valuable, consider microfilming them (especially older records) occasionally and removing microfilms from the premises. (Some offices use microfilm to store old patient records since the cost of space has risen so rapidly.)

Smoke Detectors: Inexpensive smoke detectors give effective warning before a fire gets out of hand.

Sprinkler Systems: Many large offices have built-in sprinkler systems. Smaller offices should consider installing one at the time of construction. The installation of a sprinkler system may prevent catastrophic loss by fire and pay for itself through reduced insurance premiums.

Close and Lock Patient Record Files: Although this sounds like common sense, many offices leave the files open at night. In order to minimize the risk of theft and fire damage, files should be closed each night.

Avoid Storing an Inventory of Narcotics: By not storing or inventorying narcotics, you reduce the risk of burglaries by drug addicts. Any narcotics kept in the office should be locked in the safe at night.

Electronic Burglar Alarms: Modern burglar alarms can alert the police or a private security service when anyone has tampered with or entered the office. Free-standing medical facilities in particular should consider electronic burglar alarms.

Secure and Lock Windows: Many burglars enter through open or unlocked windows. Appoint someone on the staff to make sure all of the windows are closed and locked at the end of each working day.

Keep More than One Employee on Duty in Off Hours: If your office has evening or weekend hours, be sure to have more than one employee on duty to discourage thieves and troublemakers.

Participate in Operation I.D.: Most local police departments have an Operation I.D. in which office equipment and furniture are marked with a unique identification mark or number. In the event a burglary does occur, stolen goods can be more easily recovered and the suspect incriminated.

Employee Education: Encourage employees to practice safe office procedures. File drawers should not be left open, single electrical outlets should not be overused. Point out dangers to the staff and ask staff members to be alert.

Office Design and Condition: Office design and condition should be efficient and uncluttered. The file cabinets should not be overfilled to the point of collapse. To minimize fire hazards papers should not be strewn all over the office. Old records should be properly filed or removed to a remote location and laboratories and other essential areas should be properly ventilated.

Security Service: Many medical office buildings provide a security service with watchmen who patrol the area and notify the police of any suspicious activity. Free-standing medical clinics may consider retaining a security service. Private security services make periodic visits after hours and are typically "wired" to the clinic via a burglar alarm.

Report Unusual or Suspicious Events: Any unusual or suspicious activity should be reported to the police or security service. Thieves typically check out future victims by first visiting their offices.

Keep a Close Inventory of Business Checks: Stolen checks are of prime interest to burglars. Keep track of your checks so that in the event of a burglary or theft the specific missing checks may be reported to the bank. At night, keep blank checks in the safe. Any missing, lost or stolen checks should be immediately reported to the bank.

Buy-Sell Agreements: Establish a plan for the orderly sale of the practice far in advance of the death of any members of the group. In a group practice this is often done in the form of a buy-sell agreement between the stockholders. The agreement determines when the sale will occur, and how valuation and payments are to be made. A single practitioner should explore the possibility of having another doctor or group of doctors willing to acquire the practice in the event of death or disability. In busy cities this may be impossible; in other areas where competition for patients is greater, the physician may find a group happy to enter into such an arrangement.

Legal Exclusion: When possible, draft contracts for agreements excluding you from liabilities. For example, include specific provisions in the lease agreement exempting you from liability for fire if you have discussed this with the landlord. Or, if you are a single practitioner, include an option to cancel the lease in the event of death or disability.

§ 8.03 Insurance Coverage for the Practice

A physician should be able to find insurance for almost every risk that warrants it. However, not all insurance policies cover all risks, so the physician should consult with an insurance professional to work out the best arrangement. The ideal insurance policy will be broad enough to cover unforseen losses yet specific enough to compensate the physician for a high-risk loss. Insurance for property losses should cover both direct and consequential losses. Malpractice insurance should have a realistic ceiling for both maximum benefits and premiums.

[1] Property Losses

Good property loss insurance should take into account the potential for both direct and consequential losses.

[a] Direct Losses

Your medical office should have coverage for both the direct and consequential potential property losses mentioned in § 8.01. The direct property policy usually covers office contents, such as furniture and medical equipment, and leasehold improvements under an amount based on the cost to replace them with new pieces of similar quality. You should work with an insurance professional within the following suggested guidelines to obtain sufficient coverage.

- The direct loss of property policy for your practice should be drawn up as an "All Risks" form, which lists specific exclusions for policy coverage, rather than a "Named Perils" form, which names the only circumstances under which you are covered. Although the "All Risks" form of coverage carries higher premiums, it provides you with coverage for unusual, once-in-a-lifetime losses in addition to the standard perils such as fire and theft. Exclusions on this form are few, but they usually include earthquake and flood. If your practice is situated in an area subject to these circumstances, ask the agent for a policy underwritten by a company that does not exclude those catastrophies. Check with the state and local medical associates for your specialty, since many design their own medical office coverage.

- If your office is computerized, make sure coverage for computers is included in the main policy or written in separately. Some companies cover mechanical breakdown and other broader problems as well.

- Paintings and other valuable personal items kept permanently in the office may not be covered on the policy. Check to see if coverage for these items is automatically provided or if endorsements are required.

- You should have a sufficient amount of coverage for items temporarily removed from the office, such as your medical

- bag, instruments, briefcase and items used while at the hospital, during patient visits or in transit.
- Check to see if the policy includes the cost of a professional inventory or appraisal following a loss. If not, estimate the replacement cost and if it is substantial enough to insure, add it by special endorsement.
- Provide the agent and accountant with a copy of the office lease, particularly the section dealing with leasehold improvements. Coverage depends on the terms of your lease, and the amount you have invested in improvements.

Other items that should be covered by direct property loss insurance include:

Accounts Receivable: This coverage guards against loss of income attributable to the loss of patient financial records, an insured peril. Whether or not you have such a policy, it is good risk management to keep a duplicate set of records in a different location. If your office is not computerized, a copy of the preceding month's statements would suffice as a base to start computing actual accounts receivable. Most computer systems manufacturers recommend weekly back-up, a service you should look into if your office is not already on it.

Valuable Papers: A loss of detailed patient records can cost considerable time and money to reconstruct. Even if insurance is available for such a loss, some form of duplicate record, such as microfilm or computer back-up, might be a better approach.

Embezzlement: Review the amount of fidelity insurance carried by your practice with your accountant. Having a fidelity bond (a type of employer insurance against employee improprieties) not only helps cover financial losses but excuses you from the emotional aspects of employee embezzlement: when a loss is discovered, the case is turned over to the bonding company, who can deal with it and the employee involved without prejudice.

[b] Consequential Losses

Any loss of income that results from an interruption of the practice by an insured peril (for example, a fire that not only directly destroys property but also shuts down the business) is considered a consequential loss. You should consult an insurance agent to determine the length of time it is expected it will take before your practice is running again and producing at its pre-loss income level. Most insurance policies only cover reconstruction of the practice. Coverage for income losses in the interim must be purchased as an addendum. A survey shows that 78 percent of manufacturing plants who do not have this type of coverage never get back into business after being forced to close. A medical practice is very different from a manufacturing plant, but this type of consequential loss is still an important area for review.

Business interruption insurance will reimburse the insured for losses incurred from the date of loss for a period not to exceed the time it would take to rebuild or repair the damaged property. As soon as the property has been repaired or rebuilt, the business interruption policy stops paying.

Leasehold interest also falls under consequential property insurance. This provides compensation for the difference between the actual rent on the premises and the rent payable for the unexpired term of the lease for comparable premises should the lease be cancelled as the result of an insured peril. It should also include the unamortized value of office improvements.

[2] Liability Losses

The medical profession, more so than the average business, is exposed to loss through liability. Liability losses can be broken down into a several categories, each with its own type of coverage.

[a] Professional Liability

This is essential coverage for which many state medical societies and national specialty associations have designed policies. It is a common belief in the insurance industry that this type of coverage should be handled by professional programs. Many private insurance companies that get involved get "burned" by losses, make an abrupt exit—sometimes in bankruptcy—and leave physicians with outstanding claims. Furthermore, state societies and specialty associations require physician support if they are to continue assisting the medical community through the ups and downs of the insurance industry cycles.

Regardless of the precautions you take, no physician is immune to medical malpractice suits. Whether they are meritorious or not, all suits require that you defend yourself or pay. Over the years, malpractice claims have steadily increased in both frequency and the amount of damages sought, and it would mean potential financial suicide for many physicians if there were not maximum limits to the amount payable. Each incorporated practice, as well as each physician in the practice, should have professional liability insurance. Split maximum limits of $1,000,000/$3,000,000 are common, with $1,000,000 being the maximum paid per person in a policy year and $3,000,000 being the annual aggregate, or the amount that would be paid for all claims against the practice in a single year. However, many policies are written in excess of these limits and some are written for only $100,000/$300,000. If you are in a high-risk state, you may want to purchase coverage with higher limits. (Your state medical association and your insurance agent should have information on whether your state is at high or low risk.)

Despite the fact that many physicians are employees of a professional corporation, state laws do not relieve them of professional liability. Whereas in a partnership, each physician is responsible for the actions of his partners, in a corporation the physician is relieved of responsibility for his colleagues. It is in your best interest to check your state laws before securing professional liability coverage.

[b] Public Liability

Public liability coverage guards against "slips and falls." You should purchase this coverage from a professional liability carrier to avoid potential arguments over a claim (e.g., did the patient fall off the table because she was ill and no one was watching [malpractice] or because it was slippery from overwaxing [public liability]).

[c] Employer's Liability

State legislation mandates worker's compensation coverage and rates for employers. Legislation also determines whether private insurance companies can utilize an Experience Modification Program. This program allows either an increase or decrease in the state rates, based on loss experiences of individual medical practices when compared to all medical practices in the state.

Since most physicians are small employers they do not qualify for favorable experience ratings. This means they pay a premium rate as high as 20 to 40 percent more than some practices that qualify. However, state legislation also allows a practice to join a "group" of other medical practices and pool claims to obtain dividends based on the experience of the group.

[d] Auto Liability

Even if a practice does not own a car, it should have coverage for non-owned auto liability (see § 8.01). Non-owned auto liability insurance covers the practice should an employee be involved in an accident while on practice business (e.g., the bookkeeper who has an accident in his or her own car while taking practice receipts to the bank).

However, in many instances when a case goes to court an employer's liability may be extended beyond normal limits. In a case in San Jose involving an employee who had an accident while on lunch break, the court ruled that the doctor-employer was liable because if he had provided a place for employees to eat lunch, the employee would not have been on the road at the time of the accident.

Hired auto liability coverage is normally an ancillary part of the employer's non-owned auto coverage.

Owned auto coverage is similar to personal auto coverage.

[e] Fire Tenant's Legal Liability

Here is an uncommon but possible scenario: The office building housing a medical practice burns down and is rebuilt by the landlord's fire insurance company. However, the landlord's insurance company can prove that the physician or his or her staff were negligent in causing the fire. The landlord's company can sue the practice for reimbursement of what it has paid for the rebuilding—unless the practice has a Waiver of Subrogation clause in its lease.

If the practice is without the clause, a reasonable landlord usually agrees to add one retroactively if the physician's agent can show that it will not increase the fire insurance premium. But what can be done if the landlord is unreasonable and will not add the clause?

- You can purchase an amount of fire tenant's legal liability coverage equal to the value of the portion of the building occupied.

- You can check to make sure that the property damage limit under the general liability policy at least equals the value of the rest of the building.

[f] Fiduciary Liability

There are two kinds of fiduciary liability:

- Employee benefits liability, which protects a practice if the employer fails to provide whatever group benefits are normally provided to their employees. A simple example is the employer who forgets to add a new employee to the practice's health insurance plan. When this employee becomes ill and there is no coverage, the employee has grounds for a suit.

- E.R.I.S.A. liability. Employers should be aware of the Employment Retirement Income Security Act of 1974 and its amendments. The provisions of E.R.I.S.A. require all fiduciaries and persons who handle retirement plan funds or other plan assets to be bonded for 10 percent of the aggregate amount handled, with a minimum bond of $1,000 and a maximum bond of $500,000. Bonding generally is not required of corporate trustees or insurance companies with combined capital and surplus of at least $1,000,000. Coverage is usually written on a "claims made" form rather than on an "occurrence form," so the applicability and availability of a retroactive date and extended reporting period should be reviewed with an insurance professional.

[g] Umbrella Liability

Should the maximum limits available on general, auto and professional liability policies be considered insufficient, you may have your agent purchase excess limits through an "umbrella" liability policy. Some umbrella policies profess to offer broader coverage than the underlying policies and charge a deductible for it. As there is no standard wording for an umbrella policy, you should review the options each provides with your agent.

§ 8.04 Insurance Coverage for the Physician-Employee

As an employee or proprietor of his or her practice, the physician must also consider the importance of life insurance, disability insurance and, where applicable, group insurance. Most of these policies offer a variety of compensation plans, provisions and riders that necessitate consideration of personal, family and practice needs in the event of sickness or injury.

There are three areas of employee benefit insurance the physician should consider: life insurance, disability insurance and group major medical insurance. Whether your practice is a sole proprietorship, partnership or corporation makes little difference when purchasing these types of insurance, except perhaps with regard to how premiums or benefits are taxed.

[1] Life Insurance

A life insurance policy can resolve many needs. The typical uses of a life insurance policy, or the needs which might dictate the use of life insurance include, but are not limited to: family protection; key person protection; a corporate or partnership buy-out; liquidity and estate planning; funding for prior loan commitments (i.e., repayment of education loans, repayment of loans obtained to begin a practice or for obtaining additional equipment). In virtually all situations in which an untimely death would place a financial burden on partners and/or family members, the purchase of life insurance must be considered.

Typically, the decision is not so much whether life insurance should be purchased, but rather what form of life insurance should be purchased and by what method. Although planners disagree among themselves about the relative merits of term insurance versus whole life, universal life versus interest-sensitive products, etc. they all consider the need for life insurance a given. Irrespective of its form or the way it is purchased, sound financial management of your personal and professional life demands that you have some type of life insurance. If you have been in practice for any period of time, you undoubtedly have a life insurance plan with which you are comfortable.

[2] Disability Income

The disability income, or "product," is designed to protect against the loss of earning ability caused by accident or sickness. No other financial product offers more effective protection

A physician, in particular, should be aware of the necessity for such coverage. The physician's capital value is based almost entirely on his or her earning capacity. In the physician's absence, the practice is of little value. Retained earnings, inventory, and goodwill—the basis of equity and net worth to most businessmen—are not a major part of the physician's financial life. Earned income alone compensates the doctor for his/her talent, skill, training and years of preparation.

In the not-too-distant past, most disability coverage was short-term or, at best, offered only limited long-term protection. Even though physicians have always been considered good risks and qualified for the lowest premiums and the highest amount of monthly benefits based on income, insurers typically paid relatively low amounts of disability, usually to a maximum of $4,000 to $6,000 of monthly benefits. These contracts were often subject to cancellation and/or premium increases because insurance companies were overwhelmed by the relative size of the risk. As an example, consider that if a 35-year-old became totally disabled with benefits payable to age 65 of only $3,000 a month, the total liability of the insurance company would still be $3,000 x 12 months x 30 years, or $1,080,000.

In addition, disability income by its nature contains an inherent "moral" risk not present in other products traditionally written by life insurance companies—the potential for an 'over-insured' claimant to make a personal profit. Life insurers have always guarded against over-insurance, even though it is doubtful that many people would forfeit their lives so that others might benefit financially. However, this risk is many times greater in a product where the insured is also the beneficiary.

A new breed of products from the insurance industry has recently emerged to offer the professional a solution to the protection of his or her future earning ability. A professional is most often considered a favorable risk and, since the practice of medicine represents to most physicians not only a method of earning income but also a higher calling to the service of their fellow men and women, it mitigates the insurance companies' sense of moral risk as well.

[a] **The Initial Policy**

Disability contracts offer a variety of combinations of benefit periods, elimination periods and amounts of coverage at specific income levels. All of these variables affect the cost of coverage.

The benefit period refers to the amount of time benefits will be received by the disabled policyholder. These periods can last for as little as two years or extend for life. There may be different benefit periods for disability caused by accident than for disability caused by sickness. Due to the nature of their particular skills, many physicians prefer that benefits for disability caused by an accident be payable for their lifetime, yet are content to have benefits for disability caused by illness paid only until age 65.

The elimination period, or waiting period, is the length of time between the actual disability incident and the commencement of the benefit period. Insurers offer many options, ranging from 30 days to one year. Usually, the shorter the elimination period, the more expensive the policy. It is prudent for the physician to select a 30-day elimination period, regardless of his or her earned income, unless he or she is a member of a large group. A large group can install a salary continuation plan for 30, 60 or 90 days to dovetail with an elimination period of greater than 30 days.

You should be aware of restrictions and benefits regarding the ownership and premiums of the policy you purchase. A sole proprietor or partner generally has few options available; his or her disability contract is paid for with pre-tax dollars and the benefits, when received, are tax free. However, most insurers offer a group billing discount, commonly 10 percent, if three or more persons are insured by a single billing.

[b] Sick Pay Plan

The physician who practices as an employee of a corporation has other options available. One of these options is commonly referred to as a "sick pay plan." A formal sick pay plan pays benefits to employees in the event of disability due to sickness or injury. To insure favorable tax treatment under such a plan, you must meet four criteria:

- The plan must originate and be put into effect prior to any disability.
- All employees covered by the plan must be informed about it.

- The details of the plan should be specified in a corporate resolution and should state the class of employees covered.
- The plan must be put in writing.

The employee is usually the owner and beneficiary of the policy, which means the policy can be taken with him or her to another job in the event of termination. The employer pays the premium and deducts it as an ordinary and necessary business expense. Premiums are not treated as taxable income to the employee. Disability benefits received by the employee are taxed as ordinary income. Although some relief from the taxation of benefits is available at very low income levels, most physicians should be prepared to receive benefits as ordinary income.

Another tax-effective way for the incorporated physician to purchase insurance is through the "Executive Bonus Plan." Typically, the corporation pays a bonus to the physician-employee equal to the premium and the personal tax due on the premium. The corporation treats these payments as salary/wages and claims a tax deduction for them. The physician then pays for disability coverage personally with a non-deductible dollar. Benefits payable under this type of disability contract are tax-free.

[c] **Major Contract Provisions**

Among the provisions you should consider when purchasing a disability contract are:

Non-Cancellable: This contract binds the insurance company to guarantee coverage until the insured reaches the age of 65. Many contracts are also conditionally renewable if the insured is older than 65 but still actively at work.

Guaranteed Renewable: This clause restricts the insurer's ability to increase the premium charge for coverage. A schedule of premiums payable and the duration (until age 65) is listed in the policy contract.

Dividends: Mutual insurance companies generally pay dividends on their policies to the insured. These types of policies are called "participating" policies, because the insured participates in the distribution of dividends earned on investment yields and premiums that exceed the amount used to pay claims. "Non-participating" policies issued by stock companies typically do not pay dividends to the insured.

Paid dividends can significantly lower the price of insurance. The mutual insurance company representative can furnish you with the company's past and present dividend schedules, and these will put you in a position to make comparisons with other companies and to evaluate your findings.

Your Occupation: Insurers offer three major provisions for dealing with disability in relation to the insured's occupation.

The first and probably broadest provision covers the insured's inability to perform the material and substantial duties of his or her regular occupation for the life of the contract. Typically, these contracts cover physicians for their specialty, i.e., the surgeon who loses the ability to perform surgery due to accident or sickness claims total disability, even though he or she may continue to function as a physician in some other capacity. Earnings for the surgeon's "other" occupation would in no way affect payment of the disability claim.

The second provision offers coverage in an occupation for a limited period of time (e.g., from 24 months to age 65) and requires that the insured not engage in any other occupation without a reduction of the benefits payable. Many of these contracts further state that lost earnings from the "other" or "new" occupation not related to the insured's prior occupation, education, training or economic status have no effect on benefits payable.

The third major provision concerns total disability, which insurers define as, "the inability of the insured to engage in his/her regular occupation; and not be engaged in any other occupation." Contracts with this provision, generally referred to as "loss of earnings contracts," cover all earned income from any source and pay benefits proportionately (unlike payment and earnings considerations under the second provision). Generally, loss of income contracts offer a "your occupation" rider that expands coverage to the insured's occupation for the entire benefit period, if so desired.

Sickness Defined: The contractual definition of "sickness," like the definition of "your occupation," may vary with the insurance company. The most vague and restrictive definition simply refers to "sickness commencing after the contract is in force," without actually stating what constitutes sickness. Because it is so vague, there may be difficulty determining when the insured knew of his or her condition. Other insurers choose to refer to sickness as 'sickness first diagnosed or treated after the policy is in force.' At present, the practice is generally to treat these two definitions in a like manner with regard to claim payments, although there appears to be more strength and accuracy in the "diagnosed or treated" definition as it points to a definite, ascertainable moment in time.

Specific Loss: This provides for total disability payment to begin upon the insured's loss of hearing, sight, speech or any two limbs. Total disability payments would continue for the benefit period or life regardless of any proof of loss of earnings. Variations of this provision are used to distinguish loss of use of limbs from actual severance. Some contracts waive the waiting period (the time between total disability and the commencement of the benefit period) for specific loss while others do not.

Unisex Rates: Morbidity tables have historically shown that it costs more to insure women than men for disability risk. However, many insurers now use a unisex pricing structure for their products; both men and women may be insured at the same rate.

Non-Smoker: Many insurers offer a non-smoker discount to their policy owners. Generally, they require that the insured has not smoked cigarettes for twelve months. The discount for non-smokers will range from 17 to 13 percent of smoker rates.

[d] Other Contract Provisions

Some provisions are outside the scope of the usual contract and must be added to standard contracts or, in some cases, sought from another insurer.

Survivorship Benefits: Some contracts allow for continued payment of disability benefits to a surviving spouse for a limited period of time, usually two to six months. To qualify, the insured must have been totally disabled for 12 to 24 months immediately prior to death.

Rehabilitation: Rehabilitation benefits may allow the insurer to renegotiate the amount of benefits payable when the insured enters a qualified rehabilitation program. Other rehabilitation benefits call for an additional benefit to be paid, generally limited to 200 to 300 percent of the base benefits.

Transplant Surgery/Cosmetic Surgery: As transplant or cosmetic surgery is not the result of an accident or sickness, it must usually be added to the contract specifically. Insurers may or may not require that the policy be active six months prior to these procedures for benefits to be paid.

[e] Riders

Whereas provisions are considered the "givens" of an insurance policy, riders can be attached both before and after the contract is made to personally customize the contract. Essentially, riders can be used to add provisions the contract does not already include.

Partial/Residual Benefits: Partial or residual benefits provide compensation for a policyholder who, due to accident or sickness, sustains a loss of income but continues to function in a regular occupation, although with a drop in earned income.

A rider for partial disability coverage typically does not isolate benefits payable to any specific income loss. Usual benefits would be 50 percent of the basic benefit payable for six months.

Residual benefit riders typically begin when post-accident or post-sickness earnings fall by 20 to 25 percent. Contracts vary as to the period of base earnings against which current earnings are measured. Some insurers offer more than one formula to determine the base earnings, others do not. Additionally, some contracts allow for indexing of base earnings, generally according to the CPI (Consumer Price Index). Residual benefits can be paid with or without a cap (maximum percentage increase allowable). As indexing of prior earnings—the base upon which the loss of current earning is measured—increases, benefits payable increase.

Typically, if the loss of income due to partial disability exceeds 75 to 80 percent, the total disability amount becomes payable. Some contracts also require that a partial disability claim be preceded by some period of total disability. When this requirement is a part of the residual rider, the period of total disability required may or may not be the same as the basic contract elimination period. Some companies currently offer a return-to-work provision under these residual riders. This benefit allows for a continuation of benefits after full recovery, usually for a period of three to six months.

Social Security: These riders provide for payment of additional benefits to the insured during the six- to 12-month waiting period for Social Security benefits. In the event Social Security declines to pay after this period—for example, in the event that the disability does not result in death or impair the disabled's ability to secure gainful employment—the rider provides for continuous payment of benefits until the age of 65. In the latter case, the rider usually requires that application for Social Security benefits be denied and appealed before the insurer will continue to pay the benefit. (The contract may or may not provide for the cost of the appeal.)

Own Occupation: This rider extends coverage provided by an income replacement contract to include coverage of the insured's regular occupation. Total disability is defined as the inability to perform duties of, spend time in or earn income from the insured's regular occupation, due to accident or sickness. Some of these riders limit the amount of income earned from "another" occupation to less than 200 percent of the regular occupation level.

Cost of Living: The cost of living rider provides for annual increases in the benefits payable under a disability contract. These increases may be based upon a specified percentage increase or the Consumer Price Index (CPI), up to a cap. Those related to the CPI generally have a "catch-up provision" that allows unused portions of the cap percentage to be carried forward to future years when the CPI may be above the cap rate.

Cost of living benefit increases may use either simple or compound interest. Companies may or may not limit the total benefits payable under the provision; those who do limit the cost of living increases to two times the base benefit. Many companies allow conversion to base benefit of the increased coverage after recovery; some do not.

Additional Insurance Option (Guaranteed Insurability): This rider allows for the future addition of disability income protection without medical confirmation. This option generally becomes available when the insured is in his or her mid-20's and may continue until the early 50's. Generally maximum increases available under this option are limited to two times the base purchased or the insurer's maximum issue limits. It is important to note whether the option limits the amount of additional purchases by stated dollar amounts (500 dollars per option, etc.) or whether it allows the insured to 'purchase the maximum amount he/she can

(Pub.372)

qualify for financially at any option date.' It is also important to note how frequently the option dates become available (every three years vs. every year).

Lifetime Benefits: Riders can be used to extend the benefit period for the length of the insured's lifetime. This extension of coverage is available for both accident and sickness, but variations and limitations vary with the company. For example, some require disability prior to a certain age before lifetime benefits are paid, while some scale benefits are payable based on the age at which disability occurs.

[f] Policy Exclusions

All disability income contracts contain a section that details the hazards not covered by the contract. Insurers often include some or all of the following:

- War or an act of war.
- Military service of any country.
- Pregnancy or normal childbirth.
- Self-inflicted injuries.
- Nervous or mental disorders.
- Pre-existing conditions.
- Injuries sustained while the insured is under the influence of LSD, opiates, hallucinogens, amphetamines, barbiturates or other drugs taken voluntarily without advice of a physician.

[3] Group Insurance

Most professionals' first exposure to the disability income product comes through the multitude of association group plans available to them. The pricing structure of these plans is usually "step-rated" (i.e., premiums increase every five to ten years, based on the physician's greater risk of disability with age), and it makes them appear quite affordable. The premium he or she pays is less than it would be for individual policies for the first several years. However, the premium averages out with a "private permanent" policy, so that the insured pays more in the early years but less in the later years. Eventually, the premium paid for a step-rated plan exceeds the premium a person pays for an individual policy.

[a] Questions

When deciding whether to purchase disability coverage either individually or through an association group, you need answers to a number of questions:

Is the Product Non-Cancellable and Guaranteed Renewable? Generally, association group companies reserve the right to increase premiums for their coverage. However, it is extremely rare for a medical association plan to be cancelled, and an association cannot single out individual insurers for cancellation. Some associations have plans that are guaranteed renewable as long as the association sponsors the program and does not sponsor a competing one. Association groups require continued membership in the sponsoring organization (AMA, etc.) for coverage to continue.

Does the Group Contract Offer Coverage to the Professional in His or Her Occupation? Group coverage usually offers occupation coverage for a limited period of time (24 to 60 months); however, some association group plans are now being marketed with occupation coverage given until age 65. As "your occupation" coverage increases in duration, the cost of group coverage also increases, but generally remains lower than individual coverage costs. The cost differences are easily understood in light of the earlier discussion of non-cancellable vs guaranteed renewable contracts.

Does the Group Contract Integrate Benefits? Some group contracts integrate (reduce) benefits they pay in proportion to benefits received from social insurance programs. Some also coordinate their benefits if the insured receives payment from any other group or individual disability policy.

How Much Coverage Is Available? Many group contracts limit the amount of benefits they issue. A common formula is 60 percent of compensation up to a maximum of $3,500 a month of benefit. However, the availability of larger amounts of coverage in association group coverage is on the rise. In fact, many companies now offer group coverage in very large amounts.

Some association plans may issue small to moderate benefits in addition to the maximum allowable issued on an individual non-cancellable coverage. This enables a physician to own a comfortable livable income during disability. The maximum amount companies

(Pub.372)

issue on an individual, non-cancellable basis ranges from 35 to 65 percent of the physician's net income, with the lower income receiving the higher benefit.

What Are the Policy Exclusions? Generally, group coverage offers policies with more exclusions than do individually underwritten contracts.

What Riders Are Available? Most groups offer a limited array of riders to their coverage products (See § 8.04[2][e] for examples).

[b] Overhead Expense

In recent times, the cost of doing business has risen dramatically for most professionals. A physician may have adequate disability income benefits to cover personal expenses, but that does not exclude the need for benefits to pay business expenses. The overhead expense contract is designed to help defray business expenses in the event the physician becomes disabled and suffers a loss of income.

If more than one physician is involved, each would have a pro-rata amount of the total expenses. Physicians other than stockholders, partners or other than sole owner-physicians are not eligible for this type of insurance. Premiums paid for coverage are tax deductible as a business expense and the benefits received are offset as a deductible expense. Benefits under this contract are generally paid as expenses are incurred.

Examples of overhead expenses include:

- Rent
- Heat
- Electricity
- Telephone
- Laundry
- Janitorial and maintenance
- Employee's salaries
- Interest payments
- Mortgage interest
- Taxes on business premise

- Malpractice insurance
- Casualty insurance
- Professional dues and journals
- Medical and office supplies
- Laboratory fees
- Equipment lease
- Staff fringe benefits
- Miscellaneous business expenses

Typically, this expense reimbursement contract is written for a maximum benefit period that ranges from 12 to 24 months. Multiplying the monthly benefit by the benefit period determines the maximum amount of payment due under the contract. Because of the short benefit period, in contrast to the longer benefit periods for personal expenses, premiums are substantially less.

Benefits are paid as incurred up to the monthly maximum. If expenses are incurred after disability, the benefits would continue until the maximum benefit amount had been paid. Typically, these contracts are written with waiting periods of 30 to 90 days. Many companies offer riders on their products that permit retroactive payment for expenses incurred during the waiting period. Other variations of this product include cash versus accrual accounting for expenses and partial coverage.

[c] Disability Buyout

Most partnerships and small businesses realize the importance of buy-sell agreements for preserving the practice if one or more of the owners die (although a life insurance policy for the deceased can serve the same function without interfering with cash flow). The same considerations apply to a disabled owner. Since the disabled owner is no longer able to contribute to the business, it is in the best interest of all parties to have a pre-arranged buy-sell provision in the event the disability is long term or permanent. A buy-sell agreement can be funded with a disability buy-out policy.

Generally, a disability buy-out policy insures up to 80 percent of the owner's interest. A target date at which payments will commence is selected (usually twelve to twenty-four months after the start of disability). If the insured is still disabled at the target date, the insurer pays the policy's benefits to a trustee, who in turn distributes the proceeds to the business. The policy may provide for a lump sum payment or periodic payments beginning on the target date. Of these two options, the lump sum payment is often the preferred method, since it avoids the problem of partial ownership interest which could occur if the insured recovers after the target date but prior to completion of the payments.

The premium for a disability buy-out policy is typically paid through a trustee and is not tax deductible. The benefits, when received by the trustee, are tax free but are taxed as capital gains when distributed.

[d] Medical Insurance

Medical insurance is important coverage, not only for the practitioners but also for their employees. Although some in the health care field believe in professional courtesy as a part of their ethics, once the numbers for coverage get into five digits professional courtesy may wear thin.

Major medical policies should include a "stop loss" clause, i.e., a point at which the policy pays one hundred percent acceptable to both the principals and the employees of the firm. Additionally, it is appropriate that the policy have no "inside limits", i.e., limits on the doctor's fees, limits on services provided by practitioners or limits for hospital and/or intensive care charges. An increasingly more important issue is that the major medical maximum should be at least one million dollars and preferably two million.

§ 8.05 Risk Management Checklist

A comprehensive checklist of points discussed in the chapter is provided.

__ General Risks and Liabilities

   __ Furniture

   __ Medical and business equipment

   __ Leasehold improvements

   __ Accounts receivable

   __ Patient records and valuable papers

   __ Embezzlement

(Pub.372)

§ 8.05 MANAGING YOUR MEDICAL PRACTICE

- — Post-catastrophe overhead
- — Automobile
- — Consequential losses
- — Professional and public liability
- — Worker liability
- — Fire
- — Loss of practice

— General Risk Avoidance Checklist
- — Security locks and nightly checks
- — Fire resistant safe
- — Locked files
- — Backup computer memory
- — Microfilm and remove patient records
- — Microfilm billing
- — Smoke detector
- — Sprinkler system
- — Lock up drugs and do not keep drug inventories

— Essential Insurance
- — Workers' Compensation
- — Malpractice
- — Public liability
- — Auto liability
- — Medical
- — Fidelity bond
- — Fire liability
- — Umbrella coverage
- — Life
- — Disability
- — Continued overhead

(Pub.372)

- Desirable insurance
    - Furniture and equipment replacement cost
    - Auto—comprehensive and collision
- Disability insurance
    - Non-cancellable
    - Guaranteed renewable
    - Your occupation
    - Sickness defined
    - Specific loss
    - Unisex rates
    - Non-smoker
    - Partial/residual
    - Indexing
    - Social security
    - Own occupation
    - Cost of living
    - Additional insurance option
    - Lifetime benefits
    - Survivorship benefits
- Group insurance
    - Major medical insurance
    - Overhead
    - Disability buyout

§ 8.100 Bibliography

Barosan, W.: Would Your Malpractice Defense Really Hold Up? Medical Economics Magazine. May 27, 1985, pp. 174-184.

Bostrom, H. and Ljungstedt, N. (Eds.): Unexpected Complications in Medical Care: Symposium, Sept. 26-28, 1978. Stockholm: Alnqvist & Wiksell, 1979.

Carlisle, V. G.: Protecting the Heart of Your Practice. Medical Economics Magazine. Sept. 17, 1984, p. 81.

Crane, M.: Malpractice. Will the New Premium Hikes Pull You Under? Medical Economics Magazine. May 27, 1985, pp. 129-140.

De Haon, Q. C.: Let's Stop Kidding Ourselves About Defense Medicine. Medical Economics Magazine. May 27, 1985, pp. 39-52.

Holder, A. R.: Writing DNR Orders That Won't Get You Sued. Medical Economics Magazine. Sept. 17, 1985, pp. 82-87.

Puckett, R. W.: They Said I Killed My Celebrity Patient. Medical Economics Magazine. Aug. 6, 1984, pp. 78-88.

Redish, M. H.: Legislative Response to the Medical Malpractice Crisis. Constitutional Implications. Chicago: American Hospital Association, 1977.

Appendix 8-A

MALPRACTICE AVOIDANCE CHECKLIST

(1) Do not disclose that you have professional liability.

(2) Use the x-ray as a diagnostic or confirmatory aid where it is established practice.

(3) Do not criticize the work of other physicians. To do so weakens your defense and may invite retaliation.

(4) Secure legal counsel before participating as a witness at a coroner's inquest.

(5) Maintain equipment so that it is in excellent working order at all times.

(6) Furnish proper notice of termination of services to avoid charges of abandonment.

(7) Maintain accurate records permanently. Suits are often filed years after services are rendered.

(8) Be knowledgeable about a physician's legal duty to the patient.

(9) Whenever possible and necessary, have a witness present when consulting with a patient, especially in the case of a female patient.

(10) Whenever possible, do not bring suit for fees until the statute of limitations for malpractice suits has expired.

(11) Consult an attorney about making personal assets less vulnerable to damage suit settlements.

(12) Don't guarantee results. Guarantees are uninsurable and unethical.

(13) Keep abreast of the average standards of your specialty.

(14) Be diplomatic and courteous to patients.

(15) Be certain to furnish proper instructions for the care of patients with prescriptions.

(16) Make sure patients have a clear understanding of fees, particularly if they are sizeable, before performing services.

(Pub.372)

(17) Do not give telephone prescriptions without proper verification.

(18) Keep all scheduled appointments.

(19) Assist the patient in securing the aid of consultants.

(20) Keep the patient-physician relationship strictly confidential.

(21) Inform patients of any planned absence from the practice and recommend a competent substitute.

(22) Do not practice in fields in which you are not properly qualified.

(23) Secure proper written consent in all cases. Without such documentation you can be charged with battery.

(24) Avoid any unapproved or experimental procedures or drugs.

(25) Furnish proper instructions to all assistants and monitor their follow-through.

(26) Be cautious, especially in such things as the labeling of containers, the close observation of casts for fractures, etc.

(27) Schedule patients as frequently as necessary for adequate care.

(28) Avoid admitting anything against your own interests regarding services you have performed or that someone else has performed on your behalf.

(29) Secure proper authorization before participating in an autopsy.

(Pub.372)

CHAPTER 9

Increasing Productivity Through Efficiency

> **SCOPE**
>
> The productive and efficient physician devotes every minute he or she is in the office to working with and providing services for patients. All duties other than those that can be done only by a physician should be delegated to employees: clerical staff should perform paper work, medical assistants should perform pre-examination care, outside providers and consultants should be utilized for services they can provide at lower cost and with greater efficiency. Efficient use of office time begins with the physician setting realistic goals based on costs and overhead. This includes following a schedule compatible with hours worked per week, the number of outside facilities such as hospitals and nursing homes the physician devotes attention to, the number of physicians in the practice, and the number of services a practice has the capacity to provide. Productivity goals should be revised upward as they are met and new ways of being productive should be tried. Spurs to productivity include providing cost-efficient ancillary services for patients, giving bonus incentives to productive employees and overcoming the obstacles to volume scheduling at a group practice by working split shifts. Bonus incentives should be worked out among partners to keep each member's entrepreneurial spirit alive. Once established and working within a comfortable schedule, a physician should restrict extramural services to a single hospital and single nursing home to concentrate influence and efficiency of services.

SYNOPSIS

§ 9.01 Productivity
§ 9.02 Value of Physician's Time
§ 9.03 The Work Week
§ 9.04 Production Goals
§ 9.05 Scheduling Work

(Pub.372)

§ 9.06 Facilities
§ 9.07 Utilizing Staff
  [1] Clerical Duties
  [2] Medical Duties
  [3] Other Professionals
§ 9.08 Staff Participation
§ 9.09 Incentive Program
§ 9.10 Ancillary Services
  [1] Determining Need
  [2] Types of Equipment
§ 9.11 Extramural Services
  [1] Hospitals
  [2] Nursing Homes
§ 9.12 Productivity Checklist
§ 9.13–§ 9.99 Reserved
§ 9.100 Bibliography

§ 9.01 Productivity

> Efficient use of time, staff and facilities are crucial to the success of a medical practice. The physician who works at maximum efficiency will provide quality services to patients, yet keep the costs of medicine reasonable.

Although you should always be seeking ways to better utilize time, you must be careful not to spend less time with patients. The doctor who schedules more and more patients just to fill up the appointment book often spends less time with each, and eventually alienates many. For example, some doctors adopt a full wave scheduling system (scheduling all patients to be seen in one hour to come at the beginning of the hour) so the doctor always has a patient waiting. However, many patients are unwilling to wait in the doctor's office at a considerable loss of personal time and choose another doctor.

This example illustrates why you must continually coordinate utilization of your time with patient needs. When you have extra time, it should be spent with patients.

§ 9.02 Value of Physician's Time

> Evaluating each procedure performed in your office in terms of an hourly wage, and determining the amount of yearly salary lost by

(Pub.372)

spending office time on non-medical duties illustrates areas of high productivity and those of poor or no productivity. Earning fees, rather than saving money, should be the basis for efficiency and productivity.

You determine the value of your time based on the activities you perform in a given interval. For example, a physician may earn over $1,000 an hour when performing surgery, but only $150 an hour when seeing patients in the office. The following chart illustrates how time is related to earnings.

Value of Time

Procedure	Fee	Hour	Value Per Hour
Laparoscopy	$920	1.25	$736
Limited office visit	$ 25	.16	$156
Comprehensive office visit	$ 75	.41	$183
Hospital admit	$ 60	.25	$240
Hospital visit	$ 20	.16	$125

Based on a 48-week working year, a five-day week and an eight-hour day, at $150 per hour average billing, a physician would bill out $288,000 annually. Although most physicians work more hours, many are unable to generate $288,000 a year. The reason is that they do not spend enough of their work time practicing medicine.

Inefficient use of work time may be further dramatized by calculating the value that is lost when a physician spends time on nonmedical tasks. Based on $150 an hour, one hour of unproductive (nonmedical) time per day throughout the year would come to $900,000 over a 25-year career.

In short, your most valuable commodity is the time you spend performing medical services. The first rule of high productivity is to use your time to earn physician's fees, which means concentrating on performing medical procedures. You do not generate earnings by trying to save on secretarial costs, doing clerical work, having extended lunches with salespeople or making telephone calls to stockbrokers. Likewise, the physician who hopes to set the world on fire with a new computer system, a new charting system, a system for analyzing stocks or another type of invention, often concentrates too much time on these areas at the expense of actual medical practice.

(Pub.372)

§ 9.03 The Work Week

The number of hours in the work week has a significant bearing on the physician's productivity with regard to fees generated and the image of convenience and availability transmitted to patients.

Although many physicians put in a great deal of working hours in each week, group practices and various coverage arrangements have taken much pressure off the physician and made it unnecessary for a doctor to be on call 24 hours a day, seven days a week.

However, it is important that you maintain adequate working hours. Reducing your working hours decreases the amount of time you are available and may make your practice less attractive to potential patients. From the standpoint of productivity, as dramatized in § 9.02, each professional hour is extremely valuable. The bulk of your fees come directly from production, and even when you are not working, your overhead continues to accrue.

§ 9.04 Production Goals

The physician who initially sets achievable production goals will find that, with time, the scope of those goals increases.

Management experts have observed that employees may expand their work to fit their hours, rather than seek out additional work. However, when employees are given achievable goals, and responsibilities are delegated, they become more productive and their jobs become more personally fulfilling. In the same way physicians should set goals for themselves, and then set new ones when these goals are achieved. The inability to imagine doing more work can limit achievement.

You may wish to base initial production goals on operating expenses, collection ratios, personal living expenses, etc. By evaluating the average charge per patient, you can establish a minimum patient volume. This relates patient volume to your production goals, and enables you to measure whether you are attracting enough patients to your medical practice. Because higher patient volume increases reputation and earnings, ways of increasing patient flow are important to consider.

§ 9.05 Scheduling Work

A physician should try to work out on paper a schedule for how to apportion his or her time. The number of non-patients seen, the amount of hospital work performed, and the convenience of seeing patients outside of the office should all be considered.

The physician must keep production goals in mind when planning a schedule. Although it is not always possible to carry out an exact schedule, planning a schedule so that it works out on paper is a helpful first step. To maximize the available time for patients, you must be mindful of a number of do's and don'ts:

- Do not see every salesperson who knocks on the door or sends a letter. Set aside one or two hours each month at a particular time of the month for your secretary to schedule drug company representatives, office supply salesmen, etc. who wish to show you a new product.

- Be judicious in your choice of committee and extramural work responsibilities. Measure these responsibilities carefully, in terms of how effective they are and how much of a contribution you will make to them.

- Schedule hospital work efficiently. Consider visiting the hospital at non-peak times, when more hospital staff may be available to assist you. Establish good relationships with the hospital so that the staff will help, not hinder you. If possible, schedule patients all at one hospital to avoid having to travel to many hospitals to visit a few patients. Limit the time you spend at the hospital to seeing patients and stay on time so that your office patients aren't kept waiting.

- If you are affiliated with a nursing home, try to schedule nursing patients in one quality home.

§ 9.06 Facilities

A properly designed office facility leads to smooth patient flow and increased productivity.

A busy practice will become very inefficient if there are not enough examination rooms to cover the number of patients waiting. Your practice should have a minimum of three, but preferably four, examination rooms per doctor. By making a number of rooms available to each doctor, less time is wasted waiting for staff to get patients ready, and you also have a holding space for patients waiting to see the physician after the results of laboratory or x-ray tests are processed. If your space is limited, use split shifts for group practices. This not only allows each doctor more space when he or she sees patients, it also saves money by eliminating the need to expand the facility.

§ 9.07 Utilizing Staff

Nonessential work should be delegated to staff so that you can concentrate on performing the work only you can do—caring for patients. This means having clerical staff do all patient record keeping and routing, accounts processing, transcription and patient follow-up. Medical asistants can perform examination preliminaries, such as taking the patient history, and perform routine procedures such as x-rays, EKGs and drawing blood. Hiring outside consultants who can do better work in a specialty can also increase office efficiency and productivity.

Any resource that frees you to provide medical services increases productivity; human resources are the major resource which can generate more time.

[1] Clerical Duties

You should use your clerical staff to do work that would waste your time as a practitioner, including:

Scheduling Patients: Patient scheduling should be left to your appointment secretary. Personally scheduling patients would not only use your time inefficiently, it might also disrupt the appointment schedule if what you record overlaps what the appointment secretary has already scheduled.

Charts and Filing: The clerical staff can help prepare charts for new patients and patients to be seen, and refile charts after the patient has been seen. When patient charts are immediately available, you can study the patient history more quickly.

Routing Slip or Charge Slip Preparation: A properly designed routing or charge slip simplifies your responsibility for keeping track of charges for each patient. The clerical staff can prepare the usual routing or charge slip and attach it to the patient's chart so

(Pub.372)

that you and your assistants can check off procedures performed in the course of an examination.

Hospital and Nursing Home Logs: Clerical staff can keep track of logs on your patients in hospitals and nursing homes. As long as all of the patients are scheduled in the same way as office patients, the staff will have this information available and be able to prepare daily lists on which you can indicate procedures to be performed, much like office routing slips.

Accounts Receivable Processing: Clerical staff can take responsibility for processing charges, from collecting charges marked on charts after the patient has been seen to posting charges, completing third-party billing forms, billing patients, collection follow-up, and collection posting. Competent clerical help can save you time, minimize lost charges and lead to more efficient collection.

Bank Deposits: Clerical staff should write up deposits and take them to the bank.

Accounts Payable and Payroll: When done properly and checked for accuracy, these tasks can be time consuming. A competent staff can perform them at lesser expense and generally more efficiently than can a physician.

Thank You Letters: A variety of thank you letters to consultants and referring patients can be prepared by your staff and placed on your desk for signature. This expedites processing and eliminates the time-consuming task of writing or dictating the letters. However, you should still review all letters that go out.

Recall and Reminder Systems: Clerical staff should keep track of patients who need to be recalled or reminded about appointments.

Tax Records: Use your clerical staff to assist you in keeping track of various records required for tax purposes, such as transportation and entertainment logs. Although you will have to gather most of the information for these records personally, a secretary can update them on a regular basis.

Dictation and Transcription: A good pocket dictaphone and a good secretary can save you time and save you the expense of transcribing medical charts, correspondence, insurance reports, etc. In addition, you are likely to end up with more accurate information.

(Pub.372)

By surrounding yourself with a competent, reliable and honest staff whom you can trust to take care of nonmedical work, you can free time to see more patients. Periodically review your activities to see which daily procedures can be delegated so as to allow you to see more patients.

[2] Medical Duties

A professionally trained medical assitant can perform a number of duties that will free your time for patients:

Placing Patients in Examination Rooms: An assistant may call the waiting patient, bring the patient into the examination room, and generally prepare the patient by having the patient don a medical gown and explaining the procedures to be performed.

Pre-examination: A medical assistant can record some basic items, such as patient blood pressure, pulse and weight.

Patient History: With a properly designed questionnaire and training, your medical assistant can get vital information for the patient history.

Charting: A medical assistant can record information on the medical record as you dictate it and record procedures performed for billing and forwarding purposes.

Medical Procedures: Medical assistants can perform a number of tests or preliminaries to tests in the office, including drawing blood, giving injections for treatments like chemotherapy, taking x-rays and processing the film, and running EKGs.

Screening Telephone Calls: A qualified assistant may be able to tell over the telephone whether a patient should come in to see the doctor immediately, needs hospitalization or simply needs to "wait and see."

Prescription Reorders: Working within a properly designed system, a competent assistant may be able to respond to prescription refill calls (see § 4.01[2]).

[3] Other Professionals

Other professionals, such as physician's assistants or nurse practitioners, can help free your time for patients and can also help to generate fees. A therapist working for a busy orthopedist, for example, can bring in billing for therapy services; an ophthalmologist may wish to hire opticians, ophthalmology technicians and optometrists; and it is not unusual for psychiatrists to hire social workers, sociologists and therapists to help treat their patients.

Hiring professionals should be considered an investment, since they generally are not able to pay for themselves immediately. You must consider two points when hiring a fee-producing employee: 1) what kind of work do you refer out of your practice as a consequence of not having the time or resources to provide the service? (if you refer out a substantial amount, you may be able to pay immediately for the additional employee); and 2) will the new employee be able to help you with your other work?

Utilization of outside professionals, such as practice management consultants, accountants and lawyers is a must for the successful medical practice. They can provide better services than you in work that overlaps their own specialty, be more productive per hour than you could in these areas, and probably charge less per hour than you would under the same circumstances.

Computers are tools that can help you decide whether or not outside professional help is necessary. A computer software package designed for the medical office can provide detailed information on the volume of procedures performed and the number of patients seen that would otherwise be obtainable only through sampling of accounts receivable records (see Chapter 10, Accounts Receivable Management).

§ 9.08 Staff Participation

> Employees should be encouraged to be as productive and efficient as the physician. Both merit bonuses based on increased office productivity and spot bonuses should be considered to provide incentive.

You should encourage productivity from your staff and let staff members participate in the success of the practice. Some offices have successfully adapted incentive bonuses based on the combination of production and collections: if the combined collections and production go above a predetermined level, an employee bonus is awarded. The amount to award may be calculated by using a percentage figure equal to the percentage increase in production,

(Pub.372)

multiplied by the budgeted salary expenses. This bonus is then distributed to employees on a merit basis.

An example of a bonus incentive plan is as follows:

Dr. Brown's average charges plus receipts for the past year have been $30,000 per month. Because of fee increases, Dr. Brown anticipates this average should be no less than $33,000 per month during the upcoming year. Dr. Brown sets up an incentive plan which calculates a percentage based on the following formula:

$$\frac{\text{Charges} + \text{Cash Receipts} - \$33,000.00}{\$33,000.00}$$

The percentage arrived at is used to multiply Dr. Brown's employees' base salaries. The product is the amount of a bonus paid to employees. If, for instance, charges plus cash receipts for the month is equal to $36,300, then an employees base salary would be multiplied by ten percent to arrive at the bonus figure.

You should always recognize your employees' contribution to the overall success of the office and pay periodic "spot" bonuses of $25.00, $50.00 or $100.00. Employees should be informed, however, that even in an informal program such as this, bonuses are not automatic, but a direct result of overall efficiency and success within the practice.

§ 9.09 Incentive Programs

> A physician must weigh the pros and cons of working as a single practitioner against those of working as a member of a group. Because enthusiasm can wane when a practitioner is no longer responsible for generating all of his or her earnings, group practices should consider paying productivity-based profit incentives.

The single practitioner must be an entrepreneur, since all of his or her earnings come directly from individual work and efficient operation. However, when a physician becomes an employee or takes on a partner, the entrepreneurial spirit may disappear or errode.

Group practice can lead to lower productivity if a proper incentive program is not established. For example, if profit is split equally in a two-person partnership, each partner may fall prey to the tendency to let the other partner carry the practice. As the group size increases and the percentage of profit returned from individual labors diminishes, this problem can worsen. There is simply more incentive for you to try to increase your bottom line when you are reaping 100 percent of the profits of your labor.

Some physicians in group practices fear that an incentive based split of income will result in too much competition between group members. Others feel that 100 percent incentive-based productivity does not remunerate a physician for time spent on non-income producing areas of practice development, such as business management or professional education. These physicians may be more comfortable with a profit distribution system based partially on a fixed rate of remuneration and partially on production.

However, it is important that a substantial portion of profit be divided on the basis of productivity and distributed directly to those who contribute the most to the practice. Experience shows substantial growth for practices with incentive-based compensation. If high productivity is important to you, you should practice in an incentive-based group.

§ 9.10 Ancillary Services

> Equipment purchased to provide ancillary services for patients should also turn a profit or at least pay for itself. Before buying x-ray, ultrasound or EKG machines, calculate their potential financial yield and decide whether it might be better to refer patients to the local hospital for such services. The feasibility of setting up a suborganization to provide ancillary services independent of the practice should be worked out on the same kind of basis. In addition to profitability and convenience, consider the politics of providing ancillary services and the potential for conflict of interest before making an equipment purchase.

Although acquiring a piece of equipment may provide a good service for the patient, it should also make a profit for the physician. Equipment should not be purchased until it has been determined it will break even by paying for itself or come very near to that point.

For example, a physician in a small or secluded town may find it necessary to acquire x-ray equipment. In most instances, however, this equipment is available at a nearby hospital or radiologist's office, in which case the physician may refer this procedure out until his or her patient volume justifies acquisition of the equipment.

[1] Determining Need

If your office uses a computer for billing, information on the amount referred outside the office is easily obtained. Acquisition of substantial and expensive equipment—a CAT scanner, for example—should be discussed with accounting professionals before purchase.

A simple way to calculate the feasibility of purchasing a piece of equipment is to estimate a reasonable life expectancy for the equipment (five to eight years in most cases, although a conservative estimate should be used where there is uncertainty). Then, knowing the price of the piece to be acquired, call a banker to determine what the monthly payment would be on this equipment if fully financed through the bank and amortized over the equipment's life expectancy. Add to this monthly payment the maintenance contract fee, which gives the approximate monthly cost of the equipment and maintenance of the equipment and how much revenue it will have to generate to break even; collection loss; supply costs (such as film and development for x-ray machines); and the salaries of employees who assist in the procedure to determine the break even point.

Other considerations when acquiring equipment or providing ancillary services include:

Service to the Patient: It is sometimes difficult to put a dollar amount on service to the patient. If you are able to provide laboratory and x-ray service within the office, the patient not only has the advantage of not needing to go to another office for services, but also receives a single statement. Most patients appreciate having one physician in charge of their entire procedure, and it will give your practice the image of a "full-service" organization.

Convenience for the Physician: Some ancillary services you perform in your office permit a diagnosis in the course of a single patient visit that would otherwise have to wait for confirmation from outside laboratory reports.

Politics: Sometimes "political issues" complicate the decision to acquire equipment. For example, there is a potential for conflict between a radiology office considering acquiring a CAT scanner in the same geographic area as a hospital with a CAT scanner that relies on patient volume to amortize the cost of equipment. In another instance, the relationship between a subspecialist and the primary care physician he or she refers patients to can be jeopardized if the primary care physician purchases equipment for ancillary services that the subspecialist normally provides.

Conflict of Interest: Beware of becoming so involved in providing ancillary services that you are tempted to order more work than is necessary for a patient. An example is an ophthalmologist who tells patients that prescriptions can only be filled properly at his or her optical shop. This can easily lead patients to go to another ophthalmologist with whom they feel they have greater freedom.

[2] Types of Equipment

You should always look at the volume of work you refer out when considering the feasibility of processing work within the practice. Equipment typically found in physician's offices includes:

X-Ray Equipment and Automatic Processor: Family practitioners, internists, orthopedic surgeons and other primary care physicians usually find it convenient and profitable to have x-ray equipment and processors in their offices, once their volume justifies the purchase. Until your practice becomes established, an alternative method of providing service can be arranged through a radiologist or hospital.

Laboratory Equipment: Since current Medicare regulations prohibit physicians from billing for laboratory procedures performed outside of the office and impose a $3.00 limitation for daily service and handling, many physicians have looked into buying basic laboratory equipment necessary to complete the normal range of chemistry tests. In addition to amortizing the cost of the equipment, additional staff and supply costs must be worked into your estimate.

Electrocardiogram Equipment: Since most internists and cardiologists find it profitable to acquire this equipment soon after opening a practice, the starting physician should include space for this equipment in the original office design.

Ultrasound: Many obstetricians acquire ultrasound equipment after determining the amount of work they refer to the radiologist. However, controversy has arisen over whether necessity or profit motive is the main reason that physicians order ultrasound.

(Pub.372)

In addition to ancillary services performed in the office, some physicians find it profitable to set up suborganizations related to their specialty. Ophthalmologists, for example, typically explore the possibility of opening an optic shop, while an orthopedist may consider starting a physical therapy unit. In many cases, these enterprises are set up separate from the practice. This is favorable, because it forces the suborganization to be profitable on its own. If such a venture were established as an adjunct to the practice it would be more difficult to determine its profitability and, in instances where it lost money, the more profitable practice could wind up subsidizing the less profitable suborganization without the physician knowing it.

§ 9.11 Extramural Services

> It is common for a physician to be affiliated with many hospitals and nursing homes early in private practice, but eventually productivity and efficiency are best served when he or she devotes attention to one of each. Exclusive relationships with hospitals are often mutually rewarding. Exclusive relationships with nursing homes allow the physician some influence over patient care.

While it is good to have a high availability profile, you should attempt to limit to one each the number of hospitals and nursing homes for which you provide services.

[1] Hospitals

Although many physicians utilize a number of different hospitals early in their practice, they eventually select a hospital that provides the necessary services for their specialty and limit seeing patients to that particular hospital. Although they may be on staff at a number of different hospitals, as a practical matter they use only one.

There are other advantages to working with only one hospital, besides the obvious ones. For example, the hospital administration is likely to be much more accommodating to a physician with whom they have an exclusive "sweetheart" relationship. Currently, hospitals are looking for ways to expand and protect their marketplace and they have found the establishment of joint ventures with physicians a good investment. Physicians who maintain good relationships with the hospital obviously have the best chance to enter into such partnerships.

When choosing hospitals, exclude those not well liked by the population you serve, since your reputation rests not only on your own action but also on satisfaction with your referrals and the facilities you use. The hospitals should preferably be near your office and in the middle of the community they serve.

[2] Nursing Homes

Nursing homes can pose a different problem. Although there may be a number of different nursing homes in your community, you may not feel that any are of adequate quality for your patients. Moreover, quality homes are often crowded and have long waiting lists, and you may not be able to place all of your patients in a single quality home. This may force you to work with more than one nursing home, but you should still avoid working with any homes you feel provide substandard care. Use your influence to demand nursing improvements. Aside from the obvious advantages this can bring, it will help you to develop some political clout in the nursing home.

§ 9.12 Productivity Checklist

A checklist of the important items affecting productivity is provided.

— Know the value of your time.
  — Value of each working hour = annual receipts and billing/ number of hours worked per year.
  — Calculate the amount of time lost per day to nonmedical concerns. Multiply by 5, then by 48, to determine the amount of income lost on annual basis.

— Set goals.
  — Establish minimum attainable goals based on office overhead and personal expenses.
  — Make a schedule to follow based on these goals.
  — Constantly review and raise goals.

— Use time wisely.
  — Seek ways to maximize billable services within your office hours.

(Pub.372)

- Use your time to perform duties only you can perform.
- Hire a competent staff and utilize professional advisors.
- Delegate all non-physician duties to staff.
- Have medical assistants perform basic medical duties and pre-examination procedures.

— Schedule work productively.
- Concentrate on seeing patients.
- Minimize time spent on travel by grouping visits, etc.
- Emphasize importance of scheduling productively to staff.

— Work week.
- Put in enough hours to generate profit.
- Concentrate time; minimize the number of hospitals and nursing homes visited and the time spent moving from hospital to nursing home to practice.
- Ally with one hospital and one nursing home to develop good working relationships and gain influence over care policy for patients.

— Plan efficient office.
- Make sure there are enough examination rooms and space to see a large volume of patients.
- Consider split shifts to maximize utilization of office facilities for a group practice.

— Use incentive programs.
- Compensate employees for individual productivity.
- If employed in a group, seek compensation plan that combines equal charge splits with individual productivity-based compensation.

— Provide profitable ancillary services.
- Provide services both convenient to the patient and profitable to you.

(Pub.372)

- Only perform services or acquire equipment that will pay for itself.
- Be on the lookout for items that will provide potential profits for the practice.
- Consider starting an independent suborganization to provide ancillary services.

§ 9.100 Bibliography

Laliberty, R. and Christopher, W.: Enhancing Productivity in Health Care Facilities. National Health Publishing, 1984.

McConnell, C. R.: Managing the Health Care Professional. Rockville, MD: Aspen Systems Corp., 1984.

Zoog, S. and Yarnell, S. (Eds.): The Changing Health Care Team: Improving Effectiveness in Patient Care. Seattle: MCSA, 1976.

CHAPTER 10

Accounts Receivable Management

SCOPE

> Efficient, controlled management of accounts receivable is crucial for the success of any medical practice, since poor accounts receivable management can result in substantial income loss and practice failure. Whether manual or computerized, an accounts receivable system should be simple, so that it is easy to learn and does not require an accountant's understanding to operate. It should contain automatic checks and balances so that you and the bookkeeper know that upon proper completion and balancing there are no undetected errors. It should also have built-in internal controls to discourage embezzlement and abuses of the system and permit their detection. A good system should make it possible for the office to cross check and update an account on a regular basis. An accounts receivable system must be flexible enough to (1) accommodate the billing and processing of forms and information for many different third-party insurers, such as Medicare, Medicaid, private insurance companies, preferred practice organizations and health maintenance organizations; (2) handle sources of income from outside the office, such as hospital or nursing home visits or house calls; and (3) monitor sources of extra income such as expert witness testimony and insurance company retainers. In addition, it must be able to isolate and categorize delinquent accounts and provide an efficient method for following up on them.

SYNOPSIS

§ 10.01 Types of Systems
    [1] Manual Systems
        [a] Single-Entry System
        [b] Double-Entry System
        [c] Pegboard System

[2] Computers
  [a] On-Line Computer
  [b] Batch Processing
  [c] Information Retrieval
  [d] In-House vs. Service Bureau Computerization

§ 10.02 Controls
  [1] Charge Slips
  [2] Payments
  [3] Adjustments
  [4] Balancing Accounts
  [5] Staff

§ 10.03 Third Party Billings
  [1] Medicare
    [a] Reimbursement
    [b] Terms of Coverage
    [c] Billing System
  [2] Medicaid
  [3] Medicare/Medicaid
  [4] Preferred Provider Organizations (PPO's)
    [a] Blue Cross/Blue Shield
    [b] Accounts Receivable Processing
  [5] Health Maintenance Organizations (HMO's)
  [6] Private Insurance
  [7] Worker's Compensation
  [8] Physical Examinations for Business Organizations

§ 10.04 Hospital Charges
  [1] Hospital Log
  [2] Keeping Track of Charges

§ 10.05 Miscellaneous Charges
  [1] Nursing Homes
  [2] House Calls
  [3] Miscellaneous Income

§ 10.06 Accounts Receivable Management Reports
  [1] Aging Accounts
  [2] Account Summaries

§ 10.07 Accounts Receivable Management Checklist

§ 10.08–§ 10.99 Reserved

§ 10.100 Bibliography

Appendix 10-A Financial Transaction Forms for the Medical Office

§ 10.01 Types of Systems

> Manual and computerized systems are available to manage accounts receivable for the medical practice. Manual systems, such as the double-entry and pegboard system, are often appropriate for small practices and have made the single-entry system all but obsolete. Larger practices may find computerization with either an on-line or batch processing computer to be the only efficient way of keeping track of accounts.

Although numerous accounts receivable systems are used in medical offices, all can be put into one of two categories: the manual system or the computer system. The manual system is further subdivided into the single-entry system, the double-entry system and the pegboard system. The two basic types of computer system are the service bureau (or time-share) system and the in-house system.

[1] Manual Systems

The basic concept behind any accounts receivable system is still the balancing of payments against charges on a patient's account. In manual systems, improvements have increased the ability to cross-check each step to eliminate the possibility of errors. For this reason the pegboard system is seen as an improvement over the double-entry system, in the same way the double entry was seen as an improvement over the single entry system.

[a] Single-Entry System

Years ago, the system for keeping track of accounts receivable consisted of writing down the charge for the services performed by the physician and periodically issuing patients a statement, based on those records, notifying them of the amount due. Payments received from the patient were posted to his or her account and deposited with the bank, or into the physician's pocket. Records of these charges and payments were often kept individually in the patient's file.

This simple system had neither internal controls nor any way to detect even minor accounting errors. Furthermore, the physician who relied on this system had only a checkbook balance to tell whether he or she was doing well in business or, if poorly, why, and how to make an intelligent business decision to correct it.

(Pub.372)

[b] Double-Entry System

In response to the shortcomings of the single-entry system, the double-entry system was created. Each charge and payment was posted on an individual patient ledger and in a charge and payment journal. This process provided the physician with much needed business information, greatly enhanced the billing system and allowed the office to balance the accounts receivable. By recording charges, payments and adjustments in a journal, the physician could keep track of them on a daily basis and balance the totals with the total charges for the day and the deposits in the bank. Aggregate totals could be used to compute the accounts receivable total and cross-balance the total from the ledger cards.

A major drawback to this system was that it required a basic understanding of accounting principles, particularly when figures did not balance because of an error in the system. In addition, the double-entry system was labor intense. The growing cost of labor and the need to simplify procedures in the office mandated that a simpler system be found for the medical practice.

[c] Pegboard System

Many medical offices converted to the pegboard system of accounts receivable management in the 1960's and still use it effectively. Enhancements and changes have adapted it to handle many problems faced by the modern medical office. (See Figure 10–1.)

The basic system consists of a hard board with pegs on the left side, a daysheet or journal sheet, and patient ledger cards. The daysheets and ledger cards are printed so that the financial areas of each match perfectly and so that a piece of carbon or NCR paper between them eliminates the need for dual entries. Every financial activity that is recorded on the patient's ledger card is recorded simultaneously on the daysheet. Thus, the daysheet automatically becomes a journal, and the use of carbon paper eliminates the potential for recording a number on the daysheet differently from the number on the ledger card.

At the end of the day each column on the pegboard daysheet is added up. The totals from the column are entered into a formula at the bottom of the daysheet that cross foots and checks the mathematics of the postings. If there are any errors, the formula at

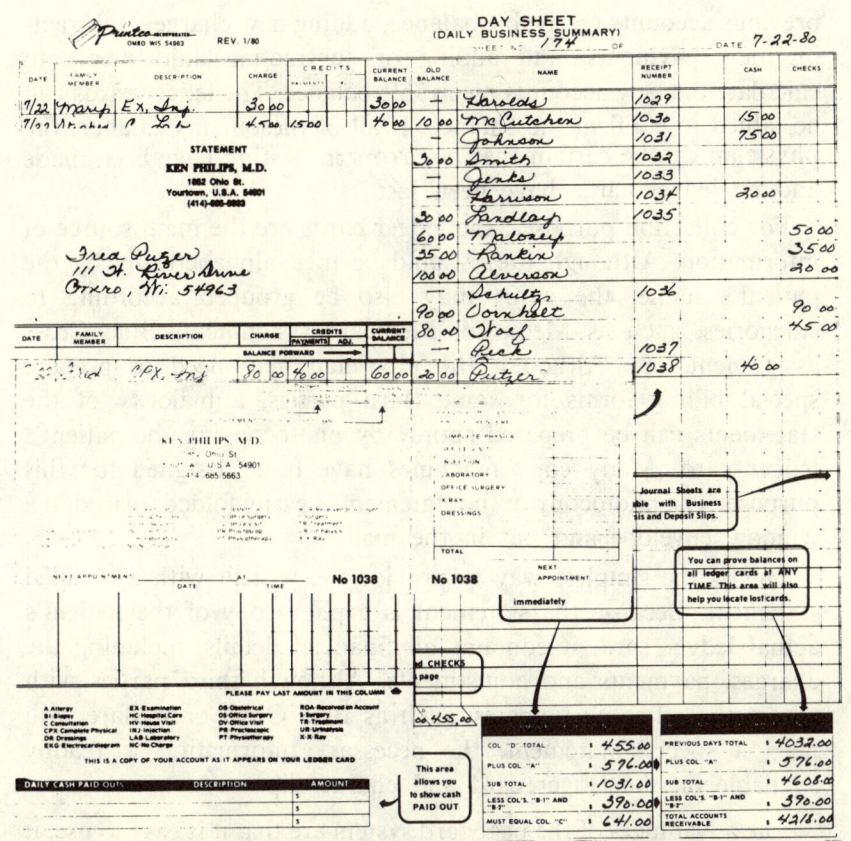

FIG. 10-1. A complete pegboard system includes ledger cards, a ledger tray with alphabetical index, an early pay envelope, color coding for ledger cards, superbill charge slips, patient statements and the actual pegboard.

the bottom will not balance. If it balances, the bookkeeper can be sure there are no mathematical errors in the daysheet or ledger cards, since they are carbon copies. Errors are easier to find since they are limited to the number of entries on any daysheet, typically thirty-six.

The daily total charges summed on the daysheets can be confirmed by adding individual totals from each charge slip. Similarly, the total payments can be balanced with the bank deposit. Any adjustments can be confirmed with a source document, such as the remittance advice from Medicaid or an authorization of discount by a physician.

Accounts receivable can be balanced through a formula at the bottom of the daysheet that calculates a running total by taking a

(Pub.372)

previous accounts receivable balance, adding new charges, subtracting new payments, and adding or subtracting adjustments to calculate the new accounts receivable balance. The ledger cards can be tallied to confirm the balance. If all of these items balance, the physician can be certain that no errors in posting have been made and no ledger cards have been lost.

For collection purposes, the ledger cards are the main source of information. Although they should be filed alphabetically by the patient's name, the cards may also be grouped according to categories, such as Medicaid, Medicare assignment, Blue Cross assignment, etc. Although the physician may need to prepare special billing forms for some third parties, a majority of the statements can be prepared simply by photocopying the patient's ledger card. Many copy machines have been designed for this purpose. The photocopy of the statement is easily folded, placed in a window envelope and put in the mail.

This is the simplest way to provide the patient with a detailed statement. Because the statement is a photocopy of the patient's actual ledger card, it contains all financial details, including the charges, payments and adjustments. Although third parties with whom the office participates, such as Blue Cross or welfare, will need a special statement, the necessary information is readily available on the ledger card and charge slip.

The advantages of the pegboard system are that it is easy to use, it eliminates a number of steps in posting, and it provides good internal control of accounts. The cost of the pegboard system is similar to other types of manual systems, so it is reasonable to conclude that any office on a manual system should be on some variation of the pegboard system.

[2] Computers

Computers began to work their way into medical offices in the 1960's. However, many physicians who purchased expensive systems to solve all of their billing problems found that the early systems could not satisfy the unique needs of the medical office. Systems were typically installed in poorly managed offices with the idea that the computer would solve the problem. Not surprisingly, medical computer systems gained a terrible reputation that persisted into the late 1970's, sustained by horror stories of physicians who converted from a manual to a computer system only to have to convert back to a manual system.

As computers became more flexible and as computer specialists learned more about the medical office, they began to develop systems that could fill many of the needs of the medical office, not the least of which was accounts receivable management. (For a complete discussion of use of computer systems see Chapter 5.)

A good modern computer system should be able to store information and sort, and keep track of and provide billing for each patient's account, regardless of type. If it is an efficient system, it should eliminate the great deal of the mathematical computations necessary in a manual system, expedite book balancing and eliminate the possibility of lost ledger cards or billing with a back-up system. A central computer with multiple terminals can allow a number of people to access and process patient's accounts simultaneously. Because the computer does all the work once information is entered into it properly, it should be able to compile vast amounts of management information that would generally be cost-prohibitive to produce on a manual system. And because all of the statements produced by a computer are printed, it gives a billing system a "professional" appearance that a handwritten statement or a photocopy of a handwritten ledger lacks. (See Figure 10–2.)

[a] On-Line Computer

There are two basic computer entry methods, batch and on-line. On-line entry refers to the processing of transactions as they occur. With a true on-line input system, a patient's charges and payments are posted into the computer as they are made. Theoretically, with an on-line system, a patient's account is kept up to date 100 percent of the time.

[b] Batch Processing

Batch processing is done in "batches." A group of charges is entered into the computer all at once, and then a total posting, as computed by the system, is compared to a batch total calculated from the charge slips. Generally, batches are small enough so that if the computer totals do not compare with the manual totals, the error can be quickly spotted. Another example of batch processing is entering all of the payments for the day into the computer to balance them against the deposit slip.

The batch entry system is the most effective, efficient and controlled system of entry because each group of entries into the computer is backed up by a batch of source documents. For a medical office, these source documents fall into four categories:

§ 10.01 [2]   MANAGING YOUR MEDICAL PRACTICE   10–8

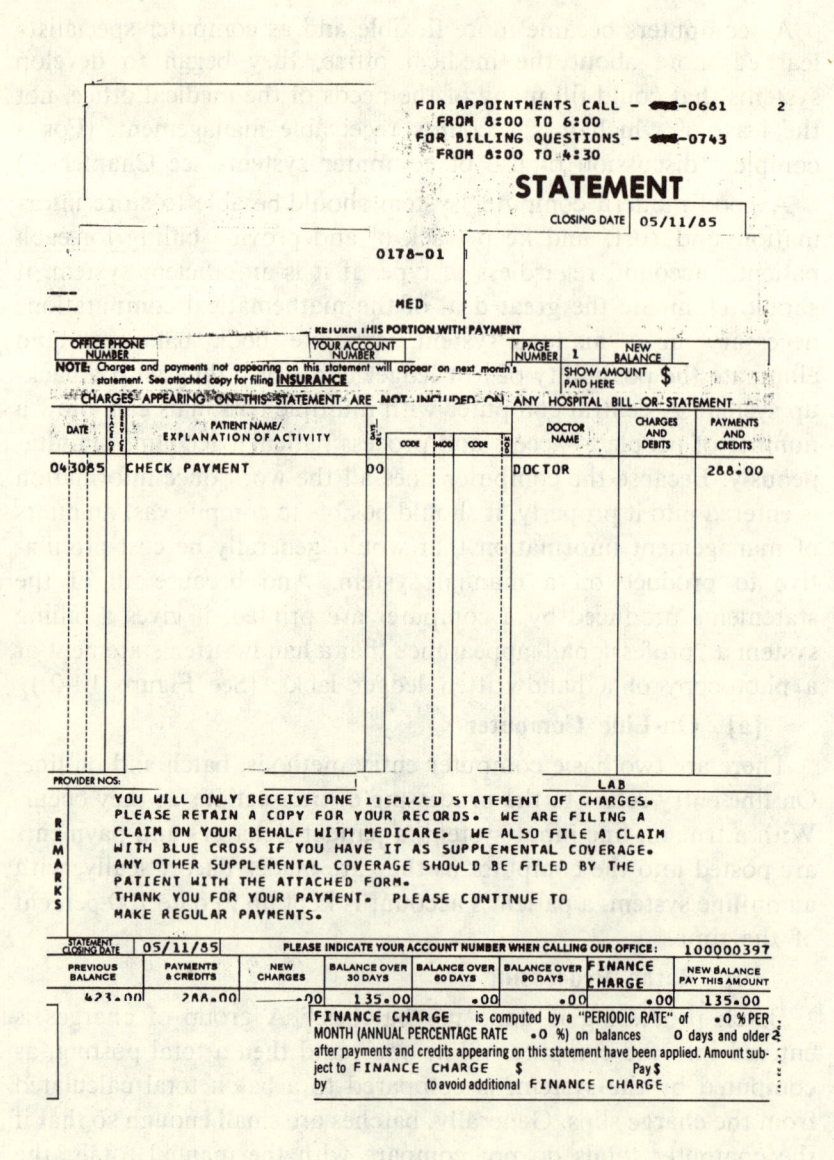

FIG. 10-2. A common computer-generated statement. The comprehensive statement includes the CPT and ICD/9 codes and all of the information necessary for the patient to complete his or her own insurance form. The "professional" printed look guarantees that numbers will not be misread.

(Pub.372)

(1) Charges. The source document for charges is the charge slip or routing slip. Each group of charges is added up prior to being entered into the computer. After the total group of charges has been entered into the computer, the computer total is balanced with the batch total. If there is a discrepancy, it is found since it is limited to that particular batch of documents.

(2) Payments. The source documents on the payment postings are the deposit slips. Each patient payment should be listed separately on the deposit form to balance any errors that could occur. Like the charges, the total payments posted, as entered into the computer, should equal the total shown as the tally of the routing slips for the batch. Both are equal to the total deposit.

(3) Debit Adjustments. Debit adjustments are those entries other than charges that increase the amount which the patient owes. An example of a debit adjustment is the penalty for a patient's check that has been returned by the bank for insufficient funds. The source document on debit adjustments should be an adjustment log. No adjustment should ever be entered into the computer without also being logged into a journal. The total debits entered into the log should balance with the total debits shown on the computer. The adjustment log should be reviewed, approved and initialed by a supervisor or, in smaller practices, by the physician.

(4) Credit Adjustments. These include any entries other than payments that reduce a patient's account balance. An example of a credit adjustment is a professional discount or a charge in excess of maximum allowed for a Medicaid patient. Like debit adjustments, the source document for a credit adjustment should be an adjustment log. All credit adjustments should have a proof source showing the adjustment is legitimate. An example of a proof source is the remittance advice from a welfare check showing the amount of disallowed charges or a signed charge slip by a physician requesting a professional discount. Each entry should be reviewed, approved and initialed by a supervisor.

(Pub.372)

[c] Information Retrieval

Demographic data—the patient's name, address, third-party information, etc.—is initially entered into a computer from the new patient information form and stored permanently. Demographic data needs to be reviewed only if the patient is new, or if information on an established patient changes.

Once the necessary basic information is entered, the computer can sort and compile all of the different accounts receivable needs. In many cases the computer eliminates a lot of paperwork since many of the third parties allow computer media for the transfer of data rather than paper.

For example, with a manual system an assistant must type out a form for each welfare patient each time the patient comes in. The information for this form generally comes from the patient's ledger card and charge slip. Once the form is properly completed and reviewed, it is batched with other forms and sent in the mail to the welfare agency, which sorts the forms and sends the the appropriate ones to their computer data entry office. The data entry people at the welfare office then take the information from the typed sheet and enter it into their computer. However, if there is any error, no matter how minor, the form will typically be rejected by the computer and sent back to the provider for reprocessing, in which case the whole process begins anew.

With a computer system the initial information is entered into the computer and then processed out in paper or into computer media format. If the latter, the information can be automatically processed into the welfare agency's computer system. Furthermore, because a computer checks the accuracy of the original information at the original entry source, any errors will be caught before they are passed on to the other party. Not only does this eliminate a fair amount of labor, but the charges can be processed more promptly because of the speed of the computer. Typically the physician's computer system can turn this whole process around in a matter of weeks, compared to a matter of months for a manual system.

[d] In-House vs. Service Bureau Computerization

The two types of office computerization are in-house and service bureau systems. An in-house computer, as the name implies, is located in the physician's office for exclusive use by the practice. A service bureau computer is at a remote location and generally processes information for many different medical offices.

[i] Service Bureau Computers. The early service bureaus handled processing by entering source documents into the computer at the service bureau. Although this method provided economy of scale and eliminated the need for capital investment by the physician, its major flaw was that the distance between the bureau and the physician's office prevented the physician from having up-to-date information on patient accounts. The result was that the physician's office appeared not to know what was going on in the event of a patient account inquiry, and in some cases collection was not possible because delinquent account information was not readily available. Good service bureaus attempted to solve this problem by periodically dating what was on the computer on at least a biweekly basis. Because of the economic advantages of this system, many offices still employ it today.

With the development of the cathode ray tube, or CRT (a device that looks like a TV set with a typewriter keyboard attached), and the development of efficient transmittal of data over telephone lines, service bureaus were able to put terminals into medical offices to allow access to records at a moment's notice. Today a well-run service bureau can provide its clients with a system in which the doctor's staff can have information available as quickly as if the computer were in the next room.

[ii] In-House Computer. The other approach to computerizing office records is bringing the computer "in-house." This entails purchasing or leasing of all of the hardware and software components of the accounts receivable system. A good in-house system runs very much like a good service bureau system. The in-house system, however, places more responsibility on the physician's staff.

For example, with an in-house system the office must process statements, insurance forms and management reports and contend with hardware breakdowns and software failures. Because of the rapid advancements in computer hardware, many in-house systems become obsolete in a shorter period of time than anticipated when their original cost is estimated.

On the positive side, the in-house system is generally less expensive than a service bureau, especially for a growing practice, and adding patients does not add cost to the computer system as it would for a charge-by-account bureau system. An in-house system generally provides the maximum amount of flexibility for "tailor designing" the office system, and can typically fill other office needs, such as word processing, electronic spreadsheets and list processing, at a minimal cost.

§ 10.02 Controls

> A system whereby every step of the billing and payment process can be recorded and double-checked is essential. This entails filling out a charge slip for each patient that records each procedure performed on the patient; splitting duties for receiving, recording and depositing any payments; having documentation to back any entry of payment or credit or debit adjustment into a patient's account; and balancing the account on a regular basis. It is important that the office be run by an efficient staff that recognizes the importance of every detail in the accounts receivable management system.

Each year a typical medical practice records a cash flow of between $120,000 to $350,000 per physician. The gross revenues of even a small practice can easily exceed $1,000,000 per year. In spite of this, a surprisingly large number of medical offices have few, if any, controls on the recording of charges, payments and adjustments in their accounts receivable processing. Without proper controls, the medical office is not only wide open to theft by one dishonest employee, it is also wide open to large revenue losses from lost charges and payments.

[1] Charge Slips

The first step for controlling accounts receivable is to minimize the potential for lost charges and the best way to achieve this is to utilize pre-numbered charge slips. A pre-numbered charge slip is prepared for each patient to be seen at the office and attached to the patient's chart. The charge slip then follows the patient, so that each procedure, whether performed by the physician or an assistant, can be checked off on the slip. It is essential that each procedure performed be checked on the form by the provider. Otherwise, even the most elaborate and rigid bookkeeping system cannot insure all charges will be entered into and remain in the billing system until paid. Employees who do not appreciate the complexities and difficulties encountered by the bookkeeping area of the office may discount the importance of the routing or charge slip and fail to make entries, relying instead on their powers of recall or assuming that someone else will record the necessary information.

If a system is established whereby a charge slip is prepared for each patient seen in the office, the bookkeepers can keep track of all charge slips and account for them at the end of the day. These charge slips can be batched and an independent total of them run to be compared with the posting totals of the batch when it is entered into the accounts receivable system. Smaller offices can sometimes post the charge to the patient's account at the time the patient is in the office. This system should, however, employ the same control of comparing the total from the independent addition of the charge slips to the posted total for the day. By observing several simple steps the physician can insure that all charges are entered into the accounts receivable system:

- Make sure a charge slip is prepared for each patient.
- Make sure the physicians, medical assistant and technicians enter all procedures they perform on the charge slip.
- Make sure all charge slips are accounted for at the end of the day by the bookkeeping department.

[2] Payments

Payments can be lost, misposted or embezzled. The best control for minimizing lost or misappropriated payments is to split duties for the employees who handle them. With a system of split duties, no one person completes the entire processing of a payment from receiving the payment to posting it to the patient's account. Under such a system, embezzlement would require collusion. It is therefore suggested that different people handle collecting money from the patient, preparing deposit slips and entering the payment into the patient's account.

All payments should be deposited with the bank so that all money received is recorded on the deposit slip. In this way the total deposit can be compared with the total payments postings for the day and if there is any discrepancy, the details of the deposit slip can be checked against individual postings.

Certain forms of payment will need additional documentation. A payment from the welfare agency, for example, generally covers more than one patient account, and it will be necessary to review the remittance advice to determine whether there have been any discrepancies. Since many different types of currency are used as payment (checks, cash, third party reimbursements), a listing of currencies can be used to balance the total cash receipts for the day.

If all of the receipts go into the business checking account, you have the confidence of at least one third party controller—the bank. When bank statements arrive, they should be reviewed by the physician or supervisor before being given to the bookkeeper to prevent accusations of employee tampering.

[3] Adjustments

Write-offs and adjustments include entries into the accounts receivable that are neither charges nor payments. Because a wide variety of entries may be classified in this category, it is essential to have a tight system of controls in this area. An embezzler may use a fictional entry in the adjustment column, for example, to balance a patient account and thereby cover up a discrepancy between the payments posted and the deposit. Another abuse of the write-off and adjustment journal occurs when a bookkeeper attempts to write off or adjust a patient's account in difficult collection situations. If the bookkeeper does not know how to pursue a particular problem with a welfare account, for example, he or she could avoid having the account appear delinquent by putting an adjustment on the account that deletes the problem charge.

To avoid some of these problems, all of the write-offs and adjustments should be posted in a separate journal to be reviewed by the physician or office supervisor. The office should have a rule that every write-off and adjustment is to be backed up with additional source documentation. For every welfare write-off, for example, there should be remittance advice from the welfare agency showing the amount of the write-off and the reason for it. Other write-offs, such as professional discounts, should be approved and signed by the physician before the discount is allowed. Any delinquent accounts to be written off should be reviewed and signed by the physician before they are entered into the system. A journal for write-offs and adjustments should be reviewed by the physician or supervisor for abnormalities or unusual entries.

[4] Balancing Accounts

Accounts receivable should always be balanced on a daily basis, otherwise most controls are rendered useless. For example, an embezzler can prevent detection of a stolen payment by posting the payment directly to the patient's ledger card but not in the payment journal or the write-offs and adjustments journal. Or, even if all charges are properly posted, a substantial amount could be lost by simple misplacement of a patient's ledger card.

Balancing accounts receivable means taking the aggregate amount of journal entries for the day and computing what the accounts receivable should be. This computed accounts receivable figure should then be compared with the actual accounts receivable figure determined by adding up the total amount of the patient accounts. Using the aggregate posting figures to compute the accounts receivable is not difficult and generally presents no problem. Daily adding of the ledger cards, however, can be a major problem for a large office with a manual system, regardless of the type of system. As a result, many offices do not add up patient ledgers more often than annually, if at all. If a discrepancy occurs, as it almost always does, by the end of a year it can almost never be located. If it is a large discrepancy, the physician may be aware a major problem has occurred but will be unable to correct it.

Before adding up and balancing ledger cards becomes unmanageable, it may be time to start thinking about computerizing the office, especially if discrepancies become common.

See the Appendix at the end of this chapter for further example of balancing sheets.

[5] Staff

The final and most important form of control in accounts receivable, as elsewhere in the office, is hiring a reliable, competent and honest staff. All employees must recognize the importance of accounts receivable and the systems employed, and not look for ways to shortcut the systems. No physician knowingly places a dishonest or incompetent person in control of accounts receivable, but many embezzlements have occurred and been detected through the years. What is not known is how many embezzlements go undetected. The point here is that even if you feel your staff is honest and competent, there is no replacement for a good system of internal controls.

§ 10.03 Third Party Billings

> Medicare, Medicaid, Medicare/Medicaid, Preferred Provider Organizations, Blue Cross/Blue Shield, Health Maintenance Organizations, Independent Practice Associations, and Worker's Compensation Boards are the major providers of third party coverage. Each practice's billing system must be flexible enough to accommodate the billing procedures required by the various third party insurers and simple enough so that it is easily understood by both the patients and the office staff.

Billings for a physician's office used to be a relatively simple matter of recording services performed and sending the patient a statement at the end of the month for the amount due. However, as the practice of medicine developed—and as medical care became more expensive—the concept of a third party providing insurance coverage to prevent personal financial catastrophe in the event of serious health problems caught on. Third-party coverage is presently available through a variety of private insurers, government subsidized programs and physician-coordinated organizations that cover almost any person, regardless of age, income or medical condition. Indeed, many patients find it difficult to obtain medical care without some kind of third-party coverage.

For the physician, the involvement of a third party usually means one more set of hands through which billings and reimbursements must pass. Physicians who adopt the philosophy that their relationship is with the patient and not with the third party often avoid filling out many of the special billing statements required by the third party. Most physicians, however, are unable to completely avoid contact with third parties, such as Medicaid or Medicare.

Because the array of services provided by physicians is vast and usually not fully understood by the layman, third parties usually implement billing systems that clearly specify which procedures patients are billed for. These systems attempt to categorize every possible procedure by description and number or procedure code, and keep track of costs by assigning a relative value to each. To determine whether a procedure is covered under the insurance contract and whether or not it was justified, third parties compare the procedure with the patient's end diagnosis, which has also been categorized and assigned a specific number, or diagnostic.

Most third party statements require the following data in addition to information shown on a physician's statement:

- Policy holder's name, date of birth, address, occupation, employer and employer's address.

- Patient's name, date of birth, address, occupation, employer, employer's address and relationship to policy holder (if different from policy holder).

- Whether the patient is covered by any other insurance.

- Attending physician and hospital if patient was hospitalized.

- Date, place and description of each service performed.

- CPT or HCPCS code.

- Amount of charge.

- Diagnosis.

- ICD (diagnostic) code.

Although the information required by third parties is somewhat standard, most have unique forms that require this information to be put in different areas. Although most third parties recognize the inefficiency of everyone having a separate form and accept a "standard" insurance form approved by the AMA, some have strayed from the standard to use forms that can be read by optical scanners and given "approval numbers." If a physician is to receive proper compensation for services, he or she must be sure the office is able to comply with such special billing requirements cost-effectively. (See Figure 10-3.)

[1] Medicare

Medicare was established by Congress to provide medical coverage for retired persons over the age of 65. It is a part of Social Security funded through the employee's and employer's share of the F.I.C.A. tax and is generally administered by the Department of Health and Human Services through private insurance carriers.

(Rel.4–2/90 Pub.372)

§ 10.03 [1]   MANAGING YOUR MEDICAL PRACTICE   10–18

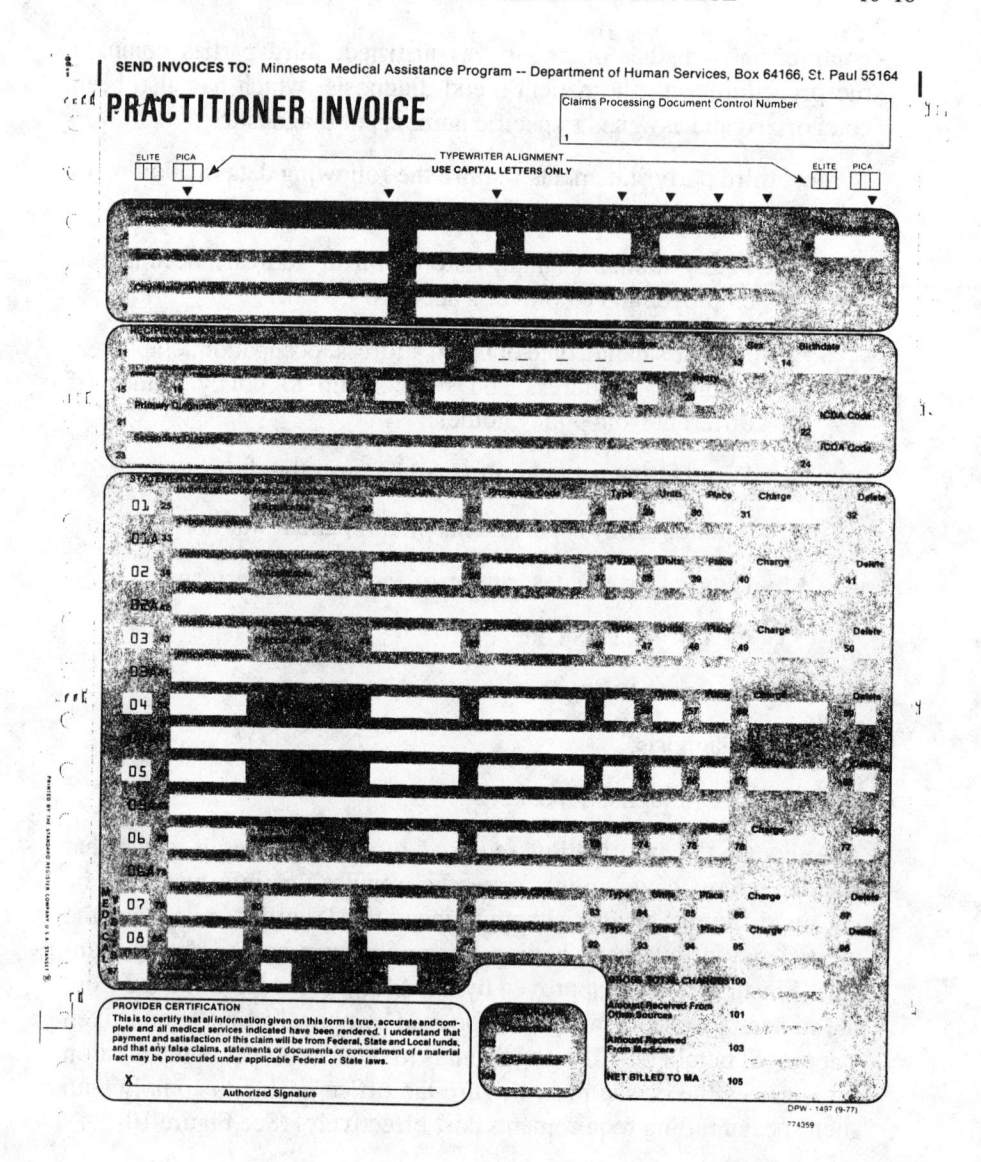

FIG. 10-3. A special billing request of the Minnesota Medical Assistant Program that does not conform to conventional guidelines. The form must be typed on a pica or elite typewriter. Failure to complete the form properly renders it "unreadable" to the program's computer.

[a] Reimbursement

Medicare is broken down into two kinds of coverage: hospital care (part A of the form) and physician's services (part B). Each year the patient pays a deductible amount under both parts of the plan, and Medicare pays 80 percent of the charges above the deductible amount subject to the maximum allowable fee.

The amount Medicare reimburses for a physician's services is determined by the lowest of three variables: the physician's fee, the physician's profile or the community profile. The physician's fee is detailed in the billing statement. The physician's profile is determined by the physician's average charge to different patients for the same procedure over a particular interval of time, based on information received by billings to Medicare directly from the physician or from the patient.

To determine the community profile Medicare breaks down the United States into many different profile sections, based on the charges by all of the physicians in that section for particular services. In this way, it is possible for one physician to receive a higher reimbursement than another for the same procedure simply because he or she lives in another Medicare profile section of the state or country.

Because of the emphasis on profiles, a physician must maintain realistic fees base on the economics of his or her practice. It is not uncommon for a new physician to set fees slightly below the community norm to help build his or her practice. Since this can mean that even once the practice has grown the physician will be prohibited by the Medicare reimbursement schedule from raising fees up to the community level, new physicians should be careful to set up a high enough fee schedule from the start. The difference between what the physician charges and how much Medicare will reimburse based on the physician and community profile is the disallowed charge. The physician must write off this disallowed charge since, under the terms of Medicare, the patient cannot be billed for it.

[b] Terms of Coverage

Under the Medicare regulations, patients have the option of seeking services from either participating or non-participating physician providers. A physician who is a non-participating Medicare provider may bill the patient directly and hold the patient financially responsible for 100 percent of the bill or the physician may bill Medicare directly. However, Medicare will not pay a non-participating physician directly, but will send the reimbursement to the patient.

The advantage of being a non-participating physician and not accepting Medicare patient assignment is that the physician is free to bill the patient through his or her normal billing method and not Medicare's. The physician does not have to come in contact with a third party and can hold the patient responsible for the balance of the bill not covered by Medicare. Another advantage is that the non-participating physician has the option to accept assignment on particular Medicare patients. If a non-participating physician arbitrarily accepts assignment, he or she agrees to the same terms and fee schedule as the participating physician, and so he or she can send the medical form directly to Medicare for reimbursement but with no further obligation to accept other Medicare patients. Under the provisions of the system, the physician cannot bill the patient for any disallowed services, but only for the deductible and the 20 percent balance not covered by Medicare.

In an effort to control the amount of reimbursement to physicians, Congress placed a one-year freeze on physicians' fees, effective July 1, 1984, that prohibited both participating and non-participating physicians from raising fees for any Medicare patient. Actually, this "one-year" freeze continued until January 1, 1987, at which time it was replaced with a set of complicated rules that allowed participating physicians to raise their fees, but limited their reimbursement. Non-participating physicians were required to adjust their fees so that they did not exceed the "maximum actual allowable charge" (MAAC). Although this permitted minor increases for many fees, in some cases the MAAC charge was less than the frozen charge and physicians were required to roll back their fees. As a result, today's non-participating physicians must be careful not to exceed their MAAC rate in charging any Medicare patient. Most physicians have had to adopt a two-tier fee schedule: the regular fee schedule and the Medicare patient fee schedule.

Congress continues to encourage physicians to become participating providers and accept assignment on all Medicare patients. Among the incentives it offers are inclusion on a list of participating physicians provided to Medicare patients and a greater reimbursement allowance. A hidden incentive is the complexity of the two-tiered fee schedules and the danger of falling out of compliance.

Effective July 1, 1984, Congress mandated that fees charged by reference laboratories for Medicare patients would be set by Medicare. Reference labs were prohibited from billing the patients for the service, and from billing the primary physician who ordered the test for the services, in effect, forcing them to become a participating Medicare provider. Likewise, on January 1, 1987, all physicians (including primary care physicians) were prohibited from billing Medicare patients for clinical laboratory testing and forced to become participating providers in accordance with the Medicare fee schedule. Effective January 1, 1990, all physicians' office labs will need to be certified.

Non-participating Medicare providers were required as of October 1, 1987 to give a surgical price disclosure form to each patient for whom Medicare is the primary insurer. This form must be signed by the patient and returned to the physician prior to any surgery with a total billing amount of over $500. (See Figure 10-3A.)

Figure 10-3A

Sample Surgical Disclosure Letter

Dear Mr./Mrs. ___(Patient's Name)___

As Dr. ___(Physician's Name)___ is scheduled to perform a ___(Type of Surgery)___ for you on ___(Date)___, Medicare regulations require that we furnish you with information regarding the amount that Medicare will be paying for your surgery and the amount you will be responsible for pying. It is our understanding that you have, in addition to your Medicare coverage, a supplemental policy from ___(Name of Supplemental Carrier)___. This policy may cover all or a portion of the bill that Medicare does not. The coverage will assist you in covering your out-of-pocket expenses according to your benefit package with them. So, after Medicare has paid their portion of this bill you will want to submit the remaining balance to ___(Name of Insurer)___ for consideration of payment. Once your secondary insurance has paid their portion, if the remaining fee is more than you feel you can financially afford, please contact our office.

Type of surgery: _____

Estimated charge: _____

   Surgeon: _____

   Assistant Surgeon: _____

Estimated Medicare Payment: _____

   Surgeon: _____

   Assistant Surgeon: _____

Physician's fees after Medicare payment: _____

It is necessary that you sign this notice prior to your surgery and return it to our office in the enclosed envelope. We have enclosed two copies, one for your records. Because this notice must accompany your patient file to surgery, a delay in returning this notice could result in postponement of your surgery. If you have any questions, please feel free to call our office.

Patient Signature:_____

Date:_____

Physician Signature:_____

Date:_____

Fig. 10-3A. A sample surgical disclosure letter. The contents of this letter can be placed on a word processor and adapted to the financial circumstance of each patient (e.g. whether or not the patient has supplemental coverage, whether the patient will complete the form while in the office or return it by mail). To fill the form out properly, the physician will need to know not only the MAAC rates for each type of surgery, but also the Medicare allowable. These should be available directly from Medicare. However, there are two precautions: the physician should ask for the allowable for a non-participating physician, as it is less than the allowable for a participating physician; and he or she should remember to deduct the 20 percent patient copayment from Medicare's allowable rates, as the patient is liable for that amount. A final signed copy should be sent to the patient prior to surgery. If the patient has only Medicare coverage, the first paragraph should be edited accordingly, and the final sentence changed to read, "Once Medicare has paid its portion."

(Text continued on page 10-21)

[c] Billing System

Billing Medicare is generally not a problem, especially in offices with computerized billings that can generate the standard claim forms. In non-assigned cases the physician may submit forms directly to Medicare on behalf of the patient, or provide forms for the patient to submit to Medicare.

If the office is on a pegboard or other manual system, a "master" Medicare form containing all of the information consistently required to file a claim should be completed for each patient. The patient's name, address and Medicare number, and the physician's name and provider numbers all would be shown on the master form so that each time a Medicare claim is to be made the form can be photocopied and the current information—the procedures performed and being billed, the CPT code, the diagnosis and the diagnostic code—can be entered.

Once the patient signs the completed Medicare form or completes the "signature on file" slip, the form can be sent directly to Medicare. A copy of the completed form should be kept in the physician's office. In the event of a non-assignment, the form can be placed in the paid-up insurance file. This is done to facilitate collecting: since Medicare payment goes directly to the patient, the physician can never know for sure whether the insurance company has reimbursed the patient; nevertheless, the physician must assume payment has been made and seek payment for services directly from the patient. In the event of an assignment of benefits (in which case the physician accepts payment from Medicare) the physician's copy of the form should be placed in a file of unpaid insurance claims.

When payment for Medicare comes directly from Medicare, there is usually one check issued for all of the procedures and patients taken care of over a given period of time. The office bookkeeper will need to review and understand the Medicare remittance advice, commonly called the EOB (explanation of benefits), to properly post payment to patients' accounts. The EOB will show the name of the patient for whom the payment is being made, the patient's account number, the specific procedure, the physician charges, the disallowed charge, the non-covered service, the portion of the bill Medicare is reimbursing, the patient's deductible amount and the patient's participation amount. (See Figures 10–4a and 10–4b.)

(Pub.372)

§ 10.03 [1]   MANAGING YOUR MEDICAL PRACTICE   10–22

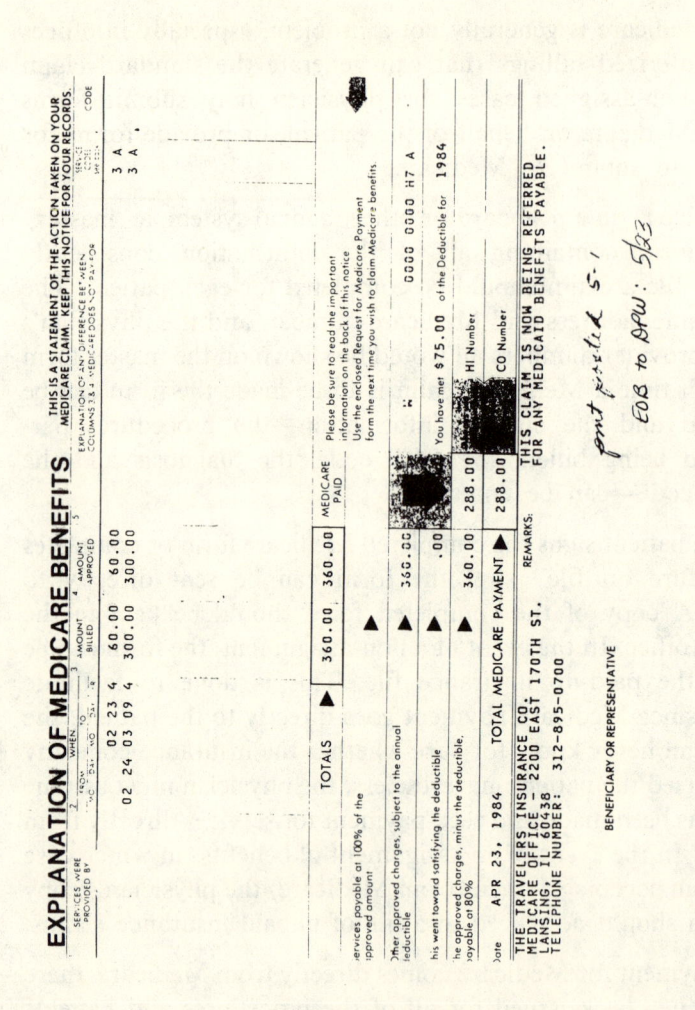

FIG. 10-4. A Medicare explanation of benefits (EOB). The advice sent to the patient (a) is markedly different from (b) the information sent in a batch to the physician.

The patient may be billed for any service not covered under Medicare (eyeglasses, contact lenses, certain kinds of medication, cosmetic surgery, etc.), the deductible amount and the 20 percent for which the patient is typically responsible.

(Pub.372)

YOUR EXPLANATION OF MEDICARE BENEFITS
Please Read This Notice Carefully And Keep It For Your Records. THIS IS NOT A BILL

| DATE 09/11/84 | PROVIDER NO | PROVIDER NAME | | PAGE 1 | SEE REVERSE SIDE FOR ADDITIONAL INFORMATION |

IMPORTANT: NOTIFICATION OF THE PROCESSING OF THE CLAIM(S) INDICATED BELOW HAS BEEN SENT TO THE APPROPRIATE BENEFICIARY.

PHYSICIAN OR SUPPLIER NAME	DATES OF SERVICE FROM / TO (MO DA / MO DA)	SEE BACK SERV TYPE	BILLED AMOUNT	AMOUNT APPROVED	(SEE **) ACTN CODE	BENEFICIARY OBLIGATION DEDUCTIBLE / CO-INS	MEDICARE PAYMENT TO BENEFICIARY / PROVIDER
	7 18 / 07 18 : A 01		25.00	16.30	101	16.30 / 0.00	0.00 / 0.00
	07 18 / 07 18 : E 01		5.00	4.20	101	0.00 / 0.00	0.00 / 4.20
	07 18 / 07 18 : E 06		10.50	10.50		0.00 / 0.00	0.00 / 10.50
	07 18 / 07 18 : E 01		7.00	5.70	101	0.00 / 0.00	0.00 / 5.70
TOTAL-CLAIM 84222022480O 4250U0			47.50	36.70		16.30 / 0.00	0.00 / 20.40

CLAIM REFERRED TO STATE WELFARE AGENCY
BENEFICIARY: NUMBER:

	08 15 / 08 15 : A 01		25.00	16.30	101	0.00 / 3.26	0.00 / 13.04
	08 15 / 08 15 : E 01		5.00	4.20	101	0.00 / 0.00	0.00 / 4.20
	08 15 / 08 15 : E 01		5.25	4.80	101	0.00 / 0.00	0.00 / 4.80
TOTAL-CLAIM o42360918100 4248G72			35.25	25.30		0.00 / 3.26	0.00 / 22.04

CLAIM REFERRED TO STATE WELFARE AGENCY
BENEFICIARY: NUMBER:

| GRAND TOTALS | | | 82.75 | 62.00 | | 16.30 / 3.26 | 0.00 / 42.44 |

```
TOTAL AMOUNT APPROVED----------------        62.00
REMAINING AFTER PHYSICAL THERAPY AND
  AND PSYCHIATRIC LIMITS------------         62.00
TOTAL AMOUNT APPLIED TO ANNUAL DEDUCTIBLE--           16.30
BALANCE PAYABLE AT 80%--------------
80% OF BALANCE PAID TO BENEFICIARY/PROVIDER---------  13.04
BALANCE PAYABLE AT 100%----------------                0.00
AMOUNT PAYABLE AT 100% NOT SUBJECT TO DEDUCTIBLE----- 29.40
TOTAL MEDICARE PAYMENT TO BENEFICIARY/PROVIDER------         0.00   42.44
```

** - EXPLANATION OF ACTION CODES:
101-SEE ITEM 5 ON REVERSE

THE TRAVELERS INSURANCE CO., PART B MEDICARE, 8120 PENN AVE SOUTH
BLMNGTON MN 554311394   TELEPHONE NUMBER - 612-884-7171

(Pub.372)

It is important to keep proper records on the patient's account in these situations. If amounts that should be written off are not, or vice versa, there will be so much confusion about the bill that collection will be greatly hampered, if not impossible. A properly designed computer system will handle these situations by applying write-offs to specific procedures within an account automatically. With a manual system each paid charge should be marked off as the payment and charge adjustment is posted to the account. At any given point the sum of the charges shown on the ledger card which have not been checked off should equal the balance of the total amount due shown on the ledger card.

After the payment has been posted to the patient's account, the original claim form sent to Medicare, filed in the unpaid insurance file, should be pulled. If all the charges on the unpaid insurance form have been paid, the form should be refiled in a paid-up insurance claim file. If only a portion of the billed procedures have been paid, unpaid claims should be checked off and the date of the payment noted. The form should then be replaced in the unpaid claim file. At the end of each month the unpaid insurance claim file should be reviewed and all Medicare forms submitted but not paid should be pulled. The bookkeeper should then call the Medicare office to inquire about the delay in payment. Because the bookkeeper will have copies of all the claim forms filed, he or she will be armed to intelligently discuss or debate any problems Medicare is having in paying the claims.

[2] Medicaid

Medicaid is designed and funded to provide a "safety net" for people in need of financial assistance for medical care. Since it is administered by the state governments, administration of the program varies widely throughout the country. Many states contribute funds in excess of the federal minimum requirements to provide expanded services; however, most providers across the country find reimbursement from Medicaid lower than what they would receive through independent billing. They provide care for Medicaid patients as a social service but try to limit the number of such patients on their rosters.

The method of Medicaid billing varies from state to state.

Requirements for statements sent to the local welfare office can range from a simple physician's statement to a detailed bill requiring all procedure and diagnostic codes to be placed in specific boxes on the form so they may be read by the agency's optical scanner.

Regardless of the state in which the physician practices, Medicaid is billed directly to and payment comes directly from the local welfare agency. Physicians are prohibited from billing the patient for any excess or disallowed charges. (Even if the physician was allowed such charges, it is unlikely they could be collected.)

A physician's copy of the Medicaid claims form should be placed in the unpaid insurance file. Like a Medicare reimbursement, the welfare agency generally pays the physician for a number of patients and procedures with one check, and the EOB will show the breakdown of the payment as applied to various patients and procedures. (See Figure 10–5.)

After the payments have been posted, the claims forms should be pulled from the unpaid insurance file and reviewed. Claims paid in full should be filed as such. If only a portion of the claim has been paid, that portion of the bill should be checked off and the claim form should be placed back in the unpaid file. At the end of each month the Medicaid claims which have gone without payment for two months should be pulled and the local agency contacted for an explanation.

[3] Medicare/Medicaid

A number of patients qualify for both Medicare and Medicaid, in which case Medicare covers the majority of charges (usually 80 percent of the maximum fee allowed) and Medicaid generally covers the Medicare deductible and the Medicare participation portion (generally twenty percent). Neither Medicare nor Medicaid will pay for disallowed charges and charges in excess of the applicable profile. (See Figure 10–6.

Since Medicare is the primary coverage for these patients, and since it is necessary to accept assignment on Medicare welfare patients (as it is for Medicaid patients who do *not* receive Medicare benefits), the initial bill is sent directly to Medicare. Medicare will process the claim and send a copy of the EOB to the local welfare

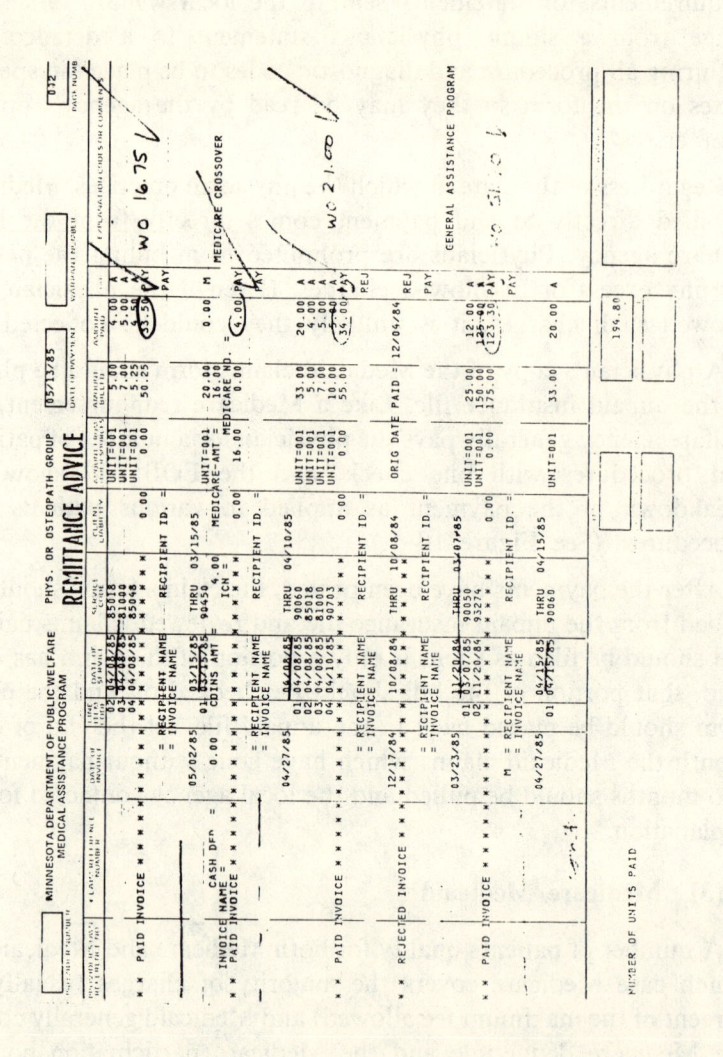

FIG. 10-5. Remittance advice (EOB) for Medicaid payments. This form contains reimbursement information for several patients that must be sorted for proper posting of charges and payments to patient accounts. Generally, the unpaid portion of the charge should be immediately written off. An exception is when the agency fails to make a proper payment on the account. Unfortunately the only way a physician can control this is to have informed bookkeepers who can detect discrepancies such as two different amounts being charged for two patients who received similar treatment.

(Pub.372)

ACCOUNTS RECEIVABLE MANAGEMENT § 10.03 [3]

agency. The welfare agency then uses this information to compute the amount due to the physician as reimbursement.

When the claim for a Medicare/Medicaid patient is completed, a copy should be placed in the unpaid insurance file. When payment is received, postings to the ledger card should be entered as they would be for an assigned Medicare account. The

FIG. 10-6. This standard billing form can be used by most Medicare and Medicaid providers.

bookkeeper should check that Medicare has reimbursed the physician for the appropriate claims and record write-offs. However, the claim should then be replaced into the unpaid insurance file until Medicaid also makes its payment.

At the end of the month all Medicare/Medicaid charges that have not been reimbursed for the Medicare portion or that have received a payment on Medicare but have not received payment from Medicaid for one month since Medicare has paid should be pulled. The Medicare office should be contacted to discuss unpaid claims, and the local welfare office should be contacted to discuss claims paid by Medicare but not yet paid by Medicaid.

[4] Preferred Provider Organizations (PPO's)

A PPO generally consists of a network of health-care providers (at least several physicians with varying specialties and a hospital) and one or more insurance companies. It may also include other types of health care facilities and providers such as chiropractors, optometrists and dentists. Members of the PPO agree to accept the PPO's fee schedule and agree not to bill patients for fees in excess of this schedule. Members generally bill, and are paid directly by, the PPO. Only uncovered charges (which vary from organization to organization but might include well-care, physical examinations, routine office calls, eyeglasses, etc.), deductibles and coinsurances may be billed to the patient.

The advantage to the physician participating in a PPO is that the PPO helps promote his or her practice (i.e., recommendations from the insurance companies that patients remain in the PPO). The other advantage is that third-party reimbursement comes directly from the PPO without going first to the patient. Furthermore, an efficiently run PPO can process billing and pay the physician within three weeks.

A disadvantage to being a member of a PPO is that the physician can no longer raise fees independently and expect full compensation. The physician is also not free to bill in accordance with normal billing procedures but must comply with the guidelines established by the PPO.

PPO's are advantageous for the patient, since the patient has the option to select either a PPO member or a non-member provider under the terms of his or her insurance policy. In the event the patient elects a PPO member, he or she need not worry about excess charges, the paperwork of billing the insurance company, or having to pay for covered services before receiving reimbursement from the insurance company. If the patient chooses not to go to a member physician, the insurance company is obligated to cover the usual and customary percentage of fees for services charged as detailed in the insurance contract. In most cases, that means the patient will only have to pay the deductible and coinsurance. Generally the patient who sees a non-member provider has to complete his or her own insurance forms.

[a] Blue Cross/Blue Shield

Blue Cross/Blue Shield functions similar to a PPO. Physicians and other providers may or may not be participating providers, and patients can go to both participating and non-participating providers (although the incentive is for the patient to go to participating providers). The option to participate is generally open to physicians on an annual basis.

Non-participating physicians need not cooperate with Blue Cross/Blue Shield or accept its fee schedules. They may bill the patient directly or bill Blue Cross/Blue Shield. However, when the claim form is processed by Blue Cross/Blue Shield, the payment is sent directly to the patient. (See Figure 10–7 for a copy of a standard Blue Cross/Blue Shield form.)

Each participating physician works directly with Blue Cross/Blue Shield and submits a fee schedule annually. Blue Cross/Blue Shield uses this data to calculate the usual and customary fee for specific procedures and the physician is informed as to the maximum fee he or she will be reimbursed for each procedure. This maximum is the lesser of the physician's fee or the usual and customary fee.

A participating physician agrees to accept this fee as payment in full and bills the patient only for non-covered services, policy deductibles and co-insurance. However, since all of the patient's charges are shown on one account, there are time lags in payment to the physician, and the patient may have additional fees charged to

(Pub.372)

§ 10.03 [4]   MANAGING YOUR MEDICAL PRACTICE   10–30

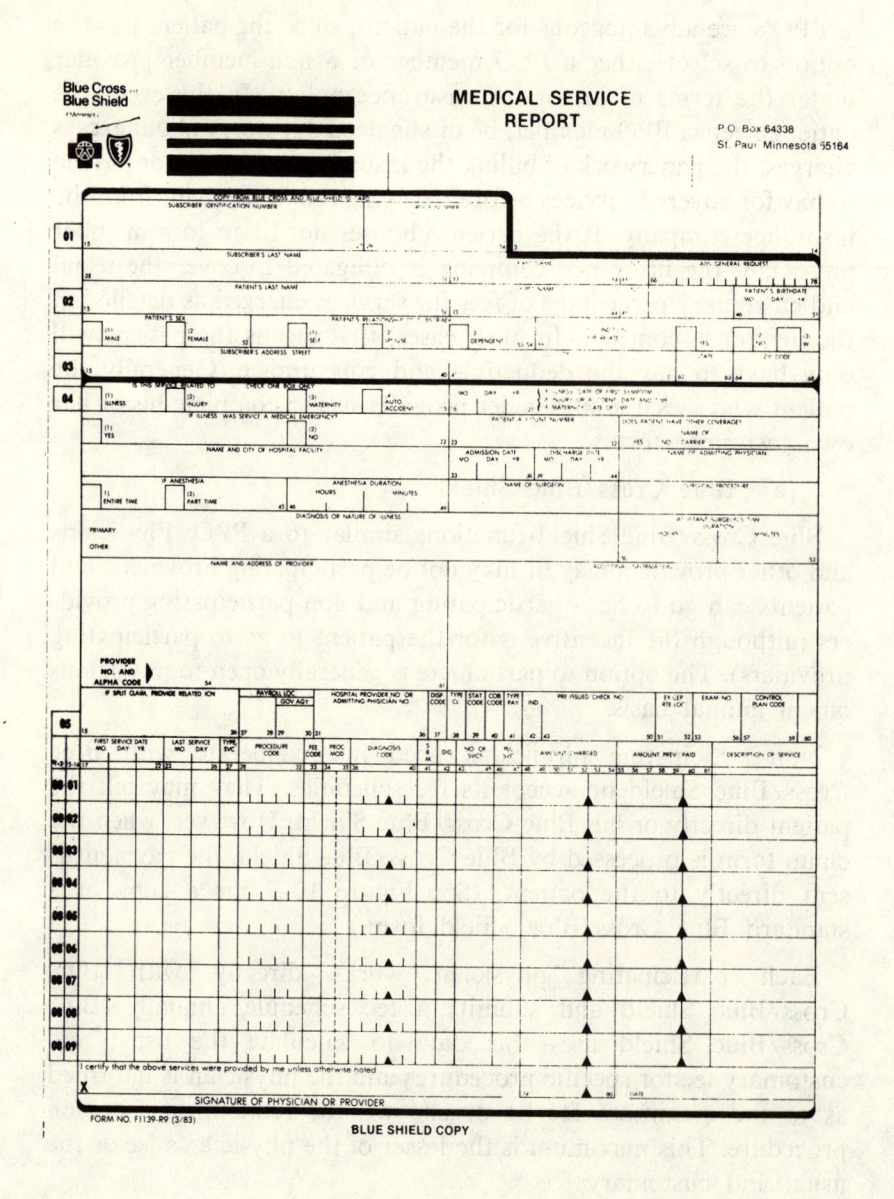

FIG. 10-7. A standard Blue Cross/Blue Shield medical service report.

(Pub.372)

his or her account before the initial fees are payed, this can cause a problem in billing. The physician's office, unable to determine the exact amount of payment to be received under the terms of the patient's insurance contract, generally sends the statement to the patient showing the entire balance due. That statement, combined with the explanation of benefits form (provided both to the participating physician and patient) allow both the patient and medical office to determine the amount the patient owes. When the EOB is received by the medical office, the patient's account should be adjusted and a statement telling the amount due by the patient should be prepared. (See Figure 10–8.)

[b] Accounts Receivable Processing

Accounts receivable processing in the PPO program can be complicated further by administrative tasks. For example, the AWARE program requires "approval" before a patient can be placed in the hospital. Also, a participating PPO physician is supposed to refer patients only to other PPO members. A physician who refers the patient to a non-participating physician must inform the patient in writing that he or she is doing so, otherwise the physician could become responsible for the entire bill. In an effort to contain or reduce health care costs, various PPO's may have other restrictions.

Since each PPO may vary in how billing procedures are to be performed and what services are covered, it is impossible to cover all the potential billing problems that can surface. For that reason, any physician considering signing up as a participant in a PPO program should carefully review the specific accounts receivable and other administrative problems that can result. While a physician should not be so rigid as to have only one method of billing that excludes him or her from all PPO participation, he or she should avoid joining up with all PPO's in the area to avoid burdening the office with a variety of different billing requirements. Computers and other office systems designed to handle the accounts receivable are often unable to handle special billing requirements and the small volume rarely justifies investment in a new billing system.

§ 10.03 [4]   MANAGING YOUR MEDICAL PRACTICE   10–32

Blue Cross and Blue Shield
of Minnesota
P.O. Box 64560
St. Paul, Minnesota 55164

PAGE 6

PROVIDER NOTICE OF CLAIMS RESOLUTION

Date: 03/04/85
Provider Number:

Patient Name Identification Number Claim Number Account Number	Service Dates From / To Group Number	Procedure Code	Charges Submitted	Less Previous Payment	Less UC&R Reduction	Less Amount Not Covered	Less Ded./Co-Insurance	BCBSM Payment	
	122784	99000	500	500	00	00	00	00	001
	121184	45300	300	1976	00	00	00	1024	001
AS22502*	TOTAL*	400	2976	00	00	00	1024	00
	010385	9CC50	2500	00	00	00	2500	00	2500
	010385	90050	2500	00	00	00	2500	00	2500
	010385	E5007	525	00	00	00	00	525	00
	010385	85018	500	00	00	00	00	500	00
	010385	61000	700	00	00	00	00	700	00
	010385	85048	525	00	00	00	00	525	00
	010385	71100	3750	00	00	00	00	3750	00
	012585	85007	525	00	00	00	00	525	00
052162C*	TOTAL*	11525	00	00	00	5000	6525	5000
	012985	85018	500	00	00	00	00	500	00
BM2640C*	TOTAL*	500	00	00	00	00	500	00
	123184	9C010	3500	2080	00	00	450	970	450
	123184	82548	750	528	00	00	45	177	45
	123184	81000	700	304	00	00	80	316	80
	123184	65048	525	384	00	00	23	118	23
Y017100*	TOTAL*	5475	3296	00	00	598	1581	598
	012585	45300	400	00	00	00	00	4000	00
	012185	53000	3000	00	00	00	00	3000	00
CSCC164*	TOTAL*	7000	00	00	00	00	7000	00
	010385	E5610	525	00	00	00	525	00	525

NOTES - Numbered messages are listed below. Alphabetic messages are found on the back of this form.
1—FULL OR PARTIAL PAYMENT FOR THIS CLAIM HAS BEEN MADE BY THE PATIENT'S OTHER HEALTH INSURANCE PLAN OR FEDERAL MEDICARE.

FIG. 10-8. A comprehensive listing of Blue Cross/Blue Shield claims, detailing the amounts paid, amounts the patient is liable for and disallowed charges. (Pub.372)

[5] Health Maintenance Organizations (HMO's)

The HMO concept has been in effect since the early 1940's. Only recently, however, have physicians in private practice begun to view HMO's as a threat to the way they have done business in the past. Owing to government support and effective marketing procedures, HMO's are growing in popularity, and since most are "closed"—meaning that once a patient elects HMO coverage he or she may not select an independent doctor for services but must go to the HMO facility—the more people who join HMO's the smaller the number of available patients for the non-HMO physician.

Physicians traditionally prefer to be reimbursed on a fee for service basis and worry only about the patient's health, rather than the cost justification of procedures. Since most of the profit in medicine is made from sick people, theoretically the more sick people there are, the more dollars are available to the health care industry under the fee for service system.

HMO's attempt to address this aspect of the economics of health care by giving health care providers economic incentives to maintain the health of patients. Instead of paying on a fee for service basis, HMO providers are paid a flat fee for each patient enrolled in the plan. This capitated fee is paid regardless of whether or not the provider sees the patient and provides services. Since the more services a physician performs means more to subtract from the capitated fees and, hence, less profit, the provider will make the most money with a group of patients who need little or no medical services. It is felt that the HMO provider will provide "wellness" programs to maintain a healthy group of patients. Thus, the emphasis of the HMO would be on preventive care, rather than on treatment.

Because the HMO assumes all of the risk for its enrolled patients, and in essence becomes an insurance company, it must be large enough to spread the risk. A provider should have at least 500 enrollees and insurance to protect itself from a catastrophic patient case involving extraordinary expenditures. In an effort to compete with HMO's, independent practitioners have formed small associations (IPA's). In IPA's, independent physicians work together to cut risk yet at the same time retain independence. For an IPA to exist, however, a third party must be involved to sell the program and handle the administration.

A practice that provides services to both HMO and non-HMO patients faces accounts receivable problems. First, proper charges must be calculated to determine the total capitation income to be received based on the number of enrollees. Although there is no additional income to be made from services performed, it is important to keep track of all procedures performed and charges to maintain control on HMO volumes.

In addition, since the patient will not be billed for services, it is necessary to keep HMO accounts separate from regular practice accounts. HMO charges to patients should be separated from non-HMO charges so that the total amount of HMO charges can be accurately written off. The amount of HMO write-offs, combined with HMO expenses for patients (such as consultant fees, drugs and hospital charges) can then be compared to the capitation income to determine whether or not the practice is making money on the HMO program. Moreover, by keeping track of charges on patients, you can determine whether or not the average charge or cost per patient is greater on the capitation program or the fee for service program.

Most of the IPA/HMO-type programs require preparation and submission of a billing form showing the patient, procedures performed and the diagnosis. This information is used to evaluate the program and have the necessary information available to determine insurance in the event of a catastrophic illness.

[6] Private Insurance

Many insurance companies provide coverage for individuals in a group (e.g., businesses). This kind of insurance, unconnected with a specific provider of medical services, is designed to prevent health problems from creating economic disaster for patients. Generally, these programs have an annual deductible of $100 to $500 and co-insurance of 20 percent. They generally do not cover routine medical services.

Although most of these companies have their own insurance forms, the same basic information as for any other third-party insurer is generally required. In an effort to reduce the number of different forms being completed in medical offices, a standard insurance form was developed. The form is approved by the AMA

(Pub.372)

and accepted by most insurance companies. In addition, the concept of the "super bill," or a form which not only details the physician's bill but all the necessary information for the insurance company as well, has become popular.

To expedite the processing of insurance forms and speed up collection, it is recommended that the medical office have a supply of standard insurance forms on hand. For doctors who refuse to deal directly with third parties, the standard insurance form may be forwarded to the patient with the patient's super bill. This eliminates the need for the patient to contact the insurance carrier for forms and can reduce the turn-around by weeks.

For physicians who don't mind dealing with third parties, a quick method of getting the insurance form completed is to have the patient sign the authorization of release of records and assignment of benefits to the physician at the bottom of the insurance form at the end of the visit. The physician's super bill can be attached to the insurance form and the form may be sent directly to the insurance carrier. If the assignment of benefits has been made, the reimbursement will go directly to the doctor.

Primary physicians who repeat services on patients can create a "master" form by completing the header information on the standard insurance form, including the patient's name, address, policy number, etc. This master may be photocopied and placed in the patient's file so that, when procedures are completed, a copy can be removed from the file, attached to the super bill and sent to the insurance carrier.

Because some third parties such as Medicare, welfare and Blue Cross require a special agreement between the provider and third party before an assignment can be made, many doctors think that accepting assignment from a private insurer results in a lower payment or agreeing to accept the insurance company's maximum fee. Unless a separate agreement is signed between the physician and third party, the physician is under no obligation to accept payment from the insurance company as payment in full. Since having the patient making an assigment of benefits directly to the physician eliminates the possibility of the patient not paying the balance due, physicians and staff should encourage patients to assign benefits directly to them. When insurance payments are posted onto the physician's bill, the balance due from the patient is less than full cost and, psychologically, the patient does not feel the service has cost as much.

[7] Worker's Compensation

To insure equitable and unilateral treatment of workers hurt on the job, legislation was created mandating that all employers provide worker's compensation insurance. The insurance covers the medical and disability expenses incurred by workers as a result of a job-related injury.

Medical services performed on patients eligible for worker's compensation should be billed directly to the covering insurance company. Although a number of companies provide worker's compensation insurance, benefits and payments are pre-determined by legislation, based on the state and the company.

Before a patient sees a doctor under worker's compensation coverage, the employer must authorize treatment. Furthermore, the employer must notify the insurance company of the injury in writing.

Since neither the patient nor the employer are responsible for the bill, the account should be treated in the same way as an insurance claim. The claim form should be filed in the unpaid claim file while reimbursement is pending and unpaid claims should be followed up directly with the insurance company involved. A separate patient account should be set up to keep track of procedures performed and covered under worker's compensation insurance in contrast to those for which the patient is responsible.

[8] Physical Examinations for Business Organizations

In many cases a business or organization contracts directly with a doctor and is responsible for the bill. A common example is the company that sends employees to a physician for periodic physical examinations. Another example is the business whose insurance company requires physical examinations before insuring an employee.

In these cases, an account can be set up in the name of the responsible party, i.e. the business, and each patient's name and the procedures performed can be entered on the statement. Generally, the physician's normal billing statement is adequate; a special statement is rarely needed. The age of the account can be controlled through the normal aging process.

§ 10.04 Hospital Charges

> New patients and consultation patients encountered at the hospital are a potential source of lost revenue if the physician does not inform the office staff of them. Use of a hospital log and a portable recording device can prevent information on charges outside of the hospital from being forgotten.

Keeping track of procedures performed and related charges for hospital patients can be a problem for a practice without a tight bookkeeping system. The potential loss of fees is greatly increased for specialists: since many of their cases are consultations, any they neglect to tell the office about are very unlikely to be recorded.

A medical staff may be aware of all patients who come into the office, yet remain oblivious to what the physician does at the hospital. Some physicians rely on receipt of the hospital list charge report for their staff to discover what services they have performed, but many cases are missed through this type of system since the hospital may forget to send the report or send it to the wrong doctor. In the case of a specialist called in for consultation, the report is often sent only to the admitting physician.

[1] Hospital Log

The first step toward getting control of hospital charges is to set up a hospital log in the office. The top of the log should show the name of the hospital and the week covered. The page for each week should be broken up into ten columns: the first for the patient's name and account number, the next seven for each day of the week the patient stays in the hospital, the ninth column to be marked when the hospital report is received, and the final column for the charge ticket number. (See Figure 10–9.)

Next, the name of every person to whom the physician provides hospital services should be entered into the log. Once the patient's name is entered into the log, it is recorded for each week thereafter until the office receives a discharge summary from the hospital or is

§ 10.04 [1]   MANAGING YOUR MEDICAL PRACTICE   10–38

                                        Week of _____
              Hospital log   Hospital_____

Patient	Sun.	Mon.	Tues.	Wed.	Thurs.	Fri.	Sat.	Diag. 1 Diag. 2	Hosp. Report	Charge Ticket Number

FIG. 10-9. A simple hospital log page.

otherwise notified by the physician. When the the bookkeeping department is notified that services have been completed, the total charges for each day are entered onto the charge slip from the hospital log and the charge slip number is entered into the hospital log to show that the charges listed have been entered into the accounts receivable system. When the hospital discharge summary is received, the ninth box is checked in the hospital log to indicate that all followup procedures have been completed.

In the event the discharge summary arrives from the hospital before the physician notifies the staff of the discharge, the staff should check with the physician to make sure all procedures have been properly recorded in the hospital log before preparing the charge slip.

(Pub.372)

[2] Keeping Track of Charges

When the physician is the admitting physician, the staff usually assists in scheduling the patient for hospital procedures and immediately enter the patient's name into the hospital log. However, in cases where the physician is not the admitting physician, the hospitalization does not originate with the physician's office, or the physician is asked to visit or give a consultative opinion on patients not familiar with the office, the staff will have no way of independently knowing the patient has been admitted to the hospital or that the physician has performed services. Therefore, it is essential that the physician have an organized and convenient method for keeping track of procedures performed at the hospital during the day, otherwise he or she is likely to forget many of them.

The most obvious way is for the bookkeeper to sit down with the physician each day and review the list of all patients in the hospital to find out what procedures were performed for the day. The physician should name any patients seen who were not listed in the hospital log (e.g., new patients, consultations). For new patients, it will be necessary for the bookkeeper to contact the business office at the hospital to obtain a patient address, third-party coverage information and other billing information. This method may appeal to some physicians who hate to pay attention to any of the bookkeeping tasks, but it is about as efficient as periodically jotting down such information on the back of napkins, envelopes and matchbook covers throughout the day.

A more efficient way is for the doctor to carry a pocket notebook or charge tablet. During the day he or she can list the names of people seen and each procedure performed. Like the hospital log, this list of charges can be tabulated on a weekly basis and then turned over to the bookkeeper. (See Figure 10–10.)

Another convenient tool for recording all of this information is the pocket dictating machine. In addition to patient and charge information the physician can record patient data right off the chart. All such information can then be transcribed and recorded directly into the hospital log after the physician returns to the office. Since it is easier for the busy physician to dictate messages to the staff rather than take the time to write them out, the dictating machine is a good way to avoid putting things off until later and possibly forgetting them.

NAME: _____

ADDRESS: _____
_____

PHONE: _____

DOB: _____

MED/WELF
BL SHIELD #: _____
HMO/PHP

HOSPITAL: _____

Inpatient or Outpatient

DOCTOR: _____

DX: _____
_____

DATE	PROCEDURE					
1	2	3	4	5	6	7
8	9	10	11	12	13	14
15	16	17	18	19	20	21
22	23	24	25	26	27	28
29	30	31				

FIG. 10-10. A monthly charge slip on which the physician can keep track of hospital patients. Once the initial procedure is performed on hospital patients, it is usually just a matter of keeping track of followup visits. Demographic data for new patients, such as proper spelling of the patient's name, age, address and third party information, can be obtained by the physician from the hospital records, although usually this information is readily available from the patient's hospital chart.

§ 10.05 Miscellaneous Charges

Sources of income such as nursing home charges, house calls, testimony fees and coverage fees must all be kept track of individually in the accounts receivable.

(Pub.372)

The medical office should be aware of miscellaneous charges made by the physician and have a method for handling them.

[1] Nursing Homes

Nursing home calls can be handled in the same way as hospital charges. A log for each nursing home is set up and patients' names are entered. The nursing home log differs from the hospital log in that many patients in the home are permanent residents. Whereas the hospital log is used to keep track of both charge postings and discharge summaries, once total charges have been tabulated and charge slips have been prepared from a weekly page in the nursing home book, that page can be removed from the book.

Once the patient's name is entered into the log the staff will know that each time the doctor visits the nursing home there may be a charge for that patient. It is still important, though, that the physician keep track of patients seen and procedures performed at the nursing home, just as is done for hospital patients—that is, with a charge pad or portable dictaphone.

In many cases it is advantageous for the physician to secure the signature of the nursing home patient on various forms. When the physician is unwilling to obtain the patient's signature it may be necessary to send a staff member to the nursing home or hospital to obtain it along with the third party forms. In some cases signatures and forms can be handled through the mail. However, this can take time and in many cases older patients are unable to interpret the information received through the mail and therefore handle it inappropriately, if at all.

[2] House Calls

It is best that any house call appointment be made through the physician's office so that a charge slip can be prepared by the office staff showing the patient's name and the date. Once the charge slip is prepared, the procedures performed during the visit and the diagnosis can be checked off when the physician returns to the office. By creating a charge slip at the time the appointment is made for the visit, the patient's name is entered into the "system" and the chance of a lost charge is minimized.

[3] Miscellaneous Income

A physician often has sources of outside income other than patient accounts receivable, such as fees from depositions, expert witness fees, coverage for other physicians and speaking fees. Generally, an account is set up for the responsible party. For example, if an attorney retains a physician to testify for a deposition or trial, an account should be set up for the attorney. If the attorney uses the physician for more than one patient, it is recommended that an account be set up to record the fee charged for each patient. The account should be kept separate from any "regular" patient account and, in this instance, be billed directly to the attorney.

Another common area for miscellaneous income in the medical office is the special charge report. Insurance companies frequently require a special report for which the physician makes a separate charge. It is recommended that all of these bills be put into an account to eliminate the question of whether or not any improprieties have occurred with regard to receipt of checks and also to allow the bookkeeper to ascertain that all charges have been billed. Generally a statement need not be sent to the insurance company; the company will automatically send the check. Because of this, one account can generally handle all of the different insurance companies.

When a physician covers for another doctor, there are a number of ways compensation can be handled. In some cases it is a simple matter of having the patient billed directly or billing the patient's third party. Other coverage arrangements call for the covering doctor to bill the attending doctor, who bills the patient and reimburses the covering physician. In this event an account should be set up for the attending physician, in which charges rendered to his or her patients are posted to be billed to the doctor. When the attending physician covers you, the charges he or she bills you would be posted to the individual patient accounts and billed to the patient or the patient's third-party insurer, as the case may be.

§ 10.06 Accounts Receivable Management Reports

To keep control of the accounts receivable and facilitate overall management, reports on account aging and account summaries should be generated as a regular by-product of the accounts receivable system.

As a byproduct of the accounts receivable, certain data should be readily available to monitor and follow up on collection problems, and to help in overall management of the office. A sophisticated, properly designed computer system can generate all of this information without additional bookkeeping work, but even a properly designed manual system can provide a fair amount of important information with a minimum amount of effort.

[1] **Aging Accounts**

There must be a system for aging accounts receivable. With a manual system, each account is reviewed by hand each month, generally at the time statements are being prepared, to determine proper collection action. The standard procedure for preparing statements in the medical office today is to photocopy the actual account cards for the private bills. Since every account is placed in the copy machine, this is the proper time for the bookkeeper to review and pull delinquent accounts for collection follow up. (Detailed collection followup information is provided in Chapter 7, "Credit and Collections.") If the number of outstanding patient accounts is reasonable, aging can be done by going through each account and categorizing the balance according to date of last payment. (Date of last payment can be used as a simpler way to age the accounts receivable since the accounts making payments generally need less attention than those with no payments, even though the original balance of the account may go back many months.)

For large offices, it is unrealistic to expect a detailed manual aging analysis of accounts. As an alternative, a random sample of accounts in the middle of the alphabet may be selected for an office to determine a sample aging analysis. For third-party aging, a review of the unpaid insurance file should be made. This is an excellent way to catch any accounts which are delinquent or lost in the third party's hands.

For offices with computers, aging information is more readily available. The computer can age reports by individual accounts and also categorize the accounts according to third parties. A computerized aging report can zero in on accounts with delinquent balances while leaving accounts in "current" status to be handled automati-

(Pub.372)

cally by the computer billing system. A good aging analysis report will give the collection department all the information necessary to follow up a delinquent account, including the patient's name, telephone number and billing address, the amount of charges and the date of last payment.

[2] Account Summaries

Another important part of management information to be provided by the accounts receivable system is a summary of the charges, payments, write-offs and adjustments. Even a good manual system can summarize monthly and daily charges by the practice, doctor and areas such as office and hospital or office/lab, special procedures, etc. A computer system, though, can generally provide a complete analysis of the production showing the dollar volume and actual volume of procedures for each of the procedures performed in the office. This can be done on both an office and per doctor basis.

This information is extremely helpful for making office management decisions. For example, the volume of procedures performed can help the physician anticipate the result of an increase in fees. If the physician is negotiating a contract with a third party, volume figures allow him or her to know the effect of a price reduction on a particular procedure.

With more and more pressure being placed on the physician to cut costs, more and more information from the accounts receivable system is required. This is one reason why larger offices are moving into computerized accounts receivable earlier now than in the past. Figures such as average cost per patient, average hospital stays for certain procedures, etc. help the physician evaluate his or her cost and effectiveness of treatment compared to the industry average.

(More details regarding the treatment reports which an automated computer system should be able to provide are given in Chapter 5, "Computers in Health Care.")

§ 10.07 Accounts Receivable Management Checklist

A checklist is provided for items to be noted when considering accounts receivable management.

Ledger Cards (Manual System)

- Patient name
- Patient address
- Type of insurance
- Date
- Service description
- Charges
- Payments
- Credit and debit adjustments
- Balance

— Journal Sheets (Manual System)
- Date
- Service description
- Charge
- Payments
- Debit and credit adjustments—balance
- Previous balance
- Patient name
- Cross footing formula
- Accounts receivable control formula

— Computer
- On-line
- Batch processing
- Service bureau vs. in-house

— Internal Controls
- Division of duties
- Adjustments approved by physician or supervisor prior to entry
- Cash postings compared and verified with bank deposits by supervisor or doctor

(Pub.372)

- Numbered charge slips for each patient; all charge slips accounted for
- Reconciliation of accounts receivable

— Charge Slips
- Patient name
- Account number
- Insurance type
- Common procedures
- CPT code
- Diagnosis descriptions
- ICD-9 codes
- Total charges

— Deposit Slips
- Depositor's name
- Amount
- Total deposit amount

— Adjustment Journal
- Date
- Patient name
- Account number
- Adjustment code
- Description of adjustment
- Approval signature

— Third-Party Forms
- AMA approved insurance forms
- Special forms for optic scanning
- Medicaid/Medicaid forms
- Blue Cross forms (mandatory if participating provider)

- Hospital Logs
  - Patient name
  - Account number
  - Box for each day of the week
  - Hospital report box
  - Charge ticket number

- Hospital Charge Slip
  - Needed to record outside charges from physician
  - May be replaced by portable dictaphone where physician will dictate all charges

- Miscellaneous Charges Record
  - HMO billing (to be kept separate from non-HMO patient billing
  - Nursing home billing (recorded similar to hospital log)
  - Insurance physical examinations, expert witness testimony, covering fees, etc. (to be entered as individual accounts receivable)

- Accounts Receivable Management Reports
  - Aging analysis
  - Unpaid insurance report
  - Delinquent patient report
  - Charge analysis report by procedure, physician, account type
  - Adjustment analysis report
  - Payment analysis report

§ 10.100 Bibliography

A.M.A. Division of Medical Practice: The Business Side of Medical Practice. Chicago: American Medical Association, 1973.

Cotton, H.: Medical Practice Management. Oradell, NJ: Medical Economics, 1977.

Lusk, E. J. and Lusk, J. G.: Financial and Managerial Control: A Health Care Perspective. Germantown, MD: Aspen Systems Corp., 1979.

McCormick, J., et. al.: The Management of Medical Practice. Cambridge, MA: Ballinger Publishing Co., 1978.

Silvers, J. B. and Prahalad, C. K.: Financial Management Institutions. Flushing, NY: Spectrum Publications, distributed by Halstad Press, 1974.

10–49   ACCOUNTS RECEIVABLE MANAGEMENT   App. 10–A

Appendix 10-A

FINANCIAL TRANSACTION FORMS FOR THE MEDICAL OFFICE

(Pub.372)

App. 10–A MANAGING YOUR MEDICAL PRACTICE 10–50

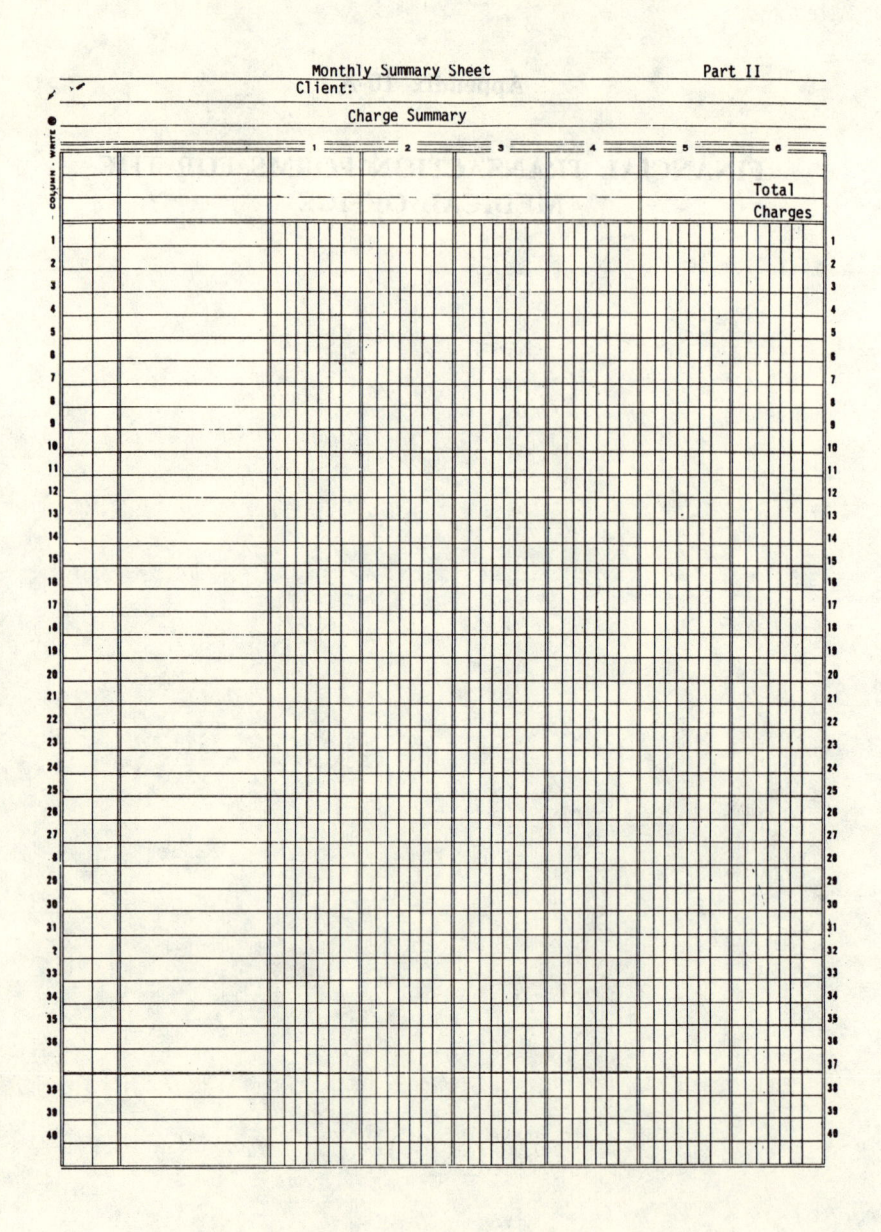

FIG 10-11. Monthly charge summary. Total charges in the sixth column should equal the total charges in the first column of the monthly receipts summary in Appendix 2.

(Pub. 372)

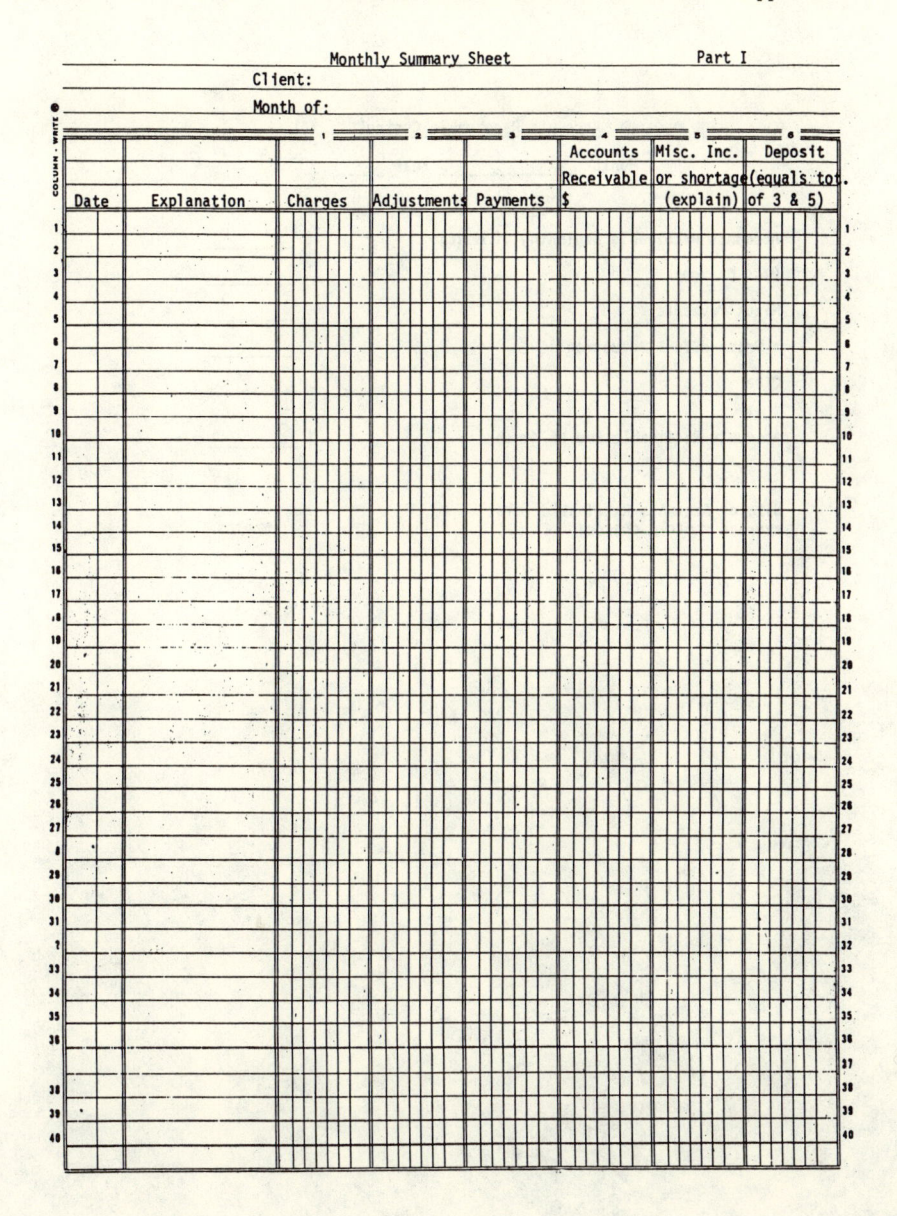

FIG. 10-12. Monthly receipts summary, showing monthly totals for charges, payments, adjustments, miscellaneous income or accounts receivable, and the amount ultimately deposited in the bank.

(Pub. 372)

App. 10-A   MANAGING YOUR MEDICAL PRACTICE

<u>Accounts Receivable Control</u>

Month _____ Year _____

Accounts Receivable Beginning of Month	$ _____
Plus Charges	_____
Minus Payments	_____
± Write-offs & Adjustments	_____
Other	_____
Accounts Receivable End of Month	$ _____
Size of Accounts Receivable relative to average monthly charges	_____ months

FIG. 10-13. An accounts receivable control form. Totals are entered onto this form from the monthly sheet. Accounts receivable at the end of the month is computed according to formula and must balance with the accounts receivable report at the end of the monthly summary sheet. This form is helpful for cross checking individual monthly balances.

(Pub.372)

CHAPTER 11

Retirement and Pension Plans

by

David L. Hicks and Michael E. Mitchell

> **SCOPE**
>
> Qualified retirement plans provide the employer with the opportunity to accumulate future retirement benefits and defer taxes on monies contributed to the plans. They also allow a means of sheltering personal income and obtaining a larger return on monies invested. Furthermore, a retirement plan for the practice enhances the employee benefit package, attracts quality employees and gives employees incentive to remain with the practice. The many plans available include defined contribution plans, which limit the deductible amount an employer can contribute; defined benefit plans, which limit the amount paid out in benefits to the participant; individual investment plans which can be held in addition to company retirement plans; plans combined to exploit the deductible and paid benefit maximums; social security integration plans; and plans that allow combined contributions by employees and employers. Most of these plans are scaled to income to prevent employees in any one wage bracket from profiting more than others. To maintain tax-favored status, these plans must be stringently regulated. The professional should have his or her retirement plan needs reviewed by a specialist on an annual basis to assure maximum benefits currently and in the future. Any and all provisions regarding qualification for participation, maximum levels of contribution or benefit payment, age at which benefits are paid and the form of such payments should be included in written plan documents and made available to all participants.

SYNOPSIS

§ 11.01 Pension and Retirement Plans
    [1] Choosing a Plan
    [2] Who Qualifies?

§ 11.02 Qualified Plans
    [1] Setting Up a Trust
    [2] Additional Benefits

§ 11.03 Types of Retirement Plans
    [1] Defined Contribution Plans
    [2] Defined Benefit Plans
    [3] Differences Between Defined Benefit and Defined Contribution Plans
    [4] Limitations on Contributions and Benefits

§ 11.04 The 401(k) Plan
    [1] Salary Reduction Agreement and Deferral Percentages
    [2] Disadvantages of 401(k) Plans

§ 11.05 Individual Retirement Plans

§ 11.06 Social Security Benefits

§ 11.07 Self-Employed and Partnership (KEOGH) Plans

§ 11.08 Disbursement of Funds and Benefits
    [1] Loans
    [2] Payment of Benefits

§ 11.09 Checklist for Pension and Retirement Plans

§ 11.01 Pension and Retirement Plans

Federal legislation has made it possible for both incorporated and unincorporated medical practices to receive substantial tax advantages for their employee retirement and pension plans. There are many different plans available, either as prototypes or individually-tailored agreements. The appropriate choice should be based on the needs of the physician(s) and made only after consultation with a pension advisor. With rare exceptions, the pension plan must be opened to all employees who meet the specifications for age, employment and vesting time.

A retirement plan is often an integral part of an employer's compensation program that attracts competent employees and provides incentive for them to remain in his or her employ. This helps reduce costly turnover and can boost morale and productivity.

In 1969 the IRS made available to medical corporations certain

(Pub.372)

tax benefits that had previously been allowed only to regular business corporations. The result was a great step forward for medical professionals in the area of tax savings, and since that time, many practices have been incorporated solely for the purpose of establishing qualified corporate retirement plans. Recognizing this, and hoping to reduce the number of medical corporations, Congress passed laws, effective January 1, 1984, to allow unincorporated medical practices the same type of pension benefits.

Many physicians are unaware of the many types of pension and retirement plans there are to choose from. Before an optimal plan can be considered, the physician must take into account his or her age and income and the number of his or her employees and their ages. One is never too young to begin thinking about retirement plans, since the longer an individual participates in one, the greater is his or her accumulation of benefits.

[1] Choosing a Plan

An employer usually consults with an accountant, attorney or pension advisor when considering a retirement plan. The plan should be chosen with the employer's needs in mind and should take into consideration current and future tax liabilities, stability and long-range retirement goals. A legal plan document is then prepared outlining the operation, the benefits of the plan, eligibility requirements and vesting schedules (individual ownership of an account or benefit). The document is then signed (adopted) and sent to the IRS for approval. Employees are notified of the plan and provided with an explanation of the plan's salient provisions.

Retirement plan documents vary in their flexibility. Individually designed programs provide more options for the employer. They are most often written and/or reviewed by an attorney. Other types of retirement plan documents include pattern or field prototypes. These plans have been previously submitted to the IRS for approval and, therefore, do not contain the options or flexibility of individually designed plans.

[2] Who Qualifies

The Internal Revenue Service and the Department of Labor have defined participation and eligibility requirements for all retirement plans. Beginning in 1985, defined contribution and defined benefit plans cannot have a minimum age requirement that exceeds age 21. If the plan has a service requirement it is most commonly one year; by law it cannot exceed two years. As an example, a plan might state that an employee must be at least 21 years old and have worked for the employer for at least one year in order to participate in the plan.

Specific classes of employees and, in certain plans, employees who have been hired within five years of normal retirement age may be excluded from participation in the retirement plan. However, these exclusions are only allowed if a minimum percentage of eligible employees continue to participate in the retirement plan. A coverage or participation test must be met each year for the continued qualification of the plan.

§ 11.02 Qualified Plans

> Qualified retirement plans are sanctioned by the IRS. They provide tax advantages to contributing employers and occasionally to employees if the plan allows them to make voluntary deductible or non-deductible contributions. A qualified plan entails establishing a trust account with trustees who will prudently invest the monies deposited. These contributions are allowed to accumulate and generate tax free interest until they are disbursed to the participants. The trustees review the plan periodically to keep an accurate account of how much money each participant is entitled to.

A qualified retirement plan is governed by a written document in which an employer agrees to provide retirement benefits for his or her employees. The purpose of such a program is to accumulate tax-deferred, interest-earning sums of money that can be used to supplement personal savings and Social Security benefits at the employee's retirement age. The IRS has approved such plans in their form and content and, thus, has "qualified" them for favorable tax treatment. Today, any employer (corporate or non-corporate) may establish a retirement plan in one form or another. It is important that the physician remember he or she is an employee for plan benefit purposes.

A primary reason for having a qualified retirement plan is the current tax deduction the employer realizes for contributions he or she makes to the plan. Moreover, these contributions accumulate on

(Text continued on page 11–5)

a tax-deferred basis in the retirement trust and, upon distribution to individual participants or their beneficiaries, the proceeds may receive favorable tax treatment.

[1] Setting Up a Trust

One of the first steps in establishing a qualified plan is to open a trust account to receive plan assets. This trust must meet both federal and state regulations and its parameters must be specified within the written trust document. Plan assets must be invested prudently by the appointed trustees, who are named by the employer in the trust instrument. The employer may select a corporate institution, such as a bank or investment firm, or may act as his or her own trustee. Plan assets must be maintained for the exclusive benefit of plan participants and their beneficiaries to be distributed upon retirement, death, disability or termination of employment.

Contributions are periodically deposited in the trust for the exclusive benefit of all participants and their beneficiaries. Annually, or more frequently, the employer or the appointed administrator reviews the retirement plan assets to keep an accurate accounting of each participant's accumulated benefit or account balance. Annual reporting forms, as required by various governmental agencies, are prepared as prescribed by law. (For a flow chart on how the retirement trust works, see Figure 11-1.)

[2] Additional Benefits

A qualified retirement plan may also provide tax-deductible disability and death benefits. In other words, personal life insurance policies, which are normally purchased with after-tax dollars, can be purchased with pre-tax dollars through a retirement trust.

A retirement trust may also allow employees to make contributions of their own, commonly referred to as either voluntary nondeductible or voluntary deductible contributions. Voluntary nondeductible contributions are attractive to some employees because they allow tax-deferred interest to accumulate on savings. The obvious benefit of voluntary deductible contributions (VDEC's or IRA's) is that they are deductible and produce a higher yield when added to the employer's contributions.

(Pub.372)

(ILLUSTRATION #1)

HOW YOUR PLAN WORKS

BUSINESS OR PROFESSION
Deposits To a Trust

PLAN ADMINISTRATOR

$ Deposits Are Tax Deductible

EMPLOYEES TRUST
ASSETS ARE INVESTED BY THE PLAN TRUSTEE(S)
- Deposits Are Not Taxed To Employee
- Funds Are Invested By The Trustee And Earn Tax DEFERRED
- Trust Is Protected From Company And Employee Creditors

Employee PARTICIPANT   Employee PARTICIPANT   Employee PARTICIPANT   Employee PARTICIPANT

Benefits Are Paid At:
- Death
- Disability
- Retirement
- Termination

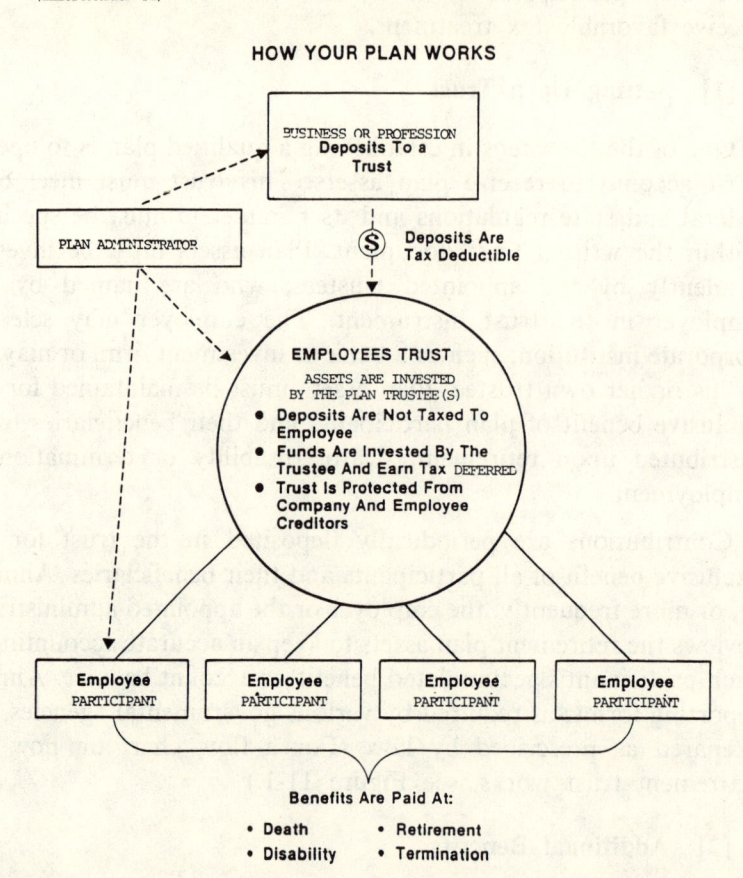

FIG. 11-1. A flow chart on setting up a retirement trust, demonstrating the accountability of the business and plan administrator to the plan participants.

§ 11.03 Types of Retirement Plans

Defined contribution plans include profit-sharing, money-purchase and target benefit plans. These plans impose a limit on the maximum amount an employer can deposit annually for participants in the plan for any one year. This limit is usually based on a percentage of the

(Pub.372)

total compensation for all participants. Defined benefit plans do not limit the amount of contributions but do limit the amount of benefits paid out to participants. Various types of qualified plans can be combined to fully utilize the advantages of each, but overall limitations must be observed if the plan is to retain its tax-deferred status.

Two types of retirement plans are available to businesses: defined contribution plans and defined benefit plans.

[1] Defined Contribution Plans

A defined contribution plan provides benefits based on employer contributions. This plan uses a specific formula to allocate the amount contributed by participants in the plan. The method of allocation cannot be used to discriminate in favor of those employees who are owners, officers or more highly compensated than others.

There are various types of defined contribution plans, the most flexible of which is the profit-sharing plan. In this kind of plan, contributions are made by the employer from current profits or earnings retained from the business. The deductible amount of these contributions may not exceed 15 percent of the total payroll for all participating employees. If an employer does not use the maximum allowable deduction in any particular tax year, he or she may carry forward that unused deduction into the subsequent tax year, subject to certain limitations. A profit-sharing plan differs from other retirement plans in that the employer is not necessarily required to make a contribution each year, even though the business makes a profit (see Figure 11-2).

The 401(k) plan is a type of profit-sharing plan that allows for deductible employee contributions in addition to the contributions made by the employer. An employee may elect to defer or reduce part of his or her taxable income and contribute the difference to the retirement plan. This feature is attractive to employees as it allows accumulation of tax-deferred personal retirement savings. (The 401(k) plan is discussed in detail in § 11.04.)

Another type of defined contribution plan is the money-purchase plan. Like the profit-sharing plan, the money-purchase plan uses a specific allocation formula for contributions. However, unlike the profit-sharing plan, the contribution formula specified in the money-purchase document is fixed. Once a percentage in the range of one to 25 percent of total employee compensation has been chosen, the employer is obligated to make that contribution each year, even if the business does not show a profit (see Figure 11-3).

The target benefit plan assumes a specific benefit will be payable to a participant at retirement age. The employer makes annual contributions to the plan to fund this stated benefit. For example, if this type of plan states that a participant will receive 50 percent of his or her annual compensation at retirement age, each year the employer is obligated to contribute to the trust the amount of money necessary to provide this benefit. The level of contribution is computed based on factors relating to the participant's salary and age. Limitations on the amount that may be contributed on behalf of any one participant are the same as for other defined contribution plans. The annual investment experience in a target benefit plan determines the ultimate benefit payable at retirement age.

[2] Defined Benefit Plans

The second category of qualified retirement plans is the defined benefit plan. In this type of plan, the employer is obligated to make contributions each year to guarantee that a specified benefit will be available at retirement age. Although this plan appears similar to the target benefit plan just discussed, the two differ a great deal in their contribution limitations. The target benefit plan limits the annual contribution for any one participant to a maximum of $30,000. A defined benefit plan has no limit on the level of contribution for a participant but rather limits the benefit payable to the participant upon his or her retirement. In many instances, the defined benefit plan offers the best opportunity for a high contribution (i.e., deduction) for the older, highly compensated professional (see Figure 11-4).

[3] Differences Between Defined Benefit and Defined Contribution Plans

Since the most common qualified retirement plans are the profit-sharing, money-purchase and defined benefit plans, we will use them to illustrate the differences in contributions and benefits, based on the following information:

NAME	AGE	COMPEN-SATION
Physician	52	100,000
Nurse	32	18,000
Receptionist	26	12,000

RETIREMENT AGE   62

Figure 11-2

PROFIT-SHARING PLAN

Contribution based on 15% of compensation

NAME	COMPENSATION	PLAN CONTRIBUTION
Physician	100,000	15,000
Nurse	18,000	2,700
Receptionist	12,000	1,800

TOTAL DEDUCTIBLE CONTRIBUTION $19,500*

*This is the maximum allowable contribution. The actual contribution may vary from year to year.

Figure 11-3

MONEY-PURCHASE PLAN

Contribution based on 25% of compensation.

NAME	COMPENSATION	PLAN CONTRIBUTION
Physician	100,000	25,000
Nurse	18,000	4,500
Receptionist	12,000	3,000

TOTAL DEDUCTIBLE CONTRIBUTION $32,500

Assuming a contribution of $25,000 is made on behalf of the physician each year for the next 10 years, and that plan earnings are no less than 7 percent, he or she will accumulate $369,500 in the account by age 62. The physician could also implement a combination of a money-purchase and profit-sharing plan so that the maximum 15 percent would be contributed to the profit-sharing plan and a 10 percent required contribution made to the money-purchase plan. This approach provides the maximum allowable deduction for defined contribution plans, yet still allows flexibility in the amount that may be contributed in future years.

(Pub.372)

Figure 11-4
DEFINED BENEFIT PLAN
Retirement benefit at age 62 is 90% of compensation

NAME	COMPENSATION	RETIREMENT BENEFIT	CONTRIBUTION
Physician	100,000	90,000 a year	71,100
Nurse	18,000	16,200 a year	1,900
Receptionist	12,000	10,800 a year	800
TOTAL DEDUCTIBLE CONTRIBUTION			$73,800

To provide a lifetime benefit for the physician of $7,500 per month or $90,000 per year at age 62, it is necessary that the plan accumulate $982,600 within the next 10 years.

[4] Limitations on Contributions and Benefits

Defined contribution plans are subject to limitations on deductible contributions made by the employer. To review, profit-sharing allows a maximum of 15 percent of the employee's rate of compensation, and money-purchase a maximum of 25 percent of the employee's compensation.

In addition to these deduction limitations, the IRS also imposes overall limits on contributions that may be allocated on behalf of the individual participant. For both profit-sharing and money-purchase, it is the lesser of 25 percent of compensation or $30,000. These overall limitations are defined in terms of an "annual addition," which is comprised of employer contributions, nondeductible employee contributions and forfeitures (amounts not distributed to an employee upon termination of employment, but rather reallocated to all remaining participants).

Under the defined benefit plan maximum allowable benefits are limited to the lesser of 100 percent of compensation or $90,000 for a participant retiring between the ages of 62 and 65. Adjustments to the $90,000 annual retirement income are made for retirement at ages earlier than 62 or later than 65. This is an annual retirement income limitation, not a deduction limitation.

(The dollar limitations mentioned above for both defined contribution and defined benefit plans are scheduled to be increased by a cost of living adjustment in 1988.)

An employer who maintains more than one type of plan must take into account contributions to and benefits from all plans when determining overall benefit limitations for employees. All plans under the same employer must be reviewed to calculate any adjustments in benefits. It is important that plans comply with these limitations to maintain their qualified status and tax advantages with the IRS.

§ 11.04 The 401(k) Plan

The 401(k) plan is a profit-sharing plan that allows the participant to defer a percentage of income into a retirement plan. This can be done through salary reduction, deferment, employer matching or employer discretionary profit-sharing contributions. An average deferral percentage test anchors contribution limitations to the deferral percentage of the lower paid two-thirds of participants so that the higher paid third does not profit from excessive deferral of monies. Disadvantages to a 401(k) plan include lack of participation among lower paid employees, linking a plan to theoretical profits and the extra administrative work involved.

The 401(k) plan is a type of profit-sharing plan that allows participants the option of receiving company contributions in cash or having the amount contributed to their plan. Under this type of "cash or deferred" arrangement, the employee does not have to include any monies contributed to the plan as part of his or her taxable income.

[1] Salary Reduction Agreement and Deferral Percentages

Another arrangement made possible by the 401(k) plan is a salary reduction agreement. An employee may elect to reduce his or her salary and have that amount contributed to the plan on his or her behalf. In this arrangement, the employee is taxed only on income received; the amount contributed to the plan is tax-deferred until it is withdrawn as a benefit.

The 401(k) option provides a vehicle for retirement plan savings at little or no cost to the employer. Unlike a typical profit-sharing plan, a 401(k) profit-sharing plan allows several types of employer and employee contributions:

    Employee: salary reduction
          cash or deferred
          employer match

Employer: discretionary profit-sharing contribution

The example in Figure 11-5 incorporates the salary reduction arrangement with a 50 percent employer matching contribution.

Figure 11-5

Employee	Compensation	Salary Reduction	Employer Match	Deferral %	Average Deferral %
Doctor	200,000	9,000	4,500	6.75	6.635
Nurse	23,000	1,000	500	6.52	(upper 1/3)
Office Manager	18,000	800	400	6.67	
Secretary	13,000	500	250	5.77	3.69
Secretary	13,000	200	100	2.31	(lower 2/3)
Receptionist	11,000	-0-	-0-	-0-	

The salary reduction column reflects the amount each employee chooses to defer. Theoretically, highly compensated employees have the potential to defer larger percentages of compensation. However, to avoid potential discrimination that favors highly compensated employees, the IRS has established strict mathematical tests that must be met. The Deferral Percentage Test must be calculated for every 401(k) Plan. All participants are grouped into an upper one-third or lower two-thirds category, based solely on their compensation. To prevent discrimination the average deferral percentages (ADP) are examined and the following guidelines are observed:

If lower two-third's ADP is:	Then upper one-third's cannot exceed
2% or less	2.5 × lower two-third's ADP
2% to 6%	3 % + lower two-third's ADP
6% or more	1.5 × lower two-third's ADP

In the illustration, the lower two-third's ADP is 3.69 percent, which falls within the limits of the second scenario listed above. Thus, the maximum deferral percentage allowable for the upper one-third under the circumstances is 3.69 percent + 3.0 percent, or 6.69 percent. Since actual deferral percentage in the example in 6.635 percent, the plan meets the test and is not considered to discriminate in favor of highly compensated employees.

[2] Disadvantages of 401(k) Plans

Although a 401(k) plan offers many advantages, there are several disadvantages that warrant discussion. Often, lower compensated employees elect not to participate in a salary reduction arrangement which, in a small professional corporation, results in the company's failure to meet the ADP test. In this case, the employer most likely would be obligated to make a contribution on behalf of the lower paid two-thirds of the staff to raise their deferral percentage and thus allow the higher paid employees to earn significant benefits (i.e., the lower the lower two-thirds ADP, the lower the upper one-third's ADP).

Another potential disadvantage is inherent in the nature of a profit-sharing plan. Contributions to and deductions from a profit-sharing plan are predicated on the existence of profits or retained earnings. In the absence of either profits or retained earnings, the employer is denied a current deduction for any amounts contributed to the plan, and the salary reduction differentials are taxed currently as income to the employee.

Periodic contributions to the plan by employer and employee must be accounted for separately. The complexity of accounting, the additional tests that must be performed to prove the plan does not discriminate and the calculation of employer and employee contributions results in increased administrative expenses. Excessive administrative costs can actually be a deterrent to implementing a 401(k) plan.

Deduction limitations under a 401(k) profit-sharing plan are identical to those under a regular profit-sharing plan. But, unlike a typical profit-sharing plan, which has a deduction limitation of 15 percent of participating payroll, a 401(k) profit-sharing plan's deduction limit is 15 percent of participating payroll after it is reduced by employee deferrals (see Figure 11-6).

[2] Valuing Liabilities

Once the total assets of the practice have been valued and totaled, practice liabilities must be determined and subtracted from total assets:

Payroll Taxes: Every pay period payroll taxes are withheld from employees' salaries. Depending on their size, payroll taxes must be

(Text continued on page 3–35)

Figure 11-6

NAME	GROSS WAGES	SALARY REDUCTION	NET WAGES
Doctor	200,000	9,000	191,000
Nurse	23,000	1,000	22,000
Office Manager	18,000	800	17,200
Secretary	13,000	500	12,500
Secretary	13,000	200	12,800
Receptionist	11,000	-0-	11,000
Total			$266,500
			× 0.15
Total deductible contribution is limited to			= $39,975

In many instances, the deduction allowed under any type of profit-sharing plan is less than the deduction allowed under a defined benefit plan (see, for example, Figure 11-4).

§ 11.05 Individual Retirement Plans

Some individuals who do not participate in company retirement plans can take contributions to individual retirement accounts (IRAs) or simplified employee pension plans (SEPs) as tax deductions. The maximum deductible contribution allowed differs with the plan, the individual's coverage under other plans and the individual's income tax filing status.

Instead of participating in a company retirement program, some employees will be able to obtain a deduction for contributions made to an individual retirement plan. Individual retirement accounts (IRAs) and simplified employee pension plans (SEPs) have different maximum contribution amounts.

An employee whose spouse, or person, is not covered under a corporate retirement plan, or whose adjusted gross income is below $25,000 ($40,000 for a married couple filing a joint return) can deduct a contribution to an individual retirement account. A nondeductible or partial deductible contribution is allowed for individuals with adjusted incomes over those amounts and covered under another plan. An IRA must be established through a financial institution that satisfies the stringent requirements of the IRS. The maximum deductible contribution to an IRA is limited to the lesser of 100 percent of annual taxable compensation, or $2000.

The simplified employee pension plan (SEP) is a type of IRA that allows a higher rate of employer contribution. This contribution is solely owned by the employee. However, both the employer and the employee can realize a deduction for the amount contributed of 15 percent of the particpant's compensation, to a maximum of $3000.

§ 11.06 Social Security Benefits

Integrated formulas are used when calculating the effect of social security benefits on retirement plans to prevent the more highly compensated employees from being discriminated against.

Since Social Security benefits are only calculated on compensation up to the current taxable wage base, highly compensated professionals do not receive Social Security benefits on compensation that exceeds the base. The IRS has recognized this inherent discrimination and thus allows the qualified retirement benefits plan to consider Social Security benefits in plan benefit calculations (see Figure 11-7).

Integrated formulas in both defined contribution and defined benefit plans help to provide all employees with retirement incomes that are relatively equal percentages of their respective compensations. Again, the IRS imposes strict guidelines when implementing integration with social security in retirement plans.

Figure 11-7

I. Defined Benefit

Employee	Monthly Compensation	40% Non-Integrated Monthly Benefit	Integrated 30% Monthly Compensation in Excess of $1,000 Plus 40% of Monthly Compensation
A	$5,000	$2,000 (40%)	$3,200 (64%)
B	2,500	1,000 (40%)	1,450 (58%)
C	800	320 (40%)	320 (40%)

II. Money-Purchase

Employee	Annual Compensation	10% Non-Integrated Annual Contribution	10% of Compensation Plus 5.7% of Compensation in Excess of $12,000
A	$60,000	$6,000 (10%)	$8,736 (14.6%)
B	30,000	3,000 (10%)	4,026 (13.4%)
C	9,600	960 (10%)	960 (10.0%)

III. Profit-Sharing

Employee	Annual Compensation	15% Non-Integrated Annual Contribution	Integrated Allocating First 5.7% of Contribution to Compensation in Excess of $12,000. Balance in Proportion to Total Compensation
A	$60,000	$9,000 (15%)	$9,469.73 (15.8%)
B	30,000	4,500 (15%)	4,392.87 (14.6%)
C	9,600	1,440 (15%)	1,077.40 (11.2%)

§ 11.07 Self-Employed and Partnership (KEOGH) Plans

KEOGH plans allow the self-employed practitioner or unincorporated partnership the same deduction limitations on defined contribution and defined benefit plans given to incorporated practices.

Prior to January 1, 1984, deductible contributions to KEOGH plans were limited to the lesser of 15 percent of compensation or $15,000 (although special limitations on defined benefit KEOGH plans at times allowed for a deduction in excess of this limitation). Since that time, all contribution and deduction limitations for incorporated businesses became applicable to the self-employed (i.e., a defined contribution plan limit of the lesser of $30,000 or 25 percent of compensation; a defined benefit limitation of the lesser of $90,000 or 100 percent of compensation at ages 62 to 65).

In calculating plan benefits and contributions for the self-employed, earned income is computed after taking into account any amounts contributed to the plan on behalf of the owner or his or her employees. As an example:

Defined Contribution of 25% of Compensation

Net Self Employment Income of $100,000
(After Business Deduction)

Net Earned Income:	$ 80,000
Contribution:	
(25% × Earned Income)	$ 20,000
TOTAL	$100,000

Earned income plus any contributions to the plan should not exceed net self-employment income.

§ 11.08 Disbursement of Funds and Benefits

Disbursements from the retirement trust before a participant is of retirement age are permitted as long as they are provided for in the plan document. Loans usually have a limit imposed on the amount, the rate of interest and the time by which they must be paid back in full. Payment of retirement benefits begins at different ages under different plans. Options most commonly available to participants include joint and survivor annuities, lump-sum payments and installment payments.

Most pension and retirement plans carry provisions to invest accumulated monies if the participant becomes disabled or dies before retirement. These "safety valves" provide a method for disbursing money to the participant or his or her survivor without violation of the plan rules and without subjecting benefits paid out to IRS penalties.

Disbursements from plans other than those described below are generally subjected to full income taxes and a 10 percent penalty. They are strongly discouraged.

[1] Loans

Employees participating in a retirement plan may withdraw money as a loan as long as there are provisions for this in the document. There are, however, certain limitations and disadvantages in borrowing money from the plan. An individual may borrow up to 50 percent of his or her vested account balance or accrued benefit to a maximum of $50,000. The employee must pay a reasonable rate of interest on the loan and the entire loan must be amortized equally so that it is paid back within five years. The interest payments on the loan cannot be deducted by physicians making payments to the plan. The sole exception to the five-year repayment rule for loans after December 31, 1986, is when the participant borrows to purchase a principle residence for himself or herself.

[2] Payment of Benefits

In money-purchase and defined benefit plans, payment of benefits may commence at the time a participant attains normal retirement age. However, in profit-sharing plans, distribution of benefits may commence at the time a participant attains age 59-1/2, even if he or she is still actively employed. In general, the business owner or professional must begin receiving distribution of benefits from the retirement plan no later than April 1 of the calendar year in which he or she turns 70-1/2.

The various options for receipt of plan benefits at retirement age or age 70-1/2 are specified in the plan document. With the exception of profit-sharing plans, all pension plans, by law, must offer each plan participant the right to elect to receive plan benefits in the form of a "qualified joint and survivor annuity." The joint and survivor annuity must be an amount not less than 50 percent of the participant's normal retirement benefit nor greater than 100 percent of the benefit. A participant may waive the right to receive his or her benefit in the form of an annuity with the consent of the non-participating spouse. In this case, distribution could then be made in the form of a lump sum or in installments. Estate planning and personal tax considerations should be carefully analyzed when selecting the mode of payment of benefits. In general, most profit-sharing plans are not required to offer plan benefits in the form of a joint and survivor annuity.

Participants in profit-sharing plans should take precautions to avoid the following distribution penalties:

- Early Distribution. A 10 percent penalty will be imposed on distributions to participants younger than 59.5 years of age for contributions made after December 31, 1984.
- Late Distribution. There is a 50 percent excise tax if the "required" amount of money is withdrawn from the plan for particpants younger than 70.5 years of age. The minimum amount of distribution after age 70.5 is based on the present value of the funds at the time and the participant's life expectancy.
- Over-Funded Plans. After December 31, 1988, a 15 percent excise tax will be imposed on "excess distributions." The excise tax is applicable to the extent that the annual distribution in the form of an annuity exceeds $112,500, adjusted for cost of living increases. A penalty tax is applicable to lump sum distributions that exceed five times the annuity distribution maximum (currently $562,500). Distribution of benefits accrued as of August 1, 1986, may have an exemption if the participant has filed an election on his or her personal income tax return for a taxable year ending before January 1, 1989.

It is recommended that a participant seek the advice of a qualified tax professional before receiving any retirement plan benefits, since each option carries with it certain tax liabilities.

§ 11.09 Checklist for Pension and Retirement Plans

A checklist of plans covered in the chapter is provided.

RETIREMENT & PENSION PLANS § 11.09

- Choosing a plan
- Consult with pension advisor
- Choose qualified plan to fit needs
- Establish trust
- Notify employees

- Qualified plans
- Defined contribution plans
    - Money-purchase plan
    - Profit-sharing plan
    - Target benefit plans
    - 401(k) Plans
- Defined benefit plans
- Personal investment plans
    - IRA plans
    - SEP plans
- Integrated plans (with social security)
- KEOGH plans

- Qualification
- Class of employee
- Age
- Vesting time

- Plan limitations on maximum deductible contributions and benefits:

Profit-sharing:	15 percent of participant compensation maximum contribution; variable annual payments
Money purchase:	Lesser of 25 percent participant compensation or $30,000 contribution; fixed annual payments
Target benefit:	Contribution limited to age and employment factors affecting payment

(Rel.3–2/89 Pub.372)

	of prearranged percentage of participant's income during retirement years
Defined benefit:	Unlimited contribution; lesser of 100 percent participant compensation or $90,000; adjustments for late or early retirement
401(k):	Deferral or reduction percentages; average deferral percentage test
IRA:	Lesser of 100 percent annual taxable income or $2,000 maximum contribution; $250 non-working spouse contribution
Social Security:	Non-integration and integration percentages for maximum contribution or benefit
KEOGH:	Same limitations as for defined contribution and defined benefit plans

__ Payment of Benefits

__ Preretirement loans

__ Joint and survivor annuity

__ Lump sum

__ Installments

CHAPTER 12

Law for the Medical Practice*

Edward Kelsay

> **SCOPE**
>
> A medical practice is a business and like any other business it must operate within legal guidelines. Some of these guidelines pertain to any business. They include using nondiscriminating employment applications; maintaining office business files and employee wage and hour files; and avoiding harassment while properly seeking compensation for unpaid client debts. Others are specific to a medical practice. These include the boundaries of trust in the physician-patient relationship and knowing when confidential information can be released to a third party; knowing whom to contact for legal consent to medical treatment; knowing the difference between rightly refusing a patient service and abandonment; and knowing the extent of liability for medical care administered under various circumstances. A physician must be apprised of all medical legislation pertinent to the practice of medicine and all general legislation applicable to the medical field. A physician should also retain, and not hesitate to consult with, legal counsel for all instances in which legal ramifications are unclear or unknown.

SYNOPSIS

§ 12.01 The Patient-Physician Relationship
    [1] Professional Obligation to the Patient
    [2] Confidentiality
    [3] Releasing Information
§ 12.02 Consent for Medical Care
    [1] Minors and Consent
    [2] Mental Incompetence

---

*Adapted from Law for the Medical Office, by Edward Kelsay. Copyright: Edward Kelsay.

[3] Child of a Divorced Couple
[4] Consent from Third Parties
§ 12.03 Good Samaritan Laws
§ 12.04 Patient Information
§ 12.05 Medical Records
§ 12.06 Medical Record Preservation
[1] Retaining Office Records
[2] Record Keeping
§ 12.07 Collecting Debts
[1] Fair Debt Collection Practices Act
[a] Provisions of the Act
[b] Common Physician Questions Regarding Debt Collection
[2] Checks, "Rubber" and Otherwise
[3] Garnishments
§ 12.08 Employment Applications
§ 12.09 Checklist for Law in the Medical Practice
§ 12.10–§ 12.99 Reserved
§ 12.100 Bibliography
Appendix 12-A Patient Discharge Notices
Appendix 12-B Acceptable Pre-Employment Inquiries under EEO Guidelines
Appendix 12-C Legislation Affecting Medical Practices
[1] Occupational Safety and Health Administration (OSHA)
[2] Privacy Act of 1973
[3] Freedom of Information Act
[4] Truth in Lending Act
[5] Equal Credit Opportunity Act
[6] Credit Reporting Agencies

§ 12.01 The Patient-Physician Relationship

The patient-physician relationship is a professional relationship that, under most circumstances, does not extend beyond the services rendered to the patient for the specific medical condition for which the physician was consulted. The crux of this relationship is the confidentiality of information given to the physician by the patient. The physician is legally and ethically obligated to respect this confidence.

Like any other business relationship, the patient-physician relationship is based on a contract between two or more persons for the rendition of a professional service: the patient comes to the physician, indicates he or she wishes to be diagnosed and/or treated, the physician offers to attempt diagnosis and treatment and the patient agrees to pay for the service. All other humanitarian and ethical attributes of the relationship are ancillary to this simple legal basis.

For the hospital-based specialist, or for the consultant, the patient-physician relationship is usually somewhat different from the scenario outlined above. In most instances the patient does not choose the specialist: either the patient is referred to the specialist, or the specialist's services are requested by the patient's attending physician. In many instances, as for radiologists and pathologists, the patient may not even see the specialist.

When a patient is admitted to the hospital, he or she enters into an "implied" contract with the attending physician and the hospital to accept and pay for all services considered medically necessary and appropriate for his or her care while he or she is in the institution. This casts the attending physician in the role of a "purchasing agent" for many of the services to be rendered to the patient, such as physician consultations, radiology, pathology, anesthesiology, etc.

[1] Professional Obligation to the Patient

Under normal circumstances, and contrary to popular belief, the physician is not required to accept anyone as a patient. He or she has the right to arbitrarily refuse any person even though no other physician is available. The one major exception to this general rule is when a physician is on emergency room call or emergency room duty at a hospital. The courts have determined that in this situation, public policy demands that the physician see the patient.

For the hospital-based specialist, there is another exception to the general rule. In most instances the hospital-based specialist has entered into a contract with the hospital to furnish his or her services to the hospital's patients. Thus the specialist, by virtue of his or her contractual relationship with the hospital, cannot arbitrarily refuse to serve a patient, except under the provisions of the contract.

After the doctor-patient relationship is begun, the attending physician is under an obligation to attend the case as long as it requires his or her attention. Again, contrary to popular opinion, the doctor-patient relationship does not last indefinitely but only as long as the particular medical condition for which the doctor's services were engaged. Thus, it has a definite beginning and a definite end.

In the usual situation, the relationship ends when the patient is discharged by the physician. The two other ways to "end" the relationship are to refer the patient to another physician or "fire" the patient. In the latter situation, the physician withdraws from the case, but only after notifying the patient of his or her intention to leave. This gives the patient a reasonable amount of time to arrange for another physician. (Figures 12-1, 12-2 and 12-3 in Appendix 12-A give several examples of notification that can be used to terminate the patient-physician relationship.)

For the hospital-based specialist, the doctor-patient relationship is limited to the services provided to the patient. Once the specialist has completed his or her work, the relationship with the patient ceases to exist.

[2] Confidentiality

The one part of the doctor-patient relationship that continues to exist long after the formal relationship has ended is the confidentiality of medical or health care information obtained by the physician or the physician's staff while attending the patient. The Principles of Medical Ethics adopted by the American Medical Association acknowledge that "A physician shall respect the rights of patients, of colleagues and of other health professionals, and shall safeguard patient confidences within the constraints of the law." It is generally accepted that the patient must trust his or her physician and know that information imparted will be kept in strictest confidence.

Disclosure of confidential information may be directly harmful to a reputation and professional standing. In almost all 50 states wrongful disclosure of patient information is declared "unprofessional conduct" and grounds for revocation of a physician's license.

Situations in which confidential patient information may or must be revealed include a disclosure made in good faith to protect third persons from a serious risk of harm, as in the case of a suicidal or violent patient, and situations where disclosure is required by law, as in the case of a patient with a communicable disease.

In instances where the physician is required by law to make a report, he or she is still protected against legal action if there is a mistake in diagnosis or in the information received and the report is made erroneously. Public policy demands that if a person is required to make a report by law, his or her status as a reporter is protected as long as the report was made in good faith. If a physician erroneously reports a patient has a contagious disease, and he or she had reasonable grounds for making the diagnosis, he or she cannot be held liable for the report.

[3] Releasing Information

The safest approach to releasing confidential information is, when in doubt, don't. It is easier to correct a failure to disclose information properly than it is to correct the improper disclosure of information after the fact.

The four steps a physician should follow to protect against legal consequences for disclosing information are:

(1) Ascertain that the person being informed is someone entitled to the information, such as the patient's parents, guardian or spouse.

(2) Do not give any information over the telephone if you do not recognize the voice of the person making the request.

(3) When responding to a request for information from an insurance company, make sure the company has a signed information release consent form from the patient and that you acquire a copy of that form to keep in your records (see Figure 12-4).

(4) If you are in doubt about someone's right to receive information, consult your attorney before you make the release. If a person requesting the information has a legal right to it, he or she will be able to produce the necessary papers (e.g., signed consent forms, a court order, proper identification that indicates the person is a public official entitled to the information) to prove that right.

§ 12.02 Consent for Medical Care

Informed patient consent is essential in the practice of medicine. It

Authorization For Release of Information

To Doctor _____.

I authorize you to furnish a copy of medical records pertaining to _____
_____ covering the period from
_____, 19_____ to _____, 19_____, or to allow
those records to be inspected or copied by _____.

I release you from all legal responsibility or liability that may arise from this authorization.

Signed _____:
Date _____:

FIG. 12-4.

may be given orally, written or be implied by the patient or, in the case of a minor or the mentally incompetent, by the patient's parents or guardians. However, under any circumstances, a written consent form is the physician's best evidence that consent was obtained.

Patient consent for diagnosis and treatment is the foundation of the practice of medicine. There are four ways in which consent for treatment may be given:

(1) It may be expressed consent, as when a patient gives consent orally or signs a consent form, or when a parent signs a consent form or gives oral consent for for the treatment of a child.

(2) Consent may be implied by action, as when a patient rolls up his or her sleeve to receive an injection, or when a parent brings a child to the doctor's office.

(Pub.372)

(3) Consent is also implied in an emergency. Whenever a patient needs immediate treatment, but is physically or mentally unable to give consent, the physician is justified in assuming he or she has consent to give treatment. However, in the emergency situation, treatment is limited to only those procedures that will save the life or preserve the bodily integrity of the patient. Procedures that could be considered "elective" may not be performed. Consent under these circumstances is sometimes referred to as "consent implied by law."

(4) Another type of consent implied by law is the consent of a parent or guardian required for treatment of a minor or for the mentally incompetent. The law assumes that the consent of a parent or guardian is equivalent to the patient's own consent.

Although consent is often given orally, a signed consent form is the best evidence of the patient's consent. However, it is only "evidence" of consent, not a contract.

With the exception of hospitalizations, most medical practice is based on consent implied by actions. If a person shows up at the physician's office at the appointed hour, it indicates that the patient is willing to undergo or continue treatment and the formal giving and taking of consent is seldom observed.

[1] Minors and Consent

Almost all states now have laws that define a minor as any person under 18 years of age, but from that point on laws differ from state to state. Although it is clear that a conscious, rational adult who has not been declared mentally incompetent is the only one who can consent to his or her own medical care, the situation for minors is not so well defined.

Many states declare that a married minor, a minor with a dependent child or an emancipated minor is an adult for all medical care purposes. An emancipated minor is usually defined as a minor separated or living apart from his or her parents or legal guardian for whatever reasons and not receiving support from them. A clarification of this definition is, "once an adult, always an adult." That is, if a minor gets married while under age and then gets a divorce while still under age, he or she is still considered an adult.

Medical treatment of a minor without parental consent could leave the physician or the physician's office staff open to a criminal complaint for "battery." (Battery is simply touching a person without consent or authorization.) In all practicality, since the treatment of the minor was for good cause, the chances of a criminal complaint are infinitesimal; however, the parents can refuse to pay the bill.

If a minor misleads the office or lies about his or her age, the physician cannot be held responsible unless he or she knew or should have known the patient's true age. Most states agree that a physician's office is not required to be a detective agency and is not liable for patient statements assumed to be true.

Almost all states have other exceptions in their laws that allow a minor to consent to medical care under certain circumstances. While these laws may be relied upon under special situations, the best rule is to always obtain the parent's consent for any treatment or procedure unless the minor falls into one of the categories where he or she can be considered an adult.

In an emergency situation the parent's consent is desirable, but usually not necessary. An emergency is usually defined as any medical situation which might deteriorate into a life- or body-threatening situation if not treated promptly. Many states have a provision that the minor may consent to his or her own emergency services.

[2] Mental Incompetence

The consent of a mentally incompetent person is not legally binding. However, mental incompetence is a designation that must be determined by a court of law. In most cases, the law presumes that a person is mentally competent until declared otherwise in a formal legal proceeding. It is safe for the physician or the physician's staff to presume that a person is mentally competent unless they are informed otherwise.

[3] Child of a Divorced Couple

If a parent brings a child for medical treatment, the physician's office may presume that the parent has capacity to give legal consent for the child's care. This presumption is eliminated only when the physician or office is given actual notice that one parent does not have legal capacity to consent, as in the aftermath of a divorce. The best rule for medical offices, however, is to always seek consent for a child's care from the parent who has custody.

The statement for services rendered to the child of a divorced couple should be sent to the parent who brought the child in for care. Since he or she authorized the services, he or she is also the only one who can attest that the services were rendered.

[4] Consent from Third Parties

A physician is occasionally faced with a situation that is not a medical emergency, but where medical intervention is still indicated and the patient is a minor or an unconscious or irrational adult. Under these circumstances, from whom does the physician seek consent?

Whenever an otherwise competent adult patient is, for some reason, incapable of giving consent, the physician must go to a third party. The general rule is the next closest kin in the direct bloodline, which simply means the physician obtains consent from the closest blood relative possible. The bloodline starts with two sets of grandparents, then comes to the parents, adult brothers and sisters, and minor brothers and sisters. In a question of consent, if you can move up and down the direct bloodline, you are almost always safe.

Some states (Texas, for example) have special statutory provisions allowing consent from other relatives: aunts and uncles, nieces and nephews, etc. Anytime a physician leaves the direct bloodline, he or she needs to be sure that state statutes provide for the deviation.

Under some circumstances, it is possible for a minor to consent for the care of another minor, an adult brother or sister or a parent. Court cases from around the United States have turned in verdicts indicating the belief that someone 13 to 14 years old has developed the maturity to make rational and reasonable decisions regarding other persons on the subject of medical care.

§ 12.03 Good Samaritan Laws

> Good Samaritan Laws vary from state to state. Most absolve the physician or trained health care individual who renders assistance at

the site of an accident or emergency of liability for any injuries sustained by the patient, provided the aid was of a reasonable nature.

Although the author has not searched the laws of all states, he has not found any state that requires a licensed health care professional—physician, RN, etc.—to stop at the scene of an accident or an emergency unless he or she is personally involved or unless he or she is requested to stop and render aid by duly constituted police authority. The Good Samaritan Act was devised to encourage physicians and other trained health care personnel to render such aid voluntarily.

In theory, if a physician stops at the scene of an accident and renders care, he or she becomes obligated to remain with the patient until another physician actively takes over care (e.g., upon the patient's arrival at the hospital). However, this led to the fear among medical personnel that if the physician rendered first aid at the site of the emergency and then left after the ambulance crew took possession of the patient, he or she might be accused of abandonment.

To alleviate this fear and its potential consequences, state legislatures adopted Good Samaritan Acts. These generally do not hold the physician or other trained health care professional who stops to render first aid at the scene of an accident civilly liable for any injury or harm suffered by the patient, provided that the services rendered were reasonable in nature. However, if the health care person does something at the scene of the accident that is unreasonable—e.g., puts a tourniquet around the patient's neck to stop a bleeding head wound—then he or she is liable for the consequences of those actions.

Most legal authorities interpret the Good Samaritan Act to apply only outside of the physician's office, clinic, nursing home, hospital or other medical institution. Although most Good Samaritan Laws are the same, they are specific on a state-to-state basis.

§ 12.04 Patient Information

A physician often needs to know a great deal of personal information about a patient before a diagnosis can be rendered. Although patients may refuse to divulge some information, such a refusal is often grounds for refusing the patient further medical services.

(Pub.372)

Before a doctor enters into a doctor-patient relationship, the doctor's office is entitled to receive all of the personal information about the patient listed on either of the two forms in Figures 12-5 and 12-6, especially if the patient is going to be extended credit.

Questions about a person's marital status, religion, ethnic background, occupation or physical disability that would not be acceptable on an employment application or in an employee interview are permissable on a patient data sheet. An individual's marital status can be of importance to a physician, both medically (i.e., next of kin, patient contacts) and from the standpoint of billings and collections. Likewise, many disease processes are peculiar to particular races (e.g., sickle cell anemia) or affected by religious practices. Obviously, a person's occupation can affect his or her health status.

With the exception of revealing a social security number, a patient's refusal to give a physician's office any information requested is grounds for refusing that patient further services. But even though federal law provides that a person does not have to divulge his or her social security number for identification purposes, both Medicare and Medicaid use the social security number as the patient identifier.

If the patient is willing to pay cash for each service as it is rendered, he or she can refuse to give the office information regarding employment and insurance. However, if the patient expects credit, then the medical office is entitled to information regarding employer, insurance or other responsible party. This information may be verified before services are rendered.

§ 12.05 Medical Records

In most cases it is agreed that the patient's actual medical record is the property of the physician while the information contained therein is the property of the patient.

There is no fixed definition of what constitutes a "medical record." A practical working definition of a medical record is anything found in a physician's file, hospital or other medical institution dealing with a particular patient. This includes not only the patient's personal history and business office information, but also clinical information, x-rays, laboratory reports, EKG tapes,

(Pub.372)

PLEASE PRINT

DATE _____

Patient introduction slip

MR.
MRS.
MISS
PATIENT _____ LAST NAME _____ FIRST NAME _____ MIDDLE

SOCIAL SECURITY NUMBER _____ DATE OF BIRTH _____ AGE _____ DRIVER'S LICENSE NO

ADDRESS _____ STREET _____ Apt _____ CITY _____ STATE _____ ZIP

HOME PHONE _____ SEX _____ MARITAL STATUS _____ REFERRED BY

EMPLOYED BY _____ EMPLOYER'S ADDRESS _____ OCCUPATION _____ BUS PHONE

SPOUSE'S NAME _____ EMPLOYED BY _____ EMPLOYER'S ADDRESS _____ BUS PHONE

CHILDREN'S NAME(S): _____ BIRTH DATE(S)

SPOUSE'S OCCUPATION

NEAREST FRIEND OR RELATIVE _____ RELATIONSHIP TO PATIENT _____ PHONE
MEDICAL INSURANCE INFORMATION

COMPANY _____ SUBSCRIBER NO _____ POLICY NO _____ COMPANY _____ SUBSCRIBER NO _____ POLICY NO

MEDICAID NO _____ MEDICARE NO

WORKMEN'S COMPENSATION _____ NAME OF COMPANY

ADDRESS OF COMPANY _____ COMPANY PHONE _____ TREATMENT AUTHORIZED BY

RESPONSIBLE PARTY
PLEASE COMPLETE THE SECTION BELOW, IF SOMEONE OTHER THAN THE PATIENT IS RESPONSIBLE FOR THE BILL

NAME _____ ADDRESS _____ CITY _____ STATE _____ ZIP CODE

HOME PHONE _____ RELATIONSHIP TO PATIENT _____ OCCUPATION

EMPLOYER _____ EMPLOYER'S ADDRESS _____ CITY _____ STATE _____ ZIP _____ BUS PHONE

SIGNATURE OF PATIENT OR LEGAL GUARDIAN

METHOD OF PAYMENT: ☐ CASH ☐ CHECK ☐ CREDIT CARD (VISA, MC)
☐ 30-DAY ACCOUNT ☐ OTHER

FIG. 12-5.

(Pub.372)

PATIENT STATISTICAL INFORMATION

PLEASE PRINT

[Form fields:]

Patient's Name _____ (Last) _____ (First) Date _____ Birth Date _____ Age _____
Child ( ) Single ( ) Married ( ) Divorced ( ) (Widowed ( ) Separated ( )
Home Address _____ Telephone _____ Zip Code _____
Religion _____ Occupation _____ Social Security No. _____
Employer _____ How Long _____
Employer's Address _____ Telephone _____ Zip Code _____

Bill To _____ Relationship _____
Address _____ Telephone _____
Zip Code _____ Social Security No. _____
Employer _____ Occupation _____ How Long _____
Employer's Address _____ Telephone _____ Zip Code _____

Name of Spouse _____ Birth Date _____ Age _____
Occupation _____ Social Security No. _____
Employer _____ Occupation _____ How Long _____
Employer's Address _____ Telephone _____ Zip Code _____

Referred to Doctor by _____
Name and Address of Closest Relative (other than spouse):
Relationship _____ Name _____
Telephone _____ Address _____

List Any Known Allergies _____
Or Drug Sensitivities _____

INSURANCE INFORMATION

Name and Address of Company _____
Type of Coverage: Group _____ Private _____ Policy No. _____
Group No. _____ Member No. _____ Certificate No. _____
Medicare No. _____ Effective Date _____

All professional services rendered are charged to the patient. Necessary forms will be completed to expedite insurance claims. The patient is responsible for all fees, regardless of insurance coverage. It is customary to pay for services when rendered unless arrangements are made in advance. Please READ and SIGN the following authorization and assignment.

INSURANCE AUTHORIZATION AND ASSIGNMENT

I hereby authorize _____ to furnish information to insurance carriers concerning my illnesses and treatments and I hereby assign to the doctor all payments for medical services rendered to myself or my dependents. I understand that I am responsible for any amount not covered by insurance.

Patient's Signature _____
Insured's Signature _____

considered as valid as the original.

FIG. 12-6.

carbon copies of prescriptions, etc. In short, a patient's medical record includes all of those things found in a physician's office or medical institution that can be traced to a specific patient.

As to who "owns" the medical record, the law is quite clear that the physician or medical institution owns the physical record (the "work product" collated and used by the physician or institution for the benefit of the patient). The information in that record, on the other hand, is the personal property of the patient and it cannot be used without the patient's specific approval.

One of the most confusing areas of ownership of medical records involves x-rays. Many persons are of the opinion that they "buy" their x-rays and cannot understand why the physician or medical institution will not give them up. However, numerous courts have ruled that the actual film belongs to the physician or institution and that the patient pays for the opinion, advice or report based upon what the x-rays reveal. In a landmark decision in a 1935 case, the Michigan Supreme Court held that x-ray films are part of the medical record, but the physician or institution cannot be compelled to relinquish them, except by lawful order from a court of competent jurisdiction.

Most legal authorities recommend that a patient be provided with a copy of the x-ray, if the physician or institution has the facility to produce such a copy. The patient requesting the copy may be required to pay the full cost of reproduction.

§ 12.06 Medical Record Preservation

A physician is required to retain medical records, employee wage and hour records, and records of all business transactions for the practice for a certain period of time past their relevance. Medical records should be kept for seven to ten years, except in the case of patients whose legal disability is removed by operation of time or law. Business records, including payroll, accounts receivable and payable, and insurance payments should be kept for four to six years and employee records should be kept for two to three years. Records should never be destroyed without first consulting a competent advisor.

Most legal authorities agree that because of the uniqueness of medical records, they should be kept a minimum of seven to ten years after the last time the patient was seen. This much time is usually sufficient to cover the various statutes of limitations on civil actions that might be brought against a physician or a medical institution.

An exception to this general rule is that anyone under legal disability at the time a cause of action occurs may bring a lawsuit within one year after this disability is removed by operation of law or time. (A minor's legal disability is removed with the passage of time; i.e., he or she can bring suit upon turning 18 years of age. Persons that have been declared legally incompetent, on the other hand, must have their disability removed by operation of law through the courts of a state.) In such cases, records should be kept for at least two years after the disability is removed, i.e., until the patient reaches 20 years of age or for two years after the person has been declared legally sane. Although the law only specifies a one-year retention after the disability has been removed, the extra year is a built-in safety factor.

It is wise to keep copies of all records in which there is an indication of some untoward event, surgical accident, an unexpected result or some other indication that legal or medical difficulties might arise at a later date.

The physician should consider using microfilm if he or she wishes to retain medical records, but finds himself or herself short on storage space. Federal law[1] specifies that records reconstituted from microfilm are to be considered the same as the original, and that retention of the microfilmed record constitutes compliance with preservation laws.)

[1] Retaining Office Records

The Federal Tax Law contains numerous references to the type of records that must be retained in specific instances. The IRS can examine a tax return and make adjustments within three years from the date of its filing. This period increases to six years if the return contains a very large understatement of income. The period may be indefinite if fraud is suspected.

The following documents must be retained permanently:

- Capital stock ledgers
- Corporate minute books
- Deeds
- Titles

---

[1] Section 1732 of Public Law 82-129.

- Abstracts and other papers pertaining to the sale of real estate
- General ledgers
- Financial statements
- Books of original entry (i.e., cash receipts and disbursements including general journal entries)
- Tax returns
- IRS audit reports
- Personnel records

The following documents must be retained for at least seven years:

- Contracts in general (after their expiration)
- Accounts receivable ledgers or cards
- Royalty statements or computations
- Bank statements and cancelled checks
- Accounts payable files (i.e., paid bills)
- Invoices for medical services rendered
- Medical insurance records

Four years is the minimum amount of time for retention of:

- Insurance policies after expiration
- Duplicate deposit tickets
- Payroll time cards

A rule of thumb should be never to destroy clinical or business records without first consulting a competent advisor.

[2] Record Keeping

The Fair Labor Standards Act requires that employee wage and hour records be kept in the physician's office. No specific forms are required. However, the employer must keep track of the hours an employee works each day and each work week, regardless of whether the employee is paid by the hour, the week, the month or on some other basis.

Although the Fair Labor Standards Act does not require a

particular form of records, it does require that whatever record is kept must include certain identifying information about the employee and data about the hours worked and the wages earned. Basic information in the record must include the employee's full name and social security number, address, birthdate (if younger than 19 years old), sex and occupation. The individual employee's record must also show the time of day and day of week when the employee's work week begins, hours worked each day, and total hours worked each work week. The wages portion of the record must indicate the basis on which the employee's wages are paid (i.e., "$4 an hour", "$200 a week", "$1,000 a month").

For office employees who work on a fixed schedule, the employer may keep a record showing the exact schedule of daily and weekly hours that the employee is expected to follow and merely indicate that the employee did follow the schedule. Whenever an employee is on a job for a longer or shorter period of time than the schedule shows, the employer should record the exact number of hours actually worked.

It is recommended that all employee records containing required information by the wage and hour law should be retained for three years. However, records on which wage and hour computations are based—e.g., sign in/out sheets and work-time schedules—may be destroyed after two years. Payroll records containing the employee identification information must be retained at least three years, and it is recommended that progress reports, evaluations, performance reviews, reprimands and firing notices be retained in the employee's file for the same amount of time.[2]

§ 12.07 Collecting Debts

A physician can collect against overdue patient debts in a number of ways: through third parties such as collection agencies or district attorneys; by garnishing the patient's paycheck; or by initiating legal proceedings. Laws against harassment and disclosure of confidential information apply to the medical office as they would for any debt collector, and the physician or the physician's agent should try to work within the guidelines of the Fair Debt Collections Act to avoid a

---

[2] This information is taken from "How to Keep Time and Pay Records under the Fair Labor Standards Act," U.S. Department of Labor, WH Publication No. 1185.

(Pub.372)

legal battle. In the interest of preserving the patient-physician relationship it is always best to use conservative collection tactics at first. Serious proceedings against a delinquent patient should not be undertaken without first consulting an attorney.

Provided the physician collects debts in his or her own name, and not by criminal means, the only practical constraints on debt collection are common sense and professional ethics. (See also Chapter 7, Credit and Collections.)

[1] Fair Debt Collection Practices Act

The Fair Debt Collection Practices Act, which became effective in 1978, establishes boundaries of proper conduct within which a debt can be legally collected. The act applies only to the activities of a "debt collector" for collecting against debts contracted by consumers for personal, family or household purposes. The term "debt collector" is defined to mean any person who uses interstate commerce or the mails for the principal purpose of collecting debts; anyone who regularly collects, or who attempts to collect, debts directly or indirectly owed to another; or any creditor who uses a name other than his or her own to give the impression or indication that a third person is collecting or trying to collect the debt.

A physician is not affected by the law if he or she collects debts in his or her own name. However, even if a medical practice is not affected by this law, there are rules or limitations in the law that should be adhered to out of common sense, courtesy and the possibility that failure to do so could be construed as "harassment" under other sections of state law.

[a] Provisions of the Act

The following points, taken from the Fair Debt Collection Practices Act, should be a part of a medical office's collection practices whether or not it is affected by the Act:

- Communicate only with the patient (or the appropriate responsible party) about his or her past due account.

- Avoid the use of obscene or profane language, or language which is designed to abuse or threaten the hearer or reader.

- Do not participate in the publication of a list of patients who refuse to pay debts, except through a consumer-reporting agency.
- Use the telephone for information and education, not to annoy, abuse or harass any person.
- Use the telephone selectively.

Any debt collector who communicates with another person other than the patient, for the purpose of finding out where the patient is, should observe the following rules:

- Identify yourself and state that you are confirming or correcting information about the patient. Identify your employer only if specifically requested to do so.
- Do not state that the patient owes any debt.
- Do not communicate with any individual for purposes of gathering information more than once, unless the individual requests you to do so or unless you reasonably believe that the person's earlier information was incomplete or that they now have correct or complete information.
- Do not communicate with anyone by postcard.
- Do not use any language or symbol on the outside of any envelope or in any telephone conversation indicating that the communication pertains to the collection of a debt. (It is all right to use standard billing envelopes, but don't stamp "final notice" on the outside.)
- If you have reason to know or believe that the patient's employer prohibits debt collection communications, then contact at the place of employment should be avoided.

If the patient informs the practice that he or she does not intend to pay the bill and has contacted an attorney, the practice should obtain the name of the patient's attorney and then cease all further communications. The physician should then contact his or her professional liability insurance company and report the incident, review records and charges to determine if there are any legal problems, and if no problem is obvious, turn the account over to an attorney or collection agency for followup.

(Pub.372)

[b] Common Physician Questions Regarding Debt Collection

Physicians commonly ask the following questions about debt collection practices:

May I ask a patient for financial references?

Yes. If you are going to extend credit to the patient you are entitled to the same kind of financial information as any other business.

Can I ask his or her previous physician about his payment history?

Certainly. Many physicians' offices routinely include a copy of the payment ledger card with the patient's record when it is forwarded to a new attending physician.

Can I give patient financial information over the telephone to other physicians' offices and to credit bureaus?

You can freely exchange information with other physicians' offices. Just be sure it really is a physician's office you are talking to. You can exchange information with a credit bureau as long as you are a member of the credit bureau or participating in its activities. However, revealing patient financial information to any other type of organization is not advisable. It is too easy to inadvertently allow confidential medical information to escape.

Can I tell a patient we are going to turn his account over to a collection agency?

Yes you can. That is not a threat, but a statement of legal fact. However, if you make the statement with no intention of ever turning the account over to a collection agency, it may be considered a threat and a form of harassment.

What is the best time to make a collection call to the patient's home?

Generally, between 6:00 and 8:00 P.M. However, the best time is whenever you can find the patient at home.

May I make a collection call to the patient's place of employment?

Yes, provided that you do not tell anyone that it is a collection call and as long as you have reason to believe that the employer does not object to outside calls.

If a patient asks us not to call his place of employment, what can we do?

If he will give you no other telephone number, call his place of employment. He should be willing to give you a time and a place where he can be contacted.

Should the doctor sign the collection letter or should the patient be told that the doctor is personally concerned about the unpaid bill?

No. Because of the importance of the doctor-patient relationship, make sure the patient understands that a particular person on the office staff is responsible for following up on unpaid accounts.

[2] Checks, "Rubber" and Otherwise

Whenever you receive a check back from the bank marked "insufficient funds," no payment at all has been made on the account. Furthermore, if your bank charges you for processing an insufficient funds check given to you by a patient, you are entitled to recover from the patient at least the bank charge.

Once a check is stamped "insufficient funds" it cannot be passed back through the federal banking system. It can be taken directly to the bank upon which it was drawn, but the law provides that a bank has the right to refuse to honor a check for a payee who is not one of the bank's depositors, because it may refuse payment to a stranger.

In some areas, usually smaller cities and towns, the local district attorney will assist in the collection of insufficient fund checks. However, this is a voluntary assistance, and not a required function of that office.

While a physician is within his or her rights to take whatever legal means are necessary to be compensated for a payment by a check drawn on insufficient funds, bringing criminal suit against the patient is inadvisable.

[3] Garnishments

Garnishment is any legal or equitable procedure through which the earnings of an individual are required by federal law to be withheld for payment of any debt (15 USCA 1672 (c)).

Portions of the federal law dealing with garnishment restrictions indicate that an individual's disposable earnings are subject to garnishment only to "25 percentum of his disposable earnings for that week, . . ." Exceptions to the 25 percent limit include those based on any order of a court of competent jurisdiction, an administrative procedure established by state law which affords substantial due process; or any order of any court of the United States having jurisdiction, or over any debt due for any state or federal tax.

Section 1675 of the law provides that no employer may discharge any employee "by reason of the fact that his earnings have been subjected to garnishment for any *one* indebtedness." The District Court of California in 1971 held, however, that an employee may be discharged if he or she has had multiple garnishments, providing that the discharge is not the result of discrimination on the basis of race, color, religion, sex or national origin.

Where there are multiple garnishments the courts have usually ruled that the first garnishment filed (i.e., first in time) creates a superior lien and is the only one that requires withholding of any said earnings by the employer. Many states provide, however, that garnishments must be refiled each month or each pay period. This means that sometimes there is a scramble to see who can be the "first in time" garnishment lien.

§ 12.08 Employment Applications

Although an employment application can be used to reveal a great deal of information about an employee, a practice can be accused of job discrimination if questions about religion, race, color, age, nationality, sex, marital status, family plans, military career and police record cannot be proven relevant to the employee's ability to fulfill job duties.

A properly filled out employment application gives the physician's office an opportunity to obtain the maximum amount of information about an applicant's educational background, skills and former employment. Because of various state and federal civil rights laws, questions about an applicant's religion, race, color, age, national origin or ancestry, sex, marital status, family plans and type and date of military discharge should be avoided unless the information can be shown to be pertinent to the job in question.

Questions about possible physical defects should also be avoided unless there is a possibility such a defect would interfere in job performance. It is against the law to deny employment because of a physical defect where the reasonable demands of the position can be met by the handicapped. An important question to ask, however, is, "Is there anything to prohibit you from performing this job safely?"

If you are using a more detailed employment application than the one outlined in Appendix 12-C, it should contain a footnote reading, "This organization does not discriminate on the basis of age, religion, race, color, national origin or ancestry, sex or marital status." As a practical matter, though, if you simply avoid asking questions about these topics either on the employment application or during the job interview, the likelihood of being accused of discrimination is lessened.

It is permissible to ask questions about a possible conviction for a felony. The question should be phrased, "Have you ever been convicted of a felony?," not "Have you ever been arrested?" It is recommended that the employment interviewer should not make any notations on the employment application form itself. Notations and evaluations based on the interview, reference checks, etc. should be made on some other form or sheet.

(For other legislation that that can affect your medical office, see Appendix 12-D.)

§ 12.09 Checklist for Law in the Medical Practice

A comprehensive checklist of points touched on in the chapter is provided.

— Physician-Patient Relationship

    — Implied contract

    — Confidentiality

    — Right to refuse services

— Informed Consent

    — Expressed consent

- Consent implied by action
- Consent implied in emergency (Good Samaritan Laws)
- Consent required by a third party for:
  - Minors
  - Mentally incompetent
  - Child of divorced couple
- Record Retention
  - Medical records: 7 to 10 years
  - Business records: 2 years to permanently
  - Employee wage and hour records: 1 to 2 years
  - Exceptions for minors and mentally incompetent
- Debt Collection Procedures
  - Fair debt collection act
  - Third party debt collector
  - Legal action for checks drawn against insufficient funds
  - Garnishments
- Laws Affecting the Medical Office
  - Fair Debt Collections Act
  - Occupational Safety and Health Administration (OSHA) Laws
  - Privacy Act of 1974
  - Freedom of Information Act
  - Truth in Lending Act
  - Fair Credit Billing Act
  - Equal Credit Opportunity Act
  - Laws for credit reporting agencies
- Formal Information Forms for the Medical Office
  - Discharge of patient from care forms
  - Letter of withdrawal

- Informed consent forms
- Patient information forms
- Medical, business and employee wage and hour records
- Employment applications

§ 12.100 Bibliography

Annas, G. J., et al.: The Rights of Doctors, Nurses and Allied Health Professionals: A Health Law Primer. Cambridge, MA: Ballinger Publishing Co., 1981.

Christoffel, T.: Health and the Law. A Handbook for Health Professionals. New York: Free Press, 1982.

Lewis, M. A. and Warden, C. D.: Law And Ethics in the Medical Office: Including Bioethical Issues. Philadelphia: F.A. Davis, 1983.

Pozgar, G. D.: Legal Aspects of Health Care Administration. Rockville, MD: Aspen Systems Corp., 1983.

Schuchman, H.: Confidentiality of Health Records. The Meeting of Law, Ethics and Clinical Issues. New York: Gardner Press, 1981.

Appendix 12-A

PATIENT DISCHARGE NOTICES

Letter to Confirm Discharge by Patient

Dear_____.

This will confirm our telephone conversation of today in which you discharged me from attending you as your physician in your present illness. In my opinion, your condition requires continued medical treatment by a physician.

If you have not already done so, I suggest that you employ another physician without delay. You may be assured that, at your request, I will furnish him with information regarding the diagnosis and treatment which you have received from me.

I am enclosing an authorization form which will allow me to release information to your new physician.

Sincerely,

_____

FIG. 12-1.

Letter to Patient Who Fails to Keep Appointments

Dear _____ _____

On_____ you failed to keep your appointment at my office. It is my professional opinion that your condition requires continued medical treatment, and I urge you not to neglect this need.

If you wish, you may telephone my office for another appointment. However, it is possible that you might prefer to deal with another physician. If this is the case, I suggest that you make arrangements promptly. I am enclosing a consent form which you should fill out and return to me if you wish me to make my knowledge of your case available to another doctor.

Sincerely,

_____

FIG. 12-2.

Letter of Withdrawal

Dear _____.

I regret to inform you that I am withdrawing from further professional attendance upon you. It is necessary for me to take this action because (Here set out reason; i.e., persistant failure to settle bill, refusing to follow instructions, etc.)

Your condition requires medical attention. Therefore, I suggest that you immediately make arrangements with another physician to provide the medical care which you should have

If you wish, I will continue to attend you for a brief period of time while you are making arrangements to retain another physician, but this period of time must not exceed seven days.

I am enclosing a consent form for you to sign and return to me. This will authorize me to release information regarding your case history, diagnosis and treatment to your new physician.

Sincerely,

_____

FIG. 12-3.

Appendix 12-B

ACCEPTABLE PRE-EMPLOYMENT INQUIRIES UNDER EEO GUIDELINES

Subject Area	Acceptable	Unacceptable
(1) Name	For access purposes, whether applicant's work records are under another name.	To ask if a woman is a Miss, Mrs. or Ms., or to ask for maiden name.
(2) Residence	a) Place and length of current and previous addresses. b) Applicant's phone number or how applicant can be reached.	None.
(3) Age	After hiring, proof of age by birth certificate.	a) Age or age group of applicant. b) Birth certificate or baptismal record before hiring.
(4) National Orgin	None.	a) Birthplace of applicant, parents, grandparents, or spouse. b) Any other inquiry into national origin.
(5) Race	Race for affirmative action plan statistics, after hiring.	Any inquiry that would indicate race or color.
(6) Sex	Inquiry for affirmative action plan statistics after hiring.	Inquiry which would indicate sex unless job-related.
(7) Religion or Creed	None.	a) Religion or religious customs and holidays.

(Pub.372)

(8)	Citizenship	a) Whether a U.S. citizen. b) If U.S. residence is legal. c) Require proof of citizenship after hiring.	b) Recommendations or references from church officials. a) If native-born or naturalized. b) Proof of citizenship before hiring. c) Whether parents or spouse nativeborn or naturalized. d) Date of citizenship.
(9)	Marital Status	a) Status (only married or single) after hiring for insurance and tax purposes. b) Number and ages of dependents and age of spouse after hiring for insurance and tax purposes.	a) To ask marital status before hiring. b) To ask the number and ages of children, who cares for them and if applicant plans to have children.
(10)	Military Service	a) Service in the U.S. Armed Forces, including branch and rank attained. b) Any job-related experience. c) Require military discharge certificate after hiring.	a) Military service records. b) Military service for any country other than U.S. c) Type of discharge.
(11)	Education	a) Academic, professional, or vocational schools attended. b) Language skills, such as reading.	

		and writing foreign languages.	
		a) Nationality, racial, or religious affiliation of schools attended.	
		b) How foreign language ability was acquired.	
(12)	Criminal Record	Listing of convictions other than misdemeanors.	Arrest record.
(13)	References	General and work references not relating to race, color, religion, sex, national origin or ancestry.	References specifically from clergy or any other person who might reflect race, color, sex, national origin or ancestry.
(14)	Organizations	a) Organizational membership: professional, social, etc., as long as affiliation is not used to discriminate on the basis of race, sex, national origin, or ancestry. b) Offices held, if any.	Listing of all clubs applicant belongs to or has belonged to.
(15)	Photographs	May be required after hiring for identification purposes.	a) Request photographs before hiring. b) To take pictures of applicants during interview.
(16)	Work Schedule	a) Willingness to work required work schedule. b) Whether applicant has military reservist obligations.	Willingness to work any particular religious holiday.

(Pub.372)

(17)	Physical Data	a) To require applicant to prove ability to do manual labor, lifting and other job-related physical requirements of the job, if any. b) Require a physical exam.	To ask height and weight, impairment or other non-specified physical data.
(18)	Handicap	To inquire for the purpose of determining applicant's capability to perform the job. (Burden of proof for non-discrimination lies with the employer.)	To exclude handicapped applicants as a class on the basis of their type of handicap. Each case must be determined individually.
(19)	Other Qualifications	Any area that has a direct reflection on the job applied for.	Any non-job related inquiry that may present information permitting unlawful discrimination.

Source: Civil Rights Act of 1964, Title VII, as amended; Equal Employment Opportunity Act of 1972; Education Amendment of 1972, Title IX; Age Discrimination in Employment Act of 1967; Equal Employment Opportunity Guidelines, 1978.

Appendix 12-C

LEGISLATION AFFECTING MEDICAL PRACTICES

[1] Occupational Safety and Health Administration (OSHA)

The Occupational Safety and Health Administration (OSHA) has promulgated regulations governing access to certain medical records, specifically, the medical records of an employee in the possession of an employer.

The OSHA regulation, found at 20 CFR 1910, applies to all employers who are in possession of medical records of their employees and is not limited to the medical profession. However, whereas most employers do not have their employees' medical records on their employees, almost all physicians, clinics and hospitals treat their own employees.

The OSHA rule states that employee medical records must be retained for at least 30 years plus the duration of employment. This is usually interpreted to mean 30 years beyond the last day the employee is employed. OSHA required medical records may be microfilmed or reproduced in other ways, "but x-rays must be kept in their original form."

These regulations give a broad range of employee access or access by a representative to all employer records relating to health. They provide that the first copy of the record requested by the employee must be provided by the employer "free" within 15 days.

[2] Privacy Act of 1973

This act, found in 5 USCA 552a, amends the Administrative Procedures Act of the United States Government. It provides that whenever information is collected by an agency of the Government concerning an individual, it is that agency's responsibility to protect the information from unlawful disclosure.

This act applies only to federal agencies and the records in their possession. It does not apply to privately practicing physicians, clinics or hospitals unless they are employed by or owned and operated by the Federal Government.

[3] Freedom of Information Act

The Freedom of Information Act was enacted by the United States Congress in 1974. Along with the Privacy Act, it was meant to assure that whenever a federal agency was collecting information about a private individual, that individual would be permitted access to that information for purposes of determining its authenticity and challenging its correctness.

This act, found in 5 USCA 552, does not apply to records held by private individuals such as physicians, clinics or hospitals.

[4] Truth in Lending Act

In 1968 the United States Congress enacted the Truth in Lending Act and then amended it extensively in 1975 by adopting the Fair Credit Billing Act. In 1980 the law was amended again.

Congress enacted the original law when it was discovered that while there were very specific statutes dealing with banks, loan companies, and savings and loan organizations, there was very little control over policies for installment purchases through retail stores. Congressional hearings revealed that many companies were consistently abusing their relationship with the public by adding service charges, delivery charges, set up charges, finance charges, past due charges and numerous other special charges to installment purchase accounts. While the amount of interest they were charging was not exorbitant, the addition of all of the special additional charges was driving the actual cost of installment-purchased items to almost unbelievable heights.

Owing to certain constitutional restraints, Congress cannot tell a company that is operating inside a single state how much to charge for its products or services. However, federal law allows Congress to enact what are called notice or information statutes. These laws require that certain information must be given under specified circumstances. In this case Congress enacted a law that said if an individual or company became a "credit lender" before finalizing a sale it was necessary for that organization to reveal certain information about its financial arrangements to the prospective purchaser.

This information is given in the form of a full disclosure of all financial arrangements. It details the amount of interest, service charge, set up charge, delivery charge, past due charge, etc. that will be added to an installment purchase contract.

The Federal Truth in Lending Act does not exclude any company, business, occupation or profession from its coverage. It states that if an individual or business become a "credit lender" (i.e., if it extends credit to customers/clients/patients and then in some way charges them for the privilege of the credit), then that individual or business must meet minimum notice obligations. In short, if a physician or physician's office is declared to be a credit lender the statement sent to every patient every month would look like the statement you receive from Bank Americard, Sears, Mastercharge, or any of the gasoline companies.

Since most physicians do not want to get involved in that kind of bookkeeping problem, they need to be aware of how to avoid the Truth in Lending Act:

- Do not charge interest.
- Do not impose a finance charge, or any other charge for the extension of credit.
- Make no formal written agreements for installment payments where there are more than four installments (excluding a down payment).
- Make no collection charge, past due charge or late charge related to the size of the bill.

Most physicians do not charge interest or impose a finance or service charge. However, many offices do establish formal installment payments, but usually not on a written basis. It is not generally viewed as an installment payment situation if the physician allows the patient to determine how much he or she is going to pay each month. It comes under the Truth in Lending Act only if it is a written agreement.

Late charges or past due charges are also acceptable, provided that they are not related to the size of the bill. If the past due charge is a fixed amount and the same for everybody, then it is excluded from the Act. However, if it is related to the size of the bill (i.e., $1 for each $100 past due), then it becomes a form of interest.

The acceptance of payments by credit card does not involve a medical office with the Truth in Lending Act. This is a matter between the patient and the credit card company. The law also deals with the treatment of credit balances. It specifies that whenever credit balances in excess of $1.00 are created then the creditor must either credit the amount of the balance to the patient's account, refund the credit upon request by the consumer or make a good faith effort to refund the amount by attempting to contact the patient at the last known address or telephone number. Such a credit balance can be retained for no more than six months before a refund is attempted.

If a physician's office wishes to charge interest or enter into formal installment payments, it should contact an attorney familiar with the Truth in Lending Act and any state requirement that might be involved.

[5] Equal Credit Opportunity Act

In 1974, Congress enacted the "Equal Credit Opportunity Act" (15 USCA 1691) with the intent of barring discrimination in all credit practices. The law provided that the Board of Governors of the Federal Reserve System could create appropriate regulations to carry out the intent of the law.

The definition of "creditor" in the act is extremely broad and includes physicians if they ordinarily grant their patients the right to defer payment for medical services rendered. This law is tied directly to the Truth In Lending Act (or, as it is now known, Fair Credit Billing Act). If a physician is declared to be a "credit lender" under that act, then he or she must comply with all of the rules and regulations of the Equal Credit Opportunity Act. This includes requiring a written credit application, giving written notice of action taken on the application, keeping copies of all applications and written notices and being subject to possible fines running as high as $500,000 for violations.

If a physician is declared a credit lender, then he or she may not consider the applicant's sex, color, race, religion or national origin, or ask about birth control practices or plans to have children when deciding to extend credit. He or she cannot exclude patient's or patient's spouse's income because of sex or marital status or exclude income from part-time employment, retirement benefits, alimony, child support or separate maintenance payments.

(Pub.372)

However, if a physician is granting only "incidental credit" he or she is relieved from the burdens imposed by the regulations. Incidental credit is primarily for personal, family or household purposes and it is neither granted under the terms of a credit card account, subject to any finance charges or interest nor granted under an agreement that permits repayment in more than four installments.

By taking advantage of incidental credit treatment, physicians can avoid the major burdens of the Equal Credit Opportunity Act and regulations.

(Adapted from "Effects of the Equal Credit Opportunity Act on Physicians in Private Practice", Texas Medicine (Journal), November, 1977.)

[6] Credit Reporting Agencies

Consumer credit reporting agencies are also controlled by federal law found in Title 15 USCA 1681-1681(t).

A consumer reporting agency is defined as any person that engages for profit in the practice of assembling or evaluating consumer credit information for the purpose of furnishing consumer reports to third parties, and who uses any means or facility of interstate commerce for the purpose of preparing or furnishing consumer reports.

A consumer report may be requested and used in response to court orders or in accordance with written instructions from the consumer to whom it relates. In addition, such reports may be furnished to other individuals for the purpose of extending credit, review or collection of an account, employment purposes, underwriting insurance, determination of the individual's eligibility for a license or other benefits granted by a government instrumentality, or for anyone else who "otherwise has a legitimate business need for the information in connection with a business transaction involving the (individual) consumer."

Certain information cannot be reported:

- Bankruptcy or Title 11 Bankruptcy cases more than 10 years old.

- Other suits or judgments more than seven years old or for which the statue of limitations has expired (whichever is the longer).

- Paid tax liens more than seven years old.

- Accounts turned over for collection which are more than seven years old.

- Records of arrest, indictment or conviction of crime which, from date of disposition, release or parole, antedate the report by more than seven years.

- Any other adverse item of information more than seven years old.

The law does provide, however, that whenever the credit transaction involves more than $50,000, the underwriting of a life insurance policy with a face value of more than $50,000 or the employment of an individual at an annual salary that equals $20,000 or more, all of the above information may be reported and considered.

Whenever someone orders an investigative consumer report on an individual, it is necessary to disclose the fact of the report's preparation. The individual being reported upon has the right to request a copy of the report. In addition to disclosure, the law also provides that every consumer reporting agency has the responsibility to allow the individual to examine the information in its files and to have placed in the files a note regarding any information with which the individual reported upon disagrees.

CHAPTER 13
Medical Practice Mergers and Affiliations*

> **SCOPE**
>
> As the practice of medicine becomes a more complex business many practitioners find themselves considering merging their solo or group practices into a larger medical entity to take advantage of the benefits available to a large corporation. The benefits of such a venture are several: larger groups can exert a greater control over third parties (such as hospitals or insurance companies), influence market forces, pool resources to purchase costly equipment and systems, diversify services, contain costs for a greater profit, control quality and spread risk. A merging of practices, though, is a complicated process that can take months to years to complete. Interested parties must first decide whether they want to form a single or multi-specialty group and choose partners with whom they will be compatible. Compatibility refers not only to personal and professional attitudes toward work styles and quality of care but also to any internal office systems or external liabilities, such as business entanglements, insurance obligations or pending malpractice litigation that will have to be absorbed into the new medical group. Pre-existing employee positions and pay levels and methods of physician compensation must be studied to determine whether they can be integrated into the new entity's practice in a way that will be satisfactory to all parties affected. Physicians interested in merging their practices

---

* Caution: Federal legislation pending in the 1989 Congressional Session may greatly restrict and/or prohibit certain joint ventures or other types of physicians' financial interests in certain entities, such as optical shops, laboratories, MRIs' CT scanners, etc. Physicians involved in such situations should consult attorneys familiar with the health care industry to review the impact of any law changes on their current situations, or situations they are contemplating entering into.

> must select advisory groups of lawyers, accountants and business professionals to help them identify and overcome obstacles to the merger and to keep the new entity functioning smoothly once the merger has been completed.

SYNOPSIS

§ 13.01 Medical Practice Affiliations: The Options

    [1] Joint Ventures
    [2] Physician Practice Groups (PPG)
    [3] Combinations

§ 13.02 The Benefits of Combined Practices

    [1] Control
    [2] Organizational Credibility
    [3] Marketing
    [4] Insurance Market
    [5] Quality Control
    [6] Cost Containment
    [7] Economies of Scale
    [8] Delegation of Business Management
    [9] Pooling Capital

§ 13.03 Consequences and Risks of Affiliation

    [1] Hospital Takeovers
    [2] Loss of Individual Control
    [3] Inefficiency of Bureaucracies
    [4] Mismanagement
    [5] Medicare and Medicaid Regulations

§ 13.04 Is an Affiliation Right for You?

    [1] Compatibility
    [2] Goal Evaluation
    [3] Approach

§ 13.05 Choosing Partners

    [1] Level of Quality
    [2] Specialties
    [3] Fees and Costs
    [4] Fee-for-Service Versus Capitation
    [5] Goal Evaluation
    [6] Work Attitudes

    [7] **Personal Attitudes**
§ 13.06 **Initial Obstacles**
    [1] **Contingent Liabilities**
    [2] **Business Entanglements**
    [3] **Antitrust Regulations**
    [4] **Integrating Offices**

(Text continued on page 13-3)

                [5]   Financing
    § 13.07   Establishing Time-Frames
                [1]   Electing a Steering Committee
                [2]   Establishing the Advisory Team
                [3]   Cost-Sharing Arrangements
                [4]   Budget and Projections
                [5]   Organizational Set-Up
                [6]   "Clean-Up" of Current Entities
                [7]   Accounting and Legal Plan to Carry Out the Merger
                [8]   Valuations
                [9]   Premerger Agreement
                [10]   Profit Distribution System
    § 13.08   Restrictive Covenants
    § 13.09   Noncorporate Legal Agreements and Documents
    § 13.10   Establishing the New Entity
                [1]   Post-Merger Advisory Boards
                [2]   Rotatation of Doctors
                [3]   Pay Levels
                [4]   Staff Evaluation
                [5]   Unified Office Systems
                [6]   Profile Changes
                [7]   Centralized Purchasing
                [8]   Telephones
    § 13.11   Public Relations
    § 13.12   Insurance Coverage
    § 13.13   Bail-Out Provisions
    § 13.14   Checklist
    § 13.100 Bibliography

§ 13.01 Medical Practice Affiliations: The Options

Physicians who wish to combine their practices and experience the benefits available to a larger medical group have several options: the joint venture, the physician practice group, or one of three possible combinations—consolidation, acquisition or merger.

Consider the following scenario: There are two radiology groups in town. Both are financially solvent but each is philosophically opposed to the other's way of practice and business. Both groups see the need for a magnetic resonance imaging machine (MRI) in their

§ 13.01[1]   MANAGING YOUR MEDICAL PRACTICE   13-4

town, yet neither feels that alone the practice has the volume to justify the expenditure and risk associated with such a purchase.

If only one of the two practices purchased the magnetic resonance imaging machine, perhaps the other group, feeling threatened, would decide to buy its own machine, making the situation unprofitable for both groups and the cost to the community excessive. However, if the medical practices consolidated or merged there would be ample volume to support the purchase and maintenance of a new magnetic resonance imaging machine, enough investors to spread the risk and a good chance that, over time, the machine would prove a profitable investment. Yet the incompatibility of the business and practice philosophies of the two groups remains, making the merger impossible.

What appears to be an insoluble problem in this case can be resolved through another possibility, a joint venture.

[1] Joint Ventures

The two groups decide that a new "entity" (business enterprise) should be created to purchase the magnetic resonance imaging (MRI) equipment. After a review of the tax situation, it is decided that it would be best to establish a partnership that would own and operate the new MRI equipment. All of the doctors in each of the groups may become partners in the new entity. In addition, the two groups may decide that it is beneficial to offer nonradiologist physicians an opportunity to participate in this joint venture.

A meeting is held and the participating physicians each contribute a predetermined sum of money. They elect a steering committee and make provisions to open a checking account. The steering committee then hires advisors to review legal and financial implications, tax consequences, financial projections, etc. of such a venture. Bank financing is arranged for the new equipment, which is purchased and enthusiastically shared by the two radiology groups and, since nonradiologists were allowed to participate in the joint venture, by other physicians in the local community as well.

Common examples of other formal joint ventures include internists who pool resources to expand their laboratory, or orthopedic surgeons who pool resources to establish a physical therapy center. Joint ventures need not be so formal: a joint venture could consist of two physicians with separate practices in the same town getting together to set up a good coverage system; similarly, in a small town where an unusual sub-specialty such as neonatology is lacking, pooling resources to hire a third physician as a specialist. Nor do joint ventures of this kind need to be exclusively limited to physicians: a physical therapist might participate with physicians, or a psychologist may decide to start such a venture with one or more psychology groups.

Today, more than before, hosptials and physicians are becoming involved in joint ventures because they are learning that working together helps both the hospital and physician to survive and prosper. The following case study illustrates a situation where a hospital-physician joint venture benefits both parties.

CASE STUDY

Physician Group A and Hospital B are located in the hub of a metropolitan area. Both the physician group and hospital are prosperous, but each wishes to expand its practice into a particular suburb.

The physician group wishes to provide services to patients outside of its metropolitan office. In addition, it feels it is missing out on some of the younger patients who tend to go to physicians in the suburban area. After examining the cost of opening up a practice in the targeted suburb, the group finds the associated cost and risk greater than it is willing to absorb at the present time.

The hospital also wishes to bring patients from the targeted suburban area into the hospital, but recognizes that this will require physician referrals since there are a number of other hospitals to which physicians currently in the suburbs make referrals.

Since Physician Group A is pleased with the services provided by Hospital B, and since Physician Group A tends to place 80 to 90 percent of its in-patient work in Hospital B, Hospital B is willing to underwrite some of the cost and risk associated with Physician Group A opening an office in the suburb. A plan is put together whereby the hospital agrees to loan money to Physician Group A for initial capital outlays and working capital. In addition, Hospital B agrees to "guarantee" a limited loss by covering losses in excess of an agreed upon amount. The deal is put together and the new office opens.

Although the hospital is out some money during the first six months of operation, the volume of new patients brought into the hospital from Group A referrals coming from the suburban office offsets the loss. After the six month period, the physicians begin to profit from the suburban office and are able to repay the amounts originally loaned them by the hospital. Thus, both the hospital and physician group are able to expand and diversify their practice and increase their profit potentials. Without cooperation, though, none of this would have been possible.

Physicians who wish to become affiliated with other physicians in a more formal way or with a particular hospital but without abandoning control or current ownership should consider the joint venture method. The joint venture is advantageous because it diversifies the risk and usually binds the parties only to a particular project. In fact a doctor could be involved in a number of different joint venture projects at the same time, with the same or different participants.

[2] Physician Practice Groups (PPG)

Physicians who wish to work on a number of projects together or who wish to carry more weight together with insurance companies, HMOs (Health Maintenence Organizations), PPOs (Preferred Provider Organizations), hospitals, etc., but without merging practices may find an affiliation of practices through a physician practice group (PPG) the ideal solution. A physician practice group is an affiliation of individual practices functioning in concert for the good of all involved.

CASE STUDY

A small town's physician pool consists of a number of group and individual practices. While this situation has worked very well for many years, the physicians recognize a new threat to the way they practice and cover their market share: the local employer, seeking ways to lower its health care costs, has been discussing with a major HMO the feasibility of opening a clinic in town. If the major employer comes to terms with this HMO and a significant number of employees are persuaded to sign up for it, the physicians currently in town will need to go along with the program or lose patients.

The physicians have a meeting, but conclude that any type of a consolidation or merging of practices is not feasible at this time. They agree instead to form a new practice, the physicians practice group or PPG. All of the separate practices agree to allow the new PPG to establish a workable HMO contract and negotiate with the local employer. In addition, each of the PPG physicians agrees that he or she will maintain a fee-for-service system for his or her regular practice, but abide by whatever compensation system is set up for patients who elect the HMO contract.

Once established, the PPG works with the town hospital and seeks out and selects an HMO program feasible for both the physicians and the hospital. The PPG then offers this service to the employer, who is thrilled because it means employees will be able to elect HMO coverage while continuing with their current physicians. Without the formation of the PPG the physicians would have been fragmented and possibly forced into contracts where they would undoubtedly have been at a disadvantage.

A PPG could also be used by physicians to facilitate joint ventures and enjoy an economy of scale, while maintaining individual practices. It might also serve as a preliminary step to the merging of practices and weeding out of physicians not compatible with the final group.

[3] Combinations

The final and most complete type of practice affiliation is one in which practices formally combine as a unit. This may take the form of a *merger*, in which one practice acquires another and does not maintain the purchased entity; an *acquisition*, in which the purchasing practice maintains both the current entity and the entity purchased (an arrangement generally used when a senior physician wishes no continued equity and is perhaps preparing for retirement); or a *consolidation*, in which two practices are acquired by a new entity.

While from a legal standpoint the specific term used to describe the combination may be important, for the purposes of this chapter the term "merger" will be used to describe all types of formal practice combinations.

§ 13.02 The Benefits of Combined Practices

> The benefits that many individual or small group practitioners consider before entering into any group affiliation generally include those that accrue to any large business organization: a greater ability to absorb risk and pool capital, greater credibility in dealing with third parties, a greater market attractiveness and ability to negotiate beneficial arrangements with insurance companies and suppliers, and centralization of internal practice concerns such as quality control, cost containment and delegation of authority.

If individual and small group practices have worked so well in the past, why has the number of larger group practices increased in recent times? Many physicians question why they should consider leaving a stable environment over which they have some control for a collective where their opinion is only a single vote.

Physicians pondering an affiliation should consider a variety of factors.

[1] Control

Traditionally, a physician was able to maintain a good patient following simply by treating patients well and earning the reputation of being a good physician. Satisfied patients referred other patients, thereby rewarding the physician with a larger practice.

However, the business end of the physician-patient relationship has changed greatly. Today, patients opt to elect insurance coverage and plans that restrict their freedom of choice when selecting physicians, hospitals, pharmacies and other health care providers to take advantage of potential cost savings, such as a competitive monthly premium and lower or no deductibles on co-insurance. The small practice may not be able to compete for these patients, since it may not be able to give the third party a broad range of services and may not be able to absorb any type of risk. The larger group, though, generally is able to provide a broader range of services to third parties in spite of risks. In addition, a large group may be able to undertake a joint venture with a hospital and offer its own health care program.

[2] Organizational Credibility

Having a large, organized group gives the practice more power in dealing with other members of the health care community, such as hospitals and insurance companies. For example, a large group that refuses to participate with a particular insurance program may jeopardize that program. The insurance company, rather than see the program fail, will be more willing to deal with the group and make changes for the physicians.

With regard to hospitals, a large group represents a significant amount of potential revenue for in-patient hospital care. The standard of competition among hospitals being what it is, a large group may be able to negotiate favorable services from the hospital and favorable terms in joint venture negotiations. The larger group may also find itself readily courted by other hospitals seeking professional loyalty.

[3] Marketing

A large group will be able to afford a larger external marketing campaign and achieve a greater return for the dollars it invests. A large regional group, for example, could take advantage of media such as radio, television and metropolitan newspapers. While something like an advertisement in a metropolitan newspaper may be affordable to a small practice, the dollars may not achieve a full return since a number of the subscribers may be outside of the group's market area. If the reputation of the group grows positively, physicians joining the group automatically gain a sense of quality and patients gain confidence in them. The Mayo Clinic is perhaps the best example.

A large group has the option to expand its hours without placing an unjust burden on any one physician. By splitting and rotating shifts, all of the physicians can have nights off. At the same time, the clinic has expanded hours that directly compete with hospital emergency rooms and critical care centers. Expanded hours will help not only from a marketing standpoint, but they will also lower the facility cost by getting more use out of the equipment and space rental.

[4] Insurance Market

A large group in a joint venture with a hospital may be able to establish its own insurance or HMO coverage and eliminate the middle man, because typically 12 percent of the health care premium goes to administration. By becoming its own insurer the group can maintain control of those dollars, and if it wishes, use a percentage of the saved premium for re-insurance for unusual risk. Because of the risk factor, there is no feasible way for a small group or individual practice to establish a health insurance plan. Having a large, diversified group of multispecialists substantially spreads out the risk, as does the greater enrollment achieved through a large group.

[5] Quality Control

When a physician refers a service outside of his or her clinic, he or she loses a certain amount of control. Although the consultant physician may wish to adhere to the standards set by the referring physician, there is really no guarantee this will be possible. With the physicians all brought under one group, the quality of medical care can be controlled more easily. Having a form of quality control helps all of the doctors maintain a high level of care. Moreover, being reviewed by one's peers encourages the attempt to keep the methods of practice up to date.

[6] Cost Containment

Having a formal review system enables the group to use certain cost containment techniques. For example, a large group of many internists is better able to estimate the average cost per patient, including the frequency of ancillary services. Comparison of patient records permits monitoring and control of outside services and hospitalization.

[7] Economies of Scale

A large group, properly managed, can take advantage of certain economies of scale. Supplies, for example, may be bulk-ordered and inventoried to secure lower prices. Vendors may be more willing to discount the price of supplies for a major purchaser than they could or would for a small group.

Legal and accounting services will generally be smaller for one large group than they would be for many small groups and the fees for these services can be put to more productive uses, such as negotiating HMO contracts or making financial projections and feasibility studies. One large group will need only one corporate tax return, in contrast to the many returns required of a large number of individual practices. Instead of several pension and profit sharing plans representing all of the different practices, there need be only one.

Benefits may be purchased at a better rate for larger groups. Group life insurance, for example, is less expensive for a large group than for any small group. A large group may benefit both the physician employee and nonphysician employees through the implementation of a plan that allows individual employees to pick their own "menu" of benefits. Generally these plans are not feasible for a small doctor group or an individual practitioner.

A large group may eliminate duplication of work and thus the cost associated with the duplication of the facility, equipment and staff training. A large group uses equipment in ways that would not be feasible for a small group. This can lower the cost of performing a procedure.

[8] Delegation of Business Management

A large group may be able to afford a higher caliber of professional management than is usually seen in an individual practice. One physician or a small group of physicians cannot afford a high-powered business administrator, and such a person would not necessarily have enough work in a small group. In a large group, though, this type of arrangement may work out to everyone's advantage. A confident and knowledgable in-house administrator greatly benefits the clinic with new insights into the workings and problems of the clinic and the application of solid business techniques.

[9] Pooling Capital

Raising capital has not been traditionally a big issue for physicians, since medicine is considered a service business; however, having more physicians available to pool capital can help to achieve certain goals. Today more money is needed to manage and expand a successful medical practice. A large group, for example, may be able to pool money from numerous stockholders to launch a limited partnership, set up an HMO plan, purchase equipment or establish a marketing campaign.

§ 13.03 Consequences and Risks of Affiliation

> The consequences of creating a large group medical entity include the physician's loss of individual control over his or her practice, direct competition from a larger hospital for patients, the frequent inconvenience or mismanagement of bureaucratic systems, and the effect that regulations posed by providers such as Medicaid and Medicare may have on the new venture's profitability.

In the early stages of medical practice affiliations or associations with other professionals or hospitals certain consequences or even risks must be considered. Evaluating such consequences must be done to determine the actual risk they incur. That is, whether they are indeed dangers or simply disadvantages or potential disadvantages of the affiliation.

[1] Hospital Takeovers

From the perspective of a hospital, it is necessary to avoid empty beds in order to maintain an economic cost per patient. The only way for hospitals to achieve this is to have a large enough physician staff to serve patients. Hospitals have traditionally solved this problem by maintaining good relationships with physicians and providing quality service, but the risk exists that the hospital may benefit more by employing the physicians and thus controlling their medical services. Indeed in many areas of the country, hospitals directly compete with private physicians by establishing extended services in their emergency rooms and by establishing critical care centers as well as in the acquisition of medical practices. Physicians who wish to avoid this must remember that the entity that administers the patient load is also the entity that controls the medical services provided.

As more and more patients surrender their freedom to choose their own doctors by becoming involved in health plans that restrict movement between physicians, the traditional stronghold of the individual practitioner is shifting to the HMO, PPO or other medical groups.

[2] Loss of Individual Control

The individual practitioner can make decisions quickly and with no other physicians to account to; he or she can order equipment, hire or fire staff, change banks, change locations and so forth, without having to call meetings, attend committees or gather votes. Similarly, in many small groups one doctor has full control or the situation is such that practices within the group are kept separate and each physician maintains maximum control over his or her practice along with responsibility for decisions.

As more physicians become involved in a project or entity, a more democratic decision-making process must be employed. Although collective participation may result in better decision-making, many physicians are unable to accept this change in control of power. Physicians who find themselves unable to act upon a decision quickly because of a committee's inability to meet at that time may also feel frustrated.

[3] Inefficiency of Bureaucracies

As an organization grows large enough to develop a bureaucracy or hierarchy, some inefficiency results. The consistency and fairness necessary for a system of orderly decision- and policy-making for a larger group may mean productive time is lost attending meetings required to implement it. A larger organization generally cannot move at the swift speed of an individual practitioner. Additional costs are incurred by hiring administrative staff people or distracting current staff members from their principle duties with additional administration. An office staff that feels compelled to please all of the doctors all of the time will cause unnecessary waste.

[4] Mismanagement

When a large group is formed as a result of a merger, mismanagement may occur. Although the physicians may have been effective managers able to run their small practices well, they soon learn that different management techniques must be employed to run the merged practice. If the group is very large or if the joint venture is unusual, it may be difficult to find experienced staff members and other outside advisors to handle the situation.

Inexperienced accountants and attorneys, for example, could end up doing excessive research in handling unusual problems. The new group may become the victim charged for all of this extra time. Worse yet, advisors may not do a thorough job of researching and thus create problems with the IRS and other government agencies by committing such errors as poorly structured buy-sell agreements.

Finding competent in-house management may also be difficult. It will take individuals who are not only experienced in health care and apprised of its current changes, but also people who are innovative and strong leaders. Current staff members unable to adapt to the new office must be helped through the changing situation in order for them to remain effective. Work must be evaluated to make sure that it is not being duplicated by different staff members.

[5] Medicare and Medicaid Regulations

A thorough review of reimbursement laws should be made to determine whether the new medical entity or joint venture would cause lower reimbursement, or worse be construed as an illegal business arrangement. Regulations on Medicare, for example, prohibit physicians from making money on services they refer. This would mean a primary care physician could not refer a Medicare patient to an outside pathology laboratory of which he or she is a partner.

§ 13.04 Is an Affiliation Right for You?

An individual or small group practitioner should give thought to a number of factors before getting involved in a group affiliation. From the standpoint of professional philosophies, these would include compatibility with other potential candidates, mutual goals and the way in which merger formation is approached.

Before deciding upon a merger or affiliation, a physician should take time to study the situation and determine whether all of the right ingredients are present. Certain issues should be reviewed to increase the probability of a good merger, and alternatives to the affiliation—such as contracting—should be explored.

[1] Compatibility

Obviously, the compatibility of the participating physicians must be carefully considered. An affiliation or merger should not even be discussed if participants do not believe they will work well together; in large groups, however, even if some members do not get along with members of another group, an overall sense of compatibility may not be absent. While it is unrealistic to expect no personality conflicts or clashes in a larger group, the new situation must be one in which the doctors will at least respect and be able to work with one another. The business plans of the participants should be reviewed for compatibility. Are the plans of the potential affiliate congruent or mutually exclusive? If the plans are not totally compatible, can they be slightly modified so that everyone's goals may be achieved? For this reason, the first step of any proposed merger should be to outline individual business plans.

[2] Goal Evaluation

In many cases, evaluating goals may be difficult if they were never clarified and clearly identified by the individual practices and physicians at the outset. Each doctor's list of goals should be specific. For example, most physicians, when asked about their professional goals, simply list providing "quality medical care." This is a laudable but rather abstract goal.

Every evaluation should spell out at least these goals:

- number of hours desired to work
- attitude toward coverage
- attitude toward personal earnings from practice
- attitude toward various third parties such as general medical insurers, HMOs, PPOs, IPAs (Individual Practice Associations), Medicare, etc.
- attitude toward types of practice, that is, single specialty, multispecialty, small, large, or medium practice, etc.
- attitude toward practice promotion and advertising
- attitude toward ratio of staff to physicians and utilization of staff, such as medical assistants, nurses and physicians' assistants

- attitude toward overhead control and spending
- attitude toward collection techniques and physicians' financial responsibilities
- attitude toward basic medical reimbursement systems, for example, fee-for-service versus capitation (per capita payment or fee)

[3] Approach

Once it appears that an affiliation will be satisfactory the best means of bringing it about should be decided. In some cases, it may be appropriate to merge the practices immediately. In other cases, it may be appropriate to approach the merger by steps in order to give all of the doctors a chance to see how they work will together. With a step-by-step approach, merger candidates start out working together in a joint venture, which could be simply a matter of setting up an efficient coverage system. The next step toward forming a merger group would be to set up a physician practice group. The physician practice group could handle the complex issues such as dealing with the HMOs and third parties while the physicians maintain their individual practices.

The final phase in the merger toward affiliation would be the gradual delegation of authority to the physician practice group while lessening the duties of the individual practice. The safety factor in this step-by-step approach is that during the early stages it allows the physician for whom the merger does not seem to be working to leave the group.

§ 13.05 Choosing Partners

A merger should not be attempted if the business interests of partners do not correspond. Specifically, interested parties should compare views on quality of medical care they hope to provide and its effect on cost containment, what specialties if any the group will offer, whether a fee-for-service or capitation arrangement is to be used for compensation, and what attitudes are held on the interaction of personal and professional life.

When developing a merger plan, the first step is to choose the physician-partners or eventual merger candidates. The potential participant should consider several criteria.

[1] Level of Quality

It is important to study the level and type of quality health care each potential participant provides. Physicians often differ in their philosophies of how to provide health care. For example, some believe that the highest level can only be achieved by conducting a full scope of laboratory tests, "leaving no stone unturned," while others believe that resorting to tests that may not yield a "highly probable" diagnosis are a waste of time and money. Another area where physicians may differ is in the delegation of work; that is, some believe that a physician must do all of the patient contact work while others prefer to utilize nurses and medical assistants whenever possible.

It is common for physicians to differ on these and other issues. And a certain amount of difference is beneficial to the group because it creates a balance. However, if attitudes and philosophies differ too greatly, then disharmony in the group is likely. An example of this is when a physician feels uncomfortable about an inter-group referral because of total disagreement with the colleagues's patient care.

[2] Specialties

Group specialties must be considered. Will the group be a single or multispecialty group? Will the group be a primary care group or simply a specialty group?

Because of the current pressure on physicians to maintain costs, primary care physicians tend to develop multispecialty groups. If the referred specialists are not part of the group, it is more difficult for the primary care physicians to control the costs after referral.

An adequate number of patients must be maintained in order for a multispecialty group to be feasible. Most specialists rely on referrals from different primary care physicians—sometimes competitors—for patients. However, the primary care physician would like to be sure that the specialist will send back the patient after the specialist services are completed. If the specialist is a member of a primary care group, the referrals from others may decrease substantially or be eliminated altogether. This results from an obvious fear that once the patient enters the practice, he or she will find all needs met in that group and may not go back to the referring doctor.

Thus, as a practical matter, before a specialist is added to a group, there must be enough patient volume among the primary care physicians. Unless the merger is substantial, it may take a number of years to build up a multispecialty group. The eventual direction of the merged group should always be considered to make sure that all of the doctors share common goals and to study the feasibility of opening the group to hire or acquire another specialty or medical practice.

[3] Fees and Costs

Review of the fees and costs of the merger candidates is essential. Although individual fee schedules generally vary, if they differ greatly it could create problems. Physicians with higher fees undoubtedly will be unwilling to lower them for fear of losing income while the lower fee doctors may not wish to raise their fees for fear of losing their patients. Physicians with lower fees also may be faced with certain restrictions in raising their fees, such as third party contracts or government freezes (for example, the 1984 Medicare freeze). Because it would not be easy to administer or justify multifee schedules, it is important that a uniform fee schedule be established for the practice. There may, of course, be different fees in a multispecialty group where the specialist's fees differ from the primary care physicians' fees.

The costs and overhead of the practices of the candidates planning the merger must also be considered when items like staffing, wage scales, equipment and facility costs are compared. Again, a medical practice with a low overhead may be unwilling to accept the high overhead figure of another practice, while the higher overhead practice may be unwilling to make necessary cuts to bring the practice into an acceptable range. If there is a huge gap in the overhead percentage of the practices, the issue should be studied carefully to detect substantial philosophical differences in spending. Comparative expense reports can help in the identification and discussion of major differences.

[4] Fee-for-Service versus Capitation

Traditionally, physicians' fees have been based on fee-for-service. In the late 1940s, began the growth of third party payments; that is, where payment was no longer made to the physician directly from the patient. During the 1970s, there was an attempt among physicians to emphasize direct payment from the patient and request that patients seek their reimbursement from the third parties.

Today with the growth of capitation reimbursement (a uniform per capita payment) for physician services, more and more physicians are facing the need to operate under a capitation reimbursement plan.

Many physicians oppose the capitation method of reimbursement citing the philosophical disagreement of putting too many financial pressures on the physician and limiting the physician's options in treating the patient. Other physicians view capitation as a method that efficiently lowers the cost of medical care by eliminating the insurer, and financially rewarding the physician for cost savings.

The economics of the fee-for-service system versus the capitation system vary and must be recognized by the medical practices that plan to affiliate or merge. Physicians unwilling to recognize or accept the economics of a particular system chosen by the group should not become involved. It would be too difficult for physicians opposed to the system of capitation to work with physicians who feel the system is an important part of the future of health care delivery.

[5] Goal Evaluation

The goals of the merger candidates should be reviewed and discussed:

- What are the long-term goals and expectations of each potential merger candidate and how will the merger help him or her to achieve it?
- Will the group be a single or multispecialty group?
- Will the group be a fee-for-service or capitation group, or a combination of the two?

- Will the group continue to grow through the recruitment of physicians or through the acquisition of other medical practices and other practice mergers?
- Do the eventual plans of the merger include acquisition of other medically-related entities, such as hospitals, pharmacies or health insurance plans, or becoming a candidate for acquisition by another entity?

Short term goals should be evaluated too, specifically:

- What are the physicians' expectations over the next two to five years?
- Will the merger get them there?
- Are senior physicians unwilling to take short-term financial cuts, since their future needs may not include remaining in practice, while younger members are more concerned about the welfare of the practice ten years hence?

All of the goals and expectations of the merger candidates should be listed and reviewed, and a master plan should be established so that everyone knows the direction in which the group plans to grow.

[6] Work Attitudes

Although most successful physicians work long hours, there is still a difference in attitude among physicians about the number of hours they will remain on call. Some physicians are able to tolerate night after night of being on call and seemingly endless patient service; others believe it is unreasonable for the physician to be on call more than one night per week. Individual practices or fee-for-service groups automatically compensate physicians who provide more services. If this compensation system is dropped in favor of giving equal shares, disagreement can occur if physicians who are on call more often feel they are carrying the lion's share of the overhead or otherwise not receiving the full benefit of their labor. Such a clash of work attitudes can lead to disharmony in the group and upset the balance between professional and personal life-styles initially established by the entire group.

The volume of services performed and the hours worked should be reviewed to identify any significant discrepancies and to see if there is an acceptable way to compensate participants who wish to work longer hours. If too many discrepancies become apparent, the merger may eventually break apart.

[7] Personal Attitudes

One of the most important yet difficult evaluations of potential merger candidates is whether or not the candidate is a "team player." Some physicians work best alone and would never be happy with or truly benefit from the merged entity. Physicians should consider how they and the other candidates will respond to other physicians, to hospital committees, medical asssociations and other bureaucracies. The physician must remember that what is best for the group may not equally benefit all of the physicians all of the time.

§ 13.06 Initial Obstacles

> Early obstacles to unifying a number of practices into a single entity usually involve the pre-existing arrangements of the individual practices. Once it is determined that a merger will violate no antitrust regulations, pre-existing practice liabilities and commitments must be investigated; also the practicality of integrating offices, combining and adapting systems and purging redundancies must be studied. Equally important is to consider how the new entity will finance any necessary changes in current office systems.

Once the merger candidates have been selected, potential obstacles to the merger must be studied. The earlier that obstacles are identified, the greater the probability they can be overcome.

[1] Contingent Liabilities

Contingent liabilities are liabilities that do not show up on the balance sheet. Contingent liabilities can range from a physician's professional association guaranteeing a bank loan on a personal yacht to a malpractice claim pending against both the physician and the professional association.

The most serious and largest contingent liability would be a malpractice claim. Each physician should fill out a questionnaire similar to the one completed for a malpractice application that inquires about any pending claims, judgments or even threats of malpractice suits. All of the business contracts signed by the physician on behalf of the physician's professional association should be reviewed by legal counsel to see if there are potential claims, such as capitation paybacks. With some health care plans, it is not uncommon for the physician to be at risk for an amount greater than unpaid reimbursement or capitation (sometimes without even being aware that such a liability is pending).

The corporate records of the practice should be examined by legal counsel for resolutions authorizing the physician's professional association to make loans or guarantee any loans. It may be appropriate to check with the authorized bank to make sure that all loans are reported on the balance sheet. In one recent case, a doctor's professional association was held liable for substantial debts that did not show up on the balance sheet. The cash created by this debt had been directly placed in another of the doctor's businesses of which the accountant was unaware.

Potential tax liabilities should be considered. Individual practices or small groups may have taken aggressive tax positions on issues that are still subject to potential audits. If the IRS disallows deductions for them, it suddenly becomes the responsibility of the new entity to "pick up the tab."

[2] Business Entanglements

In many situations, a physician's corporation and business may have been set up originally with no intent to merge but simply to benefit the owner physician or owner group. Because of this, certain "entanglements" may need to be examined prior to merger.

For example, the physicians of a small group have set up a computer billing company for the benefit of the group, Although the computer company had a number of users before the merger the major user was the small group, which is under contract with the computer company. The computer company is unable to meet the needs of the new merged group and the physician owner cannot afford the loss of the small group as a customer. Similar situations have occurred with separate and independently owned optical shops or laboratories.

Another example of a more complicated entanglement is the physician who has equipment partnerships with lease arrangements with a medical corporation. This situation is compounded by the leases having been put into a trust for the physician's children on either a permanent basis or on a Clifford Trust ten-year basis. This illustrates, again, how the needs of the new entity may not be consistent with the need of the pre-merged entity. If contracts have been weighted in favor of the trust for tax purposes, other physicians may be unwilling to accept excessive lease payments.

Other situations could include independent deals made by the practice. It is not uncommon for physicians to work out arrangements with hospitals to provide certain services. The hospitals may not be willing to either continue these arrangements with the new entity or release the small group from the contract.

[3] Antitrust Regulations

Because most individual practices are relatively small, most physicians would never think they could be subject to antitrust regulations. The merger of a medical practice, however, is not unlike any business merger and if the new entity will control a significant share of the market, the likelihood of antitrust problems arises. Therefore, it is important for the antitrust regulations to be reviewed prior to merger.

Physicians should remember that actively taking steps to create a monopoly or entering into a merger that will substantially lessen the competition violates federal antitrust laws. The merged entity will be considered in violation if, after the merger, the new entity has a 60 percent market share. The market share is based on the number of patients serviced by the new group rather than the ratio of doctors in the new group to the total community.

Legal counsel knowledgeable in the area of antitrust laws should be consulted on possibile antitrust violations or accusations of violation. If legal advisors feel there is the slightest chance that an antitrust violation could occur, it is advisable to seek further opinions from the Justice Department and Federal Trade Commission. These opinions, if favorably rendered, indicate that the government will take no action and their opinions are called "no action" letters. If the government issues a no action letter, though, this is not complete protection, since a private lawsuit could be brought against the new entity by disgruntled competitors, hospitals or third parties. The letters, however, can be used as strong evidence that the antitrust laws have not been violated.

Unfortunately, obtaining these letters can be time consuming and expensive. The physician should not be frustrated if, after the submission of full details, the government comes back to the physician's attorneys requesting more information before it will issue the letter. Physicians who fail to obtain no action letters may incur a private or government lawsuit which will cost a great deal in legal fees or may even result in breaking up the group practice.

[4] Integrating Offices

How the merging entities will integrate must be considered. For example, if physicians within a group do not receive the same hospital privileges, they will be unable to cover for each other within that hospital. If the medical group is large enough, then not every doctor needs to be on the staff at every hospital the group has an arrangement with. However, there must be enough doctors on staff to provide adequate patient coverage. With hospitals beginning to limit privileges this could become a problem. In some areas of the country, it may be best if all of the physicians receive privileges at all of the hospitals that the group will be dealing with in order to forestall any such problems.

To facilitate the integration of each office, each staff member's duties should be evaluated and detailed in a job description. Job descriptions can be compared to see where employees' duties overlap. This is not only necessary to eliminate redundancy, but also to create order and direction. For example, if two insurance clerks responsible for processing forms continue to do so in the manner to which they were accustomed in the pre-merger entity, the new entity is headed for trouble unless direction is given. In some cases, the employee's position may be eliminated and he or she may be assigned to a different position with different responsibilities. The merger makes it necessary to evaluate office staff. If a doctor wishes to "protect" any employees whose work seems redundant, the physician should provide a full explanation and suggestions for other work the employee may do.

Office systems also need to be examined. Are any of the physicians unwilling or unable to change their personal systems?

Unlike the individual or small group practice, different types of office systems as well as equipment are needed to serve a larger group entity. For example, will the current bookkeeping system meet the needs of the merged entity, or is a new system necessary? What will become of investments in areas such as office computers, typewriters, copy machines, etc.?

The new entity should be candid when identifying the the pre-merger systems that are worth continuing and those that will need to be changed because they will not work within the new entity.

[5] Financing

The new entity should also ask the following questions regarding financing of the new venture:

- Are the physicians in a position to put enough money into the new entity to cover the initial costs?
- Who will absorb the cost of previous commitments no longer needed, such as office space leases, equipment leases, service contracts, etc?

In some cases, the inability or unwillingness to finance some of the initial up-front costs could ruin the merger.

§ 13.07 Establishing Time-Frames

Since a merger often takes years to complete, it is wise to create a schedule to help transactions proceed in orderly steps. The first two steps should be to elect a steering committee to give the merger process a direction and to choose an advisory team, often from the individual practices' accountants and lawyers, to estimate budget projections, cost-sharing and profit distribution arrangements, evaluate individual inventories and generally clean up the loose ends that a gradual integration of practices may cause. An all-important part of this schedule should be the creation of a pre-merger agreement that explains what liabilities the individual practices will be responsible for regardless of whether the merger is approved.

A list of incremental steps and tentative time-frames for completing the merger should be created. Merging practices should be prepared for a long process. Only the simplest situations can be completed in less than 12 months while others, in many cases, not for years. The following list contains major items to which time-frames should be assigned.

(1) Choosing the medical specialties to be included in the group
(2) Identifing specific doctors for the group
(3) Appointing a steering committee
(4) Establishing an advisory team:
- legal
- accountant
- medical management consultant

(5) Establishing cost-sharing arrangements:
- opening a checkbook
- doctors' contributions
- appointing treasurer

(6) Entering the pre-merger agreement:
- letter of agreement between participating physicians

(7) Making budget and financial projections:
- income statements
- balance sheets

(8) Selecting an organizational set-up:
- merger, consolidation or acquisition
- new practice name
- fiscal year
- ownership ratios
- officers and responsibilities

(9) "Cleaning-up" current entities
- reviewing balance sheets
- divesting stockholder loans
- eliminating cars and other unnecessary assets
- hidden assets
- accounts receivable true-value using consistent formula
- prepaid expenses

- prepaid professional liability insurance, prepaid rent, rent deposits
- inventories
- tax refunds and credits
- future tax savings through loss carry-over deductions

(10) Evaluating the practice

(11) Entering profit distribution and buy-sell agreements

(12) Establishing personnel policy, personnel and wage scales

(13) Establishing unified systems

(14) Establishing a fee schedule while anticipating and watching profile changes

(15) Developing a system of centralized purchasing

(16) Setting up telephone systems

(17) Establishing equipment and facility

(18) Announcing merger

(19) Beginning merged practice

[1] Electing a Steering Committee

A steering committee of three to five doctors should be elected and empowered to make major decisions for the new entity. Although the idea of giving up control may not appeal to some physicians, it must be remembered that it is impossible to try to get everyone's opinion and vote on every issue.

On the other hand, the steering committee is responsible for the decisions they make and frequent reports should be sent out to the members at large. If the general membership is dissatisfied with the actions of the steering committee, a general meeting can be held and the steering committee can be asked to account for its actions or a new steering committee can be elected.

[2] Establishing the Advisory Team

It is likely that the merger candidates will have their own advisory team of accountants, attorneys and consultants and there will be some overlap of services. The new merged group will need to select an advisory team to guide them through the legal, tax and management traps of the merger.

The advisory team may consist of consultants already being used by the individual practices, or possibly hitherto unaffiliated people. The advisors should be selected by a committee on the basis of their availability, knowledge and experience in this type of medical merger. In particular, attention should be paid to the experience they have in the specific area of medical practice mergers; also what resources the advisors have available in areas in which they have the least experience. In addition to the usual problems a medical practice faces, the new entity will have the initial problems of the actual merger to contend with. In some areas of the country, consulting firms have put together specialized health care management teams that also focus on the financial, legal and management sides of practice. When possible, these firms should be sought out.

[3] Cost-Sharing Arrangements

After the steering committee has been established, it will be necessary to set up a means of funding the new entity. A checking account should be opened and a treasurer appointed. Each of the physicians should contribute an equal amount (normally, a minimum of $1000) to generate enough cash flow to hire advisors and commence other activities. The treasurer should produce a monthly report on the cash flow, that is, the receipt and use of funds. This is important because members of the group who do not know how the money is being spent are unlikely to make additional contributions.

[4] Budget and Projections

The steering committee should begin working with the accountants to make financial projections. At this time it will be necessary for the accountants to gather as much information as possible in order to do an accurate job. All of the physicians' financial reports, including summaries of charges and collections, need to be gathered. The accountants and attorneys will need to look for short-term additional costs such as the redundancy of space and equipment as the result of leases. Three sets each of income statements and balance sheets should be prepared: for best case, worst case and probable case scenarios. Based on the projections, the available distribution per doctor should be calculated so that the physicians can equate what effect the merger might have on their personal income.

[5] Organizational Set-Up

Attorneys and accountants should also be consulted to determine whether the entity would function best as a merger, consolidation or acquisition, the definitions for which are briefly recapitulated here:

Merger—when the only surviving company is one of the original companies.

Consolidation—when a new corporate enterprise is organized for the purpose of acquiring the net assets of the other companies.

Acquisition—when one firm exchanges its ownership securities for the ownership securities of another firm and both firms continue their legal existence.

These are legal definitions; in the medical field the terms are used somewhat synonymously for any type of business combination, except when there is a specific objective in identifying the specific way in which the entities are combined.

The new practice must have a new name. Undoubtedly, a generic name (Midtown Medical Group) will be more advantageous than mentioning every physician in the new entity.

A fiscal year should be selected. For tax purposes it is generally beneficial to have a fiscal year other than the calendar year. If some of the pre-merger entities work on calendar years, this too should be changed and merged into a fiscal year organization.

Ownership ratios must be determined. For example, will all of the doctors be equal owners, or will there be other considerations? If the doctors are to become equal owners, they should consider how to handle the value of different net assets.

[6] "Clean-Up" of Current Entities

The owners of the separate pre-merger entities should meet with their accountants and attorneys to identify all potential problems on their balance sheets and begin to identify all hidden assets and liabilities.

Stockholder loans should be paid up. The new entity is not going to want to inherit the assets of a doctor who owes money. Miscellaneous assets, such as office decorations and corporate cars, should be identified and removed from the balance sheet.

The proper legal documentation should be created to record all of the transactions, and minutes should be brought up to date along with corporate resolutions and documentation of any unusual items. Hidden assets of the corporation should be identified. Since most individual practices are on a cash basis, the accounts receivable carries a zero balance and does not show up on the balance sheet; likewise, inventories.

A uniform method for valuing the accounts receivable should be established by the new entity's advisors and be applied to each participant. The accounts receivable should be aged and properly valued, and uncollectable third party accounts, such as Medicare and Medicaid, should be identified and written off.

Most physicians will be surprised by the value of their inventories. The decision to "run down" inventories right before the merger date to minimize the valuation can also help eliminate the problem of each doctor carrying over different types of supplies from his or her pre-merger practice. The new entity will want to have centralized purchasing to maximize efficiency and minimize cost.

Other areas of hidden assets include prepaid expenses such as malpractice insurance, prepaid rent, rent deposits, unused tax credits, tax deposits and net operating loss carry forwards.

[7] Accounting and Legal Plan to Carry Out the Merger

Copies of the "cleaned up" balance sheets and balance sheets of the merger should be submitted to the new entity's advisors so they can prepare a strategy to allow the organization to occur under IRS Code Section 354. Under Section 354, the reorganization can be done without tax liability. Normally, the transfer of assets and interest in business entities results in a taxable gain; with proper strategy, this can be avoided.

[8] Valuations

Experience has shown that for merger purposes, there are basically two valuation approaches. The first is the casual approach in which it is recognized that all participants will contribute to the new entity and thus everyone is going to be an equal member. This may work out well if the accounts receivable, equipment, practice size, etc. of the pre-merger medical practices are relatively similar. If discrepancies exist, though, the larger the differences among the practices, the greater the chance that the casual approach will create more problems than it eliminates. Therefore, a more rational, systematic approach must be taken in most cases.

Basically, the items to consider in valuating the practice are (See also Ch. 3, for a discussion of valuation of practices):

- furniture and equipment
- supply inventories
- accounts receivable
- real estate
- leasehold improvements
- cash and securities
- miscellaneous assets (including hidden assets)
- reducing the assets and liabilities, including the following common liabilities:

    payroll taxes

    accounts payable

    equipment and other loans

    lease commitments

The steering committee should select the valuation approach formula to be followed. The accountants, attorneys and management consultants will be able to propose formulas. Direction should then be given to commence the valuation.

[9] Pre-Merger Agreement

The doctors should enter into a pre-merger agreement that contains the following items:

(1) A statement acknowledging that each wishes to merge his or her practice into a single corporation.

(2) An agreement that if the proposed merger does not take place, the pre-merger costs be shared equally. The pre-merger costs are the costs incurred to determine the feasibility of the merger and to help arrange the various merger details. They would not include any items of practice overhead or expenses which would not have been incurred had the merger discussions not commenced.

(3) An agreement that, should the merger not take place, the confidential information gained from pre-merger negotiations will not be used in any way to the detriment of the other parties.

(4) An agreement that any liabilities assessed against the previously owned corporations, including tax liabilities, contract liabilities, malpractice, etc., will be the responsibility of the original owner. Each should agree to hold the other harmless and indemnify the new entity against any final liabilities for fees, costs and expenses incurred in defending such claims. Since such liabilities should not affect the income or assets of the other doctors, each should agree to adjust to the respective compensation, dividends, assets or other benefits that result from such expenses.

(5) An agreement to split up the cost of liabilities including tax liabilities which are a result of the merger.

(6) Each should agree to free access to each the records of each physcian including accounts receivable, production records, income statements, balance sheets, malpractice insurance policies, corporate record books and contracts.

(7) An agreement that the pre-merger agreement will be a binding legal agreement.

[10] Profit Distribution System

A profit distribution method must be decided upon and a system to implement it established. Now is the time to re-think profit distribution to make sure that it meets the needs of the new practice.

Traditionally, physicians have favored incentive compensation to ensure that productive physicians are properly compensated. This has been a very successful, workable approach for many years. However, in large groups with capitated arrangements, profit distribution based on physician charges may no longer be workable. (See also Ch. 3, for various methods of profit distribution using three different criteria; also Fig. 3-5).

The new group should consider rewarding physicians who spend time on management of the practice. Without this incentive physicians will not want to spend time away from patient-care even for necessary management. Physician groups exceeding 50 physicians may need to consider having one physician as a full time "chief executive" who practices little or no medicine but monitors the profit distribution system.

For the large merged group, the following elements should be included in profit distribution:

- ownership
- leadership
- base salary for medical duties
- productivity formula
- efficiency
- cost effectiveness

Cost effectiveness and efficiency are extremely important, especially for practices with capitated plans.

§ 13.08 Restrictive Covenants

Restrictive covenants should be agreed upon in advance of a final merger in order to prevent participating physicians from spinning off and becoming competitors.

To ensure the survival of the new practice it will be necessary for the participating physicians to be fully committed to it. The doctors should consider implementing a restrictive covenant, or a covenant that prohibits member physicians from going out and competing with the group. Once these agreements have been signed, the physician has made an important commitment to the new group.

Because traditionally patients are loyal to individual physicians rather than the medical group, per se, the established physician has always had the option of leaving if he or she did not like the way things were run. The threat of financial action or injunction against a physician who leaves the group in order to organize a competitive practice increases the commitment to the present group. Once restrictive covenants are signed by all of the physicians, the goodwill or overall value of the medical entity should increase.

Having all of the physicians sign restrictive covenants also facilitates mandating restrictive covenants for the new, junior associates brought into the group. (See also Ch. 3, for restrictive covenants for associates.)

§ 13.09 Noncorporate Legal Agreements and Documents

Noncorporate agreements on distribution of income and buying out or selling the share of partners are protected from scrutiny by the IRS.

Legal agreements that would not be directly affiliated with the corporation (and thus not subject to investigation under an IRS audit of the corporation) should include:

(1) an agreement, to be signed by the shareholders, designating the way in which income is to be distributed; specifically, the agreements covered under the profit distribution section above, would be set out in a legal document available to the shareholders.

(2) buy-sell agreements among the shareholders restricting the sale of stock, creating a formula or method to value the stock and to create an orderly transition of equity in any of the following events:

- death of a stockholder
- disability of a stockholder
- a stockholder losing his or her license to practice medicine
- termination of employment with the group

§ 13.10 Establishing the New Entity

Once a merger is made final it must be approved by the Secretary of State. The entity usually acquires a new name and phone number. New systems should be established for integrating employee duties and pay levels, for evaluating staff duties and performance and for rotation of physicians through hospital and other facilities. The new entity can benefit greatly from the advice of a post-merger advisory board chosen from among the physicians' business associates to function as the merged entity's board of directors.

A corporation should be prepared to conduct the business of the merged entity. If the new medical group is a consolidation or a physicians practice group, a new corporation is created. In the event of a merger, one of the pre-merger corporations is selected to continue business.

A name for the new entity must be approved by the Secretary of State to ensure that no other business already uses it and to prevent anyone else from using it once it is approved.

A new corporation must also obtain corporate identification numbers. An application with the State Department of Unemployment must be completed for the new entity to assume the unemployment rate of the pre-merger entities, and a fiscal year must be adopted.

Corporate records must be updated to reflect all of the new corporation's events, beginning with the merger itself; the board of directors and officers of the corporation must be elected; and employment agreements must be drafted and signed by each of the participating physicians. (See Ch. 3, for the checklist on forming a general corporation.)

[1] Post-Merger Advisory Boards

With the new practice facing new and larger challenges, the doctors should consider developing an independent board of advisors different from the board of directors. The advisory board is simply a group of individual, independent advisors who will advise the practice, but the practice will be under no obligation to follow the advice of the board, nor will the board be held responsible for any actions of the corporation.

The advisory board should be made up of outside business people whom the doctors know and trust, perhaps from among candidates such as:

- the corporation's bank president
- an executive of a large industrial company
- a commercial business consultant

- a professor from a local university's business school
- an executive from a marketing consulting firm or advertising agency
- an attorney
- an insurance broker or benefit consultant

The executive advisory board members will be asked to function as an official board of directors. They will be provided with the detailed financial information, financial projections and group goals of the practice.

During the first advisory board meeting, a presentation to the board should be given to outline the history of the practice, the goals of the practice and the purpose of the advisory board. A successful presentation will excite board members about the practice and make them anxious to contribute ideas.

The second meeting should be scheduled to provide the advisory board with in-depth information including financial projections and marketing plans. Thereafter, the advisory group should meet quarterly. The well-chosen advisory board will not only help provide a wealth of new ideas for the group, it may also help the group avoid making errors.

Advisory board members should be financially compensated for each meeting.

[2] Rotatation of Doctors

Plan on the rotation of doctors through the facilities. This will allow staff and patients to establish loyalties to all of doctors and the clinic.

Another important reason for the rotation of physicians is that it helps to minimize the opportunity for a physician or group of physicians to spin off from the main group and form an independent, competitive practice. Initially, some physicians may view this process negatively, but those interested in the success of the merged practice will see how they and the group will benefit.

[3] Pay Levels

A committee should be formed to review the wage levels for staff members and to integrate personnel benefits.

Once all jobs in the clinic are defined, a comprehensive list of salaries is drawn up with a range assigned to each category. Periodically, the salary ranges should be re-evaluated and raised to keep pace with cost of living increases; otherwise salary increases should be limited to the maximum amount in the employee's job category. Once an employee is receiving the maximum salary allowed for a particular job category, he or she would be limited to cost of living raises or promoted to a position with a higher salary scale.

Next it is necessary to evaluate the fringe benefits that were provided by the pre-merger practices and coordinate them. This evaluation will prevent redundancy, and help to devise a reasonable plan that is both affordable to the clinic and not perceived as a loss of benefits to employees. In some cases it may be necessary for employees to lose benefits if one of the pre-merger practices offers excessive fringe benefits because of its small size. In the best case scenario, the new benefit package will at least equal the employees' old packages and perhaps be better.

In some cases it is possible to implement flexible benefit plans that offer the employee a variety to choose from within a certain dollar range. A benefit consultant or insurance advisor should work with the committee to reveal all pre-merger plans and set up a new combined plan. Duplication of coverage should be avoided whenever possible.

[4] Staff Evaluation

It is necessary to evaluate all current staff members and their duties and responsibilities, particularly employees whose jobs overlap or whose positions will be eliminated. Employees with overlapping jobs will need to be given new assignments or terminated. For example, employees whose job was to type up insurance forms may find their job eliminated by the merger because the clinic now uses an automated billing system. However, these employees may be well-suited to perform other business duties, such as a third-party follow up on delinquent accounts or other typing jobs.

A new office manager and administrator should be selected from within the pool of employees if possible. These key employees can then complete the task of new job assignments, duties and responsibilities. Where there is overlap of administrative or managerial duties it may be possible to make some personnel assistants. If not, it may be necessary to terminate positions.

The new entity needs to establish a personnel policy unifying all of the employees. This policy should explain the new chain of command along with all other necessary items. (See also Ch. 2.)

[5] Unified Office Systems

Since it will be necessary to establish unified office systems, now is the time to clean up any problems in the old system: outdated and awkward systems should be thrown away, old charting systems should be replaced with new ones, antiquated bookkeeping systems should be up-dated with computerization, unified routing slips should be adopted by all departments. In particular, the following systems usually need to be reviewed and adopted:

- telephone answering and message systems
- appointment scheduling systems
- uniform patient charting
- standardized billing system
- standardized routing slips
- standardized collection policy
- standardized dictation processing
- standardized information systems
- standardized recall systems
- standardized letterhead and business cards

[6] Profile Changes

Each practice has a pre-merger profile against which the new merged practice profile can be checked. At present, a substantial portion of fee reimbursements come from third parties, making it important that profiles given after the merger be correct.

The new profiles should generally be weighted as an average of the previous profiles. Inquiries should be made into any fee charged at a lower rate than allowed by the weighted average.

Generally, a copy of the profile may be obtained from third parties upon request. (See also Ch. 7, which provides an overview of profiles and their impact.)

[7] Centralized Purchasing

A system of centralized purchasing helps the new enterprise maximize efficiency, avoid duplication and take advantage of volume discounts. A staff member should be delegated the authority to negotiate purchases within the guidelines established for the quality of supplies. Although it may seem like a minor detail, a specific supplier can make a significant difference in the overhead of the group or merged practice. It should be one of the goals to reduce costs through implementation of proper systems.

An example of the type of problem faced by the new, larger clinic is the situation in which one of the participating physicians prefers the most expensive items for his or her patients, because the physician believes the less expensive ones are not of adequate quality. High quality surgical gloves or specimen cups may seem reasonable and affordable for a small practice, but it can pose a problem for a larger, merged practice. If the person responsible for supplies, tired of constant complaints from the physicians and working without budgetary guidelines begins ordering top-grade supplies for all items, the result is high overhead rather than the decrease anticipated through the merger.

[8] Telephone.

A new merged practice may overlook installing an adequate phone system. The receptionist will be swamped by the multiplicity of calls, and as is often the case in a new multispecialty practice, their complexity. Moreover, previous phone configurations may prove inadequate for the new merged group and because most physicians own or lease their phones rather than rent them, additional cost may be incurred in disposing of pre-merger systems.

Phone needs of the new office should be anticipated early. For example, it may be necessary at the new office to have an operator answer phones and route calls to the proper departments. Interdepartmental conference systems may be desirable, so may phone-line hook-ups that perform computer billings and receive information from remote offices, or access to data banks such as research libraries.

Once these needs are defined alternative proposals and bids should be sought from at least three firms and the trade-in value on old phone systems considered. Once a number of proposals that meet all of the clinic's requirements are defined, the choice of which phone system should be chosen is based on the following criteria:

(1) price amortized over five years.

(2) phone service contracts and how quickly needs can be responded to if there is a breakdown.

(3) the flexibility of the system for future expansion (can the phone be upgraded without substantial cost and, if not, can the phone be traded in without substantial loss).

Since the clinic will have to choose a new phone system, pre-merger phone numbers need to be phased out. Considering that patients probably have the old numbers recorded in various places, a phase-out period of one to two years in which dialing the old number will give the user the new one is recommended.

§ 13.11 Public Relations

Because a large medical entity has greater resources for publicity, some thought should be given to advertising the new medical affiliation in the local business community. Publicity should be timed so that no one will be unduly surprised by the merger; also it should not be so early that embarrassment would result if the merger were not approved.

An initial decision must be made as to whether or not merger talks will be kept secret or announced to the staff and general public. In making the decision consider the advantages of keeping communication open:

- The doctors will not feel they are involved in a "cloak-and-dagger" operation. They will be free to discuss nonconfidential details with key staff and business people.

- If the merger is completed, the doctors will not have to worry about accusations from staff or other doctors that they were kept uninformed.
- People radically opposed to the merger will be able to share opinions prior to the merger consummation.
- If the staff feels they have been informed and involved in the merger their cooporation in making it work is likely to be greater.

However, the disadvantages of keeping an open line of communication should also be considered:

- Individuals or entities threatened by the proposed merger (a hospital that fears a physician group will wield too much power) may take steps to undermine it.
- Practices not involved with the merger could feel threatened and take steps to aggressively compete, perhaps deflating some of the potential impact of the new merged entity.
- Possible embarrassment in the event that the merger talks fall apart and the merger never takes place.

Once the merger is near completion, it is important that a public relations strategy be developed and set in motion. The first step is to prepare the medical community for the merger. Participating physicians should begin seeking support for the merger from influential members of the health care community, hospital administration and staff, nursing homes, etc.

Five to seven days before the actual merger, it should be announced to members of the health care community and other leaders. If the physicians have done their job, the news, at this point, will not be a surprise and will be supported by most of these people. Once the medical community is adequately informed, press releases should be mailed to the local media, particularly to the community papers. Unless the merger is of a tremendous magnitude, the news release may receive little or no attention but at least it will have been publicized.

Finally, a warm, descriptive letter should be sent to all of the clinics' patients, active and inactive, explaining the basic details of the merger and how it will affect them. Obviously, the letter should stress all of the positive aspects of the merger and point out all of the ways in which they, as patients, will benefit.

Depending on the size and market area, the clinic may wish to purchase media exposure to its opening. (See also Ch. 1, for some basic advertising areas open to medical practices.)

§ 13.12 Insurance Coverage

The new entity must have basic forms of insurance. Lawyers and accountants should be consulted on the best type of policies for a large group and to identify any difficulties pre-merger entities will have terminating individual policies.

Just as it is important that the benefit packages of the merged practices be carefully integrated, so is it important that the business insurance of the practices be carefully reviewed and smoothly integrated.

The first important business insurance that comes to mind with any physician is professional liability insurance. A merger can sometimes create unusual problems in this area, since it is likely that the individual practices were covered with other carriers. If some of the doctors have to switch insurance to new carriers the clinic may find additional premiums for the so-called "tail" attached to the claims-made policies.

Basically, there are two types of malpractice insurance, claims-made and occurance. While occurance packages were the most common prior to the malpractice crisis of the '70s, most policies today are on a claims-made basis. A claims-made basis means that the insurance covers only those events in which claims are made during the period of insurance enforcement, and only those events which occurred while the physician was covered by the same company. To terminate coverage, the insurance companies sell a final policy called a tail.

The insurance expense in this area can become a burden during the first few years of practice and must be included in initial budgeting. It is also important that comprehensive coverage is obtained for the clinic so that there are no gaps. The best way to ensure this is to have a single professional liability insurer.

Because of the increased size of the group, it is likely that extra or key insurance will not be necessary for all participating physicians.

That is, the intensified workflow caused by the death or loss of a physician in the group could probably be absorbed by the rest of the group on a short-term basis. Exceptions to this, however, should be examined. If certain physicians are key people in their specialty, it may be appropriate to identify these doctors and have "keyman insurance" taken out on them, with the clinic as beneficiary. The same applies to any specialist in the group who could not be easily replaced and whose services could not be absorbed into the practice of the other doctors.

The whole area of insurance needs to be reviewed, since insurance previously taken out may no longer be needed in some areas, and in other areas new needs may be created. (See also Ch. 8, for a checklist of essential areas of business insurance.)

§ 13.13 Bail-Out Provisions

Allowing physicians to remove themselves from becoming entirely committed before the merger is approved is a practical way to attract participants and weed out those whose interests may not be good for the long-term life of the merger.

Early in merger talks, it may be necessary to have "bail-out provisions" to persuade physicians to participate in the initial concept of merging of the practices. A physician may be unwilling to make any type of commitment unless he or she feels there is a way to "bail-out." At a certain point, however, any type of bail-out provision can become detrimental to the group as a whole, since it ultimately discourages the concept of working together. By the time the merger is completed, all bail-out provisions should be eliminated, the idea being that the doctors who have pursued the idea this far should be committed to making the merger work. Any lack of commitment will be detrimental and very likely lead to a merger failure.

The elimination of bail-out provisions may be very specific through direct measures such as restrictive covenants, or through less subtle measures such as the rotation of doctors among offices. It would also include the elimination of old systems and the centralization of new ones. Buy-sell agreements should be very specific to treat the terminated employee equitably, but not to encourage termination or to encourage someone from leaving and launching a competitive practice. The contract should provide for equitable arrangements for senior physicians to work with the practice in a way which would encourage patients to stay with the practice, rather than switch to another after the senior doctors retire.

§ 13.14 Checklist

A comprehensive checklist of points discussed in the chapter is provided.

— Decide on the type of affiliation
  — Joint venture
  — Physician practice group (PPG)
  — Business combination: merger
— Choose partners on the basis of
  — Level of quality
  — Specialty fees
  — Overhead
  — Philosophy on reimbursement
  — Business goal evaluation
  — Work attitude
  — Personal attitude
— Appoint a steering committee
— Establish an advisory team
— Establish cost-sharing arrangements
— Enter pre-merger agreement
— Make financial projections
— Select organizational set-up
— Clean up current entities
— Value the practices
— Set up a profit distribution system
— Set up buy-sell agreements
— Establish personnel policy
— Establish wage scales

- Select personnel and appoint to positions
- Establish unified office systems
- Establish a fee schedule
- Determine current practice profiles and establish a method to track profiles assigned to the new practice
- Establish a system of centralized purchasing
- Set up a telephone system
  - Phase out old numbers
  - Coordinate Yellow Pages advertisement
- Establish the equipment and facility
- Announce merger
- Check list of potential merger and pre-merger problems
  - Hospital takeovers
  - Loss of individual control
  - Inefficiencies of bureaucracies
  - Lack of experienced management
  - Medicare and Medicaid regulations
  - Contingent liabilities
  - Business entanglements
  - Antitrust regulations

§ 13.100 Bibliography

Anders, Geoffrey T., et al.: Merger: Means to Meet Your Practice Goals? Pennsylvania Medicine, Feb. 1986, p. 64.

Beck, Leif C.: So You Want to Merge Your Practice, Do You? Group Practice Journal, Mar.-Apr. 1985.

The Health Care Group. Structuring Your Practice in the Changing Medical Environment. Seminar and Material.

CHAPTER 14
Succeeding in a Prepaid Health Care Program

> **SCOPE**
>
> As more and more patients seek out low-cost health care, it is almost inevitable that a physician will become involved with some form of prepaid health care program, whether a preferred provider organization or, more likely, a health maintenance organization (HMO). These programs may benefit the physician by securing the patient base and eliminating the third-party insurer as a middleman. However, unless a medical group is large enough to incorporate itself as an HMO, the physician will have to deal with a third-party organizer. The physician who considers joining a prepaid program must devote the same attention to a contract with this third party as with any other third party. The physician must check the reputation of the third party and make sure every offer discussed with the third party is included in the contract. The physician must be satisfied with both the type of health care provided under the plan and the patient population served. Before signing, the contract must be examined for any potential restrictions on referral to outside sources, for the quality of medical care and for other potential problems. It must also be studied in relation to the plan's cost containment policy. The physician should also know under what terms the contract can be altered or terminated when the agreement is no longer satisfactory.

SYNOPSIS

§ 14.01 Prepaid Health Care Programs
    [1] History of Prepaid Health Care
    [2] Types of Program

- [a] Health Maintenance Organizations (HMOs)
- [b] Preferred Provider Organizations (PPOs)
- [c] Insured Health Products

§ 14.02 Reasons for Participating
- [1] Potential Economies
- [2] Control

§ 14.03 How a Prepaid Program Works: Pros and Cons
- [1] Cost Containment
- [2] Incentives

§ 14.04 Preparation: Evaluating Program Viability
- [1] Reviewing Strengths and Weaknesses of the Practice
- [2] Joining a Program
  - [a] Experience and Tenure
  - [b] Financial Strength
  - [c] Reputation
  - [d] Market Share
- [3] Economics of the Program: Who Gets What?
  - [a] Distributing the Capitated Dollar
  - [b] Timing Capitated Payments
- [4] Bookkeeping and Reporting Requirements
- [5] Dispute Resolutions
- [6] Expanding to Handle New Patients
  - [a] Facility Planning
  - [b] Patient Flow and Budgeting
- [7] Arrangements for Outside Services

§ 14.05 Federal and State Laws
- [1] General Federal Laws
- [2] Variable Restrictions

§ 14.06 The Specific Contract
- [1] Established Standard of Care
- [2] Joint and Several Liability
  - [a] Hold Harmless Clause
  - [b] Contractual Restrictions
  - [c] Physician Services
  - [d] Referrals
- [3] Peer Review Liability
- [4] Cross-Liabilities: Sharing the Blame
- [5] Anti-Trust Concerns
- [6] Points to Note When Reviewing a Contract
  - [a] Open-Ended Utilization Review

        [b] Arbitration Clauses
        [c] Termination
        [d] Confidentiality Requirements
        [e] Entire Agreement Provisions
        [f] Open-Ended Grievance Procedures
        [g] Restricted Referral
        [h] Professional Liability Insurance Requirement
        [i] Medical Records and Confidentiality
        [j] Peer Review
        [k] Assignable Contract
        [l] Amendment/Modification Provisions
        [m] Billing and Payment Issues
§ 14.07 Monitoring Profitability
        [1] Accounting: Accrual Versus Cash Basis
        [2] Anticipating Growth
        [3] Profit Distribution and Changing Incentives
        [4] Monitoring Costs
§ 14.08 Checklist for Prepaid Health Care Programs
§ 14.09 Glossary of Terms in Prepaid Health Care
§ 14.100 Bibliography

§ 14.01 Prepaid Health Care Programs

Alternative health care programs command a large share of the modern medical marketplace. In particular, prepaid programs offer strong competition to traditional fee-for-service practices. Among the more popular prepaid health plans available today are the health maintenance organization (HMO), the preferred provider organization (PPO) and innovative programs devised by traditional third-party insurers.

Before 1980, fee-for-service practices were competing with alternative health care programs in only a few parts of the country. These programs, health maintenance organizations (HMOs), were begun specifically with the encouragement and support of a government concerned with the spiraling cost of medicine, the rising expense of the Medicare program and general lobbying for national health insurance. Interstudy, a Minneapolis, Minnesota, think tank, concluded that the answer to all of these issues was a health care program that would give physicians economic incentives to contain costs.

(Rel.2–2/88 Pub.372)

[1] History of Prepaid Health Care

HMOs began appearing during the 1970s. Given the small market share the famous Kaiser Permanente Plan in California made between 1940 and 1980, few physicians felt the prepaid program would ever affect the fee-for-service practice.

The prevailing attitude has since changed. After years of working with HMOs through cost and risk contracts, federal legislation (TEFRA) encouraged the development of more prepaid programs by creating a new organization, the Competitive Medical Plan (CMP). A qualified CMP may contract with Medicare to provide coverage. This is a desirable program for Medicare providers, since it defines the cost per patient, in contrast to a fee-for-service program based more open-endedly on the number and type of procedures performed.

At the same time, employers began seeking ways to lower employee health costs. HMOs offered employers opportunities to obtain coverage for their employees at costs lower than traditional fee-for-service policies. Furthermore, the government mandated that employers at least offer HMO coverage to employees as an option. In addition to lowering the employer's premium costs, prepaid programs reduce or eliminate out-of-pocket costs to the employee, a very appealing feature for young families.

After more than ten years of development, what once seemed an insignificant form of alternative medical coverage has clearly had a major impact on public health care. Physicians who have ignored prepaid programs are finding their patient bases shrinking, not so much from patient dissatisfaction with medical care as from a simple matter of economics. Although in some cases patients return to private practitioners after becoming disgruntled with an alternative system, many younger and healthier patients elect to stay with the prepaid program. Younger physicians with newer practices are finding it more difficult to build a fee-for-service practice since many prospective patients have committed themselves to prepaid programs.

[2] Types of Program

The kinds of prepaid programs available to physicians vary with the location of the practice. These days, a number of different programs may spring up within a single area. Although many of them do not survive, they at least offer the physician in search of a prepaid program a broad range of choices to consider.

[a] Health Maintenance Organizations (HMOs)

HMOs are based on the idea that the costs of medical care can be kept low if the physician is given incentive to keep patients healthy, rather than just cure those who are already sick. The economics of an HMO are structured so that the physician is paid equally for each patient assigned to him or her, regardless of the number of procedures each patient requires. This is in direct contrast to the fee-for-service approach, which pays the physician on a "work done" basis. Implicit in the HMO approach is the rationale that healthy patients require fewer costly medical procedures than sick patients, and so it will be more profitable for the physician to maintain the patient's health.

There are presently four basic HMO models: the group model, the staff model, the independent practice association (IPA) model, and the mixed model.

Group Model. In the group model, one or more medical groups contract with the HMO to provide services. The group model HMO may be exclusive or nonexclusive. Under an exclusive contract, provider groups may not offer services to patients outside the HMO plan. A nonexclusive contract would permit such outside medical care.

In the group model, the physician group contracts with the HMO, and after receiving a capitated payment (a set reimbursement based on the number of patients treated under the plan), it is responsible for all of the health care needs of patients enrolled in the program, including physician costs, hospital costs, supplies, drugs, etc. In some cases, the group may choose not to be responsible for certain risks in return for a lower capitated payment.

Generally, patients are permitted to select among the medical groups participating in the plan to find the one that best suits their tastes. Once the patient selects that group, though, he or she may not have the option to switch, except at certain pre-arranged times.

Staff Model. The staff model HMO employs the individual

physician like a staff member to provide medical service. This model carries the greatest chance of personal gain or risk of personal loss for the physician owner.

Independent Practice Association (IPA). The Independent Practice Association (IPA) is similar to the nonexclusive group-model HMO. However, it is generally open to private practices and its enrollees do not make up the bulk of the physician's patient base. Unlike the group model HMO, IPA physicians are generally paid on a fee-for-service or modified fee-for-service basis. That is, the physician generally agrees to a fee schedule from the IPA that is lower than his or her current fee schedule. Reserve witholdings may be used to reward cost-efficient providers.

Mixed Models. In an effort to appeal to a larger market, today many HMOs use a mix of the three types of program.

[b] Preferred Provider Organizations (PPOs)

The Preferred Provider Organization (PPO) was established to compete with the HMO. A PPO is a group of independent practices working together to keep the cost of health care down. The PPO generally contracts with employers, unions, insurers or other third party administrators in an effort to provide lower medical costs within a fee-for-service program.

The lower costs may be a result of discounts negotiated between physicians and hospitals or through more economic utilization of services. Ideally, the PPO is tightly monitored to terminate arrangements with providers who charge excessive amounts.

The advantage of the PPO to the patient is that he or she can have medical costs defined under a PPO provider, but still receive some reimbursement from a third party insurer if he or she seeks treatment from a provider outside the program. A modified version of the PPO, the Exclusive Provider Organization (EPO), requires that patients see only EPO physicians unless they are referred outside the EPO by one of its providers.

[c] Insured Health Products

Traditionally, insurance companies have acted as "middle men," collecting premiums from the insured and paying out claims to physicians, hospitals and other providers. This adds the insurance company's cost of administration and profit to the general cost of medicine and makes the amount of the deductible the only incentive for limiting the use of medical services.

However, with the proliferation of competing HMOs and other prepaid medical organizations, insurance companies are finding their market share in the health care industry rapidly shrinking. HMOs have replaced the outside insurance company as the middle man. They can offer more services to the insured at lower premiums as a result of economic incentives used to control the participating health care providers.

In an effort to compete with HMOs and to protect or expand their market share, insurance companies have devised a vast variety of new products. Generally, these products offer the consumer more options than does the HMO. For example, an insurer, like an HMO, may employ a network of physicians who provide low-cost medical services based on discounted fees or controls such as restricting referrals or pre-admission requirements for hospitalization. The insurer may then offer the consumer the option of using a provider within its low-cost network, or a provider outside the network for higher-priced services that will still be partly covered under the terms of the insurance policy.

§ 14.02 Reasons for Participating

Prepaid health care programs appeal to many physicians because they protect the shrinking base of patients and allow the physician to retain some control over the practice that might be lost through affiliation with a hospital or by joining a large medical group. By eliminating the third-party insurer and discounting supplies and services, they also open up new potential economies.

Even though a physician may be doing a good job and getting referrals from other patients, his or her market share in the fee-for-service area may be shrinking for the simple reason that HMOs can usually offer patients basic health care at a lower price. With this in mind, it makes sense for a physician to look into prepaid programs from two marketing standpoints: to protect the current patient base and to expand potential market share.

[1] Potential Economies

In the usual fee-for-service approach to health care, it is the middleman—in this case, the third-party insurer—that benefits from any cost reductions and is penalized by excessive costs (which are eventually passed on to the patient). The physician benefits only if additional or larger fees are charged. By eliminating the middleman, the prepaid medical program can realize a potential economy. This may not be a practical expectation for a new, inexperienced HMO that realizes it does not have the necessary actuarial and administrative expertise. However, it may be perfectly feasible for a large HMO with experience, rating, and a large enough patient base.

In a capitated program (a set reimbursement) where the physician receives capitated payments based on the number of patients in the practice, the physician benefits directly when the amount of necessary care is less than anticipated. Physicians with large practices further benefit by contracting for services at a discount rate with other health care professionals.

[2] Control

Given the competitive environment of modern medicine, few physicians are able to risk opening a private practice. Established physicians in small groups are also finding it difficult to compete with larger groups. The alternative is finding employment in a large group where the individual physician has little or no control over operations.

The prepaid medical program is one way in which the physician can maintain control over his or her practice. Although there will always be a fee-for-service market, its continual shrinking means there will be fewer medical organizations able to work exclusively on a fee-for-service basis. By deciding to participate in a prepaid program many physicians feel they will be able to maintain a fee-for-service practice as well as control over their business.

§ 14.03 How a Prepaid Program Works: Pros and Cons

The profitability of a prepaid health care program depends on the ability to contain costs and to enroll a sufficient number of patients.

Many physicians resist entering the area of prepaid health care for ethical reasons. They feel that it is unfair to put the physician in the position whereby he or she may profit by witholding care.

Others have tried prepaid plans that have ended in failure and left them with bitter feelings toward such programs, even though most failures are a direct result of inexperience on the part of the HMO administration, the physician group or both.

One can debate the ethics or the incentives for participating in these programs. However, it is an unavoidable fact that prepaid health care programs are a significant part of modern medical care, and the physician needs to know how they operate before deciding whether to practice in one or not.

[1] Cost Containment

The profitability and success of a prepaid program depends on its ability to contain costs. Cost containment should include careful evaluation of all services provided. Its focus is as much active as reactive patient management. This means that the prepaid program should include patient education programs and routine diagnostic screening, with the idea that the cost of prevention or early diagnosis is less than that of treatment.

Once a patient has reached the treatment stage, the prepaid provider may feel pressure to reduce costs, and so a physician may feel he or she cannot order tests, get a consulting opinion or hospitalize a patient without making an economoic evaluation.

Profitability of the prepaid program also counts on the ability to enroll a sufficient number of members to make it actuarially sound. Proponents of the prepaid method contend that the quality of services must be kept high if one is to build up and maintain a sufficient number of members. Opponents argue that the incentives are for the prepaid provider to give service only to healthy patients, since the capitation fee paid them is the same whether the patient requires medical services or not. Furthermore, they argue that there is incentive not to provide services for the patients in the program who need them, since the loss of such patients would enhance the profitability of the plan.

[2] Incentives

Every program offers incentives to the physician to convince him or her of its profitability. Some questions the physician should ask about these incentives before entering the prepaid program include:

- Is there sufficient enrollment to guarantee sufficient capitated income? Actuaries agree that there must be a minimum enrollment of 500 patients assigned to the clinic.

- Assuming a satisfactory number of enrollees, what risk groups are they in? If a new program offers open enrollment, it may attract an above-average amount of patients who would normally be uninsurable. If the physician is assigned a patient group with a higher ratio of high-risk patients than the capitated payment is based on, the plan is doomed to failure. As a rule the physician should endeavor to attract a higher ratio of healthy patients.

- Are the program's methods the least expensive way to provide the best necessary care.

After the initial review, some physicians may determine that they are happier with a fee-for-service program than with the risk sharing prepaid health care entails. They may feel the business aspect of medicine should be left to the insurance companies, and that by making it the physician's concern will only compromise the quality of care. Physicians who have tried prepaid programs and found they had become an "invasion" of the way they practiced medicine may feel the same way.

However, many physicians will decide to join a prepaid program because they believe such programs enhance the quality of medical care while reducing its cost, and because they see in the program a means of achieving financial success.

§ 14.04 Preparation: Evaluating Program Viability

The physician considering joining a prepaid program should first check the reputation and economic stability of the third party organizer. Fee schedules and distribution of capitated fees should be discussed. The physician must also take into account the type of patient enrolled under the plan, whether the contract is exclusive or allows involvement with outside contractors, whether there are restrictions on referrals and whether the practice can accomodate a potential surge of new patients without compromising standards of care.

Many physicians panic at the thought of a shrinking base of patients or a loss of control of their practice. As a consequence, they jump immediately into as many prepaid programs as possible with the idea that, even if some of the programs do not survive, they will still be involved with the ones that do. This can be a serious mistake.

Involvement with a financially unstable prepaid program can cause serious, even devastating financial problems for a medical practice. Even if the practice overcomes these problems, the experience may sour the physician on future participation in prepaid programs. Perhaps most important, though, many patients of the physician will join whatever program his or her practice joins. If the practice later decides to drop the program, the physician risks "giving away" patients to a prepaid program in which her or she no longer participates.

[1] Reviewing Strengths and Weaknesses of the Practice

Joining a prepaid health care program out of fear of a shrinking patient base or simply the need to acquire new patients is a weakness the practice should resist. Rather, a medical practice should deal from its strengths. Some of these strengths might include:

- the practice's reputation in the medical community and public eye
- the practice's patient base, since many patients would never be lured from the practice and into a prepaid program otherwise
- the practice's location and hospital connections
- the practice's current marketing system, even if it includes nothing more than referrals from other physicians and patients
- the practice's demonstrated ability to treat patients

Evaluating the practice's strengths should reinforce a physician's awareness that his or her practice is an asset to the program under consideration. It should make a physician selective about which program to join.

It is possible for a medical group, especially a large group, not to join a program and establish its own HMO or prepaid program. However, the administrative assistance and expertise this requires is beyond the means of most small practices. Most likely, the small practice will get involved with a prepaid program administered by a third party, such as Blue Cross or Blue Shield, or a local or nationally run HMO.

[2] Joining a Program

A physician should begin by making a list of all potential programs and consider which will best fill the needs of his or her practice. For example, if the main reason for joining a program is to attract new patients, the physician should evaluate the program's current market share and growth history. Other aspects of the third party to investigate include its experience and tenure, financial strength and reputation.

[a] Experience and Tenure

How long has the third-party organization behind the program been working in the prepaid health care market? If it is new, as many are today, find out how long it has been involved in health care insurance. Avoid inexperienced new entries to the field.

Check on the carrier's commitment to health care. Do not get involved in a situation where the third party is "bailing out" by selling a health care product line to another insurer, or abandoning it altogether.

Check the references of other physicians cooperating with the third party. Contact them to discuss their satisfaction or dissatisfaction with the third party. Ask whether they have been able to make the prepaid program successful and how it compares with their experience in fee-for-service from an economic standpoint.

[b] Financial Strength

Check to determine if the premiums charged by the third party are adequate to compensate participating physician groups and to generate potential profit. Some programs, in an effort to compete with other HMOs, charge premiums based on market expansion regardless of actual cost. Lowered capitated payments may attract new patients, but they can break the backs of the individual providers. Ultimately, this leads to financial disaster felt most strongly by the participating health care providers.

[c] Reputation

Is the program's reputation congruent with the type of care your practice wants to provide? For example, if your main patient base has been business executives, and the prepaid program's main market is the blue collar worker, will this be compatible with your practice? Does the program have a reputation for excellence in care, or for lower premiums? Does it attract an older or younger population base, or a mixed base?

[d] Market Share

Review the third party's current market share and its ability to attract new patients. Also review how patients are assigned within the program and which patients would be assigned to the practice. A program often attracts new patients less through its own efforts than by inheriting patients who join because their physician is one of the providers. This can be good for the program, but not for the participating physician. If these are the only patients assigned under the program, the profit margin the physician enjoyed before joining may be lowered. Furthermore, since patients only periodically have the option to change health care programs, a patient whose physician drops from the program may be reassigned to another participating practice.

In addition to the third party's ability to attract new patients, check the type of patients attracted and the revenues they produce. The health care costs for a younger, healthier patient population are far less than those for Medicare patients. A program with a greater number of high-risk patients should be charging adequate premiums to offset the risk. It is also important that the program assign healthy patients on an equal basis so that no one physician provider absorbs the full risk of the less healthy patients. If the program is new, it is important that it have enough patients to make it actuarially sound: 500 patients is considered the minimum for a fiscally sound program.

[3] Economics of the Program: Who Gets What?

Once the programs in general have been evaluated, program economics should be considered. In a capitated program, the physician is paid a flat dollar amount per enrollee. The amount of capitation, based on the age and sex of the patient, is obviously a

§ 14.04[3]   MANAGING YOUR MEDICAL PRACTICE   14–14

product of the premium charged to the patient. The premium includes the entire scope of health care services, such as:

- the physician's services, including primary care, consultants, sub-specialists and surgeons
- hospital costs
- pharmaceutical costs
- specific supplies
- x-ray and laboratory fees
- out of area costs
- dental and optometry costs (although this may be optional)
- outpatient and emergency care (see Figure 14–1).

[a] **Distributing the Capitated Dollar**

The physician must be aware of what portion of the capitated dollar his or her practice will receive and the services for which the practice will be responsible. Generally, unless a huge multi-specialty organization is involved, the program will have to contract out for certain services. For example, it may not have surgeons on staff and it would never be able to provide in-patient hospital care.

In some cases, it is advisable and acceptable for a practice not to accept that portion of the capitated fee relative to certain aspects which the primary group cannot provide, such as hospitalization or referrals. Generally, however, the third party organization is hesitant to do this because it feels that the physician controls these expenses and should have economic incentives and rewards for handling them in a cost-effective way.

Unlike what the physician was used to previously, under a prepaid program he or she may be responsible for many, if not all, components of a health care budget. This is mentioned for two reasons. First, physicians' fees are generally only a small part of a total health care budget. Second, an individual physician's costs typically increase once he or she becomes responsible for more expenses in a health care budget. Whereas office overhead may have been the physician's only concern for breaking even in private practice, once in a prepaid program substantial portions of revenue have to be allotted to outside vendors.

(Rel.2–2/88 Pub.372)

WHERE THE HEALTH CARE PREMIUM GOES

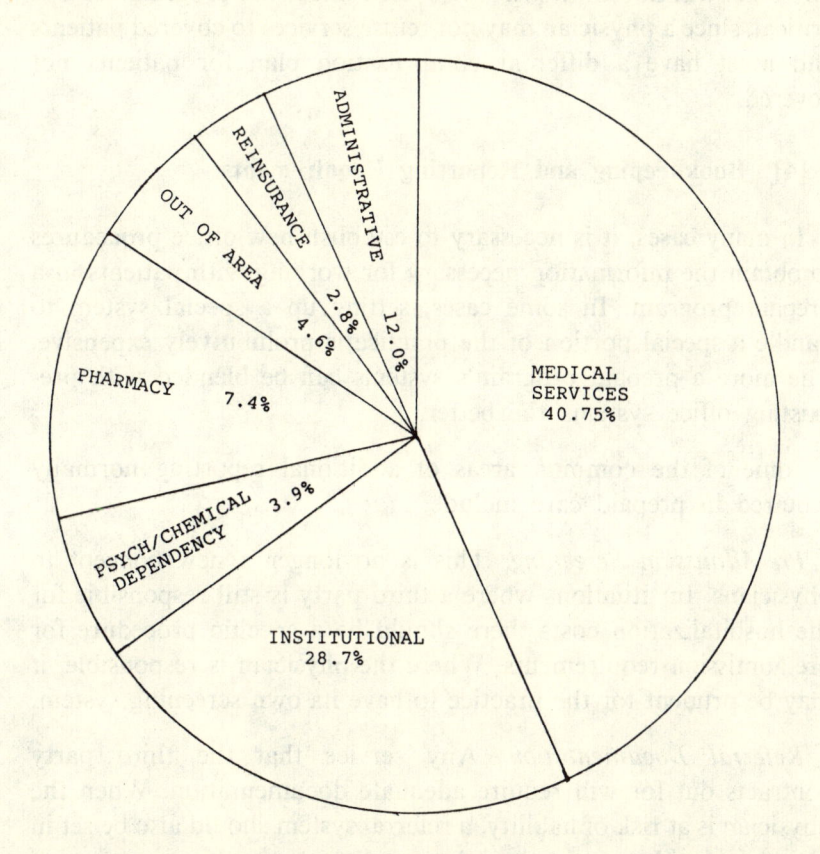

- ADMINISTRATIVE 12.0%
- REINSURANCE 2.8%
- OUT OF AREA 4.6%
- PHARMACY 7.4%
- PSYCH/CHEMICAL DEPENDENCY 3.9%
- INSTITUTIONAL 28.7%
- MEDICAL SERVICES 40.75%

Fig. 14–1. The prepaid health care "pie," and the slices into which the premium is divided.

[b] Timing Capitated Payments

The timeliness of capitated payments are another important concern. Physicians who are used to being paid after services are rendered will obviously have to adjust in a prepaid program. The time value of money in a capitated program is critical and late payments are not acceptable.

It is also important upon receipt of the capitation check that a complete list of patients enrolled be provided. Without this, the physician will not know who is covered under the program. This is critical, since a physician may not refuse services to covered patients and must have a different compensation plan for patients not covered.

[4] Bookkeeping and Reporting Requirements

In many cases, it is necessary to establish new office procedures to obtain the information necessary for working with patients in a prepaid program. In some cases, setting up a special system to handle a special portion of the practice is prohibitively expensive. The more a prepaid program's systems can be blended with pre-existing office systems the better.

Some of the common areas of additional reporting normally required in prepaid care include:

Pre-Admission Screening. This is no longer a new concept to physicians. In situations where a third party is still responsible for the hospitalization costs there should be a specific procedure for pre-admission requirements. Where the physician is responsible, it may be prudent for the practice to have its own screening system.

Referral Documentation. Any service that the third party contracts out for will require adequate documentation. When the physician is at risk of liability, a referral system should also be set in place to provide protection and serve as authorization for referring physician to perform services. It should also be used to determine outstanding liabilities in order to determine the profitability of the program (see Figure 14–2).

Claims Processing. How will the claims by outside providers such as hospitals and consultants be processed? In many cases, the third party may be in a good position to process them. In others, the participating practice is responsible for the bill, in which case it will be important to match referral documentation with bills from the consultants. It will be necessary to screen charges to make certain that authorized or unnecessary procedures were not performed. It will also be important for the physician to review hospital charges to ascertain that the practice is not being billed excessively.

SAMPLE REFERRAL FORM--U.S.A. MEDICAL CENTER
_____

1. Patient Name _____ 3. Date _____

2. Identification Number _____

4. Referred to _____
               _____
               _____

5. For _____ Consultation Only   6. Schedule Date of
       _____ Treatment Only   Appointment _____
       _____ Other

7. Description of Problem _____
   _____

8. The following test results are available _____ Laboratory
                                            _____ X-ray
                                            _____ Other

9. Note: a. The referral is for one visit only.
          b. All laboratory and radiology tests must be performed
             within U.S.A. Medical Center.
          c. No further referrals are possible without the
             written approval of the medical director.

10. Signed by

    _____
    Primary Care Physician

    _____
    Medical Director

Distribution of copies:

    Original - Referral Physician
    Copy 1 - Referral Physician - Return with report
    Copy 2 - Claims Tickler File
_____

A referral slip should be used to authorize work to be done by outside physicians. It will control how much work must be done and may be used to determine outstanding claims.

Fig. 14–2. Referral documentation. Such documentation can be used to ascertain pre-authorization for referred services and explain expenses that will and will not be covered under the terms of the health care plan.

[5] Dispute Resolutions

In the event that a dispute arises between the physician and the consultant or hospital, there must be an orderly process for handling the situation. A common dispute occurs when a consultant does more work than the prepaid physician authorized or felt was necessary. There must be a good working relationship to minimize problems in this area, since it will be different from the normal relationship between the primary care physician and the referral physician: the primary care physician is now "the gatekeeper" who must pay careful attention to services contracted.

[6] Expanding to Handle New Patients

If the program is successful and brings a substantial number of patients into the practice in a short period of time, the clinic must be able to handle the accelerated demand for patient care. A successful prepaid program, unlike a fee-for-service program, can grow rapidly and the burden on the individual physician can be substantial. If, for example, another provider of services drops out of the program, a large number of new patients may suddenly be assigned to the practice. The same would be true if the prepaid program succeeds in attracting a new major employer.

[a] Facility Planning

Facility planning is a critical issue. It must include not only the patient care for the new prepaid portion of the practice, but also for the current and future fee-for-service portion of the practice because it will affect the following factors.

Physician Staff. The maximum productivity for each physician should be examined to determine the practice's capacity to take on additional patients. This should be viewed in terms of increasing the individual practice's productivity through more effective management and better utilization of staff. (See also Ch. 9, Increasing Productivity Through Efficiency.) The specialties of participating physicians should be reviewed to determine which patients will have to be referred to outside providers. The feasibility of adding certain specialties to the staff should be weighed against the cost of referring out for the same services so that appropriate arrangements can be made with outside providers.

Nonphysician Staff. The use of nonphysician staff should be studied to determine if there is a sufficient number employed and whether the clinic can recruit sufficient staff in the event of growth. The type of staff needed should be reviewed to enhance overall productivity. Business staff must be able to handle extra paperwork and reporting requirements so that managing physicians will have accurate information with which to make prudent business decisions.

Office Space. Will there be adequate space to handle an influx of new patients? In some instances, this can be taken care of through more efficient scheduling or expanding office hours. However, the physician planner should not overlook less obvious office areas that will be affected, such as the business office, the patient reception area and storage. Once space is utilized to capacity, other options must be available. In some cases, this may mean leasing of convenient extra space; in other cases, it may mean moving the office to a completely new location. A third option could be the opening of a satellite branch or office.

Equipment. Steps must be taken to ensure the office is adequately equipped. On the technical side this means adequate basic equipment such as examination tables and instruments. The physician may also want to look into the feasibility of acquiring more sophisticated equipment, in which case he or she should determine whether the acquisition of such equipment, when combined with associated labor and supply costs, would be lower than the cost of referring procedures out. The need for nontechnical equipment and furnishings such as computers and software for the business portion of the practice, and comfortable furniture for the waiting room should not be overlooked.

A practice's ability to take on new patients must be balanced with the prepaid program's goals and expectations. Unlike the fee-for-service practice, it is unlikely that a provider in a prepaid program will suddenly be able to "stop" accepting new patients.

[b] Patient Flow and Budgeting

Physicians will need certain data to be able to make intelligent planning decisions based on the prepaid program's effect on patient flow. First, the number of enrollees in the program and the estimated growth of enrollees must be determined. This information must be obtained from the administration of the program. Unfortunately, even if the administration has a good track record, it will not be able to determine with certainty whether certain major employers will sign up with the program or how many employees will register as patients.

Physicians not used to dealing with capitated income should realize further that the number of enrollees will not correlate with current data on fee-for-service patients. The number of patients in fee-for-service is measured by the number who have come in and received services. The number in a prepaid program is meausred by the number assigned to the practice and for which the clinic is receiving capitated payment. Since this will include patients who may never need services, the number of capitated patients enrolled could be larger than is immediately apparent.

As the practice becomes involved with a program, operations should be monitored so that in the future facility needs can be more efficiently related to the number of enrollees. In the beginning, at least, a practice may have to rely on projected utilization information based on the prepaid program's history, rather than on direct experience.

The physician should also make a financial budget that projects associated revenues and expenses to clarify certain financial goals from the outset and make certain they can be realized under the prepaid program. There may be additional costs up front—for example, when a new employer is enrolled, patients may take quick advantage of "free" services, such as annual physicals—that the capitated income does not immediately offset.

[7] Arrangements for Outside Services

Outside services such as hospitalization and consultants can be arranged for on either a capitated or discounted fee-for-service basis. Whatever the arrangement, it is good if economic incentives for the provider of these services can be established to balance with cost-containment goals of the clinic.

However, it may be difficult to place an outside specialist on capitation. It is difficult to obtain adequate actuarial information to determine what portion of the capitated premium the specialist should receive. Further, the specialist may resist taking a capitated fee, since he or she may feel that it gives the primary care physician incentive to take advantage of the arrangement and immediately send them patients with conditions associated with their specialty, regardless of how much specialized care these patients really need.

Capitation (a set reimbursement) for hospitalization is more common, since it is easier to determine what portion of the premium dollar generally goes towards hospitalization. However, many physicians elect not to use capitation for hospitalization, reasoning that, through careful control, they can reduce the average hospital stay and reap greater financial gain. In these cases the physicians negotiate a discounted fee-for-service rate with the hospital or perhaps some sort of DRG arrangement (the type of arrangement through which Medicare currently reimburses hospitals).

It is important that referring hospitals and physicians be informed of the program and its arrangements ahead of time. Otherwise, there is a potential for the loss of numerous dollars. For example, an orthopedist who sees a patient, unaware that the patient is in a prepaid program or uninformed of the rules of that program, could perform services not authorized by the primary group or place the patient in a hospital with which the program has no prearranged agreement.

§ 14.05 Federal and State Laws

The physician should ascertain that the contract is in compliance with federal and state regulations for HMOs before signing the contract.

When the physician decides to enter a prepaid program, the bottom line is that he or she has entered into a contract and must uphold the obligations specified within the contract. Any physician contemplating such a move should seek the help of a competent attorney. This is not as easy as it may sound, since few attorneys specialize in health care law; most are unfamiliar with what is "normal" in these situations, what governmental regulations exist and what the overall economic ramifications will be for the physician. Most attorneys who specialize in health care law represent hospitals and what's good for the hospital is not always good for the individual physician. So it is important that the physician find an attorney who specializes in the health care field and who represents principally physicians.

There are basically two areas of legal concern for a physician entering a prepaid program: a general understanding of applicable federal and state laws governing HMOs, and the obligations and risks a physician may incur by entering into a contract.

[1] General Federal Laws

To meet federal qualifications for HMOs, a prepaid plan must fall under the definitions of federal HMO laws and the federal employee health benefit program. The purpose of HMO legislation is to license and certify HMOs and to authorize government agencies to purchase prepaid health services. Physician concern with the government as a purchaser of care, centers mainly around Medicare, but it can also include Medicaid and the federal employees' health benefit program. A federally qualified HMO must also satisfy the provisions of the federal HMO law, which mandates that certain employers offer an HMO option for employees.

Federal law defines an HMO as a provider of a comprehensive range of health care services to a voluntarily enrolled population in a geographic area on a primarily prepaid basis. TEFRA legislation created an organization called a Competitive Medical Plan (CMP). A CMP does not have to be a federally qualified HMO, but it can contract for Medicare beneficiary health coverage. Thus, a CMP, although it must be approved by the Health Care Finance Administration (HCFA), has broader parameters than an HMO.

[2] Variable Restrictions

Laws vary with particular states, but there are several general areas of legislation the physician entering a prepaid program needs to know:

Insolvency. The financial stability of the HMO is a matter of great concern. To protect the consumer in a failed program, insolvency laws in some geographic areas may require a plan to maintain certain reserves. In other cases, the law may allow the plan to cover the reserve requirement through indemnification by participating physicians.

Advertising Limitations. As a general rule, advertising of HMO progams is permitted providing the ads do not identify, refer to or make any qualitative judgment concerning any physician who provides services to members or subscribers in the program, in accordance with the American Medical Association position on advertising.

Corporate Practice of Medicine Restrictions. Laws prohibit the corporate practice of medicine to prevent the potential conflict of interest that could arise from a physician-employer relationship. If there is no specific legislation permitting the HMO to avoid problems in this area, the prohibition of corporate practice of medicine must be carefully evaluated.

Certificate of Need Requirements. Some states have enacted Certificate of Need Statutes that conform to federal criteria. If applicable, compliance with state requirements are important, since such compliance may be a pre-requisite for obtaining an HMO license or becoming operational. The state Health, Planning and Development Agency generally makes final approval.

Limitations on the Use of Certain Health Providers. State laws may prevent an HMO from utilizing certain health professionals, such as physician's assistants, nurse practitioners and other paraprofessionals that the HMO intends to rely on for cost containment. Regulations restricting the services performed by these professionals and other salient laws should be reviewed.

§ 14.06 The Specific Contract

As with any contract, the physician entering a prepaid program should consult a legal advisor about the provisions of the contract. Major points to be evaluated include distribution of liabilities between the physician and third party, ascertaining whether the standard of care will be compromised by cost containment policies, utilization reviews or referral sources, participation in peer reviews, confidentiality of medical records, and determining the physician's power to alter or terminate the contract.

Physicians are exposed to a liability risk far greater than the average business person, namely having to compensate a patient for injury that results from a treatment or the failiure to provide proper treatment. Many contracts for prepaid health care programs contain provisions concerned with physician liability in two areas:

liability incurred through the physician's failure to provide a standard of care not equal to established standards of care, and joint liability incurred through association.

[1] Established Standard of Care

The established standard of care is an ever-changing measurement that reflects current local practice, technology and teachings of medicine. The practice of defensive medicine that relies on tests and procedures to minimize risk and make diagnoses more precise has, over the last 20 years, influenced the standard of care. This has created a higher standard, but one that is also more expensive to attain and not always cost efficient.

[2] Joint and Several Liability

Joint and several liability describes a situation in which a person is harmed by the action of two or more parties. If those parties are found jointly liable and only one has the means to compensate the injured party, the more financially secure of the two parties can be held responsible for the entire amount. The bottom line of such a law is that it is better to increase one wrongdoer's burden than decrease the victim's compensation.

Two exposures to liability are commonly increased by contracts with third parties. One is the use of "hold harmless clauses" which may appear in the contract. The other is restrictions in the contract which conflict with the physician's standards of care.

[a] Hold Harmless Clause

To protect itself, the HMO may attempt to limit liability by including provisions in its contract that shift most or all of the liability onto the physician. Such provisions typically appear in the form of "hold harmless" clauses or implied indemnification clauses.

The hold harmless clause says, in essence, that the physician agrees to hold the third party "harmless" as to any liability that arises; if anything bad or negative happens, the physician agrees to assume full responsibility for the actions that caused it. While it is true that the physician ultimately makes the medical decisions that affect the patient's course of treatment, in many contracting situations issues such as prior authorization restrictions, utilization limitations, administrative mistakes and other restraints imposed in an effort to contain costs may have a direct or indirect impact on the physician's medical judgment. Thus, the physician who signs the hold harmless provision should realize that he or she is not only accepting the responsibility for patient care, but also agreeing to cover the cost to the third party in the event of a malpractice suit. This includes legal damages, investigative costs, attorney fees, etc.

The physician should also be aware that by signing a contract with a hold harmless clause, he or she may be going into assumed contractual liability "bare." Most professional liability insurance policies for physicians specifically exclude liability assumed under contract from their coverage; therefore, the physician will not be able to rely on malpractice insurance for help in the event of lawsuits that arise as a result of the hold harmless clause. The physician would thus need to defend and indemnify the third party out of pocket.

[b] Contractual Restrictions

There are potential dangers in contractual restrictions imposed on the quality of care and treatment, since the standard of care owed to the patient remains the same regardless of these restrictions.

If the standard of care achievable under the contract differs from the community standard, the physician is put in an uncompromising situation: if on the one hand the physician adheres to the community standard, he or she will be in breach of contract; if on the other hand the physician complies with the contract's standard of care and the patient comes to harm or an unsatisfactory outcome, the physician may be held liable for the patient's injuries.

[c] Physician Services

Most prepaid contracts require some type of prior authorization before they will cover costs or reimburse the physician for services. The physician should make sure before signing the contract that the third party's authorization policy is compatible with good medical practice. If authorization is denied for treatment that is consistent with the physician's best medical judgment, the physician should challenge the decision. The contract should provide for an appeals procedure to address this possiblity, since a third party's refusal to authorize or pay for care which ought to be rendered in good medical practice does not excuse the physician from providing the care.

If a situation arises in which the physician deems necessary medical care not approved or covered by the third party, the physician must take certain steps for self-protection and to protect the patient as well. The California Medical Association, which has reviewed many such cases, recommends the following:

(1) Document disputes and any appeals in the patient's chart and in letters to the third party and to the patient.

(2) Inform the patient of the reason for any procedures, treatments or recommended tests and the potential risk of foregoing such medical care. This too should be documented on the patient's chart.

(3) Provide assistance to the patient in seeking authorization or care from other sources.

[d] Referrals

Many third-party contracts restrict referrals to within a network of participating physicians with the intention of keeping the money in the program. From the standpoint of liability this may pose a special risk to the physician.

Physicians have a legal responsibility to refer patients to appropriate specialists. If the third party has neglected to contract with a sufficient variety and quantity of specialists, adverse consequences may result. Physicians must first satisfy themselves as to the adequacy of referral sources under the contract. If the physician feels referral sources within the network are not adequate, the contract must allow referrals to outside the network. It should be noted that physicians using a group of specialists outside the network for their general fee-for-service patients and a different network for the prepaid patient could be setting themselves up for a lawsuit by a patient dissatisfied with the results of treatment.

Physicians who refer prepaid patients to nonparticipating physicians or hospitals need to ensure that the patient both understands and approves the ramifications of such an action. Since this referral may result in uncovered or extra expense to the patient, the patient must be apprised of this prior to services. Furthermore, the physician should assist the patient in forcing the third party to provide coverage under such circumstances.

[3] Peer Review Liability

The physician is also liable for involvement in the peer review process. Fortunately, as a result of strong public policy favoring physician peer review, most states provide significant legal protection for physicians engaged in peer review activities. The protection provided by these laws, however, is typically granted to physicians serving on hospital staffs or in medical societies. Because some third party health care contracts may require the physician to serve on a peer review committee whose interest is cost containment rather than quality of care, immunity may not be applicable.

Physician exposure to peer review liability comes from two possible sources: the patient hurt by a physician decision who sues on grounds of professional negligence; and colleagues who sue because a peer review decision affects their economic interests. Professional liability insurance may not extend to cover peer review liability. If it does, the physician should determine whether the coverage is limited to hospital medical staff committees and medical society committees or also includes third-party organizations.

[4] Cross-Liabilities: Sharing the Blame

Under the provisions of joint and several liability, liability for compensating the injured party can be shifted to the partner who is more financially secure. In a situation where the physician has signed a hold harmless contract, it is possible for the physician to assume responsibility for liabilities for which the third party would otherwise have taken the blame. Even if the contract does not appear to shift liability, the third party may seek to blame the physician for injury to a patient. Administrative mistakes or deficiencies that deny or limit care can leave the third party open for a lawsuit for negligence, misrepresentation, breach of contract and bad faith.

[5] Anti-Trust Concerns

Anti-trust law is an important area of concern whenever any type of joint business venture takes place, and the federal government has used anti-trust regulation against the medical community a number of times. In 1983, the Federal Trade Commission ruled that the Michigan State Medical Society unreasonably restrained competition by conspiring with its members to influence the reimbursement policies of Blue Cross of Michigan and Michigan Medicaid.

Physicians' groups such as medical societies or medical staffs should not try to discourage membership in any specific contract or third party soliciting physicians for contracts; neither should an individual physician support any group decision of this nature. Physicians in group programs face the greatest risk of anti-trust violation in the area of fee-setting. The individual physician should also be careful to decide on his or her own whether to sign a contract, as a group action establishing the terms of the contract could result in anti-trust charges.

[6] Points to Note When Reviewing a Contract

The physician should pay attention to several basic points before signing a contract. These points should encompass the terms of agreement, the mutual obligations of participants in the contract and the option to break the contract if the arrangement does not work out satisfactorily.

[a] Open-Ended Utilization Review

This provision restricts the way in which the physician may provide services. It might include forcing the physician to employ certain cost-containment methods, rejecting certain types of patients or obtaining authorization before treatment is rendered.

In addition to increasing the administrative burdens of the physician, such a provision increases the physician's liability by making it more difficult to balance patient care with contractual obligations. Physicians should be aware of and comfortable with any utilization review procedure and certain that it is congruent with the standard of care in the community and the physician's own standard of care.

[b] Arbitration Clauses

The contract may contain provisions referring all disputes to arbitration. This can be a slow process with built-in limitations on the number of appeals and no chance for peer review. In some cases this agreement may preclude litigation entirely without avoiding legal fees and other expenses. Arbitration should not be presumed an inexpensive and easy solution to disagreement with the third-party provider.

[c] Termination

Termination agreements should be reviewed very carefully. It may be difficult for a physician to leave a prepaid program once patients are enrolled. Ideally, a termination agreement should contain provisions that permit the physician to continue seeing current patients for a period of time and allow the physician to reject new patients under the program.

In general the contract may restrict the physician's ability to terminate the contract. It may be tied to the patient's contract expiration, which could pose a problem in the event the program proves completely unprofitable for the physician. Another provision may call for automatic renewal of the contract without allowing the physician the opportunity to renegotiate terms or fees.

[d] Confidentiality Requirements

Many contracts have confidentiality requirements that require the physician not to disclose any patient information to any person not authorized by the third party. So ambiguous a provision could be interpreted to justify the witholding of information from staff, colleagues and patients themselves in a way that is not congruent with the physician's standard of care. A physician's failure to abide by this agreement could result in breach of contract and liability for damages. The physician should always be clear with regard to which items are considered confidential under a contract and assess how keeping such information confidential might affect patient care.

[e] Entire Agreement Provisions

Some contracts may carry a provision to the effect that the written agreement can change all terms and conditions and that any prior agreements, promises, negotiations or representations, either written or oral have no weight. In essence, this nullifies any promises, sales pitches or statements and solicitations not found in the contract proper. Since presentation is often a large part of selling a prepaid program to the physician, this provision can be extremely important.

[f] Open-Ended Grievance Procedures

The contract may have grievance procedures that are either unspecified or refer to another agreement or policy that is not part of the actual contract. For the physician, this turns the contract into a blind agreement to follow unclarified procedures and may constitute a waiver of impartial grievance hearing. The grievance committee may not be impartial and the physician may have given up his or her right to litigate.

[g] Restricted Referral

Restrictive referral provisions may bind the physician to making referrals within the third-party network. This may disrupt the physician's established referral patterns and force the physician to refer patients to sources with which he or she is not familiar. Should any adverse consequences arise, the physician could be blamed for them and be held liable for the patient fees in the event of referral to a physician outside the network.

The physician can avoid this by ensuring beforehand that referral services are up to his or her own standard of care. If he or she deems that referral to a noncontracting hospital or physician is in the patient's best interests, the patient should be made aware of this and the information documented on the patient's chart.

[h] Professional Liability Insurance Requirement

Many contracts require that the physician maintain a certain amount of general and professional liability insurance at his or her own expense. The contract may further require that the physician name the third party as an additional insurer. In this case, the physician should make sure that the amount of coverage can be obtained, and assess the additional cost that results from naming the third party.

[i] Medical Records and Confidentiality

Contracts generally provide the third party reasonable access to medical records maintained by the physician. This provision is often described in broad language authorizing disclosure of *all* medical records, and the physician could wind up bearing the cost of reproducing voluminous medical records and liability for damages caused by unwarranted disclosure of those records. In this situation, contractual requirements do not supersede existing laws protecting the confidentiality of medical records. The physician should determine in advance whether the contract is congruent with laws protecting against improper disclosure.

[j] Peer Review

If the contract calls for compliance with peer review systems established by the third party, the physician should check whether the review is subject to any standards or procedures. Peer review that is conducted solely for the purposes of cost-containment can have an impact on the standard of patient care and the physician's liability risk.

The physician who is required to review other physicians will face an additional liability: he or she may be sued by a dissatisfied patient for failure to take proper action and by the physician under review for loss of income.

[k] Assignable Contract

Provision in the contract dealing with assignability addresses the issue of whether contract obligations and rights may be transferred to other parties. Some contracts allow the third party, but not the physician, to assign these obligations and rights to another third party. Under such a contract, the physician may discover that his or her rights have been assigned to a third party to whom they object. The physician may wish to negotiate limitations on assignability.

[l] Amendment/Modification Provisions

Contracts may give the third party unilateral power to modify the agreement through notice to the physician. As a result, the physician may be obligated to comply with changes in fee schedule, utilization standards, etc., or be forced to terminate the entire contract.

[m] Billing and Payment Issues

The contract may be structured to give the third party maximum use of money and physician compensation, regardless of whether the program is 100 percent capitated or a mixture of capitation and fee-for-service. A third party that makes only large, single payments to the physician can seriously affect the cash flow crucial to the functioning of a prepaid program.

§ 14.07   MANAGING YOUR MEDICAL PRACTICE   14–32

Furthermore, some contracts permit third parties to withhold compensation, even in the form of capitation, until the physician can provide a full report of procedures performed. It may be very difficult for the physician's business staff to provide this information, and in some cases it may be impossible to comply without reprogramming the office computer. The physician should request specific, detailed, contractually-required billing information and formats and make sure the obligation of the third party to make payments is specified.

§ 14.07 Monitoring Profitability

> The economics of a prepaid program usually necessitate shifting from the usual cash basis of accounting to an accrual method. Since physicians in a prepaid program are not at liberty to increase profits by increasing charges or expanding their market, they must closely monitor the efficiency of individual physicians or responsibility centers and not hesitate to revamp or eliminate practices detrimental to the program's existence.

The physician who has entered the prepaid market needs to accumulate data to prepare simple financial reports for the purpose of monitoring the profitability of various programs. A simple summary report the physician should consult on a monthly basis might look something like this:

U.S.A. CLINIC, P.A.
1988 HMO SUMMARY

	CAPITATION INCOME	HMO* CHARGES	OTHER (EXPENSES) INCOME	HMO GAIN (LOSSES)	CUMULATIVE GAIN (LOSS)
FEBRUARY	$5,510	$6,011	$300	$ -800	$ -800
MARCH	4,449	4,715	412	-678	-1,478
APRIL	5,962	3,396	680	1,886	408
MAY	10,455	3,883	751	5,821	6,229
JUNE	6,385	6,903	890	-1,708	4,521
JULY	6,883	5,303	910	-729	3,792

*MEASURED AGAINST WHAT THE CHARGES WOULD HAVE BEEN UNDER FEE-FOR-SERVICE.

[1] Accounting: Accrual Versus Cash Basis

Physicians traditionally have used a cash basis of accounting to reflect income and expenses: the physician reports cash as it is collected and expenses as they are actually paid (an exception being capital expenses, which are amortized over the life of the equipment purchased in accordance with depreciation guideliness). This simplifies accounting and provides tax benefits for the physician, since taxes do not have to be paid on accounts receivable.

Under the accrual system of accounting, the practice reports income based on charges after write-offs and bad debts have been subtracted, regardless of whether money has actually been collected. Under this accounting method, expenses are reported when they are actually accrued, rather than paid for. The accrual method of accounting is used by publicly-held corporations and is considered to accurately reflect an organization's financial position.

As a practical matter, cash-basis accounting gives an accurate picture of the financial management of a mature fee-for-service medical practice, since cash receipts generally equal net charges (gross charges less write-offs and adjustments). However, for a medical practice involved in a prepaid program, the accural method may be preferable to the cash-basis of accounting for two reasons.

First, the prepaid clinic may receive substantial amounts of "unearned" income in the form of capitated payments. These payments are received in advance and require the clinic to provide services for a period of time. This income must be allocated over the period of time in which the physician is obligated to provide services before it properly reflects the financial results of the prepaid program. The inexperienced medical practice may make the mistake of treating these early payments as income and use the money to pay expenses or physicians' salaries.

On the other side of the coin, certain expenses will accrue under a prepaid program, even though they have not been paid for. These could include outside referrals, ancillary services such as lab and x-ray, hospital care, etc. If the clinic does not have a system to "reserve" a portion of the capitated income for these expenses, it could lead to insolvency.

Therefore it is essential for managerial purposes that the clinic

REFERRAL COSTS: ANALYSIS OF CLAIMS RECEIVED/PAID
MARCH 1987

Month of Incurral[1]	
March	$ 9,650
February	9,875
January	1,972
December	1,380
November	1,065
October	170
September	420
August	590
Total claims processed in March	$25,222

[1] Month that service was actually provided.

Fig. 14–3. Accrual vs. cash basis accounting. This illustrates how the reporting of expenses would differ between the two systems. Under the cash basis of accounting the referral expenses would be reported as $9,650. Under the accrual method, the expenses would be reported as $25,222, since the accrual method matches expenses with the period in which they occur regardless of when they are paid.

maintain accurate accrual accounting on the prepaid portion of the practice. As a greater and greater portion of practice income comes from prepaid programs, the overall accounting system should shift to the accrual method. While the cash basis method gives the fee-for-service physician a tax advantage by requiring that the physician only pay taxes on income collected, the accrual method may provide reciprocal tax advantages for the physician in the prepaid program by allowing him or her to avoid paying taxes on capitated income paid in advance and allowing the physician to deduct accrued expenses which have not been paid (see Figure 14–3).

[2] Anticipating Growth

In the past, physicians have been able to meet increases in expenses by increasing fees and productivity correspondingly. This is difficult, if not impossible, for the single practice to do under the terms of the prepaid contract. If the practice becomes more a prepaid than a fee-for-service provider, it will become more important for the physician to be aware of expenditures and costs.

To keep costs under control, it is necessary to identify them as they relate to a particular department or "responsibility center," defined as that part of the practice responsible for certain activities. In a large medical clinic, each physician or each specialty may be considered a responsiblity center, as may each ancillary department (such as laboratory and radiology), shared support activites (such as reception, appointments, business office, etc.).

Since a prepaid practice knows what its income will be, it will have to decide how to allocate expenses. A budget can be prepared for each responsibility center to establish performance guidelines and to allow the clinic to determine its collective costs and cost per patient (see Figure 14–4).

[3] Profit Distribution and Changing Incentives

Fee-for-service practices are usually production-oriented, or concerned with generating fees. This by itself is not consistent with prepaid health care, as the generation of charges does not affect the income of the clinic. Rather, the economic motivation under a capitated plan is to keep patients healthy to minimize the cost of medical care.

As a result, most prepaid medical groups need to shift from being production oriented to compensating physicians with a base salary and incentives. The incentives must center largely around utilization, referral and other forms of cost control.

After a practice moves into prepaid health care it is important that profit distribution and incentives to the individual physician employees remain consistent with the profitability of the overall clinic. Basic criteria given for profit distribution in Chapter 3, section § 3.50, would not change, except perhaps in certain areas. It is also important to remember that as a medical practice moves into the prepaid health care arena all of the information necessary to make these decisions may not always be available. It will be helpful, for example, to develop data to evaluate the physicians' total productivity measured in terms of procedures performed, and to evaluate the average cost of treatment for the physicians' patients. This data will allow the clinic to evaluate each physician based on

§ 14.07[3]　　MANAGING YOUR MEDICAL PRACTICE　　14–36

Description of Cost	Amount $	Total Patients	Average Per Patient	Clinic Average	Budget
In Patient Hospitalization					
Out-Patient Hospitalization					
Outside Referrals					
Lab					
X-ray					
TOTALS					

PHYSICIAN'S NAME

FOR 12 – MONTH PERIOD ENDING

This report should be filled out for all patients.
It should also be filled out by diagnosis.

Fig. 14–4. An example of a simple budget form that can be used to monitor a prepaid health care system's responsibility centers.

both productivity and the physician's ability to treat patients cost-effectively. Once an average for total physicians in the clinic is established, comparisons become easier.

[4] Monitoring Costs

Under a prepaid program, a clinic may increase total revenues by increasing the number of enrollees, but the income per patient will not be increased. The only way net income per patient can be increased is to decrease the cost per patient.

Some per-patient costs can be decreased by optimizing the ratio of fixed expenses to patient volumes; for example, by increasing the number of enrollees to a point where it is not necessary to take on more rent expenses decreases the cost per patient alloted to rent and occupancy.

The more direct expenses must be monitored for comparative and planning purposes, both on a per-physician and per-diagnosis basis. Individual cost analyses can then be compared with aggregate costs to determine which physicians are practicing cost-effectively and which are exceeding average costs. However, these figures alone will not tell the whole story. It will be necessary to review those physicians' practices where apparent costs-per-patient are high in order to see if there are any unusual cases or circumstances that warrant such excess. Where there are not, it will be necessary to determine why the physician's style of practice is causing the higher cost-per-patient.

Some of the data that the clinic's computer should keep track of include:

- average length of hospitalization and average cost
- referrals to outside physicians and costs
- average cost of ancillary services, such as lab and x-ray
- total average cost listed by diagnosis

This information can be extremely valuable in helping the clinic evaluate each physician's method of practice. Successful providers will need to point out to their less successful associates where they can perform better. Although such feedback is difficult, it is critical for the overall success of the program.

§ 14.08   MANAGING YOUR MEDICAL PRACTICE

The clinic as a whole should be concerned with finding ways to lower costs. This can range from maximum utilization of facilities to getting discounts on supply purchases and negotiating favorable fee arrangements with outside physicians and hospitals. As more medical practices enter the field of prepaid health care and more practices become sophisticated managers, more of this information will become available on an industry-wide basis. Practices able to beat the averages will be more profitable; those unable to do so may end up going out of business.

§ 14.08 Checklist for Prepaid Health Care Programs

The following is a list of points the physician should consider before signing a contract to participate in a prepaid health care program.

— Type of Prepaid Program
  — Health Maintaneance Organization (HMO)
    — Group Model
    — Staff Model
    — Independent Practice Association (IPA)
    — Mixed Model
  — Preferred Provider Organization (PPO)
  — Insured Health Products

— Pros and Cons of Prepaid Health Care
  — Pros
    — Control of practice
    — Preserving patient base
    — Eliminating middleman
    — Lowered costs translating to greater profits
  — Cons
    — Cost containment vs. standard of care
    — Loss of patients if contract is terminated
    — Instability of program or organization

— Assessing the Third Party
  — Ownership
  — Names under which third party operates
  — Experience and tenure
  — Reputation
  — Board of directors and officers
  — Financial strength for last five years
  — Goals
  — Market share
  — Geographic area in which it conducts business
  — Is third party licensed in your state
  — Has third party ever been investigated by Department of Justice or Federal Trade Commission (FTC)

— Evaluating the Plan as a Contract

— The Contract in General
  — State laws under which the contract will be governed
  — Is contract standard for all participating physicians
  — Does contract allow physician's name to be used on brochures and other advertising media
  — No blank spaces
  — Review all documents incorporated into or referenced in contract
  — Can third party reassign the physician's contract
  — Are all oral offers made included in the contract

— The Plan in General
  — Check references of participating providers
  — Obtain copies of all different contracts offered to physicians in the plan
  — Which employer and employee groups receive benefits
  — Application fees or dues

- Costs for which physician will be responsible
- Distribution of premiums or capitations

— Enrollees

- Number of patients physician may or must serve in a specified period of time
- Must physician serve all patients referred
- Responsibility for identifying which patients qualify under the contract

— Physician Liability

- Will contract affect the physician's professional liability insurance coverage
- Extent of third party's obligation to carry liability insurance
- Does professional liability insurance carried by the third party extend coverage to physicians
- Is it necessary to name third party as additional insured under professional liability insurance
- If third party subcontracts for utilization review, peer review, or related activites does liability insurance extend coverage to activities of the subcontractors
- Is it necessary to maintain a specific dollar amount of professional liability insurance
- Has third party been a party to professional liability litigation or dispute
- "Hold harmless" or indemnification clauses: is physician solely responsible for anything that goes wrong
- 24-hour liability: is physician required to make arrangements for another physician to cover in the event of absences or vacations

— Exclusivity and Referrals

- Does contract prohibit physician from contracting with competing third parties

- Does contract restrict referral patterns:
  - Are permissable referral sources adequate
  - Limitations on referrals to laboratory or other ancillary facilities
  - Limitations on involvement with professionals, such as assistant surgeon, anesthesiologist, etc.
- Does physician have right to examine contract referral physicians

- Cost Containment vs. Standard of Care
  - Do procedures require preauthorization from organization
  - Is preauthorization congruent with standard of care
  - Utilization review and standards of review
  - Are services not covered defined and must patient pay for those services

- Capitation Payments and Fee Schedule
  - How is fee schedule determined
  - Contractual obligations made on the third party for payments
  - Outline of time limits for payments
  - Changes in fee schedule: unilateral or must physician be consulted

- Confidentiality
  - Compliance with state laws regarding medical records and confidentiality
  - Are provisions requiring the physician to keep proprietary information confidential specific and reasonable

- Peer review
  - Reviewed by physicians or nonphysicians
  - Qualifications of review coordinator

- State laws for peer review: does immunity extend to third party or to physician

- Grievances
  - Does contract address grievance procedures
  - Do arbitration provisions preclude possibility of pursuing corporate actions through the courts

- Altering and Terminating Contract
  - Are contract amendments unilateral for third party
  - Does contract rollover from one year to the next
  - Can physician renegotiate fees
  - Can physician terminate contract
  - Amount of advance notice to be given before termination
  - Is physician responsible for telling patients of contract termination
  - Must physician continue to provide services after contract has been terminated
  - Physicians right to terminate in the event of third party insolvency and extent of liabilities

- Monitoring Economy of the program
  - Cash basis vs. accrual basis of accounting
  - Growth
    - Physician incentives
    - Monitoring responsibility centers
    - Cutting cost per patient

§ 14.09 Glossary of Terms in Prepaid Health Care

Following is a glossary of terms and their definitions used frequently in discussions of prepaid health care.

Alternative Delivery Systems (ADS). Health care delivery systems other than fee-for-service. Alternative delivery systems include HMOs, CPMs and PPOs. New products developed by insurance companies that do not offer the normal fee-for-service type of reimbursement are also considered alternative delivery systems.

Capitation. Refers to the method of payment in which the service provider is paid and is based on the number of registered patients, rather than on the number and type of services performed. The amount of capitation is based on the number of services and other factors such as the patient's age and sex. Clinics receiving capitated income provide all defined services at no additional cost to the patient, although patient co-payment may be enforced to prevent overutilization of services.

Competitive Medical Plans (CMP). Created by the federal government to broaden the type of medical entity that could contract with the government to provide health care for Medicare patients. The CMP is a capitated plan that defines the costs of Medicare patients on a per-head basis rather than on a fee-for-service basis.

Co-Payment. The out-of-pocket payment required from a patient in a prepaid health care program. This is usually a nominal, flat charge, such as $5.00 per office visit. The general purpose of such co-payment is to discourage overutilization for frivolous purposes.

Covered Services. Refers to all of the medical services the patient may receive at no additional charge or incidental co-payment charge under the terms of the prepaid health care contract (see fully-covered charges).

Dual Choice Option. Refers to an insurance product which offers indemnity insurance as an alternative to HMO or PPO coverage at the same premium. Benefits differ under the two types of plan.

Fee-for-Service/Prepaid (FFS/PPD) Medical Group. Refers to a medical group providing services to patients on both a fee-for-service level and in a prepaid program. This type of practice is becoming more and more common as fee-for-service practices enter prepaid programs and prepaid programs offer alternative care to their usual health care package.

Fully Covered Services. The services which a covered prepaid patient can use without having to make any type of payment other than a possible co-payment.

Health Maintenance Organization (HMO). Comes from the

original concept that the organization is designed to maintain health rather than treat illnesses as they occur. Today, this term refers specifically to an organization whose business is to provide medical services to patients who pay periodic premiums to cover specific medical and health services.

Independent Practice Association (IPA). A legal entity formed by a group of individual practices which can contract with other organizations for business purposes. For example, the IPA may include a group of physicians, hospitals, pharmacists, etc. This group can function as an HMO for business purposes. The attractive feature is that the patient enrolled under an IPA-type HMO may move freely among member practices.

Insured Services. Services which may be covered under the patient's HMO contract, but not as part of the capitated income received by the medical group. As such, the medical group is able to bill the third party at an additional contracted fee for these services.

Joint Venture. May refer to any combination of effort between two or more legal entities to form a third organization. A joint venture could become a partnership, but remain simply a "project" of mutual benefit for two or more parties.

Managed Health Care. The concept of cost controls employed through utilization reviews, required second opinion for surgeries, pre-admission authorization for hospital admission and other efforts to control costs. These concepts, originally employed by HMOs to contain costs, are spreading to most health insurance programs, whether fee-for-service or prepaid.

Medicaid Prepaid Plans. Refers to an HMO or CMP contracting with the state to provide services to Medicaid patients on a capitated basis. Under these plans, the prepaid program generally needs to provide a report to the state for services rendered.

Medicare Supplemental Plans. Patients receiving benefits under Medicare may be covered one of three ways under an HMO plan:

(1) If the Medicare patient is still employed, he or she may be covered under the employer plan; however, a portion of the medical care bill will be reimbursed by Medicare, either through billing or through capitation. Noncovered

charges will be paid for by the employer, representing the patient's supplemental coverage.

(2) Individuals may enroll in supplemental plans offered through an HMO. The patient then pays a premium to the HMO to cover expenses not paid by Medicare, such as the patient's deductible and participation portion. The HMO may then bill Medicare on a fee-for-service basis or may receive a capitated portion based on the number of patients registered.

(3) Medicare patients, where eligible for Medicaid, may have their supplemental benefit paid for by the state through Medicaid.

Member Months. The number of prepaid patients enrolled for one month, generally used to measure the enrollment and determine the capitated income risk.

Negative (Adverse) Selection. A situation where an identified group, such as a geographic area, employer group, etc., has a higher than average rate of utilization.

Noncovered Charges. Services not covered as part of the premium paid by the employer or patient. Examples of common noncovered services might include cosmetic surgery, or dental care.

Participating Medical Group (PMG). A medical group contracting with a third party to provide medical services.

Positive Selection of HMO Members. Positive selection reflects a population of member patients with better health and lower than average utilization.

Preferred Provider Organization (PPO). A network of health care providers forming an organization to provide services to patients at pre-arranged levels of compensation. Generally the patient has the option to move about freely within the PPO network. In some cases, the patient may leave the PPO network and still enjoy insurance coverage, though not without financial penalties. Generally, physicians in the PPO group will be compensated on a modified fee-for-service basis.

Prepaid (PPD) Only Medical Group. A medical group that provides services on a capitated basis only.

Prepaid Patient. A patient covered under an HMO or other prepaid plan.

Premium. The monthly amount paid to the HMO or other third party by the covered patient or employer.

Reinsurance. The concept of having the medical group purchase insurance to cover unexpectedly high, catastrophic costs for a prepaid member. The purpose of reinsurance is to avoid the economics of havng one catastrophic patient wipe out all the revenues of the entire capitated program.

Self-Insurance Prepaid Plan. Allows an employer to contract with an HMO to establish a fund to cover medical treatment for employees. If the treatment costs exceed the funded amount, the employer pays the balance. If the treatment costs are less, some of the excess is refunded to the employer. In this way, the employer shares some of the benefit and risk and is thus encouraged to promote health maintenance.

Shadow Pricing. Refers to the idea of setting an HMO premium for an employer group slightly below the indemnity insurance premium, even though the cost of treating the employer's HMO members may not justify the premium.

Shared-Risk Services. Applies to the concept of a risk-sharing arrangement between the third party and medical group. They usually apply to such services as inpatient medical care, ambulance costs, inpatient hemodialysis and extended care facility costs. The fund is calculated on an enrolled member basis for the medical group. If the amount spent for the shared risk services is less than estimated, the medical group generally receives part of the surplus. If the costs are higher than expected, the medical group may be required to pay into the fund part of the additional costs. The concept is to literally "share" the risk and share the economic savings.

Stop-Loss Limit. Estabishes a maximum dollar amount of coverage per patient which the actual capitation covers. If the patient's cost runs higher than the stop-loss limit, the third party could cover the additional costs. The third party might seek reinsurance (which see) to fund this additional risk.

Triple-Choice Option. An insurance plan offering an HMO, PPO and indemnity coverage as alternatives under the same insurer for the same premium. Benefits under each of the plans vary to balance off the fact that premiums are equal.

§ 14.100 Bibliography

Michaels, Joel L.: Legal Issues in the Fee-for-Service/Prepaid Medical Group. Denver, CO: Center for Research in Ambulatory Health Care Administration, 1982.

Neal, Patricia A.: Management Information Systems for the Fee-for-Service/Prepaid Medical Group. Denver, CO: Center for Research in Ambulatory Health Care Administration, 1986.

Robinson, Richard and Snelson, Elizabeth A.: Revised Physicians Contracting Handbook, 1982.

Schafer, Eldon L. and Cocke, Michael E.: Management Accounting for Health Maintenance Organizations. Denver, CO: Center for Research in Ambulatory Health Care Administration, 1984.

Schafer, Eldon L., et al.: Management Accounting for Fee-for-Service/Prepaid Medical Groups. Denver, CO: Center for Research in Ambulatory Health Care Administration, 1985.

Schafer, Eldon L., et al.: Evaluating the Performance of a Prepaid Medical Group: A Management Auditing Manual. Denver, CO: Center for Research in Ambulatory Health Care Administration, 1985.

CHAPTER 15

COMMUNICATION IN THE MEDICAL OFFICE

> **SCOPE**
>
> Poor communication between physicians, staff and patients can impede the efficiency of even the most carefully organized medical practice. Good communication entails treating seriously all forms of written and oral communication, whether letters, memos, reports, one-on-one conferences, presentations or meetings. The person initiating communication must always formulate the objectives of the communication and determine the best way of delivery to get his or her points across. He or she should be able to define a specific audience and determine whether that audience will respond best to a direct or indirect approach to an intended subject. Written communication allows a person to organize, edit and record thoughts. Oral presentations and meeting can be more spontaneous but often require planning and organization. Presentations should be outlined in advance; the speaker should talk clearly and always summarize points at the conclusion. The person who chairs or leads the meeting should write up an agenda in advance. He or she should choose participants selectively, brief them if necessary and conduct the meeting so that it accomplishes its objectives without wasting time. Good communication skills can only improve the efficiency of a medical practice; bad communication skills can have disastrous consequences.

SYNOPSIS

§ 15.01 The Problems of Poor Communication

§ 15.02 Types of Communication

    [1] Oral Communications

MANAGING YOUR MEDICAL PRACTICE

    [2] Written Communication
§ 15.03 Formulating Objectives
§ 15.04 Managerial Style
    [1] The Tell Style
    [2] The Sell Style
    [3] The Consult Style
    [4] The Joint Style
    [5] Selecting the Appropriate Style
§ 15.05 Analyzing the Audience
    [1] Personality Types
    [2] The Thinker Personality
    [3] The Intuitive Personality
    [4] The Sensing Personality
    [5] The Feeling Personality
§ 15.06 Structuring Your Message
§ 15.07 Putting a Message in Writing
    [1] Planning
    [2] Format
    [3] Editing
§ 15.08 Making Presentations
    [1] Planning the Presentation
    [2] Outlining the Presentation
    [3] Delivery
§ 15.09 Effective Meetings
    [1] Planning the Meeting
    [2] Type of Meeting
      [a] Consultative Meeting
      [b] Recommendation Meeting
      [c] Delegation Meeting
      [d] Information Meeting
      [e] Instructional Meeting
    [3] Selecting the Participants
    [4] Creating the Environment
    [5] Briefing Participants
    [6] The Agenda
    [7] Leading the Meeting
      [a] Before Starting the Meeting
      [b] Starting the Meeting
      [c] Directing the Meeting
      [d] Coming to a Consensus

(Rel.3–2/89 Pub.372)

                [e] Concluding the Meeting
                [f] Recording the Meeting
    § 15.10   Checklist for Office Communications
    § 15.100   Bibliography
Appendix 15-A   Daily Report
Appendix 15-B   Memorandum
Appendix 15-C   Meetings

§ 15.01 The Problems of Poor Communication

Good communication between physicians, partners, staff and patients is essential to the management of a medical practice. A lack of communication can upset even the most efficiently organized office routine.

Good communication in the medical office will lead to better practice management. Poor communication can lead to problems that seriously affect practice efficiency.

Here are three examples of typical communication problems that can occur in the management of a medical office:

Case 1

Dr. Jones, a very busy practitioner, hired Judy to increase collections at his office. Judy had worked for Doctor Nelson, a practitioner Dr. Jones had spoken to many times throughout the year and whose high collection percentage and low accounts receivable he had always envied. Three months ago, when Dr. Jones learned that Dr. Nelson was retiring and that Judy would be available, he hired her immediately.

On Friday morning, Dr. Jones arrives at his office to find Judy's letter of resignation on his desk. Consulting his afternoon schedule, Dr. Jones sees that he is booked solid and that there are patients in the waiting room who have been waiting for an hour already. Dr. Jones realizes the importance of discussing the matter with Judy, but does not feel that he has time. He has to put it off until Monday morning.

While Dr. Jones sees his afternoon patients, Judy sits at her desk fuming. For the past three months she has attempted to meet with Dr. Jones to discuss the collection policies and procedures. Judy is well-versed in collections and has some very good recommendations to make, but she has been very frustrated as a result of several

§ 15.01   MANAGING YOUR MEDICAL PRACTICE   15–4

things. The final issue that led to her decision to quit surfaced when Betty Hanson, an established patient, told Judy that she had no business discussing her account with her. Betty Hanson went to Dr. Jones. Dr. Jones told Betty not to worry about her account, he knew that she was a good patient and that she could pay whenever she wanted to.

Case 2

Dr. Nelson is not scheduled to see patients Friday afternoon, and needs only to spend an hour at the office to dictate a couple of charts before picking up his paycheck. He is then going to take the rest of the afternoon off to go shopping.

Betty, Dr. Nelson's office manager, comes into the office with a frustrated look on her face. "Dr. Nelson," she says, "I have all of the payroll checks for you to sign, however, if the doctors cash their checks today, there won't be enough money. I'm afraid that none of the doctors are going to be able to cash their checks until we get some more money in."

Dr. Nelson is incredulous. How could the office be in such dire shape so suddenly? Only last month the physicians met and discussed the profit with their accountant. Based on excess profits, they had decided to purchase a new x-ray machine this month. Now Betty is telling him that he will not be able to take his salary today!

Case 3

Dr. Kesler likes to get to the office before his patients do so that he can review the morning mail and review the charts of the patients he will be seeing that afternoon. Since he has a busy Monday morning lined up, he has arrived at his office 30 minutes before his first scheduled appointment.

A brown envelope from the government sitting in the mail catches his eye. Upon opening it, he discovers that it is a letter from the Internal Revenue Service. It states that he is in violation of reporting requirements for his retirement plan. The IRS is proposing a penalty equal to $25 a day for each day the return is late. From the letter, it appears that the return should have been filed six months ago. Dr. Kesler remembers reading an article last month in one of the practice management journals where one doctor's retirement plan was disqualified because he did not file the necessary reports with the IRS. The liability to the doctor in the article came to hundreds of thousands of dollars. Dr. Kesler immediately begins to fumble through the phone book for his accountant's phone number.

In reviewing each of these three scenarios, it can be shown how the office communication process broke down to cause, or exacerbate, the problem and transform it from something calling for attention to a matter of urgency.

Case 1

Judy is leaving mainly as a result of poor communications. When she arrived at her job she was excited by the challenge of helping Dr. Jones increase his collections and cash flow. Her many years of experience with Dr. Nelson gave her assurance. She originally had set up Dr. Nelson's collection system, and worked hand-in-hand with him in coordinating the collection policy for the office and following up on delinquent collections.

However, working for Dr. Jones proved to be an entirely different situation. When she arrived on the job, Judy discovered that there was no policy on collections nor any type of follow up procedures outlined for employees. As a result, Judy immediately set up a proposed policy of collections and procedures to be followed. After working on the policy between attempts to get the cash flow sped up, Judy eagerly presented the completed plan for Dr. Jones' approval. When she asked to set up a meeting to discuss it with him, he suggested that she give the material to him for his review. In spite of Judy's frequent inquiries about the recommendations, Dr. Jones' only response was that he had not gotten around to reviewing them yet, but would in a few days. One day last week, while looking for a lost ledger card, Judy found the report in the file on Dr. Jones' desk buried between some medical journals and advertising brochures. It was obvious that Dr. Jones did not consider his review of her recommendations a "top" priority.

Lacking the authority to implement her policies and procedures without approval, Judy had limited success improving Dr. Jones' collections. As she waited for the changes to be approved, she had to try to follow the "way things have always been done." When Betty Hanson went to Dr. Jones last week and Dr. Jones went over Judy's head (and failed to discuss it with Judy afterwards) she knew that she could never be effective in Dr. Jones' office. As a result, she decided to take a job offered to her by another doctor, even though the position paid slightly less.

Case 2

Dr. Nelson's cash shortage should have come as no surprise. Although his practice is doing well, the cash was short for the month because of the substantial amount diverted to the purchase of the new x-ray machine. Had Dr. Nelson been receiving weekly cash flow reports from the office, the problem would have been flagged earlier on. He could have discussed the situation with his office manager or accountant, and he would have learned that an appropriate solution to the problem was to finance the purchase of the x-ray equipment and amortize it over a few years. All of the financing could have been pre-arranged and the doctors would have been able to cash their checks on time.

Case 3

When Dr. Kesler reached his accountant, Jim Quinlan, Jim reminded him that the pension administrators would undertake all of the necessary filing requirements as part of their annual fee. Since Jim always charged extra for these reports, Dr. Kesler was happy to delegate this job to the pension administrators. After three years with the pension administrators, however, Dr. Kesler decided to turn the entire pension over to his insurance company, which would provide a guaranteed return and "handle all of the administration." Dr. Kesler quickly phoned the insurance representative, Frank Glassman. Frank informed Dr. Kesler that his company felt it was the accountant's responsibility to prepare the IRS reports. Frank had not communicated with Dr. Kesler's accountant because he assumed that Dr. Kesler would handle this. It was beginning to look like the reports simply had not been filed. Dr. Kesler called Jim back to try to determine the best course of action.

The above examples are proof that it is essential for the medical practitioner to establish excellent interoffice communications, specifically in the following areas:

- with patients
- with the office staff
- with the hospital administration

- with fellow physicians, particularly with partners or those with whom the physician is sharing patient care
- with physician advisors, for example, accountants, attorneys, insurance representatives, pension administrators, etc.

§ 15.02 Types of Communication

All forms of oral and written communication are important. They include meetings, presentations, one-on-one contact, reports, letters and memos.

There are a number of different aspects of communication within the medical office, both formal and informal.

[1] Oral Communications

Oral communications can take the following forms:

Meetings. Meetings can be conducted in a conference room, or through telephone conference calls that allow each participant to stay in his or her own office. Meetings can be held with staff, fellow physicians, hospital administration or patients and their families.

Presentations. Presentations can be made to fellow physicians, patients during educational programs and sometimes the public through a hospital-sponsored event. Physicians who are prominent and sought out by the news media may end up giving presentations for press conferences.

One-on-One Contact. Like group meetings, one-on-one contact can be conducted in person or over the telephone. One-on-one contact can entail communication with patients, other physicians, staff members, advisors, hospital people, suppliers, etc. It may be the most common form of communication used by the physician.

[2] Written Communication

Written communication can take the following forms:

Reports. The managing physician should receive a number of readable, informative reports. An example of a daily financial report prepared by the bookkeeper is shown in Appendix 15-A. This simple report helps keep the physician informed on a daily basis about the cash situation and the office production, outlining both charges and the number of patients seen. All of this information is readily available to the staff members who compile the report. Other routine reports include the financial reports prepared by the accountants.

Memos. A memo is an excellent form of communication that can be used to establish a record. Memos can be dictated at any time of the day or night, in the car or at the hospital—in other words, whenever and wherever the thought occurs. An example of memo format is provided in Appendix 15-B.

Letters. Letters can be an extremely efficient way to communicate with advisors and other physicians. In addition, letters are excellent practice builders when used to communicate with patients.

§ 15.03 Formulating Objectives

For any communication to be effective, its objectives must first be defined. Objectives encompass what is to be achieved by the communication and how it is to be achieved.

The first step in organizing inter-office communications and becoming an effective communicator is to calculate objectives. The objectives of communications can be broken down into three areas:

General Objective. The general objective is what a person hopes to accomplish through communication, a comprehensive statement about what is being done or what problem is being solved.

Action Objective. The action objective specifies what action should be taken to accomplish the general objective. The action objective (or objectives) should state specifically the action to take place.

Communication Objective. The communication objective is the specific outcome expected as a result of the communication.

Attention to all three objectives will ensure that the ideas have been delivered. The following scenarios are offered as illustrations.

(1) The *general objective* is to make patients feel important and better served when calling the office. The *action objective* is to have the staff answer the phone in three rings. *The communication objective* is that as a result of reading this memorandum, the staff will make sure every phone call is answered within three rings.

(2) The *general objective* is to eliminate lost charges. The *action objective* is to prepare a charge slip for each patient seen during the day, making sure that at the end of the day a charge slip has been returned to bookkeeping for each of the patients registered during the day. The *communication objective* is that as a result of the meeting, the bookkeeper will make sure that there is a charge slip for each patient registered at the end of each day.

(3) The *general objective* is to make certain that all necessary tax reports are timely, completed and filed. The *action objective* is to make sure that the accountant prepares the necessary returns and notifies the office of proper filing dates. The *communication objective* is that as a result of reading this letter, the accountants will understand that they are responsible for completing or to at least notifying us of any filing requirements.

§ 15.04 Managerial Style

Once communication objectives have been defined, it is necessary to determine the most appropriate managerial style for delivering them.

Once the objective of the communication is determined, the management style in which it is to be delivered should be considered. In her book *Guide to Managerial Communication,* Mary Munter describes four different managerial styles: tell, sell, consult and joint.

[1] The Tell Style

The tell style of management communication is used in situations where information is being delivered and there is no need for audience involvement. For example, the tell style would be used by the office manager explaining to the bookkeeper how to balance the cash with the daily deposits.

[2] The Sell Style

In this situation, the communicator attempts to persuade his or her 'audience.' An example is the physician who has researched the need for and types of buy-sell agreements and determines that it is extremely important that they be in place in the office. He or she calls a meeting with associates to persuade them of the importance of these agreements and authorizes agreements to be prepared by the corporate attorney for review and signature.

[3] The Consult Style

The consult managerial style depends on obtaining information or opinions from the audience. An obvious example of this are physicians consulting each other on patient care. It would be foolish for one physician not to share the information on a patient with another physician working on the same case.

[4] The Joint Style

With the joint managerial communication style, there is a high level of audience involvement and joint action by the communicator and the audience. One example is when a physician calls a meeting to discuss ways to better handle the patient flow in the office. This might include input from the receptionist, nurses and assistants, as well as from other physicians.

[5] Selecting the Appropriate Style

An effective communicator may automatically select the proper style. In many cases, however, signals may get mixed. For example, the physician who employs a joint managerial communication style when telling a staff member to do something a particular way may produce only frustration and a lack of communication: the physician becomes annoyed when the staff member does not appear to be accepting and implementing the recommendations, while the staff member wonders why the physician will not listen to his or her ideas on the subject.

§ 15.05 Analyzing the Audience

> Differences in personality may sometimes cause communication problems. Although each person's personality is a blend of various traits, he or she can generally be characterized by one of four dominant personality types: intuitive, sensing, feeling or thinking.

Whether the physician intends to call a business meeting, have a one-on-one conference or give a presentation, he or she must consider the audience, or recipient of the message, in order to determine the best method of communication. The following points need to be considered:

How much common knowledge is shared? A physician will communicate with a physician of the same specialty differently than with the bookkeeper. The physician must consider how much background information to give so that the audience will be able to understand the situation and not be bored with redundancies or information that they already have. Professional education, business experience and age are among the many factors that must be kept in mind.

How can the message be made to appeal to the audience? The physician should determine what benefits will accrue to the group receiving the message when he or she is deciding how to communicate it. One communication consultant recommends the use of "you statements": for example, the statement "I want the daysheets balanced everyday before you go home. I think the deposit slips must be balanced with the daysheet because I feel we have been losing money around here," is much less likely to be welcomed or acted upon than a statement like "After a discussion with our accountant, I was convinced that you would benefit substantially by making sure that the deposits balanced with the cash sheets before you went home each night. If you balance the sheets each night, you won't have to worry about the accountants bothering you at the end of the month; you will have the pleasure of knowing that everything is right when you go home. You will appeciate the feeling that your work is done right because you take pride in your work." Obviously, the second message is much more likely to fall upon receptive ears.

[1] Personality Types

To communicate effectively, a person should be aware of different personality types. Understanding personality types can sometimes help explain what appear to be problems in communication. Consider the following example:

Case 4

Dr. Mellin, a urologist in a small office, employs Sharon on a full-time basis and has one other employee come in to do bookkeeping twice a week. Sharon has been working for Dr. Mellin for two months. At first Dr. Mellin was delighted by Sharon's cheerful behavior and her willingness to greet the patients and treat them very hospitably. She was very aggressive in implementing new ideas and pointing out errors of the office which needed to be corrected. Dr. Mellin was happy that Sharon had felt comfortable doing this, and he was quick to praise her for the good work she had been doing and for the new ideas she had presented to the office.

During the last few weeks, however, things seemed to have changed. Feeling that Sharon has become familiar with office procedures, Dr. Mellin has been spending less and less time with her. But Sharon doesn't seem to accept the fact that Dr. Mellin will not be available to answer all of her questions forever, and she has been very demanding of his time. Dr. Mellin finds this frustrating, as he feels that Sharon shouldn't need so much guidance. He has been trying to ignore her requests, and has been more curt and formal with her for fear that she was perceiving their relationship as too personal. Instead of helping, however, Dr. Mellin's approach has made the situation worse. Sharon seems to be mad at Dr. Mellin all of the time and Dr. Mellin is starting to dread coming into the office.

This is a problem common to small offices: personality conflicts surface quickly and can lead to termination if they are not resolved expediently. In a larger office, friction between physician and staff, physician partners or staff members can usually remain hidden for a longer period of time.

The problem outlined above does not result from anything in particular that either Dr. Mellin or Sharon are doing wrong. Sharon's strong initiative type of personality demands recognition and appreciation. When she first started the job, Dr. Mellin invested substantial time working with her, in the hope that management of the practice would improve once she began to set things right. Thus, Dr. Mellin was satisfying Sharon's needs and she was pleased to work hard for him. As Sharon become more confident and familiar with her job, though, Dr. Mellin began to pay less attention to the office and stopped meeting her recognition needs. When Dr. Mellin became more formal with Sharon, with the idea that it would help, it only resulted in further alienation. Eventually, Dr. Mellin realized what was wrong with the situation and made an effort to recognize

Sharon and compliment her performance. The situation improved because Sharon, feeling more important and appreciated, was back to a good level of performance, obviously pleased with her job.

Psychologists and consultants have recognized different personality types for many years. Psychologist Carl Jung conceptualized eight different personality types, broken into four functional types. They can be summarized thus:

- 1 and 2: Extroverted Thinking and Introverted Thinking;
- 3 and 4: Extroverted Feeling and Introverted Feeling;
- 5 and 6: Extroverted Sensing and Introverted Sensing;
- 7 and 8: Extroverted Intuitive and Introverted Intuitive.

A basic understanding of the traits of these four functional types of personality can help to identify individuals.

Thinking Personality

Extroverted	*Introverted*
Dominant	Analytical
Practical	Independent
Bold	Quiet
Disciplined	Disciplined
Objective	Curious
Analytical	Adaptable
Conscientious	Clear-Thinking
Logical	Intellectual
Decisive	Organized
Energetic	Logical
Confident	Keep Trying
Responsible	Efficient
Determined	Thoughtful

Feeling Personality

Extroverted	*Introverted*
Friendly	Modest
Tactful	Cooperative
Warm	Sincere
Cooperative	Loyal
Enthusiastic	Understanding
Cheerful	Tolerant

Agreeable
Understanding
Considerate
Loyal
Idealistic
Sympathetic
Gracious

Sensitive
Sympathetic
Committed
Independent
Controlled
Soft-Spoken
Patient

Sensing Personality

Extroverted
Realistic
Factual
Persuasive
Open-Minded
Easy-Going
Tolerant
Efficient
Quick
Calm
Considerate
Tactful
Diplomatic
Friendly

Introverted
Dependable
Stable
Thorough
Factual
Systematic
Painstaking
Persevering
Reliable
Practical
Objective
Serious-Minded
Effective
Conservative

Intuitive Personality

Extroverted
Innovative
Enthusiastic
Imaginative
Confident
Persistent
Involved
Stimulating
Perceptive
Persuasive
Forward-Looking
Mature
Serious
Energetic

Introverted
Creative
Persevering
Ingenious
Understanding
Soft-Spoken
Reserved
Intelligent
Sincere
Observant
Determined
Patient
Keep-Trying
Frank

Although people cannot be simplified into four separate categories and, in reality, are a blend of these various types, generally one or two categories dominate the personality of each individual. Some individuals have a personality type which is extreme and obvious while others are more difficult to observe.

[2] The Thinker Personality

An individual with a predominant thinking personality is very analytical and logical. He or she is a great planner and expects things to go according to those plans. He or she likes to make sure that everything has been considered and that the best option has been selected. This type of person has to see the proper conclusion being developed or things will not be acceptable.

The thinker type personality is prone to a number of errors in communication. He or she often:

- over-explains
- is too noncommittal
- speaks in a monotone
- doesn't express feelings enough
- is too pedantic
- lays out his or her presentation in too rigid of a fashion

In communicating with a thinker type personality, a person should:

- lay out all of the facts
- convince the person that all of the options have been explored
- re-cap the presentation in writing, if possible

In persuading the thinker type, one must be careful not to 'overload' them. Although a thinker must feel that all of the facts have been considered, too much data can render them incapable of drawing a conclusion. If unable to draw a conclusion, he or she may demand more information, which only compounds the problem.

(Rel.3–2/89 Pub.372)

[3] The Intuitive Personality

The individual with an intuitive personality type is a promoter. Generally speaking, this person thinks in terms of the future. A major problem with a strong intuitive personality is that by the time the person begins to reap the benefits of his or her ideas, he or she has moved on to another project. Recognition is important to the intuitive personality. This type of individual likes being associated with celebrities and the most "in" things. Whereas a thinker personality may buy a car based on a careful analysis and which will best fulfill his or her needs, an intuitive type personality may buy a car if he or she feels it is the most fashionable or "the latest."

When it comes to implementing a new system in the office, the person with the thinker personality type needs to be convinced the system was selected only after all of the options had been reviewed and it was concluded that it would be the best system for the office. The intuitive personality, on the other hand, must be convinced that it is "the latest technology" and is indeed being used by "leading" physicians.

People who are predominantly intuitive tend to:

- be too scattered in comments and jump about in their presentation
- raise too many issues
- appear ego-centered
- run on at length
- appear rigid
- appear too judgmental
- appear condescending
- be too abstract
- concentrate too much on the concept, and not enough on how to implement it

In communicating with an intuitive personality type, the other person often must do the footwork. The intuitive personality tends not to pay attention to details; to keep this type of person interested and excited, it is important to have a continual source of new ideas.

The intuitive personality will become bored and disenchanted in a static situation.

The worst thing one can do to the individual with an intuitive personality type is ignore them or take them for granted.

[4] The Sensing Personality

A person with a strong dominant sensing personality type is an action person, a doer. The person is concerned exclusively with the present situation. The sensing personality type does not want to waste time studying a problem; he or she wants immediate action. If the computer being looked at seems to do the job, the sensing type will want to order it. It doesn't matter whether the other systems will do the job or not; that's not relevant.

In communicating with an individual with a strong sensing personality, one must get to the bottom line fast: "We're getting a new computer system on Monday. We'll want to have it installed right away so that we don't get behind with our postings or billings. Plan on spending some overtime next week so that we can get the job done."

A predominant sensing personality type tends:

- to be less willing to take the time to listen to the other person's side of the story
- not to ask enough questions from the other person
- to control the conversation
- to interrupt, and not let the other person finish a statement
- to come on strong and put the other person on the defensive
- not to take the time to learn the person's viewpoint or objections

In communicating with the sensing personality type, one must show results and progress. This type of individual hates "try-hards" (a person who always tries hard but never gets things done.) A sensing personality is not interested in efforts, but in results. A physician who has a sensing personality won't care if the staff re-did his or her coding systems, but will be very pleased at the increased reimbursements from third parties as a result of the work. For this kind of person, if something does not achieve results, it is a wasted effort. When communicating with a sensing personality, one should know what results they want and when they want them. They should be given as much latitude as possible to determine how to do the job.

[5] The Feeling Personality

A feeler uses feelings and past experiences to evaluate and make decisions. He or she is very nostalgic and slow to change, and might give the following type of excuse: "I don't see why we need a new computer system, the pegboard has been doing a fantastic job for the last 20 years."

Feelers often:

- spend too much time talking about the past
- forget to cite facts
- over-simplify
- rely too much on personality and not enough on data
- tell too many anecdotes or stories
- take too long to get to the main point
- do not push to bring objectives out into the open
- avoid bringing up any unpleasant facts

One must be very sensitive to this type of person's feelings and understand that his or her decisions are based heavily on past experience. "It's true the pegboard has lasted for 20 years and achieved positive results. It was very difficult to abandon our old system which worked very well up to that time; however, once we implemented the pegboard, we all benefited. Based on our past experience, I feel that now is the time to switch our office to the computer." Feelers are much more loyal and open to ideas if they believe the other person cares about them.

§ 15.06 Structuring Your Message

> Oral communications must be tailored to fit the audience's personality type. The audience personality type will determine whether a direct approach or indirect approach is more appropriate.

When communicating, it is important to analyze the members of the audience and adjust to them, rather than expect them to adjust to you. A good communicator will be aware not only of the audience's personality type but also of his or her own personality type and compensate for personal weaknesses. By doing so one becomes a much more effective communicator and develops a better understanding of why things were not communicated when it is clear that they should have been.

When communicating verbally, one must keep in mind the audience memory curve, which is that an audience will remember most things said at the beginning and end of the presentation. It is important to determine what points are to be emphasized so that one can determine where to put them in the presentation. Obviously, the important points should be put in the beginning of the presentation and/or at the end to increase the probability that the audience will remember them.

There are two basic strategies one can employ when presenting a point, the direct strategy and the indirect strategy. When the audience is likely to agree, interested in results or very busy, one should use the direct strategy, giving the generalization or conclusion first before proceeding to examples that offer specific support. For example:

The telephone committee recommends the purchase of the XYZ phone system for the following reasons:

    Reason One

    Reason Two

    Reason Three

The direct strategy gets the decision out front while the audience is listening. Sensing personality types appreciate this "bottom line" approach and individuals who want supporting information will listen to find the appropriate data supporting the conclusion.

The indirect style can be used when one anticipates that the audience will disagree with the conclusion or argue with the conclusion. If the audience has a strong thinking personality, it may also be appropriate to use the indirect approach to outline the facts before the conclusion.

When employing the indirect strategy, one should save the

strongest argument supporting the conclusion for last. At that point, the disagreeing audience may be more likely to be persuaded.

§ 15.07 Putting a Message in Writing

Putting a message in writing creates a formal record and gives the person writing it a chance to evaluate and edit it before it is sent. A written communication should be planned, outlined and put into an organized format that calls attention to the main points.

There are a number of advantages to communicating in writing. It gives the writer the opportunity to evaluate and study what he or she is trying to communicate to the audience. It also creates a record of the communication that will prevent an audience from saying "you never told me." Generally, unless transmitted as a form letter, a written communication also is perceived as more serious and personalized.

Because writing creates a record that can be studied and reviewed, it is important that nothing in what is written is erroneous or confusing. Nevertheless, much written communication within and going out of the office is often poorly constructed because not enough time is devoted to its planning and organization.

[1] Planning

Initial planning of written communication can range from carefully organizing one's thoughts before beginning dictation, to dictating ideas, creating an outline and basing the entire writing on the outline. Generally a person can communicate much more powerfully and effectively simply by organizing his or her thoughts first. He or she may wish to jot down a few major points on a note pad in order of importance.

When writing, remember that much correspondence is not read thoroughly. If the writer doesn't get his or her point across early, the reader may not take the time to finish the correspondance. Unrelated points must be identified clearly,. Because the reader may lose interest in what is written early on, and assume he or she has grasped the contents of the message before completing the entire correspondence, it may be appropriate in some circumstances to prepare separate letters or memoranda for each topic.

[2] Format

It may be appropriate to adopt basically standard formats for some correspondence. When done with thought and purpose, this can result in positive long-term effects. A physician dictating letters to referring physicians regarding a patient may want to use a standard format. For example, a specialist might dictate such letters according to the following format:

Harold Nelson, M.D.

2345 Webster Street

Anywhere, USA 12

Jane Brown, M.D.
300 Medical Building
USA Town, MN 5511X

RE: John Hampten

Dear Dr. Brown:

Diagnosis
Based on my examination of Mr. Hampten . . . . (give diagnosis, etc.).

History

(Give patient history, exam results, basis for diagnosis.)

Thank You

Thanking you for your confidence . . . .

Sincerely,

Harold Nelson, M.D.

Note that in the above format, the subject's name is clearly listed. In the next section, the diagnosis, probable diagnosis or a list of probable diagnoses is outlined. This is given first because it is the reason why Dr. Brown is referring Mr. Hampten to Dr. Nelson.

The next section of the letter outlines the history, exam results and the basis for the diagnosis. The last section of the correspondence is a thank you. It is likely that the reader will pass over the thank you. From a marketing standpoint, it is probably better to send thank you letters separately and periodically to good referral sources; this increases the likelihood that they will be appreciated.

When the thank you is part of the main letter, it is usually considered an irrelevant formality.

When writing memoranda, reports and correspondence, use highlighting to draw attention to particular sections of the material and to dramatize key points. Highlighting can be in the form of bold lettering, indentation, capitalization, underlining, or any other method that draws attention. For example:

MEMORANDUM

TO: Julie Fritz
FROM: Dr. Miller
DATE: February 15, 1989
RE: Staff Meeting on February 14, 1988.

TARDINESS

At our meeting it was pointed out that employee breaks are frequently running beyond the 15-minute period allotted. This is putting unnecessary stress on the employees not on break. Effective immediately, <u>employees will be docked on their salaries if they are not back in their station by the end of the break time.</u>

CASH RECEIPTS

As a result of the additional attention being paid to collections by the bookkeeping staff, cash receipts for the past month were up 5 percent. It was decided that <u>a $50 bonus will be paid to Sue Anderson and Sherry Nelson.</u> You should give the bonuses to Sue and Sherry personally, and let them know that <u>the bonus is a direct result of their good performance.</u>

APPOINTMENT SCHEDULING

The patient flow has improved enormously during the past month with the implementation of our new wave scheduling system. <u>Twenty-five dollar ($25) bonuses should be paid to Sally Walker, May Hanson and Debbie Smith for their contributions in making the system work. The waiting time of patients is down</u> and we were able to see <u>an average of two or more patients per day</u> as a result of the new scheduling system.

The memoranda outlined above are easy to read because the points requiring action are easy to spot and leap out at the reader.

The same type of technique can be used in writing letters, reports, etc.

A number of different correspondence formats can be used in the medical office. Generally speaking, the physician should select a favorite style and use it for all of his or her correspondence. It is recommended that physicians in a group practice all use the same standard format for correspondance. Some groups use different formats depending on the individual doctor's preference, and this not only breaks up the unity from an appearance standpoint, but also makes it difficult for secretaries to determine which style should be used.

The remainder of this section gives the standard elements that should appear in any letter and several possible formats for organizing them.

Standard Elements of a Letter

(1) Heading: Sender's address, followed by date, either on printed letterhead or typed out.
(2) Inside
Address: Receiver's name, title and address, e.g.:.
   Ms. Rachel Worth
   Street Address
   City, State, Zip Code
(3) Salutation:
   Formal: My dear Ms. Worth
                  Dear Ms. Worth
   Semi-formal: Dear Ms. Worth
   Informal: Dear Rachel
(4) Subject line (optional):
   Used as a headline for the reader's benefit.
(5) Closing and Signature:
   Formal: Very truly yours,
                  (Sincerely yours,)
                  ABC Clinic
                  John Morrell, M.D.
                  Medical Director
   Semi-formal: Yours truly,
                  (Sincerely yours,)
                  John Morrell, M.D.
                  Medical Director

Informal: Cordially,
                  John Morrell

Semi-Block Format

  Date
Name
Address
Address
Salutation:

_____
_____
_____
_____

  Closing,
  Signature

Modified Block Format

  Date
Name
Address
Address
Salutation:

_____
_____
_____
_____

  Closing,
  Signature

Full Block Format

  Date
Name

Address

Address

Salutation:

_____

_____

_____

Closing,

Signature

[3] Editing

With word processors and memory typewriters, people have come to expect "perfect or near perfect" correspondence. Because modern equipment has made editing easy, physicians should take every advantage to enhance their correspondence. Whereas moving a paragraph or changing a sentence used to require the complete retyping of a letter, the word processor can "cut and paste" paragraphs, sentences, words, etc., and insert sentences, words and paragraphs or delete them with a stroke of a key. Thus, there is no reason for the physician not to edit written communications for clarity while he or she is reading them back, particularly those communications leaving the office. When editing, a person should:

(1) Edit for communication:
- Are the objectives accomplished?
- Is the appropriate style being used?
- Is the correspondence appropriate for the recipient?
- Are the main ideas emphasized?

(2) Edit for organization:
- Are ideas grouped together in clear order?
- Are the ideas logical?
- Do the major points get across fast enough?

(3) Edit for good writing:

§ 15.08   MANAGING YOUR MEDICAL PRACTICE   15–26

- Look at the document in its entirety, paragraph by paragraph, sentence by sentence, for good utilization of words.

(4) Check the grammar and punctuation.

§ 15.08 Making Presentations

> When making a presentation, the speaker should first choose a subject on which he or she can speak knowledgably and then outline the important points he or she wants to make. The speaker should tailor the terminology of the presentation to the understanding of the audience, speak positively, vividly, and where possible use visual aids.

Although a physician may not consider himself or herself a public speaker or orator, most physicians will need to make presentations in front of other people at some point in their careers. Presentations can range from a meeting with the office staff, to a formal presentation to other physicians at the hospital to a public presentation done to generate goodwill and promotion.

Physicians should not shun giving presentations since they are an excellent tool for communication and can also be used as a practice builder. Physicians who are shy or uncomfortable about making presentations might also look into joining a local chapter of the Toastmasters, an organization devoted exclusively to helping members build confidence through public speaking.

[1] Planning the Presentation

To make a good presentation, the speaker must know his or her subject. In addition, the speaker should pick a subject that he or she is excited about and enjoys. While an orthopedist might do a presentation on how he or she developed a series of exercises to help patients with back problems, a cardiologist might discuss how patients who adhere to certain diet and exercise programs have experienced one-year full recoveries. Too often, people believe that the topics they know best will be uninteresting to others, leading them to select topics which they know less about.

The physician should know that people are intrigued by the practice of medicine and, generally, are very interested in what they have to say. When a physician talks to nonphysicians, technical medical terminology should be avoided.

(Rel.3–2/89 Pub.372)

Personal interest in the subject will make the presentation stand out as something special. A physician interested in jogging, for example, might develop a presentation on the risk and benefits of jogging. The presentation could emphasize how to minimize and avoid the risk while maximizing the benefits. Even subjects that are less specifically health-related can be addressed in a medical presentation: a physician very interested in renovation of old houses, for example, could develop a presentation on the health hazards of home repairs and renovations.

[2] Outlining the Presentation

It is important to determine the objective of the presentation. Generally a presentation will have one or more of the four objectives:

- to inform
- to convince
- to get action
- to entertain

In outlining the talk and points to be addressed, consider what needs to be presented in order to achieve the objectives.

Use samples and comparisons to "paint pictures" for the audience. A statement like: "Stop, look around you. The probability is that one in five of us will die from cancer" is much more vivid than "490,000 Americans die from cancer each year." The statement "Every pound of fat puts additional strain on your heart" is not as powerful as "For every pound of fat, your heart must pump blood through 100 miles of capillaries." When descriptive examples are used, the audience will become more interested in the presentation; this increases the likelihood of getting the point across.

Visual aids can be an excellent tool for getting the point across. Visual aids can take the form of slides, overheads, flip charts or chalk boards. Overheads and slides can be made in advance to ensure that they illustrate that proper points. Drawing on the blackboard or using a flip chart will give the impression of spontaneity or personalization. Visual aids should also be geared toward the audience. Do not use the same technical slides which were well received by a group of physicians when addressing a group of nonphysicians. A drawing that diagrams how a specific medical procedure is performed is much more appropriate for the public than a slide showing the actual procedure.

When preparing a presentation, put together an outline organizing and covering all of the points which are to be presented. Do not try to memorize the entire speech word for word. Worse yet, do not make a draft of the presentation which will be read. Plan on speaking to the group audience in basically the same way that one would speak to a small group or an individual. If the topic is well-known, and an outline is available to help the speaker remember the points he or she wishes to make, the presentation will go well.

[3] Delivery

The introduction to a presentation should be positive and designed to get attention. It should not contain apologies like: "I'm not quite prepared to cover this topic, but I am going to give it a try."

One good way to start a presentation is with an example: "In our practice, we have diagnosed X cases of colon cancer each year. Of those, X percentage lead to fatalities. This saddens us because we know that of the X number of patients who will die, Y of them could have been saved by treatment if they had come in a year earlier for diagnosis. This is just one reason why we recommend annual examinations after age X.'

Stress can be an enemy or an ally. Too much can rattle the speaker, but a certain amount of stress can keep the speaker alert and bright. "Stage fright" is a normal part of the process of giving a presentation. Even the most experienced speakers continue to have stage fright before giving presentations. The best way to maintain control over fright and to have confidence is to be prepared. If a speaker knows his or her topic and is well-prepared, the fright usually disappears as soon as the presentation begins.

A speaker should not try to imitate the techniques or style of another speaker. He or she should try to act natural and give the presentation in a way that is most natural for him or her. All too often speakers feel that they must incorporate jokes into the talk to be effective. The probability of successfully introducing humor into the talk is far exceeded by the probability that the humor will not have its desired effect. A quick cost-benefit analysis should demonstrate the wisdom of not incorporating jokes into the presentation.

During the presentation, the speaker should make each point vividly. He or she should call attention to a new point with a new example or with a new visual aid. When emphasizing points, the speaker should make every effort to show how the audience benefits from the knowledge of the points.

At the conclusion of the presentation, the speaker should summarize the major points and benefits he or she has covered. This leaves the audience feeling enriched by the presentation and refreshes their memory on the points made. As the memory curve illustrates, audience memory increases at the end of a presentation.

§ 15.09 Effective Meetings

When planning a meeting, the leader should make every effort to avoid wasting the participants' time. Meetings should be organized in advance: the leader should determine whether it is to be a consultative, informational, instructional, delegational or recommendation-type of meeting. Objectives should be outlined and written down on an agenda. Participants who can give positive input should be chosen and, if necessary, briefed in advance of the meeting.

Physicians attend many meetings in the course of their career. Although the physician may leave some meetings feeling excited and informed, many times he or she leaves feeling inadequately informed and believing that a major portion of the meeting was a waste of time. In this, the physician is not alone. In his book *We've Got to Start Meeting Like This,* Roger K. Mosvick states that over 50 percent of the productivity of billions of meeting hours is wasted.

While the average physician cannot control many of the meetings he or she must attend, he or she can take command of the physician and staff meetings within his or her own office. Many times meetings become such time wasters that they are avoided altogether in a physician's office. Since office meetings are a critical part of inter-office communication, this must be avoided.

[1] Planning the Meeting

Most meetings in the medical office are hastily organized without a clear focus on their purpose. Not surprisingly, the staff often leaves the meeting feeling frustrated and disorganized. If the physician does not personally plan the meeting, he or she should make sure that the meeting planner (normally the officer manager) has planned it adequately. The person planning the meeting should keep in mind the following goals:

- The meeting should have clearly defined goals and should stay focused on these goals.
- The group attending the meeting should understand the objectives and stay focused on the goals.
- The agenda should avoid needless conflicts.

The first step in organizing the meeting is to define its purpose and objectives. The purpose and objective should be written down with a brief summary, preferably one sentence. For example:

- The purpose of this meeting is to introduce the new CPT codes and discuss how we will implement them.
- The purpose of this meeting is to discuss the new Medicare Fee Allowance and to make sure that the office complies with the new Medicare law.
- The purpose of this meeting is to discuss the importance of phone answering and make sure that all employees know precise procedures to handle the different situations which may arise in our office.

Examples of memos designed to record meeting objectives and agendas that can be used to inform in advance of the meeting are given in Appendices 15-C, 15-D and 15-E.

[2] Type of Meeting

The purpose and objective of the meeting determine the type of meeting which should take place. In the medical office, several types of meetings take place:

- consultative meetings
- recommendation meetings

- delegation meetings
- information meetings
- instructional meetings

Although there are numerous variations, for the most part, all meetings in the medical office fall into one of the above categories. The meeting planner should recognize the type of meeting that is being set up and endeavor to run the meeting in this format.

[a] Consultative Meetings

The purpose of a consultative meeting is to obtain the group's suggestions for a specific problem or issue. The problem should be described by the meeting leader (usually the physician or office supervisor) and the group should explore the problem thoroughly and arrive at a solution. The consultative meeting is usually called on an "ad hoc" basis to get additional information to solve an immediate problem. The meeting is consultative in the sense that the group is called together to give counsel or advice to the decision maker, that is, the physician or the supervisor. The leader should make a specific effort to listen and minimize speaking to optimize the groups' suggestions. Individual participation will be spontaneous, usually without the benefit of lengthy consideration, but it can be valuable in helping the physician or supervisor to make a decision.

[b] Recommendation Meeting

The recommendation meeting, like the consultative meeting, is called to seek staff input. Unlike the consultation meeting, however, the recommendation meeting is more formal. It may appoint a committee of staff members to study a problem over a period of time and to make a recommendation. The leader should meet with the group to outline the problem and make it clear that it is the group's task to make recommendations to the manager. Group members should be made to understand that while they have full discretion in making recommendations, the final decision will be left to the leader. Nonetheless, recommendations of the group will be influential in the decision process.

[c] Delegation Meeting

As for the recommendation meeting, the purpose of the delegation meeting is to solve a problem or problems. Unlike the recommendation meeting, however, responsibility for making the final decision is delegated to the group. The leader should be specific when defining the problem to be solved, and specific on the group's authority to solve it.

It should be stressed that once the decision is made, there should be no intervention or later modification on the leader's part. This is a common error in the medical office that should be avoided. It is better to avoid the delegation of decision-making altogether if the manager is unwilling to give up that control. Generally, delegation of the decision process in the medical office is given to trivial items (color of the new patient information forms), or avoided altogether as a result of the leader's fear of loss of control. Delegation of the decision-making process can be a valuable tool however, when authority is delegated to the proper group.

[d] Information Meeting

Information meetings provide the staff with certain types of information. Without the proper use of information meetings, office communications can be limited to the office "grapevine" that spreads distorted or confusing information.

The information meeting can take the form of a "briefing" where the staff is updated on an immediate event, such as the termination of an employee, or it may be something more involved, such as a conference to explain a new office policy or new Medicare regulations that require a change in traditional office billing practices.

Unlike the consultation, recommendation or delegation meetings, the information meeting does not seek out the opinion of the group members, nor does it seek counsel with regard to any decision; with an information meeting, the decision already has been made.

[e] Instructional Meeting

Instructional meetings, like information meetings, are used to provide the staff with information. The instructional meeting differs from the informational meeting, however, in the sense that it provides information to specific staff members relating to how they do their job on a day-to-day basis. The instructional meeting may be run by the physician, office supervisor or an outside person. For example, the implementation of a new computer system may require training with experts from outside of the practice. An instructional meeting could also be called to train staff skills in answering the phone and handling patient phone calls.

[3] Selecting the Participants

When planning a meeting, the organizer must give adequate thought to who should attend and why each person invited should be there. Having individuals present who are not going to contribute productively to the meeting can make a meeting frustrating and unproductive for everyone. The inappropriate attendee may steer the direction of the meeting onto the wrong course. In addition, the larger the meeting, the more difficult it is to be productive. In many cases meeting leaders invite individuals for no other reason than to prevent the individual from feeling "left out."

When deciding who should attend the meeting, the physician should consider the following factors:

- Whether the person has direct responsibility for or authority over the topic of discussion.
- Whether the person has the information necessary to make an effective decision regarding the topic. (If the information can be easily obtained elsewhere, such as from a management report, use the report rather than waste the individual's time and having an unnecessary participant.)
- Whether the individual has the responsibility to implement the recommendations of the meeting group.

There should be a limit to the number of participants who attend the meeting. The fewer who attend, the less likely for the meeting to drift from its purpose and the easier it will be for the participants to focus on the purpose of the meeting. The organizer should also try to have an odd number of attendees at a decision making meeting to avoid deadlocks. Groups of five and seven are considered ideal.

[4] Creating the Environment

The meeting environment—specifically, the date, time and duration of the meeting—can strongly influence the outcome.

The time and date of the meeting is critical for obvious reasons.

The meeting must be held at a time in which all of the members can attend. Since the meeting may have to be scheduled at a time the participants would normally attend to other responsibilities, every effort should be made to minimize such interruptions. If the meeting is to run short, it may easily be squeezed in during the working day. If the meeting will run long, however, it may be necessary to schedule it at a time other than working hours, or adjust the normal working hours (not schedule patients during the meeting and have the answering service cover all phone calls). Morning meetings can be good because people are typically at a high energy level. In addition, the meeting can be started an hour before office hours begin or first appointments can be delayed.

The length of the meeting should be determined in advance. Meetings that "go on until we finish" will become less and less productive toward the end of the meeting, and may self-destruct as participants lose energy. Meetings that begin and end at designated times allow participants to perform efficiently at the meeting and schedule other work efficiently as well.

The ideal site for a meeting is related to the duration of the meeting. If, for example, the meeting is to be short, it may be appropriate to have a "stand up meeting," in a place without seating. This type of environment encourages a quick meeting; the meeting can be finished in the same amount of time it would take participants to "get comfortable" in a normal meeting environment. This kind of environment is usually appropriate for briefing meetings.

At the opposite extreme, physicians might meet at a retreat, or remote location for a meeting that will extend for an entire day or longer. This type of meeting may be held at a resort or hotel that provides all of the necessary amenities. If the meeting is to be an ambitious office meeting, consider a late afternoon or early evening meeting in a private room at a local hotel, where food and refreshments can be served. If a lengthy meeting is to be held at the office, consider having someone other than a meeting participant responsible for refreshments.

When planning a meeting, always consider the possibility of interruptions. While the doctor's consultation room or the employee lounge may appear to be a good place to hold a meeting, they may also be subject to frequent interruptions that take meetings off track and extend them unnecessarily.

[5] Briefing Participants

To maximize the effectiveness of the meeting, each participant should have a clear understanding of the objectives and goals. Each individual invited to the meeting needs to be told why he or she is being invited, what he or she will need to present or bring and the anticipated result of the meeting. If an individual needs only to attend a portion of the meeting, this should be clearly communicated along with the specific time he or she should be at the meeting and the amount of time he or she will be needed. This is courtesy and it will allow meeting participants to use their time more efficiently. Many productive hours are lost by having participants sit through a portion of the meeting where they are not involved.

Another briefing technique is to give the participants questions in advance of the meeting. If there are specific questions that the meeting participants will be expected to respond to, the participant should be given advance notice, when possible, so that he or she can best prepare ways to communicate the answer to the group. This gives the participant an opportunity to prepare visual aids when appropriate.

With briefings, participants can prepare properly for meetings. Meetings at which participants are adequately prepared can resolve the greatest number of problems in the shortest amount of time. Participants should be told in advance who else will be at the meeting (at least in the sections in which they will participate). A copy of the tentative agenda should be given to participants when possible, along with the time, place and anticipated duration of the meeting.

[6] The Agenda

Meetings without an agenda will be called together hastily with no clear definition of objectives and goals. Meetings should always have an agenda to keep the group on track with respect to the subject and the allotted time. The agenda should list the topics, name who is responsible to cover each topic, the time each topic is to be started and the time at which discussion of the topic will end.

Topics may need to have individual points listed for clarity, or to ensure that the topic is adequately covered.

The agenda should be realistic, and not overly ambitious. The number of items on the agenda should correlate with the expected length of the meeting. A common error is to underestimate the amount of time necessary to adequately cover the topic (although a more common error is to allow discussion time to exceed the allotted time on the agenda.) The following is an example of an agenda:

U.S.A. CLINIC

AGENDA

STAFF MEETING ON DECEMBER 14, 19XX

Item #	Topic	Responsible Participant	Time
1	Phone Answering	Sue Ellen	7:00 a.m.
2	Medicaid Bulletin	Jane	7:20 a.m.
3	Missing Files/ File Check Procedures	Sue Ellen	7:45 a.m.
4	Meeting End		8:00 a.m. Sharp

Note that in this example, the starting time of the next item implies the ending time of the current topic. The meeting leader should make certain that each topic is wound up on time and that the next topic is started on time.

[7] Leading the Meeting

The person leading the meeting is responsiuble for keeping the meeting moving along on schedule. He or she must solicit input from everyone at the meeting. Although the leader must not dominate the proceedings, he or she must know when to intervene to keep the meeting from getting sidetracked by irrelevancies, interruptions or arguments between participants.

[a] Before Starting the Meeting

Before starting the meeting, certain guidelines should be followed to help make the meeting as productive as possible (if the meeting is simply an informative or briefing meeting, some of these principles will not apply).

The leader should remember that his or her purpose is not to dominate the meeting, but rather to solicit participation from the attendees. The meeting leader must be prepared to do more listening than talking.

The leader should prepare to remind the group that participation is needed and that everyone's input is valuable. The meeting leader determines the influence of the meeting group. Will the group's decision become policy, or simply be used as information to be consulted by someone else making the decision?

The leader should realize the importance of reporting back to the group members the impact of the meeting. It is important that the participants know which of their recommendations were followed, which are under consideration, which have been rejected and the reasons for the rejections. The leader should also be prepared to encourage dissenting view points and minority views. The unpopular opinion should not be discouraged or frowned upon since, in many cases, it may offer the best solution.

[b] Starting the Meeting

After the meeting is called to order, the leader should apprise the group of the purpose, objectives and goals of the meeting. Although participants should have been informed of these before the meeting, it is important to start the meeting by restating the objectives and goals.

The leader should give a summary of the background of the problem and the topics to be discussed. He or she should then define the boundaries of the meeting; that is, determine which specific topics will be covered and which topics will not be part of the meeting discussion. For example, if this is a meeting on appointment scheduling, it should not drift off to discussion of office collections (even though office collections are important and not entirely unrelated).

The agenda should then be presented for approval by the

participants. At this point, the participants have an opportunity to seek clarification of any of the agenda items, or suggest modification of the agenda. Once a consensus has been reached on the agenda, the leader should point out that the meeting will not be allowed to deviate from the agenda. At this point, the agenda should not be modified any further except for extraordinary circumstances.

Finally, the leader should appoint a recorder. It is extremely important that this be done to prevent confusion and misunderstanding of what occurred at the meeting. The recording of the meeting should not be left to the leader, whose attention should be directed toward running the meeting. During the meeting, the recorder should periodically state the specific items agreed upon, particularly with regard to major points. How the agreement is recorded should be read to assure agreement of the group.

[c] Directing the Meeting

From the time it begins until the time it ends, it is the leader's task to guide the meeting. When directing a meeting, the successful leader will keep the following points in mind:

Stay on Agenda. Letting the meeting drift to interesting, but irrelevant topics will prolong it unnecessarily and hinder its effectiveness. Allowing nonagenda items to surface and be discussed is sometimes excused because the nonagenda items are "important." Good planning, however, will already have organized items on the agenda by order of priority so that they are sure to be covered. "Important" items should be left off the agenda if they are less important than those items on the agenda, and there is not enough time to discuss them. It may be better to put them on the agenda of the next meeting.

By forcing the meeting to stay on agenda, the leader and the group will have the satisfaction of having discussed the items which they set out to address and tabled those things which were not on agenda for the next meeting. A meeting that ends this way will leave the participants feeling good about the meeting, and eager for the next one.

Involve Participants. The meeting leader should make every effort to involve each of the participants. The key to insure participation by each member is to assign each participant an issue prior to the meeting. Having properly forewarned the participants, the leader should feel comfortable in asking each participant for his or her specific presentation.

Protect Minority Opinions. Part of the key to encouraging open participation is to respect minority opinions. If minority opinions are ridiculed or ignored, full participation cannot be expected. All participants will become more self-conscious about what they say and avoid presenting ideas which they feel may not be accepted. The creativity of the group will disappear and new ideas will cease to surface. Also it is frequently the minority opinion which presents the best ideas. Physicians should be particularly careful in this area. In employee meetings, employees are not only naturally hesitant to disagree with their boss, but in general, easily intimidated by physicians because of their title. Being aware of this, physicians should not use their status to intimidate but rather to make efforts to encourage participation, not "punish" contrary ideas which are presented.

Seek Clarification. During the meeting, the leader should seek clarification for vague or incomplete statements. For example, during an office meeting, Sue states, "I think that the office would function more efficiently if employees had more respect for each other's position." While this is a statement that could easily be agreed upon, it is rather vague and does not solve or address any particular problem. The leader might respond to a question such as this by stating, "Sue, could you cite some specific examples or observations you have made where you feel we are weak in this area?" Sue might go on to state, "When I am on the second lunch shift, I find it very difficult to keep my mind on work when I'm hungry and the first lunch shift is late from returning. In that situation, I really can't leave my post until the first shift has returned to cover for me. I think that this is an area where we should all be sensitive to make sure that we all return from lunch and other breaks on time." Here is a situation where the leader has taken a vague statement and elucidated from it a very specific issue. While everyone might have agreed with the first statement, it was not likely to solve any problems without having been clarified.

Evaluate Generalizations. The number of generalizations that are made but never evaluated at meetings is surprising. In many cases, not accepting generalizations and probing deeper can uncover solutions to problems which otherwise might have been considered unsolvable. For example, during the meeting to discuss large write-offs, Jane exclaims, "Most of our write-offs are from Medicaid patients, and we all know that there is nothing we can do about it." While everyone might agree with that statement, letting it go unexamined will not solve any problems and may end up costing the physician money. Further investigation should be carried out to determine why the reimbursement from Medicaid is low, and to determine if anything, in fact, can be done to improve it.

Avoid Irrelevant Conflict. It is the leader's responsibility to identify irrelevant conflicts at the meeting and step in and separate the combatants. Irrelevant conflicts can take the form of debating old business, issues not on the agenda, or worse, personal items. While genuine subject-related conflicts should be encouraged, irrelevant conflicts waste time and energy and may discourage group participation.

Listen. Although it is the leader's job to inform and brief participants, he or she should not dominate the group. The leader's function is to solicit orderly input from all of the attendees. The leader who is too domineering will only discourage participation from other members and make them reluctant to present ideas other than those they feel will be accepted and approved by the leader.

[d] Coming to a Consensus

When possible, the leader should steer the group to a consensus on all of the important issues. While it is not always possible to come to unanimous agreement on all issues, when it can be achieved it has a number of advantages. A consensus decision which has been reached without coercion and in a systematic fashion is more likely to yield the best solution to the problem under discussion. Furthermore, group members are much more likely to "make the decision work" if they agree with it and had a part in coming to the decision.

[e] Concluding the Meeting

All too often meetings come to a hasty conclusion with no time left to summarize and make a final clarification of the salient points. Generally, this is a consequence of the meeting running longer than scheduled because the group did not stick to its agenda.

To ensure a successful close to the meeting, the leader should:

Budget Time for the Conclusion. Scheduling the conclusion on the agenda will leave enough time to review briefly what has been accomplished, to answer any final questions and to outline expectations. Five to seven minutes should be sufficient for summarizing a one-hour meeting.

Repeat Items of Consensus. It is important to review those items which were agreed upon to ensure that everyone leaves the meeting with the same understanding. Any action steps should be outlined and the person responsible for carrying them out identified.

End the Meeting on Time. Meetings that do not end on time disrupt schedules and decrease peoples' willingness to participate. They generally disrupt the office schedule, leaving the doctor behind schedule and frustrating patients and staff alike. Meetings that run late on personal time, such as evening meetings, create poor feelings and possibly personal conflicts among the staff.

[f] Recording the Meeting

"Say, didn't we talk about this a few months ago? What did we decide?" "Say, wasn't someone supposed to follow up on that?" "I thought we were supposed to implement those changes last year." These statements are commonly heard at the *next* meeting. All too frequently, decisions are made and forgotten, or never followed up on. Sometimes action items are not followed up on because no one can remember who was responsible for them. Rehashing issues and decisions only to toss them on that useless heap of good ideas never implemented is a waste of energy and time. Drafting minutes of the meetings prevents this. It makes clear the responsibilities of various individuals, thus making it easier to hold people accountable for their responsibilities.

Copies of the completed minutes should be distributed to each of the participants. The original copy of the minutes should be filed in the office with the minutes of other meetings.

The following guidelines can make recording the minutes easier:

- Generally speaking, meetings need not to be tape recorded. Tape recording can inhibit discussions and result in lengthy notes and transcribing time and high costs. If it is an important "high-level" meeting, it may be desirable to tape the meeting and have the tapes transcribed for editing and reduction to minutes.

- The chairperson should not also be the one recording the meeting. This duty should be delegated to a meeting attendee.

- The recorder should have experience. An inexperienced recorder should "practice" recording the meeting in a back-up capacity before taking full responsibility for recording the meeting.

- The recorder has the ultimate responsibility to ask for clarification of vague, disorganized statements, seek internal summaries on major conclusions and seek rank order of consensus decisions, including reasons and rationale.

- The recorder should record major conclusions. He or she should make sure that a recording is accurate by asking for precise phrasing or rephrasing that is acceptable to all. The general rationale for a specific decision, including reporting arguments and facts, should be recorded. Specific actions which are to be taken and the person responsible for them should be recorded. Due dates of projects should be listed.

- The minutes should be kept as brief as possible. Unnecessary verbiage should be kept out or removed in the final draft.

- After the meeting, the notes should be organized and submitted to the meeting leader for corrections or additions.

- After the final notes are completed, copies should be distributed to the attendees.

§ 15.10 Checklist for Office Communications

A comprehensive checklist for perfecting communication skills is presented.

—Forms of Communication
    —Oral
        —Meetings
        —Presentations

- —One-on-one contact
- —Written
  - —Reports
  - —Letters
  - —Memos

- —Formulating Communication Objectives
  - —General objective
  - —Action objective
  - —Communication objective

- —Style of Delivery
  - —Tell
  - —Sell
  - —Consult
  - —Joint

- —Assessing Personality Types
  - —Intuitive
  - —Thinking
  - —Feeling
  - —Sensing

- —Presenting Oral Communication
  - —Direct Approach
  - —Indirect Approach

- —Presenting Written Communication
  - —Plan
  - —Dictate
  - —Edit
  - —Put in appropriate, consistent format

- —Giving Presentations
  - —Choose subject with personal interest
  - —Choose words carefully for the specific audience
  - —Outline points and objectives
  - —Use vivid, "visual" examples
  - —Use visual aids

—Speak positively
—Avoid humor
—Summarize points at conclusion

—Planning Meetings
　—Define general purpose and objectives
　—Determine type of meeting:
　　—Consultation
　　—Recommendation
　　—Instructional
　　—Informational
　　—Delegation
　—Choose format (stand-up, in-house, etc.)
　—Select participants
　—Select chairperson and a meeting recorder.

　—Schedule the time, place and duration of the meeting.

　—Determine the best method for briefing participants
　—Cause as few disruptions to schedules as possible:
　　—Consult participants' schedules
　　—Inform in advance
　—Determine the physical needs of the meeting
　—(visual aids, refreshments, etc.).
　　—Delegate to assistant
　—Prepare tentative agenda
　　—Outline all points to be covered
　　—Provide attendees with copy
　—Prepare and rehearse orientation speech

§ 15.100 Bibliography

Carnegie, Dale: The Quick and Easy Way to Effective Speaking. NY: Simon and Schuster, 1962.

Frank, Milo O.: How to Get Your Point Across in 30

Seconds or Less. NY: Simon and Schuster, 1986.

Johnson, Bonnie McDaniel: Getting the Job Done.

Glenview, IL: Scott, Foresman & Co., 1984.

Mosvick, Roger K. and Nelson, Robert B.: We Have Got to

Start Meeting Like This. Glenview, IL: Scott, Foresman & Co., 1987.

Munter, Mary: Guide to Managerial Communications.

Englewood Cliffs, NJ: Prentice Hall, Inc., 1982.

APPENDIX 15-A
DAILY REPORT

Checkbook Balance	$_____
Savings Balance	$_____
Bills to Pay Total	$_____
Approximate Payroll Due on 15:	
Staff	$_____
Dr.s	$_____
Approximate Payroll Due on 30th:	
Staff	$_____
Dr.s	$_____
Payments Posted This Month Thru———	$_____
Charges Posted This Month Thru———	$_____
Accounts Receivable Balance	$_____
New patients Seen This Month	_____
Total New Patients Seen This Month	_____

APPENDIX 15-B
MEMORANDUM

TO: _____

FROM: _____

DATE: _____

§ 15.100   MANAGING YOUR MEDICAL PRACTICE   15–46

RE: _____
MESSAGE:
_____
_____
_____
_____
_____
_____
_____

APPENDIX 15-C
MEETINGS

TO: _____
FROM: _____ PHONE: _____
DATE: _____

MEETING NOTIFICATION
DATE: _____
TIME: START: _____ END: _____
LOCATION: _____

AGENDA
_____ _____ _____
_____ _____ _____
_____ _____ _____
_____ _____ _____

MEETING OBJECTIVE: _____
_____
_____
_____
_____
_____

(Rel.3–2/89 Pub.372)

PRE-MEETING PREPARATION

CHAPTER 16

Marketing Your Medical Practice

> **SCOPE**
>
> Physicians need to market their medical practices to make themselves standout among the competition. A well-planned marketing strategy will increase the size of a medical practice and supply a growing practice with a plan for accomodating future expansion. A coherent marketing strategy calls for analyzing a practice, planning short and long-term objectives, implementing strategies for achieving those objectives, and constantly assessing whether the practice is meeting those objectives within the established time frame and budget. The physician must determine what the strengths of his or her practice are, and then target the audience to whom those strengths will be promoted. The means by which the physician can market a practice include: creating a practice brochure, publishing a newsletter, mounting a public relations campaign, accepting public speaking engagements, promoting special events, presenting a dynamic image through the practice sign and logo, advertising the practice in print and audiovisual media, starting a direct mail campaign and implementing a patient education program. At the same time the physician markets a practice, he or she should be careful not to de-market the practice. The physician must maintain a pleasant and efficient office environment for the benefit of the patients and must never neglect physicians and colleagues who refer patients.

SYNOPSIS

§ 16.01 Why Physicians Need Marketing

§ 16.02 What is Marketing?

MANAGING YOUR MEDICAL PRACTICE

§ 16.03 Developing a Marketing Plan
- [1] Research
- [2] Planning
- [3] Implementation
- [4] Evaluation

§ 16.04 Targeting Your Market
- [1] Analyzing Your Service
- [2] Patient Profile
- [3] Studying the Community

§ 16.05 Choosing Your Marketing Strategies
- [1] Types of Practices
- [2] Developing a Budget

§ 16.06 The Practice Brochure

§ 16.07 Creating a Newsletter

§ 16.08 Public Relations
- [1] Press Kits
- [2] News Releases
- [3] Media Interviews
- [4] Publicity Photographs
- [5] Feature Articles
  - [a] Explain New Developments
  - [b] Share Success Stories

§ 16.09 Public Speaking

§ 16.10 Special Events

§ 16.11 Creating an Image
- [1] Logo
- [2] Signs

§ 16.12 Advertising
- [1] Newspapers
- [2] Yellow Pages
- [3] Radio and Television
- [4] Coupons

§ 16.13 Direct Mail
- [1] Guidelines for a Direct Mail Campaign

§ 16.14 Patient Education
- [1] Consultation
- [2] Patient Information Cards

- [3] Standardized Materials
- [4] Patient Instruction Cards
- [5] Audio Tapes
- [6] Note Pads
- [7] Staff Education

§ 16.15 Patient Relations
- [1] De-marketing
  - [a] Long Waiting Periods
  - [b] Patient/Physician Communication
  - [c] The Office Environment
  - [d] Staff Attitude
- [2] Internal Prospecting
- [3] Follow-Up Visits
- [4] Waiting Room Resume

§ 16.16 Professional Relations
- [1] Complimentary Practices
- [2] Networking

§ 16.17 Marketing Checklist

Appendix 16-A Marketing Resources

§ 16.01 Why Physicians Need Marketing

Marketing is a fact of life for the physician who wants to have a competitive and successful practice.

Physicians were not allowed to advertise or promote their practices until 1978, when the United States Supreme Court overturned the ethical codes of professional societies that had prohibited such marketing. As a result of this extraordinary decision, physicians were allowed to advertise and, perhaps more importantly, solicit patients directly. This constituted more than a change in law: it signaled a change in tradition.

The surge in medical marketing over the past 12 years has been a response both to changes in legislation and to changes in the health care system. The growing surplus of physicians nationwide, and competition between private practitioners and health maintenance organizations, have reduced the workload of the average physician. At the same time, patients are consulting physicians less frequently. Thus, in today's health care environment, the physician who prefers the autonomy of private practice must learn to market his or her services.

§ 16.02 What is Marketing?

Marketing is a tool you use to identify a target market, identify the benefit you can provide for that market, determine a strategy for communicating with that market and implement that strategy to achieve marketing goals.

Marketing is both a science and an art; a process that combines research, proven communications techniques, and creativity to bring your services to the market effectively and profitably. It involves four basic elements:

- defining your market;
- defining your service;
- defining your marketing strategies; and
- implementing your marketing stategies.

The most fundamental action of marketing is to determine whom the practice will serve, and in what ways. Shrewd marketing takes into account the packaging and promotion of medical services that will fill the needs of both current patients and prospective patients. To be able to do this, you must take a careful look at the present and future characteristics of the patient population you want to serve. The information gathered through analyzing patient and market data can help direct your practice towards its most profitable group of patients and mix of marketing strategies.

There are two kinds of marketing: external and internal. External marketing encompasses all of the activities that extend to the outside world. Internal marketing involves the activities that occur within a practice. An external audience may include current patients, professionals, prospective patients, or the community and the media. Internal audiences are usually limited to current patients and staff.

§ 16.03 Developing a Marketing Plan

A marketing plan is a flexible operating mechanism that can help you manage your practice and work toward its success. The four steps for developing a marketing plan are: (1) researching the health care market and your practice's position in it; (2) planning short and long-term objectives for your practice based on market research; (3) implementing protocols for achieving those objectives within a specific

time frame and budget; and (4) establishing criteria for evaluating your practice's progress in achieving its objectives.

In the past, the only marketing tool a physician needed was a good reputation. Times have changed. Due to increasing competition from within the medical profession and from without, a physician must be persistent in marketing his or her talents if he or she is to attract patients. This calls for a coherent marketing strategy.

Developing and monitoring a marketing plan is an ongoing process. It invoves more than just placing an advertisement in the local newspaper, redecorating the waiting room or direct mailing to potential referral sources or residents in the community. In fact, occasional random efforts like these may only succeed in draining the practice budget without increasing revenues.

You must plan for growth. A good marketing plan will outline realistic steps for both establishing and expanding your practice. A marketing plan is not something that you write up and then put away on the shelf to gather dust. Rather, it is a blueprint you can use to guide your efforts and monitor your practice's progress. Ideally, you can adjust and revise your marketing plan as your practice grows. (See Figure 16-1.)

Marketing Plan Outline

- Statement of purpose
- Analysis of the practice
- Description of services
- Profiles of current and prospective patients
- Analysis of the competition
- Short-term and long-term goals
- Specific marketing strategies for achieving each goal
- Statement of implementation including scheduling, budgeting, staff responsibilities
- Plans for monitoring, evaluating, and adjusting the marketing plan

Figure 16-1

§ 16.03[1]   MANAGING YOUR MEDICAL PRACTICE

There are four phases in the development of a comprehensive and ongoing marketing plan: (1) research; (2) planning; (3) implementation, and (4) evaluation.

[1] Research

Before you can devise a marketing plan, you must analyze your practice in detail. Collect as many facts about your practice as possible in order to accurately assess its current position in the marketplace. A practice analysis should answer the following questions:

- What is the background and history of your practice? What is its current status?

- What are the strengths and weaknesses of your practice? Are there problems with scheduling, cancellations, insurance or reimbursement management?

- Who are your current patients in terms of age, sex, race, income, insurance coverage, chief problems, current living situations, etc.?

- Who is your competition? How many other physicians in your specialty are treating similar problems and practicing in the area? How long have they practiced in that location?

- What services do you provide and which patients need them?

- Is your current location desirable? How many people live in the area? Is the population expected to grow or shrink? What are the demographic characteristics of the population?

- What is your image? How do your current patients perceive your practice? How are you perceived in the community? Are you known in the community?

- Who are your potential patients? What are their wants and needs? What must the practice do to meet those needs?

Intuition, judgment, and experience by themselves cannot accurately answer these questions. A practice needs hard data to plan for the future. By analyzing the demographic information marketing research yields, you can identify your practice's present problems and future opportunities. (*See infra* § *1.04.*)

[2] Planning

Once you have gathered facts through market research, you must transform them into a comprehensive marketing plan. The research will help you identify the wants and needs of your current and potential patients. You may then use the marketing plan to determine how to shape the practice to satisfy those needs, profitably.

A marketing plan demands that the physician define his or her practice in terms of what it does for patients. Analysis of the practice will reveal its strategic advantages (for instance, whether its competitive edge lies within the physician's specialty or range of services). An important goal is to determine which elements of your practice can best be used to create an image of its special value in the minds of potential patients. The key lies in targeting te patient groups— which your practice can serve better than its competitors— and communicating its intentions to provide services tailored for these groups.

The next step in developing a marketing plan is setting realistic short-term (within one year) and long-term (within one to three years) objectives. This process will help you crystallize your expectations for your practice. Such goals might include increasing the number of patients you serve, building a wider referral network, amassing a higher gross income, or improving your practice's professional image.

Once you determine which goals your practice can achieve within one year, and which will take longer, you can set priorities for realizing those objectives based on their anticipated benefits.

[3] Implementation

Once you establish goals for your practice, you can begin working out individual protocols for achieving them. A marketing plan should explain in detail how these protocols will be implemented, by whom, and when.

It is important to develop a time frame for achieving each goal step-by-step. In this phase of the marketing plan, you should also develop a budget for the year which itemizes the cost of each marketing strategy implemented to achieve an objective. A commitment of 15 to 30 percent of the projected gross earnings for the coming year is a reasonable range for investment in the growth of a practice. (*See infra* § 1.05.)

[4] Evaluation

A marketing plan should outline how you will evaluate the program. You should establish standards of performance as criteria for assessing results. This permits you to review the marketing plan on a periodic basis by comparing actual progress against the goals of the implementation schedule.

There are several tools that can be used to measure the results of a practice's progress: patient surveys, voluntary feedback, tracking referral sources, income generated, increased usage of services, and patient complaints. If necessary, the marketing plan can be adjusted and your goals modified, based on evaluation.

§ 16.04 Targeting Your Market

Before you can define and achieve your practice's objectives, you must first know the market you serve. Targeting your ideal market involves analyzing the benefits your practice provides, developing profiles of patients who use your services, and studying the community in which your practice is located.

A physician would never advise a course of treatment without first reviewing a patient's history, gathering information about the patient's complaint and performing a physical examination. If he or she did, the consequences could be disastrous, even fatal.

Likewise, random efforts to increase your patient-base, made with little understanding of who your patients are, could prove fatal to the financial health of your practice. If your practice is to be successful, you must formulate, "package," advertise, and provide health care services with the idea of satisfying one major goal: winning the acceptance of a clearly defined market segment. Targeting a market segment enables you to understand who your patients are based on demographic, geographic, psychographic, and other factors. Through marketing research, you can develop a realistic picture of his or her services, patients, and community.

[1] Analyze Your Service

When targeting a market, it is essential that you perform a detailed service analysis. By collecting as many facts as possible about your practice, you can accurately assess its current position in the marketplace.

A service analysis should describe:

- the background and history of your practice;
- the practice as it currently operates;
- the range of medical services the practice provides, including a breakdown by specialty or complaint;
- the practice's medical and support staff;
- the practice's facilities and equipment;
- the practice's competition, both free-standing and hospital-based; and
- the practice's reputation in the community.

The service analysis may also cover intangibles, by answering questions such as:

- What benefits does your practice offer to potential patients?
- What real or imagined needs do your services fulfill?
- How do your patients and the community perceive your services?

[2] Develop Patient Profiles

Although a physician must consider his or her patients as individuals, certain groups of patients share basic needs and wants. By creating profiles based on those needs and wants, you can target and develop strategies for reaching patients who match them.

You can use many different sources of information to develop patient profiles. For example, you may want to draw on personal knowledge of who comes to your practice or rely upon patient surveys or health care industry studies. The most common types of information used in the development of patient profiles include:

- *Demographics*—These include such variables as geographic location, income, age, sex, education, religion, race and social class.
- *Geographic*—Although geographic location is a subset of demography, it merits special attention. You will want access

to markets in close proximity to your practice, metropolitan, or rural markets, and perhaps regions with different climates or cultural/sociological actors.

- *Psychographic*—Psychographic factors are concerned with the different "lifestyles" of your targeted patient groups. One aspect of psychographics is individual patterns of practice usage. Another psychographic approach clusters patients according to their "AIO's"—Activities (work, hobbies, sports), Interests (families, home, community, recreation), and Opinions (politics, religion, health).

- *Practice Benefits*—Through analysis of practice benefits, you can identify the reasons why different patients seek your medical care. Characteristics of a practice that may influence a patient's choice include: size, appearance, convenience, speed, reputation for quality care, and price.

- *Rate of Usage*—Analysis of the rate of usage provides information on the volume of services various patients use. Classifications might include "present heavy users" and "present light users." Usage rate classifications are valuable only if the reasons for variation between groups are spelled out and analyzed. Differences in usage can usually be traced to demographic factors such as age, income, employment status, etc.

[3] Studying the Community

If your practice is to be successful, you must analyze the local population to target potential patients. Demographic reports and other variables used in the development of patient profiles provide valuable information regarding:

- the age, type of family and household, race, and income levels of people in the community;

- the local population's consumer lifestyles in terms of social, economic, demographic, and housing characteristics;

- the number of people in the community likely to carry medical insurance, and the source of their insurance; and,

- the kinds of media most effective for reaching the people in your community.

Once you have identified key characteristics of the local population, you can determine the best means for matching services you provide, with the needs of prospective patients. Consider the benefits of your services and ask yourself: Who needs these services? Who may be persuaded to need them? What essential prerequisites exist with regard to potential patients?

§ 16.05 Choosing Marketing Strategies

> **Choosing a marketing strategy entails determining the type of patient you wish to attract to your practice based on the services your practice provides, choosing a means of communicating with those patients, and developing a budget for your marketing goals.**

When choosing a marketing strategy, you must decide whether you only want to attract patients similar to those your practice already serves, or to expand into other markets. Market research may identify a new target group your practice has not reached before, yet can adequately serve.

If you want to reach more patients of the type your practice currently serves, you can develop a patient profile based on yor current patient load, and search for concentrations of potential patients who match this profile.

If, on the other hand, you want to target a previously untapped market, you can use market research to select the segment of the population with the greatest potential. Once you identify these desired patients, you can pinpoint the geographic areas in which they are highly concentrated and determine the media (direct mail, advertising, etc.) most likely to reach them. Community demographic information of this sort is useful for long-range planning, developing new services, and tailoring existing services for target markets.

Once you have identified the market segments you wish to reach, you are ready to choose the marketing strategies that will "expand" your practice. This entails weighing the benefits of various communication channels and approaches that will make your practice better known to the targeted market segments. Knowing the nature of your practice will help you choose the most effective and economical strategies for reaching patients.

(Rel.4–2/90 Pub.372)

[1] Types of Practice

A community-based practice is built on self-referrals and referrals from persons in the community. The foundation of a hospital-based practice, on the other hand, is the professional community. (See Figure 16-2.) Certain specialities tend naturally to either be community-based or hospital-based. The type of practice defines the marketing messages, channels and methods most effective for promoting it. (See Figure 16-3.)

REFERRAL METHODS

	HOSPITAL-BASED	COMMUNITY-BASED
SOLO		self referral
		lay referral
GROUP	professional referral	

Fig. 16-2. Chart showing the different referral methods for hospital- and community-based practices.

TYPES OF PRACTICES

	HOSPITAL-BASED	COMMUNITY-BASED
SOLO		primary care, family medicine, obstetrics/ gynecology, plastic surgery
GROUP	radiology, anesthesiology	

Fig. 16-3. Chart showing the different specialties of hospital- and community-based practices. The nature of the practice will determine the marketing message and the means for communicating it.

There are many methods at your disposal for communicating information about your practice. (See Figure 16-4.) The key to determining the communication method best suited to your practice is to consider each marketing channel and method in relation to your practice's objectives. (See Figure 16-5.) Questions you should ask yourself regarding the most appropriate channel of communication include:

- Does your audience use this channel?

- Does your audience believe this channel?

- How can each method be used to bring your message to your target audience?

- How can you use a combination of methods to develop a coordinated marketing program?

MARKETING METHODS

PERSONAL CONTACT	PUBLICATIONS
☐ Public Speaking	☐ Brochures
☐ Seminars	☐ Newsletters
☐ Speaking Engagements	☐ Patient Education Materials
☐ Word-of-Mouth	☐ Direct Mail
☐ Telephone Contact	☐ Press Kit
☐ Personal Correspondence	☐ Business Cards, Letterhead

PRINT PUBLICITY	BROADCAST PUBLICITY
☐ Hard News	☐ News Coverage
☐ Feature Stories	☐ Interview Programs
☐ Photographs	☐ Slides/Videotape/Film

ADVERTISING	OTHER
☐ Yellow Pages	☐ Literature displays
☐ Coupons	☐ Exhibits
☐ Newspaper	☐ Signage
☐ Radio	☐ Give-aways

Fig. 16-4. A list of the many methods a physician can choose to communicate a marketing message.

OBJECTIVE	CHANNEL	METHOD
PUBLICIZE PRACTICE EXPANSION	MEDIA	News releases Feature stories Announcement
	PUBLICATIONS	Direct mail Newsletter article
	PERSONAL CONTACT	Letter to patients, professionals
	SPECIAL EVENT	Open house

Fig. 16-5. A physician must consider the proper channel and the proper means within that channel of achieving the practice's objectives.

[2] Developing a Budget

How much should a physician spend on marketing: three percent, five percent or seven percent of gross? There is no simple answer to this question; since it doesn't make sense for physicians who have different goals and competitive situations to spend the same percentage on marketing, there are no simple formulas for calculating the percentage of budget that should be allocated for marketing activities.

A marketing budget should be based on your goals for the growth of your practice. These goals should be expressed in terms of specific monetary figures. One way to determine how much of the budget to allocate on marketing is to determine projected gross collections for the coming year based on the trend of previous years, then set a goal for the practice that surpasses the projected collections. The marketing budget should be between 15 and 30 percent of the goal amount. For example, if you wish to bring in $100,000 over projected collections, then you should plan on spending at least 15 percent ($15,000) on marketing to achieve that goal.

To plan a budget, you should select your marketing strategies and estimate the costs involved in implementing each one over time. (See Figure 16-6.) It is necessary to get specific quotes from printers, marketing consultants, the media, and then determine which ones will bring in the most patients for the dollars spent.

MARKETING STRATEGIES AND BUDGET				
	MONTH 1	MONTH 2	MONTH 3	TOTAL
EXTERNAL STRATEGIES				
INTERNAL STRATEGIES				
TOTALS				
PROJECTED BUDGET				

Fig. 16-6. Example of a chart the physician can use to assess marketing strategies in terms of time and budget.

§ 16.06 The Practice Brochure

Your practice brochure is an important tool for establishing and reinforcing the identity you wish to present to your patients.

Sooner or later, almost every physician must deal with producing a practice brochure. This inevitably raises questions such as:

- Should the practice brochure be a simple flier, or many elaborate booklets printed in a variety of colors?

- Should it be designed to attract new patients or to explain your office's policies and procedures?

- Should it emphasize one special service or provide an encyclopedia of information on your specialty?

Whatever the answers to such questions are, the goal of the practice brochure should be to effectively and efficiently communicate a message that "sells" the practice. Brochures produced within the following guidelines will attract attention, invite readership and save money by avoiding unnecessary or wasteful steps.

(1) *Determine your objective.* Ask yourself these questions: What do you want your brochure to accomplish? Do you want it to convince more people to try your services? Do you want it to reinforce ties with existing patients? Do you want it to create a sense of identity for your practice?

(2) *Identify your target audience.* If your objective is to convince more people to use your services, determine who your potential patients are. What are their wants and needs?

(3) *Spell out your strategy.* List the reasons why you think patients should choose your practice over the competition. Determine what makes your practice special, then determine the one benefit or selling quality that is most important to your target audience. By stressing this benefit in your brochure, you will appeal to the reader's natural self-interest.

(4) *Support your benefit.* Give the reader convincing reasons for believing your message. Include a strong biography, examples of successes, quotes or photographs of satisfied patients.

(5) *Choose your style.* What is the "personality" of your practice? Decide what tone and manner to use in your brochure. A distinctive personality may be the quality which sets your practice apart from your competition. This personality should be congruent with the character of your target population.

(6) *Put your benefit on the cover.* If you want your brochure to sell your practice, the cover must have a headline which promises your strongest benefit. Remember: your name or the name of the practice is not your headline; it promises readers no direct benefit.

(7) *Use one illustration or photograph on the cover.* One large illustration is more effective and dramatic than several small ones or none at all.

(8) *Choose artwork that tells a story.* Use an illustration or photograph that shows your benefit to its best advantage. People are interested in people, so be sure to choose photographs of scenes with people in them.

(9) *Communicate clearly.* To ensure that readers understand your message, answer the following questions: Is the message on the brochure simple and straightforward? Does the copy follow a logical flow? Does it reinforce the benefit you set out on the cover? Does it interest and intrigue the reader?

(10) *Spotlight important information.* To make your brochure easier to read and more visually interesting, use subheadings, bullets, and bold type faces where appropriate. Also, a little well-placed color helps draw the attention of the reader.

(11) *Motivate the reader to take action.* What do you want the prospective patient to do after reading the brochure? It should contain a clear call to action. For example, if you want readers to contact you for more information, include a mail-in post card, or invite them to call your office.

(12) *Develop a design concept.* Your brochure should look professional, or it shouldn't be done at all. Work with a graphic designer and have him or her develop two or three different layouts that amplify your content. Then, select the one that is most visually appealing and appropriate.

(13) *Make the size appropriate to the way(s) you'll distribute the brochure.* Do you want to use the brochure as a self-mailer, mail it in a standard envelope, or display it in your office? The size and shape of your brochure will effect every aspect of the layout, so make these decisions first.

(14) *Choose paper and ink which enhance your image and please your target population.* To convey a state-of-the-art practice, choose glossy paper and electric colors. Textured paper and a subdued palette suggest a more traditional image.

(15) *Keep it simple.* Don't pack every inch of your brochure with pictures or copy. White space gives the reader's eyes a chance to rest and prevents your brochure from looking cluttered and "grey."

(16) *Save money with stock photographs.* When you want an unusual

§ 16.07   MANAGING YOUR MEDICAL PRACTICE

or specific photo, use a photo from a stock house. This can reduce your costs significantly.

(17) *Make your brochure readable.* Choose a typeface which calls attention to your message, not to itself. Avoid clever or unusual typefaces, and stick with one throughout the brochure. To save on typesetting charges, be sure your brochure's copy is accurate and complete before type-setting begins

(18) *Make changes on the mechanical before it goes to the printer.* The mechanical is a clear indication of what the printed page will look like. Once the type is set, the type proofs are pasted down on lightweight cardboard. The area for the artwork is indicated, and the original artwork or photographs are attached to the mechanical.

(19) *Ask for several print bids.* Draw up specifications describing the size of your brochure, number of pages, weight and type of paper stock, ink colors, and number of photographs or illustrations. You will be amazed at the variation in bids between different printers. Select a printer who has experience with brochures and can handle colors, as well as black-and-white jobs.

(20) *Be consistent.* If you develop more than one brochure, insist that they resemble each other to maintain your identity. Follow the same format and use familiar graphics to develop a family of brochures

Once you have successfully developed your practice brochure, use it. Give it to new patients to create a powerful first impression, send it to current patients to reinforce ties, mail it to prospective patients and referral sources, and use it to boost the morale of your staff by creating a sense of identity for your practice.

§ 16.07   Creating a Newsletter

Newsletters are useful tools for improving rapport and increasing loyalty between you and your patients. They let patients know you are concerned about their health all year round.

Physicians who neglect to strengthen their relationships with their patients create an opening for competitors. By issuing a newsletter, you can periodically reinforce the quality of the services your practice offers in a very positive, personal way.

A newsletter is a periodical publication distributed regularly to established patients, prospective patients, and new residents in the neighborhood. It may be an inexpensive typed bulletin or a more expensive and elaborate publication. A well-written and edited newsletter that deals with matters of concern to patients and that provides really useful information can enhance the reputation of your practice. It can also serve as a source of material for publicity.

Newsletters are very popular, but they are not effective if they fail to communicate to their audience. Before producing a newsletter, you must determine the identity of your audience, what the newsletter is trying to accomplish, how it will be delivered and the desired audience response.

It's important to develop a newsletter's style, format, and content to support communication goals. A newsletter is counterproductive if it is poorly planned, written or designed, or issued on an irregular basis. The appearance and message of the publication influences the patient's perception of the practice.

Ideally, a newsletter for patients should present information that is of interest to them, in addition to promoting the practice's services. The editorial content should balance articles geared to the various segments of the target population. For example, it might include different articles on topics relevant to older people, women, men or people who work at a specific occupation with a high community profile. A typical newsletter may include:

- A letter from the physician. A friendly letter in a personal style conveys that the physician is accessible and concerned about patient satisfaction.

- Patient profile. A success story about a patient who is pleased with his or her recovery or care. For example, a section on parents of newborns is appropriate for a pediatrician.

- Practice news. Include information about new associates or staff, new services, conference attendance, seminars, speaking engagements, news coverage, or other activities.

- Identity box. List personal information on the practicing physicians' credentials. Don't forget the basic information that tells people how to reach you, name, address, telephone number, and a brief description of your practice.

(Rel.4–2/90 Pub.372)

A newsletter must be readable and attractive. It should be printed on quality paper and designed to have an open, uncluttered look. A standard masthead should be designed for consistency and easy recognition. The format of any periodical publication, such as a newsletter, should be designed so that the recipient recognizes it instantly by the third or fourth issue. Desktop publishing makes it possible to create attractive, professional materials in a timely and cost-effective manner. (See Figure 16-7.)

A common newsletter format is a tri-fold self-mailer, with space for a mailing label and a pre-printed return address. This eliminates the need for an envelope. Newsletters can be mailed to selected households within the community. For distribution purposes, you may wish to engage a mailing service, which will keep your mailing list on file, print and affix mailing labels and distribute the newsletter after it is printed. An alternative is an in-house computerized mailing system.

Of course, you should also display the newsletter at your office. It makes excellent reading material in the waiting rooms and patients can take it home to friends and relatives.

§ 16.08 Public Relations

Shrewd public relations can help establish your reputation as an expert in your field. The tools of a public relations campaign are the press kit, the news release, interviews with the media, publicity photographs and feature articles.

You can develop name recognition and attract new patients through a well-planned, consistent, and ongoing public relations program. If area residents read about your practice's services and specialty in the local paper, they will remember it when they have a problem.

A public relations program will:

- build the professional reputation of your practice in the local and professional community;
- give the public a better understanding of your specialty;
- inform referral networks of your expertise;
- generate inquiries about services; and,
- increase your patient volume.

(Rel.4–2/90 Pub.372)

CONNECTIONS

Volume 1, Number 1

Helpful information on the problems of everyday life
from CONSULTATION ASSOCIATES

THE LONELINESS OF MOVING

You don't have a single friend or neighbor to write on the emergency information card at your child's new school. Your weekends seem empty without meeting your best friends for pizza on Friday night. You walk up and down the local mall almost every day just to be around people. You recently moved.

Relocating your family and possessions may be one of the most difficult things that you will ever do. Moving to a new home, however exciting, is a wrenching, emotionally stressful experience.

Unfortunately, people often think there is something wrong with them if they can't cope with the upheaval of moving. They make the mistake of underestimating the impact of saying good-bye to familiar places and faces.

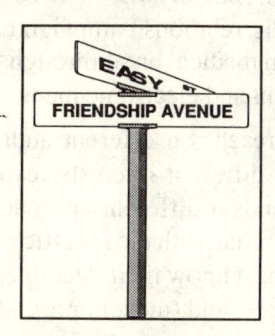

People who have just moved to a new area have to cope with the loneliness of establishing new ties for everything from finding a babysitter to choosing an auto mechanic. They have temporarily lost their support network.

It's normal to mourn the loss of a familiar home, family, and friends. Once the frenzied activity of moving is over, a period of "grief" may set in. The feeling of being alone and depressed may take hold two weeks after the move or four months later.

Studies have shown that people have a basic need to feel rooted or related to others in order to enjoy a feeling of well-being. We need to know someone who will give us help if we need it; we need close friends with whom we can exchange confidences; we need the feeling of self-esteem that is given by friends who respect us; and we need the sense of community provided by knowing people who share our social concerns.

When we move, these needs are frustrated until we can make new connections. Sometimes, it's hard to allow yourself to relate to people in your new community. It may seem impossible to make the effort to introduce yourself to new neighbors, to reach out and find activities and people that interest you.

If you're having a difficult time settling in a new home or making friends, talking to a supportive professional can help you with your feelings of isolation.

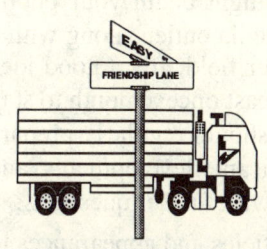

SUGGESTIONS FOR MOVING

Don't avoid saying good-bye. It may seem easier at the time, but in the long run, it can create a greater sense of loss. Resist the temptation to sever ties with your old neighborhood. Maintain relationships. Allow yourself to go through the emotions associated with moving.

Before you move, find out about your new community. Write ahead to get information on schools, community organizations, and churches. Introduce yourself to your new neighbors. If they don't invite you over for coffee, you can invite them to your new house — even if you're not completely unpacked.

Establish family traditions that move with you. Doing things together as a family makes you feel at home, no matter where you live.

Fig. 16-7. Sample newsletter

Public relations involves communicating a message to the public, or a selected audience, through the media. This necessitates supplying reporters, editors, and program directors with medical news on a regular basis. At the same time that you provide valuable, accurate

§ 16.08[1]   MANAGING YOUR MEDICAL PRACTICE

information on current health topics or interpret the latest health care issues and trends, you will create an image of concern and competence for the practice.

Typically, a public relations campaign targets the health editors of local newspapers and magazines, as well as the program direcors of local radio, television and cable stations. These editors and program directors need experts who will serve as a source of new information for their readers or listeners, who they can turn to for an opinion on a topical news item or trend, or who will be guest speaker on a talk show. A planned public relations campaign can help you become the main source of news on medical breakthroughs and new and interesting information for the print and electronic media.

Each media outlet reaches a dfferent audience, employs different technologies, and has different interests, capacities, and limitations. Therefore, each demands a different approach, tailored to its unique needs. You must be familiar with the specific requirements of the media you plan to use. You must know their deadlines, formats for submitting materials, contact people, and (most importantly), the interests of their readers or listeners.

Public relations only works in the long term if it's consistent. To become a recognized expert, you should periodically contact the media.

There are a variety of strategies you can use to enhance the way people think about a practice including: press-kits, news releases, feature stories, and media interviews. You might begin your public relations efforts by sending press-kits to all media outlets along with a letter introducing yourself as an expert in your field. It's a good idea for you to study the professional literature at least once a month to stay on top of new trends and developments. You should regularly prepare news releases or feature articles on significant developments and distribute them along with instructions to call with further questions.

Sending out announcements on personal articles and appearances to media contacts to let them know that colleagues consider the physician an expert, is also a good idea. You can send a postcard on articles, talks, and appearances to your patients to suggest they read, listen to, or watch the upcoming media coverage of your practice.

[1] Press-Kits

It's very important to develop a press kit about your practice that includes the following elements:

- your curriculum vitae;
- a black-and-white photo of yourself;
- a practice profile or brochure;
- a list of topics with which you are conversant; and,
- a list of past appearances or articles.

You should send this press kit to all local newspapers, magazines, radio, and television stations.

[2] News Releases

You can get your message into print by providing local newspapers with informational news items. The primary vehicle for communicating with the media is a news release that provides an accurate and concise description of your new development or event. (See Figure 16-8.)

The information in a news release should be presented in straight news style, with the most important facts at the top of the story, followed by the less significant details. The first paragraph should answer who, what, why, where, when, and sometimes how. Often, a busy editor or reader won't look beyond the first line, so make sure your opening sentence counts.

A news release can discuss specific services, techniques, a new associate or a noteworthy event such as an open house. To be sure you have included all the necessary information, you may want to end the release with a brief paragraph describing the practice. (See Figure 16-9.)

Don't express personal opinions in a news release, unless they are in a quotation that can be attributed to a hysician or patient. Also, be judicious in your use of adjectives. A newsletter should be factual.

Before distributing it, check to be sure that the release is accurate in every detail regarding names, titles, dates, and times. A release should never contain typographical errors, misspellings or cross-outs.

The following guidelines can help you prepare a release:

- Use 8 1/2 x 11-inch paper. Either your letterhead or plain white bond paper is acceptable.

NEWS RELEASE

FOR IMMEDIATE RELEASE

> For further information,
> Contact: Rebecca Anwar
> 215-649-8770

LOCAL SURGEONS PRACTICE HOSPITALITY

(PORTSMITH, VA, November 11) Professionals from throughout Portsmith County attended an open house at the new offices of Valley Spring Surgical Associates on Sunday, November 9th. Many physicians on the staff of General Hospital as well as local accountants and attorneys toured the spacious facilities of surgeons, James Brown, M.D. and John White, M.D.

"We are celebrating two important new developments for our practice today:," said Dr. White, who is a specialist in vascular surgery and Director of Trauma Services at York Hospital. "They include our recent move to Valley Spring Drive where we have the space and equipment to perform many outpatient diagnostic tests and surgical procedures. We are also happy to announce that a new associate, Dr. Brown, has joined the practice.

Designed for patient comfort and convenience, the new modern office includes a non-invasive laboratory on the premises that enables the doctors to perform non-invasive diagnostic tests using state-of-the-art equipment and technology. It is also stretcher and wheelchair accessible, with free parking.

Valley Spring Surgical Associates moved to the new location from Wedgewood Road. The practice, which specializes in vascular problems, also diagnoses and treats problems of the bowel, stomach, gallbladder, rectum, and breasts.

Fig. 16-8. Sample news release

- Type or word-process your release on one side of the paper only, always double-space, and leave wide margins for the editor to write notes.

- In the upper right hand corner, include the name of a contact

TEN STEPS TO A GOOD NEWS RELEASE

(1) Tell who, what, when, where, why and how.

(2) Give the name, address and telephone number of a contact person.

(3) Include all of the interesting information.

(4) Put the most important facts in the first paragraph. Keep your story brief and to the point.

(5) Explain medical terms or jargon in everyday language.

(6) Remember newspaper deadlines—mail releases 10 days to two weeks before the event.

(7) Do not pester editors. Unless you pay for the message to be printed verbatim, do not expect it. News and advertising are seperate operations of the paper.

(8) Direct your information to the health care reporter.

(9) Send photos of local people on the staff along with the release.

(10) Check your release for accuracy.

Figure 16-9

person and telephone number. In the upper left hand corner, include the date that the information may be released, or simply put "For Immediate Release." Also, be sure to include the name of the practice and its address.

- Summarize the story in the headline, which should be typed in capital letters.
- Try to limit the release to one page.
- If you use more than one page, type the word "MORE" at the bottom of the page, and a few key words from the headline at the top of the following pages with the page number.

[3] Media Interviews

One benefit of establishing your reputation as an authority in a given area is that you may be called upon to comment on news events that pertain to your specialty. Local newspapers and television stations are always looking for ways to "localize" national events. For example, an interesting segment may focus on your practice as an example of a national trend. Public affairs programs also need experts to interview on interesting topics. You might inform local stations that you are an authority in special areas. Media interviews have a tremendous impact on community awareness of your practice.

The following are suggestions for talking to the press:

- Prepare for an interview. Have someone conduct a practice interview with you. Pick two key points that you want to make. Decide exactly how you want to define your practice in just one sentence.

- You don't have to answer every question. If a reporter gets into a personal area, such as asking you about your income, it's fine to say "I'd rather not discuss it." Try to keep the interview focused on the topics you want to talk about. Make your key points even if the reporter doesn't ask about them.

- You may not see your name in print. It sometimes happens that you are interviewed, but not mentioned in the article. Reporters go to many people when they are gathering information. Although you can't do anything once the article has been printed, you can take action while it's being prepared. After you give an interview, call the reporter back, and ask if he has any additional questions. Don't ask if you'll be quoted. Just offer more insight and information.

[4] Publicity Photographs

Sooner or later, every physician needs a good photograph for publicity purposes. The following are guidelines for having one taken:

- Look professional.

- Have the photographer shoot both color and black-and-white prints.

- Have the photographer take your picture in a number of poses: with patients, without patients, reviewing x-rays, smiling, looking concerned, etc.

- Try to relax so that the picture does not look posed.

[5] Feature Articles

"Publish or perish," the famous maxim of the academic world, may be applied to the practice of medicine. Publishing articles in your local newspapers and professional publications is essential to ensuring a constant flow of patients to your practice.

Printed articles put your practice in the public eye. A by-line article, or an article written by you or a member of your medical staff, educates the public about health issues, develops trust in your expertise, reassures current patients of your skills, and ultimately, attracts new patients.

The benefits of by-line articles are well worth the effort you put into writing them. Keep in mind, though, that one article is not enough. You must write and place articles at regular intervals to keep the public aware of your practice.

Finding time to write articles can be difficult, but if you understand the process of preparing by-line articles, your efforts won't be wasted. You'll know just how much material you need and what format to use. There are three basic approaches which you can use in preparing by-line articles: you can give advice, explain new developments in your field, or tell a success story about a patient.

As a medical expert, you are in a perfect position to provide patients and prospective patients with useful information. Getting a second opinion, choosing a surgeon, preparing children for their first dental examinations, or simply explaining the benefits of psychotherapy are all excellent topics for this type of educational article.

While the article will be perceived as a public service piece which offers authoritative, accurate medical information, it will actually convey a very important message about you to readers. Essentially, this type of article says, "I understand your worries and concerns about your health. As a caring and solicitous physician who is interested in your welfare, I am going to give you some expert advice."

It is important to pay close attention to the tone and style of the article as well as its content. Ideally, the reader will perceive you as a physician who is empathetic and helpful. You can accomplish this by addressing common concerns which patients have expressed to you in the past, and by offering reassurance.

Be careful in your use of language. People tend to mistrust experts whom they cannot understand. Simple, straightforward language will make it easier for people to believe in you.

Remember, the general public tends to be frightened of illness and invasive procedures. In a by-line article, you can establish yourself as a physician who understands and alleviates their anxieties. Ultimately, your article will communicate that the solution to dealing with their anxieties is to consult a caring and accessible professional: you.

[a] Explain New Developments

You can demonstrate your professional expertise to potential patients by explaining new developments in your field with language which the general public can understand. Technical advances and new procedures are examples of good topics for articles. You may also choose to write about developments that are not so new, but which have not yet become common knowledge.

Another approach to the "expert" article is to localize an event in the national news. For example, if a well-known celebrity is having a pacemaker inserted on an outpatient basis, you can take advantage of the celebrity's spotlight by writing an article explaining why ambulatory surgery is a good choice for this type of procedure.

By making a difficult, complicated subject comprehensible to the reader, you will show that you are knowledgeable in your field. In writing an article of this nature, you should provide sound, relevant background information and discuss risks and benefits of a treatment or procedure. Remember to discuss medical procedures in terms of how they benefit people. Your language should be detached, omniscient and rational.

To get the most benefit from this article, you should come across as an experienced authority. You can do this by giving examples from your personal experience and mentioning the number of years which you have been in practice. Sound like an expert. Choose words which are crisp, authoritative and definite.

[b] Share Success Stories

People love to read about other people. Medical stories have an inherent drama which is always of interest to the general public. Telling the stories of patients, who found that their treatment was a positive experience, will calm the fears of prospective patients who feel anxious and worried.

If you're interested in writing a human interest story, you have to make an effort to identify patients who have interesting stories to tell and surgeons who have demonstrated unusual achievements. Don't forget to obtain the patient's approval and cooperation.

In developing a human interest story, you should write about the patient's background, medical problem, successful recovery, and positive feelings about your practice. It's also a good idea to include generic information about the procedure and the benefits of your approach. Always tell the story of your practice, explaining specific features that should make it the patient's first choice. You may choose to emphasize your medical specialty, your philosophy of care, or even the attractive design of your facility. If possible, send along a photograph of the patient leaving your office. For example, photographs of young children holding stuffed animals are always heart-warming.

Don't forget to include a brief biography at the conclusion of the article with information on your credentials and follow-up information.

To get the maximum benefits from your articles, send copies to patients who have used your service in the past, and to professional colleagues who refer patients to you. You should also leave copies in your waiting room for patients to take home to read.

§ 16.09 Public Speaking

A planned public speaking program will develop your reputation as a medical expert, enhance your image as a concerned health care provider, and increase your practice's patient volume.

Through the power of the podium, you can spread the positive reputation of your practice. A planned program of public speaking is a direct and personal way of reaching potential patients and increasing referrals from the professional community: it is not a professional activity which is reserved only for "star" performers. By following a few simple guidelines, you can feel comfortable and confident about giving presentations. With practice, you can be as adept at public speaking as you are at providing medical care consultations.

Develop your own speaker's kit. Put together presentations on your areas of specialty or interest. For example, a child psychiatrist may want to discuss new treatment modalities for autism, or an orthopedic surgeon could talk about coping with arthritis. When you talk about a subject which you know very well, your enthusiasm and knowledge will outweigh your nervousness. Avoid esoteric subjects. The audience wants to be entertained as well as educated. Develop a "menu" of interesting presentations to offer professional groups and community organizations.

Make your presentations dynamic. Your conviction and the force of your personality must dominate your speech. If you want to keep the audience's attention, do not memorize your speech or read from a script. These styles of speaking lack life and spontaneity, making you seem like a mechanical robot. Instead, use index cards to organize your information and speak naturally.

Empty your pockets of change and keys. Then, if you feel the urge to hide your hands in your pockets, at least you will not distract the audience. Another tip that is seemingly self-evident, but necessary to keep in mind, is not to chew gum. These two nervous habits can ruin the best speech.

Make sure your presentation has an opening which captures your audience's attention. Begin your speech by arousing their curiosity, offering a benefit, or giving a warning. Convince the audience that you are worth listening to by establishing your expertise.

Try to develop a personal rapport with the audience. Make the people you are addressing feel like you are talking to them personally. Make eye contact with members of the audience. Also, speak their language. If you are giving a presentation to your colleagues, it is appropriate to use medical terminology. In speaking to the general public, avoid medical terms and use words which are more easily understood by the lay person. Involve the audience in your presentation by asking them questions.

Remember, the purpose of the presentation is to "sell" your service. While it is important to provide medical information, you also want to convey the benefits of your practice. Tell stories about patients you have treated to illustrate your main points.

Close your presentation with a brief summary of your most important points. You may want to tell a story about a patient which confirms and reinforces the benefits of your care. Invite the audience to call your office for additional information. Be prepared to answer questions after your presentation. This is your opportunity to get to know your audience, and to show them that you are truly responsive to their concerns. Finally, always have ample copies of your practice brochure to distribute to the audience, so they have something about you and your practice to take home, and hopefully, will share your message with family and friends.

Polish your presentation. Practice it in front of colleagues, friends, family members and in front of a mirror. Record it and listen to the tape, not only for substantive content, but for enunciation, grammar, and intonation. If possible, hire a public speaking consultant to help develop speeches and coach you. Besides making you feel more comfortable with the subject, practice improves your delivery, and develops your poise in front of a group.

Target your audience. To maximize your efforts, arrange to speak to groups who may need your services in the future or who can refer patients to you. For example, if older people make up a large proportion of your patients, then you may want to target senior citizen organizations in setting-up speaking engagements. On the other hand, if adolescents are a major portion of your practice, then speaking at high schools and youth groups should be your main goal.

When speaking to referring colleagues, think about how you can help them help their patients. For example, as a psychiatrist, you will want to inform the medical community about exactly what psychiatry is: its suitability, benefits to patients, how follow-up is dealt with, the availability of adequate long term care for patients who require it, and the importance of continued reports to the referring physician for the overall care of their patient.

Visual Aids. In the process of developing a speech, you may find it useful to employ visual aids. This is particularly helpful in simplifying a complex treatment or a concept too far removed from the common knowledge of your audience. It is also a way to increase attention and retention. Visual aids range from the familiar blackboard to charts and slides. In addition, there is an almost unlimited variety of new media, including videotape (which you can use to show a process in slow motion or to stop motion at points of special interest), and film strips which provide step-by-step descriptions. However, the use of visual materials may open the speaker to certain potential hazards: like all good things, these aids can be misused. Failing to use them correctly may detract from the effectiveness of your speech rather than increase it. Do not let your visual aids reduce you, the speaker, to a secondary role.

Book your presentations. Assign the responsibility for setting-up speaking engagements to one individual. A good place to start booking lectures is with the organizations you belong to, such as hospitals, libraries, school associations, or health clubs. Other groups always looking for good speakers include: alumni, educational, religious, civic, social, benevolent, and fraternal groups, as well as trade and labor organizations. Find out the name of the program chairman, and write to him or her explaining that you are available to speak on a variety of mental health topics. To pique their interest, enclose your list of presentations, then make follow-up telephone calls to set up speaking engagements.

When you begin your public speaking program, you will have to actively pursue speaking opportunities. Once you have a solid track record, organizations will call you.

§ 16.10 Special Events

Publicizing special events lets members of your community know your interest in interacting with them.

Special events to promote your practice—like an open house to show off a new office, a wine and cheese party to introduce a new associate to the professional community, a holiday party to thank staff for a job well done—play an important role in the marketing plan. Whether they arise naturally from the growth of a practice, or are created specifically to draw attention, special events can be used to put your practice in a favorable light.

A special event should have a special result. Since an event requires extensive preparation, it is important that it has a clearly defined purpose which will benefit the practice. Your first step in planning an event is to determine your objective. Consider whether the purpose of the event is to create awareness, emphasize accomplishments, or honor an individual. Details to consider when planning your event include:

- Type of event: formal or informal;
- Guests: professional community, general public, staff;

- When: time of year, date, time of day;
- Who is in charge: office manager, marketing consultant;
- Budget.

You must promote your event. Send out a news release describing it, and hire a professional photographer to take photos that can be sent out to community newspapers. Make sure brochures on the practice are exhibited where guests can easily take copies. (See Figure 16-10.)

You are cordially invited to an
OPEN HOUSE
at the new office of
VALLEY SPRING SURGICAL ASSOCIATES
on Sunday, November 9th from 3 to 5 P.M.

25 Valley Spring Road   R.S.V.P.
Portsmith, Virginia   *215-649-8770*

Fig. 16-10. Sample advertisement for a special event.

§ 16.11 Creating an Image

Creative signs and logos will give your practice a dynamic image.

The visual representation of a practice is essential to creating a positive reputation and attracting new patients. A mundane letterhead, business card, or an undistinguished sign or advertisement in the telephone directory, conveys that your professional approach is uninspired. An artistically-designed logo or sign will draw attention to your practice and convey a dynamic image.

(Rel.4-2/90 Pub.372)

[1] Logo

A well-designed logo establishes a distinctive and dynamic professional identity. An attractive graphic image can communicate a specific message about your practice. Depending on your goals for the practice, a logo can target a specific demographic group, develop name recognition, or publicize a specific area of your expertise.

Not every practice needs or should have a logo. If a physician prefers not to expand his practice, and is content with an occasional referral, then a logo may be unnecessary. However, a logo is a must for physicians who plan to promote their services. If you use the Yellow Pages, newspapers, or direct mail to communicate with current or potential patients, you need a logo to identify your practice.

Image and identity should be consistent. Before investing in a logo, it is important to define your identity and decide the image you want to project. Ideally, a logo portrays the definition, direction, and distinction of a practice.

To crystallize your professional image, begin by determining the attributes by which you presently identify your practice. For example, your image might consist of a combination of the following characteristics: competence, expertise, quality of care, professionalism, progressive, or family oriented.

Your logo should always be current. If you change the name of your practice, you should change your logo to reflect that change. Consider redesigning your logo if you expand existing services or simply want to change your reputation. A new logo has the power to dispel an existing image.

A logo has several elements: a symbol, a logotype or distinctive typestyle, color, and a tagline. Ideally, the symbol communicates your message at a glance: it may be a realistic illustration of the instruments of your profession or specialty, or a representational symbol (for example, of a family,: to convey that you are an expert at working with families); or it may be an abstract design that conveys an image of growth, stability, or other characteristic that sets the tone for your practice.

The style of your logo should be consistent with the nature of the practice and your personality. While a surgeon may choose a formal abstract symbol to depict his or her practice, a pediatric dentist may prefer a light-hearted caricature of him- or herself treating a patient.

The colors of a logo evoke emotion. By carefully choosing shades, you can create the desired feeling in your target audience.

The tagline is a four- or five-word statement that reinforces the strong point of your practice.

The following are practical suggestions for developing a logo:

- To build name recognition, incorporate the practice name into the design or have the name printed close to the symbol.

- Make sure that your logo will be effective when it is reduced to a small size for business cards and small ads, or enlarged for your sign.

- Choose your colors carefully, but don't use many: each color increases the printing price for stationary and direct mail. The logo must also work well in black and white.

- Use your logo everywhere your name appers: on letterheads, business cards, advertisements, newsletters, statements, publicity and promotional materials. A logo works through constant exposure.

[2] Signs

In the old days, a physician put out a "shingle" with small lettering to advertise his or her practice. Today, physicians have to consider every avenue available to them for recruiting patients, including the one outside the front door.

There are several factors to consider in planning and purchasing a sign. Remember that sign companies are experts on construction, not marketing. They should not decide what the sign should say.

A sign should do more than simply announce the name of your practice and your specialty. It should convince people to call you. To accomplish that, the sign should let them know what you offer by listing the symptoms or problems that you treat. The sign should also explain why people should come to you, rather than going to someone else, by spelling out what is so special about your practice: use, emergency care, friendliness, etc. Finally, the graphic image on the sign must invoke trust.

From a practical standpoint, plexiglass is a good choice for a sign: it is easier to change a plexiglass face and less expensive than purchasing an entirely new sign. You should place the sign on your property in a position of maximum visibility. Go for a walk down your street to study the best location. Make your sign is as big as the law and the landlord will allow to ensure that it will be noticed. Finally, light your sign so that it can be read at all hours of the day.

§ 16.12 Advertising

Advertising in newspapers, over radio or on television is a way of reminding your target audience of the services and benefits you provide. The character of your audience will determine the advertising medium most appropriate for your purposes.

Advertising can increase your patient volume and help you hold on to your current patients. Through advertising, people come to know you better. And it is only natural that people will choose your practice or stick with it if they know what you provide.

When advertising your practice, you should put every effort into choosing the right words to convey who you are, and what makes your practice unique. Whether you use newspapers, the Yellow Pages, radio, television, or coupons, advertising provides you with an opportunity to say much about yourself and your practice — in few words — to a large audience.

The size and type of your practice, the group you are trying to reach, and your advertising budget all will determine the most appropriate advertising media for your practice. Many physicians use more than one medium to saturate their geographic area.

[1] Newspapers

A newspaper ad should be big enough to deliver your message without too much clutter, and attractive enough to be noticed. Photos make even more impact. Key elements for a good ad include:

- a good visual to attract attention;
- a strong headline that gets your message and image across;

- a clean layout with enough white space to rest the eyes;
- the right typeface; and,
- a border to make it stand out from the rest of the page.

The newspaper's advertising department can help you with the design and layout of your ad. They can also make recommendations on print style.

You should decide whether you want to place your ad in a small local newspaper or a large city paper. Always consider the geographic area realistically possible to draw your future patients from, or continue to reach your current ones. Weekly community papers may also attract newcomers to your area or let current patients know about a new service or a new partner. It may be more cost effective to buy ad space for several weeks at a time.

[2] Yellow Pages

Many people use the Yellow Pages of the phone directory as a handy reference for health care. Physicians and surgeons are among the services most often sought out through the Yellow Pages. If you are listed by profession and specialty, your name will be chosen by those looking for a doctor near work or home. Newcomers to a community who need a doctor may turn to them in an emergency or as their only source for referral.

Your Yellow Pages ad has to sell in a small space, and convince people to use you for your services out of the many other names that appear on the same page. Any technique that makes you stand out on the page provides the opportunity to attract more patients to your practice. For example, display ads and alphabetical listings in bold print automatically catch the eye.

Any extra information gives the reader added incentive to call you. If you choose to list only under the general heading, you can add information such as your specialty or some procedures you provide in a few lines following your name. If you use a display ad, you can cross-reference to your listing or to a specialty guide that follows these listings.

Use the Yellow Pages coupons in the back of the directory to encourage more response to your ad by offering a discount on the initial examination or another incentive.

[3] Radio and Television

Depending on the size and nature of your practice, radio and television ads can be very effective. However, these are also among the most expensive forms of advertising, so you must know whether it will be worth your while, in terms of profit, to use them.

Most radio stations are aimed at a particular audience. They can provide you with demographic information (such as their audience's age, sex, income, and other traits) that will help you decide where to place your radio ad and how to present yourself to a particular audience. Radio stations cover broadcast areas of varying sizes, and some may be too large for your particular practice.

"Drive time," or the hours when people commute to and from work, is considered the optimum time for reaching people through radio advertising. However, slots in this time period are generally more expensive.

Since radio gets your message out quickly and has the emotional power of spoken words, going directly to the listener's ear, you can deliver strong messages about yourself and the quality of your practice. The radio station can help you create your commercials, write a script, or recording it yourself if you have a good voice. Some have talent departments that will do all the work for you.

Television is the most powerful advertising tool because it attracts large numbers of people who see and hear about you while they are relaxing at home. It's also the most expensive of the media. However, air time on a local cable station may be more affordable than network television. Since cable can cover a smaller market, such as your particular county or town, you may want to consider this form. Make sure you are represented through a professional high quality commercial.

[4] Coupons

Coupons are issued in many formats and through many sources: the back of the supermarket register tapes, in shopping cards, on Welcome

Wagon flyers, in free magazines distributed in many stores, and in Val-Pak type mailers to the home. There are also coupon ads in the Yellow Pages.

You should carefully consider the value of offering discounts or other free incentives when advertising your services. It is generally better to make a moderate offer and give strong reasons why you are the best provider, than to imply that you offer the cheapest service: at some point, people may decide that they get what they pay for, and a cheap image can damage your professional reputation.

Coupons yield uneven responses and may work differently at various times of year. About once a year, you should change the look of your coupon and the offer.

§ 16.13 Direct Mail

> A direct mail campaign allows you to market yourself to a specific audience by stressing specific aspects of your expertise. Whether you work from a personal or professionally prepared mailing list, you must follow up a series of direct mailings with phone calls to see if you are communicating your message effectively.

Direct mail is used to create a "direct" response. A well-planned campaign of personal letters sent through a direct mail plan will introduce you and your practice to new residents of your community, generalists and specialists who will refer patients, and even local business. Provocative letters or mailers are cost-effective ways to develop new relationships, "sell" your expertise and services and pave the way for face-to-face meetings.

Traditionally, direct mail campaigns generate a one to two percent return. However, you can increase your response through follow-up telephone calls and additional mailings.

Choose your targets. Direct mail allows you to carefully define and select your target audience within the tightest possible parameters. Begin your campaign by compiling a specific prospect list. This list is essential to the growth and development of your practice. In generating a list, try to define your targets in terms of location, age, income, type of specialty and other characteristics.

Several sources may be helpful for compiling your direct mail list including the Yellow Pages, the membership directory for the local

Chamber of Commerce, and commercial directories. You can also buy a prepared mailing list for as little as $30, to as much as $,000 dollars for a thousand names. (If you are interested in purchasing a list, the *Directory of Mailing List Houses* [Todd Publications, New York] may be helpful in locating a supplier.) Each month "new resident" mailing lists are available for purchase through various list companies. On the average, there are approximately one to two percent new residents in most areas, per month.

Define your service. Direct mail offers you the flexibility to focus on the distinctive capabilities of your service. It's particularly useful for selling a specific service as the answer to a problem, such as injuries on the job, stress reduction, or screening programs. Try to identify a problem which your clinical expertise can solve for your prospects.

Outline your strategy. Develop a written plan of action which describes your objective, the timing and mechanics of the mailing, and the follow-up. For example, your objective may be to set-up appointments to meet with personnel directors of major companies in your community.

Be sure to control the follow-up process. You should take the initiative in contacting physicians or executives. Call each person on the list within seven days after your letter goes out. If you are taking the responsibility for following up, then it is a good idea to send the letters out in small batches of five or ten, depending on how much time you have to devote to responses. If you sign the letter, then you should be the one to deal directly with the response.

Develop a hook. Before you put your pen to paper, you must decide how you are going to get the attention of your readers. Do you want to stir curiosity by sending a short note stressing a specific point? Do you want to give the prospect an opportunity to sample your services by offering a free physical? Do you want to describe your brochure in glowing terms and then offer to send it in the future? Do you want to offer to give a free health informtion talk to interested groups?

Write your letter. Never hint: be direct, and get to the heart of the matter. Explain how your services will benefit the prospective client and briefly describe your services and your qualifications to perform the services. Then, tell the reader what the next step is: either ask the reader to call you for more information or let him or her know that you plan to make a follow-up call.

Be persistent. Don't try to tell your whole story in one letter. Your goal is to pique the reader's interest. You'll either wear the reader down, or win him or her over by sending a letter with a different angle month after month. Ideally, your prospects should receive at least two mailings a year.

The best test of your direct mail campaign is the telephone follow-up. You'll know if it was successful by the response to your calls. If the campaign has been effective, the telephone calls should reveal familiarity with your practice, recall of the letter, and willingness to set an appointment or arrange a personal meeting that can lead to a business contract or a new referral source.

[1] Guidelines for a Direct Mail Campaign

Launching a typical direct mail campaign may involve:

- sending households in your targeted area an introductory letter with a brochure (This letter should specify that you are available to discuss any questions or assess any problems.);
- mailing a welcome letter and the practice brochure to new residents each month;
- sending current patients personally signed letters expressing that you enjoy having them as patients and are available to care for their family and friends;
- sending holiday greeting cards to patients;
- writing a letter to previous patients whom you cared for over the past five through eight years. This letter should convey interest in their progress, emphasize that you're available to provide care for their family and friends or to offer any help necessary to maintain their health; and,
- sending sympathy cards when you become aware of a severe illness, sudden disability, or death of one of your patients or his or her relatives.

You can make the most of direct mail by:

- mailing often;
- varying your format: using self-mailers, letters, article re-

prints, newsletters, post cards, greeting cards, announcements, etc.;

- updating your mailing list;
- riding on coattails of current events: cold winters, flu season, holiday depression, etc.;
- sending personalized letters;
- focusing on a specific service.
- concentrating on special groups (For example, if you're an active member of a synagogue or church, send low-key letters about your practice to the members.);
- using a P.S. on every letter;
- encouraging people to act now; and
- following up.

§ 16.14 Patient Education

A patient education program will show paients that you respect their intelligence and are concerned about their ongoing welfare. At the same time, private consultation, patient information cards, audiotapes and standardized material reinforce instructions regarding follow-up health care, assuage patient concerns regarding health care procedures and compliment risk management procedures.

Today's patients are knowledgeable health care consumers who no longer blindly trust the authority of the physician. They think of themselves as customers who can walk out of "the store" if they don't like the service.

Patients today demand to be informed and involved in their health care. A patient education program designed for such purposes can bring a multitude of positive results: your patients will enjoy greater satisfaction and peace of mind; you will benefit through improved patient cooperation, decreased stress, reduced risk of malpractice claims, and increased repeat or referral business.

Quality patient education increases patient satisfaction significantly. Yet, it takes time to give each patient a short course on his or her specific condition and, when necessary, to explain follow-up care in detail. Large segments of practice time may be spent explaining and repeating instructions. By developing the necessary teaching tools, though, a practice can easily provide correct information in a way that promotes patient understanding to the benefit of both the patient and physician.

Teaching tools include patient information and instruction cards, audiotapes, note pads, and a library. You may want to make some provision for teaching materials that patients can take home with them. Patients often have difficulty paying attention to verbal instructions so, by providing them with material they can take home, you give them an opportunity to learn about appropriate response and follow-up care for their conditions at their leisure, when they may be more receptive.

[1] Consultation

The best teaching tools reinforce the information provided to the patient during private consultation. There are several points you should remember when speaking with patients:

- Be brief. Provide the smallest amount of information required to make the point.

- Use everyday English. Avoid complex medical terms or jargon.

- Provide information in order of importance. Also, give instructions in the chronological sequence to be followed by the patient.

- Be specific. For example, say "Take the medication at 8 in the morning, 2 in the afternoon, and 8 in the evening," rather than "Take medications three times a day."

- Repeat important information. Restate the message in different words.

- Make sure the patient understands. Encourage patients to ask questions. Ask them to repeat your instructions.

[2] Patient Information Cards

Patient information cards are an important marketing tool. Ideally, these cards present personalized information from the physician along with a few sentences describing the practice and its name, address and telephone number. They may provide information on specific health problems or procedures. Information cards should be focused communications on specific topics that the physician frequently discusses with patients, or on issues patients repeatedly bring up.

Patient information cards should be easy to read. Written materials should be presented on a fourth- or fifth-grade reading level and accompanied by clear illustrations. A simple question and answer format is ideal for patient information cards. For example, a card on cataract surgery may ask (and answer) the following questions:

- What are cataracts?
- Will I be able to see clearly after surgery?
- How should I care for my eyes following surgery?
- Will the cataracts grow back?
- Pros and cons of laser surgery.

Cards should be prepared with the patient base in mind. For example, if the practice treats many senior citizens or persons of Hispanic origin, cards should be printed, respectively, in large type or in Spanish.

Information cards can be both attractive and inexpensive to produce. Choose a different color for each card to achieve a pleasing rainbow effect when the entire series is displayed in the waiting room.

Distribute patient information cards both inside and outside of the office. Exhibit them in your waiting room with a sign instructing patients to "Take One," and distribute them at seminars, speeches at civic organizations and other special events. When patients take these informational cards home to share them with family and friends, they become an easy means of spreading your name around the home and community.

[3] Standardized Materials

Customized high quality information cards are ideal. However, patient education materials relevant to various specialties are also available through most professional associations. For example, the American Psychiatric Association provides the "Let's Talk About" series. These cards should be affixed with gold or silver foil self-adhesive labels with the name, address, and telephone number of the practice.

[4] Patient Instruction Cards

Patient instruction cards on specific health problems should be given to patients during initial consultation and again when they are discharged. For example, you may want to give a woman who has undergone a breast biopsy at an outpatient surgery center, a card on how to do a monthly breast self-exam.

These cards are an essential component of the discharge process. They help to ensure that patients understand what to do at the time of discharge, and thus are vital to risk management. (*See also* ch. 8.) It is imperative to document that the patient actually received specific written discharge instructions. A signed document listing the discharge instructions that the patient received, and any further instructions, should be included in your records.

[5] Audiotapes

It's very reassuring for patients to be able to listen to their physician explain their health problem and follow-up care. You can develop a series of take-home audiotapes for patients on topics that you discuss with them most often. These tapes, which reinforce what the physician has told the patients in the office, are relatively inexpensive to reproduce once the message script has been written.

[6] Note Pads

It's a good idea to have a supply of pencils (imprinted with the practice name, specialty, and telephone number) and note pads (also imprinted) on hand in the waiting room and examination rooms. Encourage patients to jot down questions they may want to ask during their visit. This also provides patients with something constructive to do while they are waiting to be seen.

[7] Staff Education

Every member of the staff should communicate the high quality of care provided by the practice. A patient education program often begins with educating the staff. Providing staff education is an important way of showing patients that you care about them.

Make sure the staff is aware of:

- the causes and treatments of the health problems addressed by the practice;
- the impact of these problems on patients and families;
- the opportunities for resolving these problems and improving the quality of life.

In many practices, physicians delegate patient education responsibilities to nurses who spend time with each patient, answering their questions and clarifying instructions.

§ 16.15 Patient Relations

Long waiting periods, inadequate facilities, lack of physician/patient communication, and poor staff attitude can de-market your practice. Your practice will benefit if you maintain a good office environment, prospect your patients for referrals and promptly schedule follow-up visits.

It's a well-known fact that it is much less expensive to keep current patients than to attract new ones. Physicians can't take their patients for granted. If they want people to return year after year, they have to work to retain their goodwill.

[1] De-marketing

De-marketing is the process of creating a negative image. Poor patient relations, long waits, abrupt treatment, or an unpleasant environment, de-market your practice in a way that no marketing campaign can make up for. Slick advertisements and glossy mailings used as part of your marketing plan also can de-market your practice if you fail to live up to the promises they make.

Word of mouth is still the best form of advertising. In most cases, people make decisions about where to seek medical care on the basis of personal recommendations and experiences. If your patients are dissatisfied with your care, or if they become disgruntled and walk out before being seen, they will share their complaints with family, friends, and co-workers. You will rapidly develop a reputation for poor services and patient care.

De-marketing will undermine your efforts to increase your patient load. Before you even consider marketing, you need to focus on your existing services.

There are several steps which every practice should take to avoid de-marketing. First, you should analyze your operation for potential problems and implement preventive strategies. Second, you should address any patient complaints immediately and take corrective actions. Third, you should periodically assess your practice in an effort to improve the quality of the services.

[a] Long Waiting Periods

Waiting is the number one de-marketing problem. If patients are not seen soon after they arrive, they become annoyed. If they become frustrated enough to walk out, they will tell their family and friends, give a detailed account of the long wait, and of negative aspects of your practice.

Today, the general public is aware of the method of patient processing many health care providers use, in an attempt to create the perception that patients are attended to rapidly. This method involves making patients wait successively in the waiting room area, the treatment area, the x-ray area, even the lab area. Patients are not deluded into thinking that they are being taken care of quickly because they are undressed and waiting in a treatment room or a different lounge. To avoid creating a situation where such waiting periods are necessary, do not block-schedule patients, but stagger appointments. (*See also* ch. 4.)

A time study can help prevent long waiting periods for your patients. By analyzing your patient flow, you can determine how many patients you can see realistically in an hour. A time study will establish a patient-per-hour rate for both the physician and staff and provide vital information for staff scheduling. For example, if your busiest periods are evenings, then you may want to schedule more coverage or a different configuration of coverage during those hours. A time study will also help you determine if patients are consistently held up at a particular stage in their visit.

The layout of your facility may also play a role in the delay of attending to patients. A practice should have enough examination rooms, consultation areas, and secretarial and technical space. Otherwise, the physicians and staff will always be waiting for each other. But having enough space is not sufficient in and of itself: the space must also be designed to maximize efficiency. If a physician has to waste valuable time walking several minutes from one location to the next, not only does the patient wait but the entire process of patient care attenuates.

Identifying all space requirements is an essential planning task you should undertake prior to building or renovating your practice. You can speed up patient flow by assigning a non-clinical staff person the responsibility for moving patients through the office. This individual should not have any clinical responsibilities. His or her only function should be to accompany (i.e., move) patients to the examination room, x-ray room, or lab.

[b] Patient/Physician Communication

To keep the patient flow moving, you must keep your consultations brief. At the same time, though, patients should not feel they are being rushed. The key to patient satisfaction in these circumstances is "quality time." It is essential that you give patients your full attention. Make eye contact with them and talk to them during the examination and treatment. Even if you are simply suturing a small laceration in a patient's hand, it is important that you attend to the person and not just to his or her hand. Patients feel well taken care of when you sit and talk with them face-to-face, even if only for a few moments in the examination room.

You can save time during consultations by working in tandem with a scribe. The scribe writes out the chart, while you examine the patient. This frees you of clerical duties to concentrate on medical tasks, and allows you to devote your attention completely to the patient.

[c] The Office Environment

Long patient waits and lack of doctor/patient communication are only two of the problems that can de-market your practice. The third is the office environment itself: make your office as pleasant as possible. Provide a variety of up-to-date magazines and other reading materials in your waiting area and examination rooms. Be careful not to abuse patients by subjecting them to loud music or blaring television sets.

Cleanliness is extremely important in all health care facilities. Take a walk through your office, and try to imagine how it looks to a patient. Messy vending machine areas, overflowing trash cans, dirty linoleum and stained carpeting create an immediate negative impression. Make sure that you have adequate storage space, and do not use your corridors as closets or observation areas. Your ffice should have wide corridors with ample navigating room for gurneys, as well as for people on crutches or in wheelchairs.

[d] Staff Attitude

If, in spite of all your efforts, a patient complains about your services, respond to the complaint immediately. When you receive a letter describing an unhappy experience at your office, call the patient to discuss the problem. For good measure, do not send a bill or submit an invoice for reimbursement. If a patient complains during a visit, make sure everyone is aware of the complaint and responsive to eliminating its cause, no matter how minor it seems. A positive, problem-solving attitude on the part of all staff members can go a long way toward resolving patient complaints, and relieving patient frustration.

De-marketing prevention is vital to the health of your practice. Have a marketing consultant give your practice a regular check-up to diagnose current and potential problems and to offer a plan of treatment.

[2] Internal Prospecting

The most effective and least expensive way to get new patients is to ask your current patients for referrals. Motivating referrals often involves as little as letting patients know that you're interested in providing care for their friends and relatives.

One effective way to let patients know you are interested in referrals is to put up a sign in the reception area that says: "New Patients Always Welcome." You may also want to print this phrase on business and appointment cards, in the practice brochure and in patient newsletters.

Reinforce your interest in referrals through conversations with patients. Physicians often find it difficult to ask for referrals because they don't want to give patients the impression that they need business. Patients, however, will be interested in doing a favor for a doctor who has taken good care of them.

(Rel.4–2/90 Pub.372)

If a patient pays you a compliment, you may say," Thank you. I enjoy hearing good things about my work. I'd appreciate it if you'd tell your friends about it." It's also a good idea to give patients extra business cards to share with friends who may need your services.

If you get a referral, make sure that you thank the person who gave it to you. Take the time to make a personal telephone call, and then follow it up with a letter and a small gift. This process can be incorporated into the daily functioning of the office. For example, when a patient telephones for an appointment, the receptionists should ask who referred him or her to you. This should be noted on the patient's chart and a letter should be prepared for your signature. This can be a standard letter, written for this specific purpose and entered into a word processor for easy access and retrieval. If appropriate, send the patient several copies of the practice brochure or patient newsletter to pass along to friends or relatives.

[3] Follow-Up Visits

Repeat business is the cornerstone of any practice. A few strategies can help you fill your appointment book in advance.

Be specific about the importance of the follow-up and return visits. Many patients do not return for the follow-up examination because they do not understand the potential consequences of ignoring it. Explain the risks involved in skipping the follow-up in detail. For example, an ophthalmologist will want to let patients know that the follow-up exam can detect glaucoma, which may lead to blindness. Make sure people know why they should come back.

Let patients know as soon as possible about the follow up appointment. During their first or second visit, explain why they need to return for follow up. Ask them to promise to come back so you can prevent any potential problems from happening.

Walk patients to the front desk and ask your receptionist to pencil in the follow up visit in the appointment book, even if it's a year away. Ask the patient to address a special reminder postcard which should be mailed several weeks before the appointment. It reminds them to come back, and in their own handwriting.

Finally, call the patient to confirm the appointment. Then, when he or she leaves, start the process all over again.

[4] Waiting Room Resume

A waiting room resume spells out your expertise for patients. It's an excellent way to inform them of your credentials and special achievements. You may display your resume in a plexiglas stand, or hand it directly to patients when they enter the office for their first appointment.

To be effective, the waiting room resume should be easy to read. Remember to include:

- your professional credentials;
- your education;
- hospital affiliation;
- honors and awards;
- consulting activities;
- volunteer/community activities; and,
- published articles and medical appearances.

§ 16.16 Professional Relations

You can expand your referral base by letting colleagues who refer patients to you know how much you appreciate their help, by seeking out fellow physicians whose practices compliment your own, and by networking with other practitioners in your community.

A vital referral base can be the key to the success of a medical practice. There are a variety of techniques for gaining valuable referrals through other physicians.

Keep a computerized list, card file or notebook with the names and numbers of your current referral sources. You must constantly nurture your relationships with these important colleagues. The following are suggestions for how to use your list:

- Send a supply of your practice brochures along with other materials. Then, the referrer doesn't have to write down your name, address, and phone number, or draw a map each time he or she sends a patient. All he or she has to do is give the patient your materials.

- Pick up the phone. After treating a referred patient, call the referring physician and let him or her know how things went. The act of making the call shows that you want to work with the physician.

- Send thank you notes to referring physicians. This is a simple gesture that reminds them you appreciate referrals. Consider including the note as a cover letter sent with your examination notes on the patient.

- Recognize the loyalty of referrers. Send them a restaurant certificate for two at the holiday season or some other suitable gift. This is an acceptable and appreciated gesture, one that you also can make to physicians outside your current referral network as new sources develop.

- Develop a reciprocal arrangement where you and physicians whose specialties are related to yours display each others' newsletters in their offices. For example, a pediatrician may want to cooperate with an obstetrician.

- Produce a joint newsletter with other physicians or swap columns. This cuts production costs and can lead to referrals.

- Invite your referrers out socially, for example, to play tennis or golf. Don't make your relationship all business.

[1] Complimentary Practices

It is important to continually try to develop new referral sources. Concentrate on specialities that are most likely to compliment your own. Identify physicians who also treat your patients. Then provide them with useful information about mutual patients. This is particularly useful for specialists whom patients seek on their own without referrals from their family doctors. This practice demonstrates your concern and establishes a common ground between the specialist and primary care physician.

Develop relationships with practitioners new to your community. Write a congratulatory letter welcoming them to the area. Invite the new physician to lunch or to your office to get acquainted.

Try a similar approach with established physicians. Read your local medical publications, and keep your eyes open for recurring names or for physicians who are doing interestig work in their fields. Call or write them, inviting them to lunch to discuss both of your practices and recent advances in your field. You may invite them to a professional seminar or lecture, and then to lunch or dinner afterwards.

[2] Networking

You may want to hold a networking lunch to meet fellow professionals. Invite about eight guests to an excellent local restaurant. Explain to them that the purpose of the lunch is to meet new people and update everyone on their activities. Ask each guest to bring enough business cards for an exchange. When lunch begins, ask everyone to introduce themselves and give a brief description of their practices. Then briefly comment on what is happening in your practice, and discuss new equipment or procedures in your field.

Your networking group may evolve into a multispecialty marketing cooperative that shares marketing ideas and experiences. The group may plan joint marketing activities, such as health fairs or open houses.

When you receive a patient from a first-time referring doctor, the referrer will probably ask the patient how the visit went. So make sure the patient is treated well. This means giving him or her an early appointment, a longer than average examination and good follow-up.

§ 16.17 Marketing Checklist

A comprehensive checklist for marketing your practice is provided.

__ Developing a Marketing Plan

    __ Research health care market and your practice's position

    __ Plan short- and long-term objectives for your practice

    __ Implement protocols for achieving objectives within a time frame and budget

    __ Establish criteria for evaluating practice's progress

__ Targeting a Market

    __ Analyze your practice

    __ Develop patient profiles

(Rel.4–2/90 Pub.372)

- __ Demographic factors
- __ Geographic factors
- __ Psychographic factors
- __ Practice benefits
- __ Rate of Usage
- __ Study your community

__ Choosing Marketing Strategies
- __ Target patients
- __ Establish budget
- __ Choose mode of communication

__ Marketing Tools
- __ Practice brochure
- __ Patient newsletter
- __ Public relations program
  - __ Press kit
  - __ News release
  - __ Media interview
  - __ Publicity photographs
  - __ Feature articles
- __ Public speaking
- __ Special events
- __ Practice image
  - __ Logo
  - __ Sign
- __ Advertising
  - __ Newspapers
  - __ Yellow pages

-     ___ Radio
-     ___ Television
-     ___ Coupons
- ___ Direct mailings
- ___ Patient education program
  - ___ Consultation
  - ___ Patient information cards
  - ___ Standardized materials
  - ___ Patient instruction cards
  - ___ Audio tapes
  - ___ Notepads and pens
  - ___ Staff education

___ Maintaining Patient Relations
- ___ Hold patient consultations
- ___ Prospect patients for referrals
- ___ Schedule follow-up visits
- ___ Display professional resume

___ Maintaining Professional Relations
- ___ Make list of referral sources
- ___ Compose standardized thank you note for referrers
- ___ Seek out complementary practices
- ___ Attend networking parties

Appendix 16-A

Marketing Resources

These resources provide useful information an practical advice on important factors in the marketing of your medical practice.

Reading List

Books

Adler, Mortimer J.: How to Speak, How To Listen. New York: Macmillan Publishing Co., 1983.

Brown, Stephen W. and Morley Jr., Andrew P.: Marketing Strategies For Physicians. Oradell, NJ: Medical Economics Books, 1986.

Carlson, Linda: The Publicity and Promotion Handbook. Boston: CBI Publishing Co., 1982.

Freitag, Joan: Designing The Perfect Logo and Brochure For Your Practice. Atlanta, GA: American Health Consultants, 1988.

Kelly, Kate: The Publicity Manual. Larchmont, NY: Visibility Enterprises, 1988.

Milone, Charles L., et al.: Marketing For The Dental Practice. Philadelphia, PA: W.B. Saunders Company, 1982.

O'Brien, Richard: Publicity, How to Get It. New York: Harper and Row, 1977.

Producing Practice Newsletter. Madison, WI: Professional Communications, Inc., 1984.

Sachs, Laura: Do-It-Yourself Marketing for the Professional Practice. Englewood Cliffs, NJ: Prentice-Hall, Inc., 1986.

Seltz, David D.: Handbook of Innovative Marketing Techniques. Reading, MA: Addison-Wesley Publishing Company, 1981.

Periodicals

Dental Economics. Tulsa, OK: PennWell Publishing.

Healthcare Marketing Report. Atlanta, GA: Jan Michael Lok.

Medical Economics. Oradell, NJ: Medical Economics Co., Inc.

Physician's Marketing and Management. Atlanta, GA: American Health Consultants.

The Physician's Advisory. Plymouth Meeting, PA: MCA Publications.

Sources of Demographic Information

Government

Each state has a health data center which is part of the state health department. These centers offer the best source of data for a modest price.

U.S. Department of Commerce
Bureau of Census
Washington, D.C. 20233
202-763-5020

Information Services
CACI
8260 Willow Oaks Corporate Drive
Fairfax, VA 22031
800-292-2224

Donnelly Marketing Information Services
70 Seaview Avenue
P.O. Box 10250
Stamford, CT 06904
800-527-DMIS

National Planning Data Corporation
20 Terrace Hill
Ithaca, NY 14850
607-273-8208

Urban Decision Systems, Inc.

West: P.O. Box 25953
       Los Angeles, CA 90025
       213-820-8931
       800-633-9568

East: P.O. Box 551
       Westport, CT 06881
       203-226-8188

CHAPTER 17

Understanding Medical Office Coding

SCOPE

Procedural and diagnostic codings are major determinants of third-party reimbursement for physician services. CPT codes are used to report most cognitive procedures and procedures concerned with surgery, anesthesia, radiological studies and pathology and laboratory reports. HCPCs codes elaborate some CPT codes and are much more specific with regard to physician supply coding. The ICD–9–CM manual supplies the physician with codes for the diagnosis of most injuries and diseases. It is essential that the physician be familiar with these basic coding systems and train the medical and billing staff accordingly. To achieve maximum reimbursement for services, the physician must know which coding system local carriers adhere to and how to interpret the coding texts for each system; understand the difference between consultation, referral and acceptance of patient care; appreciate the different levels of service provided for established and new patients; and know how to use coding modifiers and explanatory statements to justify procedures performed under circumstances not accounted for in the standard coding texts. Failure to meet these minimal requirements can result in improper billing, inadequate remuneration and, in some instances, an audit of the physician's records.

SYNOPSIS

§ 17.01 Overview of Coding Systems
    [1] Coding Terminology
    [2] Which Codes to Use
    [3] The Importance of Relative Value

§ 17.02   Supporting Office Coding
§ 17.03   Using the CPT Text
    [1]   Format
    [2]   Symbols
    [3]   Deleted Codes
    [4]   Notations
    [5]   Introduction
§ 17.04   CPT: Medicine
    [1]   Hospital Charges/Initial Hospital Care
    [2]   Subsequent Hospital Care
    [3]   Hospital Discharge Services
    [4]   Nursing Home and Skilled Nursing Facility Charge
    [5]   Emergency Department Services
    [6]   Immunization and Injections
    [7]   Preventive Medicine
    [8]   Psychiatry
    [9]   Ophthalmology
    [10] Echocardiography
    [11] Allergy and Clinical Immunology
    [12] Chemotherapy Injections
    [13] Case Management Services
    [14] Handling Codes (99000, 99001 and 99002)
    [15] Postoperative Follow-Up Visits
    [16] After-Hours and Holiday Charges
    [17] Other Location
    [18] Supplies
    [19] Prolonged Services
    [20] Critical Care
§ 17.05   CPT: Surgery
    [1]   Surgical Packages
    [2]   Separate Procedures
    [3]   Nonpackage Surgical Procedures
    [4]   Incision of Lesions
    [5]   Repairs
    [6]   Grafts and Flaps
    [7]   Orthopedic Services
    [8]   Vascular Injection Procedures
    [9]   Maternity Care and Delivery
§ 17.06   CPT: Radiology
    [1]   Complete Procedures
    [2]   Professional and Technical Component
    [3]   Miscellaneous
§ 17.07   CPT: Pathology and Laboratory
    [1]   Multichannel and Group Tests
    [2]   Individual Chemistry and Toxicology Test

[3] Surgical Pathology and Consultations
§ 17.08 Modifiers for CPT Codes
§ 17.09 Other CPT Appendixes and Index
§ 17.10 HCPC Coding
    [1] Alphanumerical Coding
    [2] HCPC Modifiers
§ 17.11 Levels of Service
    [1] New Versus Established Patients
    [2] Defining Services
        [a] Minimal Service
        [b] Brief Services
        [c] Limited Services
        [d] Intermediate Services
        [e] Extended Services
        [f] Comprehensive Services
§ 17.12 Consultations
    [1] Consultant Visits
    [2] Intermediate Consultation
    [3] Extended Consultation
    [4] Comprehensive Consultation
    [5] Complex Consultation
    [6] Follow-up Consultations
§ 17.13 Relative Value Indexes
§ 17.14 ICD-9-CM Diagnostic Coding
    [1] The ICD-9-CM Text
        [a] Volume Three
        [b] Volume Two, Section One
        [c] Volume Two, Section Two
        [d] Volume Two, Section Three
        [e] Volume One
    [2] Alphabetical Index
    [3] Punctuations
    [4] Symbols
    [5] Instructional Notations
§ 17.15 Checklist for a Coding Library
    [1] Ancillary Texts
    [2] Third-Party Manuals
§ 17.16 Tips for Proper Coding
§ 17.17 Coding Checklist

§ 17.01 Overview of Coding Systems

The procedural and diagnostic codes physicians report on routing slips and patient records determine the amount they will be reimbursed by third parties for their services. CPT and HCPCS codes are the two current procedural coding systems. The ICD-9-CM is the diagnostic coding system. Reimbursement also may be affected by relative value index adjustments. Physicians need to be aware of which coding systems are used by third parties in their areas, and they must keep up to date on any changes made in these systems.

CAUTION: Medical office coding is currently going through enormous changes. The new Harvard-based Resource Based Relative Value Scale (RBRVS) will radically change the way Medicare and presumably other third parties reimburse physicians. The RBRVS will undoubtedly institute some changes in coding. In addition, new codes are constantly being issued. Readers must stay abreast of all bulletins and guides given to them directly from the third parties in which they are participating.

Hospital coding for services rendered is currently based on a single system of coding, Diagnostic-Related Groups (DRGs). Essentially, hospitals are paid based based on an amount that has been assigned to a specific DRG code. Hospitals have an economic incentive to treat the patient efficiently and in the least expensive way, as they are entitled to the "profit" when the DRG reimbursement exceeds their actual expenditures.

At the present time, there are two basic systems for the coding of physicians' medical services: procedural coding and diagnostic coding. As it does not appear that a DRG-type system will be developed for physicians in the immediate future, physicians will continue to be paid according to the amounts assigned to these procedural and diagnostic codes, and third parties will increase their monitoring of the appropriateness of a procedure by cross-checking it against the diagnosis.

[1] Coding Terminology

It is important for physicians and their staff members to understand the terminology used in coding. (*See Figure 17–1.*) The following is a quick synopsis:

CPT Codes. CPT is an acronym for the American Medical Association's text *Physicians Current Procedure Terminology.*

HCPCS (pronounced "hick-picks"). An acronym for the Health Care Financing and Administrations Common Procedural Coding System.

FIG. 17-1.

- HCPCS Level One. Refers to CPT procedural codes.
- HCPCS Level Two. Refers to codes developed by the Health Care Financing Administration to supplement CPT. These codes often are referred to as HCPCS. These codes were developed to provide more specific identification of such items as medical supplies, injections and dental services.

(Text continued on page 17–5)

BASIC CODING SYSTEMS

- **CPT (90050, 93000, 45300 Etc.)**
  - Visits
  - Procedures
  - Lab
  - X-ray
- **HCPCS (A4550, J0190 Etc.)**
  - Injections
  - DME
  - Supplies
- **ICD-9 (465.9, 79.9, 401.1, 250.0 Etc.)**
  - Diagnoses

COURTESY OF PROFESSIONAL CONSULTING

FIG. 17-1

- HCPCS Level Three. Refers to local codes. Each local Medicare intermediary has the freedom to create codes and modifiers for use within the geographic region it administers.

ICD-9-CM. An acronym for the *International Classification of Disease, 9th Edition, Clinical Modifications,* which is published by the World Health Organization. This text assigns codes to all the different diagnoses.

Relative Value Index. Refers to a text that assigns a nonfinancial relative value to each of the different procedures. First developed in the early 1950s in California, use of the relative value index declined during the 1970s, when the federal government became concerned that the index could be used as a tool for price fixing by physicians. Notwithstanding such concern, third parties have continued to use relative value indexes, a number of which currently are available to physicians.

RBRVS. An acronym for Resource Based Relative Value Scale, which refers specifically to the Hsiao Harvard Study completed by William C. Hsiao and presented to Congress in 1989. Medicare reimbursements will be based on the RBRVS beginning in 1992.

[2] Which Codes to Use

In general, the physician should apply the following rules when determining salient coding for services provided by his or her practice:

(1) Local codes (HCPCS Level Three) have the highest priority. Since the local carrier is responsible for administering a particular health plan, local coding always should be used first. As a practical matter, local codes are diminishing in utilization as HCPCS and CPTs standardize items.

(2) The national HCPCS Level Two codes should take the second priority. For example, while the CPT text has the one code (99070) for supplies, the HCPC codes specifically identify supplies through a separate set of codes (A4200 through A4927).

(3) Finally, HCPCS Level One codes (CPT codes) should be used. Although level one codes are the last codes to use in areas where there is potential for conflict, as a practical matter, they comprise the bulk of most physicians' coding.

The ongoing changes in the coding field warrant monitoring. Attention should be paid to bulletins and newsletters from all third parties, particularly those from Medicare and Medicaid, as it is obvious that the federal government, through Medicare, sets the method for the billing of physician services that other third parties follow. Updated CPT texts should be ordered each year, and all changes should be noted. Medical office charge slips should be updated to include these changes, and the physician, medical staff and business staff should be kept abreast of these changes.

[3] The Importance of Relative Value

The RBRVS will not change the methodology of physician billing (i.e., procedural codes and diagnostic codes), but it will change the relative value and amount paid for the different procedures. In general, cognitive procedures (e.g., office visits, hospital visits, consultations and critical care) will receive greater reimbursement, while other types of surgical and more specialized procedures will receive less reimbursement. Emphasis will be placed on paying physicians for their own cognitive and surgical procedures while removing the financial incentives for ancillary services, such as laboratory and x-ray studies. Legislation may soon prohibit physician ownership in other types of medical business ventures, such as those involving magnetic resonance imaging, CT scanning and lithotripters. Therefore, physicians should focus on fine-tuning their procedural coding and being aware of what the maximum reimbursements will be paid for the various procedures they perform themselves.

Since physicians were told in the 1970s that relative values were illegal price fixing tools, many considered them a snare to be avoided. Physicians must understand, however, that relative values have in the past played an important role in determining how much a physician is reimbursed for a particular procedure and will continue to do so in the future. As such, the physician should pay particular attention to the relative values assigned to procedures they commonly perform as well as to the potential impact of the new RBRVS as it begins to phase in.

§ 17.02 Supporting Office Coding

Third parties may audit physician records to ensure that the diagnostic and procedural codes reported are consistent with the services rendered. Physicians must be able to support their coding practices with proper documentation.

Once third parties began to limit the amount they reimbursed for various procedures and physicians began to understand the concept of relative value, third parties began to see "CPT inflation" or "creep." CPT inflation describes the practice by which physicians simply report a code with a higher relative value in order to procure a larger reimbursement from third parties. Third parties—Medicare, Medicaid and Blue Cross, in particular—have reacted by exercising their right to "audit" physician records to determine if a physician is "overcoding." Obviously, auditors will not be able to review the actual procedure performed; they will have to rely on the medical record to support the billing claim.

Because audits often are conducted at random, physicians should always be prepared to back up their billing procedures. Reliance on the business staff to do coding does not relieve the physician of ultimate responsibility.

As a practical matter, most audits are either the result of unusual coding patterns as compared to the norm for a particular specialty or based on patient complaints. *Figure 17-2* illustrates the type of documentation a third-party auditor looks for. In order to avoid allegations of fraud and abuse, the physician should:

- Be considerate of complaints from employees who are doing the billing.

- Respond immediately to patient complaints. Patients who feel they are not receiving proper attention from office staff are likely to bring their grievances to their Medicare carrier.

- Avoid an attitude of "getting even." Sometimes frustrated physicians will decide that they can compensate for poor reimbursement rates and delays by overbilling a little.

- Be mindful that the government appears to be watching the following:
    - misuse of billing codes;
    - billing for services not rendered;
    - billing for a higher level of service than was rendered or documented;
    - billing for unnecessary services without appropriate certification of medical necessity.

§ 17.03 Using the CPT Text

In order to use the CPT text efficiently, the physician and staff must be familiar with the book's contents, heading/subheading format, use of specific modifying symbols and notations for each code.

AUDIT FORM

OFFICE VISITS	LEVELS OF SERVICE					
	MINIMAL	BRIEF	LIMITED	INTERM.	EXTENSIVE	COMPHENS
NEW PATIENT		90000	90010	90015	90017	90020
ESTABLISHED PATIENT	90030	90040	90050	90060	90070	90080
Code Criteria	1 of 2	3 of 4	4 of 6	5 of 7	8 of 11	10 of 13
Blood Pressure Ck, Suture Removal, etc.	|X|				|X|	|X|
Temperature						|X|
Pulse					|X|	|X|
Primary Complaint / Symptoms		|X|	|X|	|X|	|X|	|X|
Secondary Symptoms				|X|	|X|	|X|
Duration and/or Course of Illness			|X|	|X|	|X|	|X|
Review of Systems					|X|	|X|
Past Medical History					|X|	|X|
Family History						|X|
Physical Exam (One Area)		|X|	|X|			
Physical Exam (Two or More Areas)				|X|	|X|	
Complete Physical Exam (May Include Pelvic Exam)						|X|
Lab and X-ray Values and Findings			|X|	|X|	|X|	|X|
Diagnosis / Problem		|X|	|X|	|X|	|X|	|X|
Treatment / Interpretation of Patient Test Results / Education / Conference	|X|	|X|	|X|	|X|	|X|	|X|

WHEN THIRD PARTY PAYERS AUDIT YOUR RECORDS, THEY USE FORMS LIKE THIS ONE. DO YOUR PATIENT CHARTS CONTAIN DOCUMENTATION OF THE LEVELS OF SERVICE FOR WHICH YOU HAVE BILLED, AND THE APPROPRIATE TEST RESULTS?

COURTESY OF PROFESSIONAL CONSULTING

FIG. 17-2

Each physician (as well as all members of the physician's medical and billing staff) should be familiar with the CPT text. The CPT book is organized as follows:

1. Table of contents
2. Introduction
3. Guidelines and procedures listed by separate section:
    Medicine
    Anesthesiology
    Surgery
    Radiology
    Pathology and Laboratory
4. Appendixes
5. Index and instruction on index utilization

In using the CPT text, it is helpful to be familiar with its basic organization:

(1) Within each of the five main sections, the codes are grouped into subsections. A review of the Table of Contents will facilitate immediate access into a particular section and subsection.

(2) The subsections are divided into groups of codes, called headings. For example, the subsection "Office Medical Service" includes separate headings for new patients and established patients.

(3) Depending on circumstances, headings sometimes are broken down further into subheadings.

(4) The specific CPT code is listed along with a description of the procedure.

[1] Format

The format of the CPT text is designed to group procedures on the basis of their shared elements.

For example, at the beginning of the "Medicine" part of the CPT text, the code number 90000, "Office Medical Service, New Patient; brief service," is an umbrella heading that encompasses a group of procedures. Under code section 90010, one finds the indented heading "limited service," indicating that it is a more specific subheading. The indentation signals the user to read the main heading from above and automatically include before the words "limited service" the phrase "Office Medical Service, New Patient." As such, the complete description for 90010 is "Office Medical Service, New Patient; limited service." Likewise, for code 90015, which also is indented, the complete description would be "Office Medical Service, New Patient; intermediate service." It is important to note that the semicolon indicates the end of the shared description for the indented services listed immediately below.

[2] Symbols

A number of symbols are used in the CPT text, and the physician should be familiar with what they stand for. The following is a summary of the salient symbols:

Circles. A circle (●) is printed to the left of codes that have been added recently to the CPT system. This makes it easier for the user to identify new procedures and services that do not appear in the previous year's volume.

Triangles. A triangle (▲) to the left of a code indicates that the description of the procedure has changed since publication of the previous CPT text. In order to avoid billing problems, it is important to make sure that these changes are noted and the codes utilized properly.

Stars. Stars or asterisks (*) appear to the right of several codes in the surgery section of the text. When a star appears to the left of the code, it indicates that the surgical package concept does not apply.[1] In other words, the procedure denoted is simply the surgical procedure and does not include any pre- or postoperative care.

[3] Deleted Codes

When codes are deleted from the CPT text, a parenthetical notation generally is placed in the area where the code had previously been located. Usually the note refers the user to another code to be used in place of the deleted code.

---
[1] *See* § 17.05[1] *infra*.

[4] Notations

There are numerous notations throughout the CPT text. These notations facilitate proper utilization of the codes and point out various exceptions. Users of the text should take time to read all the notations surrounding codes being used. It is highly recommended that in addition to reading and studying the entire introductory section of the text, physicians and staff should review the codes salient to the physician's speciality and all the notations surrounding those particular codes. By doing so, the physician will learn how to use the coding system efficiently, increase reimbursements and lower the risk of an audit.

[5] Introduction

Physicians, staff (medical assistants, lab technicians, nurses, etc.) and insurance clerks should read the introduction section of the CPT book for a proper introduction to the text. The introduction is approximately 15 pages long and contains general information on how to code, along with the levels of service for office visits, hospital visits and consultations.

§ 17.04 CPT: Medicine

> Codes used for the "Medicine" section of the CPT text cover most cognitive services, such as patient visits and hopsitalization. They also cover basic noninvasive procedures performed in several specialty areas, including ophthalmology, psychiatry and cardiology. Physicians seeking maximum reimbursement must be aware of which codes are time-driven, which cover single procedures, which cover a constellation of procedures and which will not be paid for by local carriers.

The "Medicine" section of the CPT text covers all medical specialties, and its codes range from 90000 to 99199. Codes for cognitive services, such as office visits, hospital visits, consultations and critical care, are found in this section. In addition, noninvasive procedures and services for several specialties, such as gastroenterology, ophthalmology, otolaryngology, cardiology, dialysis, physical medicine and dermatology, are included. (Invasive procedures and services for the specialties can be found in the third section, "Surgery.")[2]

---

[2] *See* § 17.05 *infra*.

[1] Hospital Charges/Initial Hospital Care

Hospital initial care is billed using one of three levels of service: brief, intermediate or comprehensive. Initial hospital care is used to bill the summary history and the physical admitting of the patient to the hospital. Services provided under this code should take place in the hospital rather than in the office. Intermediate hospital admissions are used for patients with previously documented evaluations that are still considered current, e.g., readmissions within 30 days. The brief hospital admission code is used for admissions in which neither intermediate nor comprehensive services are performed. It involves an abbreviated history, pertinent examination and plan of investigation and/or medical management.

Separate coding has been created to bill the history and examination and establishment of hospital records for the *normal* newborn. This code is used for birthing room deliveries as well as evaluations taking place in the delivery room or the nursery. The 90225 should not be used to bill initial examinations of babies who have difficulties and require a more extensive evaluation; in these cases, the standard hospital initial care codes should be used instead (90200–90220). For newborn care in other than a hospital setting, including the physical examination of the baby and conference(s) with parents, code 90757 can be used. It should be remembered that the newborn admission is not a global code, encompassing all hospital newborn care.

[2] Subsequent Hospital Care

Subsequent hospital care after the patient has been admitted falls within the range of codes 90240 to 90282. A review of the subsequent hospital care services indicates that subsequent hospital care is based on each day of care, not each service. As such, a claim for services will be rejected if the third party receives a billed for two services on the same day. To receive full reimbursement for multiple services rendered on the same day, the physician should code for a higher level of service.

For example, instead of listing a limited level of service twice, the physician should consider listing an extended level of care for that day. Again, the patient's medical record should note the two visits and what services were provided during those visits. Some local Medicare intermediaries employ modifiers that can be used to indicate that the patient needed to be seen more than once on the same day.[3]

[3] Hospital Discharge Services

Code number 90292, Hospital Discharge Day Management, is used to bill for the final examination of the patient, discussion of the hospital stay, instructions for continuing care and preparation of the discharge records. As it includes the examination and education of the patient, it *may not* be billed along with a hospital visit. If the services delivered on the final day of hospitalization are more extensive than a standard discharge, bill the appropriate level of service for the services actually delivered instead, e.g., a critically ill patient for whom critical care services were delivered and who subsequently dies.

[4] Nursing Home and Skilled Nursing Facility Charge

Patients receiving services in a skilled nursing facility (SNF), an intermediate care facility (ICF), a long-term care facility (LTC) or a transitional care unit (TCU) are billed using either Initial Care or Subsequent Care nursing home admission codes (90300–90370). A nursing home admission must be conducted in the nursing home rather than in the office or as part of the discharge from a hospital.

Medicare now requires that visits made to nursing home patients carry a modifier notifying the intermediary whether the physician saw a single patient (SP) or multiple patients (MP). Both the diagnostic codes submitted with the single visit and the nursing home notes should indicate the rationale for the acute care visit. It is important to recognize that although transitional care units are often part of the hospital, visits are treated as if they were nursing home visits. The number of visits permitted in a time period, and reimbursement for those visits, is therefore significantly more restricted.

---

[3] *See* § 17.08 *infra.*

[5] Emergency Department Services

There are currently three sets of codes used for billing emergency department services: 90000 to 90080, 90500 to 90580 and 99062 to 99065.

The first set of numbers, 90000 to 90080, is used to designate physicians who have not been assigned to the emergency room for the service rendered. The accompanying description indicates that the physician has a formal relationship with the hospital in which he or she is responsible for seeing patients in the emergency room during a specific time period (e.g., a physician specializing in emergency medicine). An agreement between physicians in

(Text continued on page 17–15)

which going to the emergency room to provide care is part of the on-call services is not the same as an agreement between a physician and a hospital. When a physician is working under an agreement with other physicians, he or she is not considered *assigned* to the emergency room.

If a physician is assigned to the emergency room of a hospital, the emergency department service codes 90500 through 90580 can be used. Physicians also should bill for surgical or diagnostic services rendered in addition to cognitive service. For example, monitoring blood gases, reading an EKG, laceration repair or fracture treatment can be billed in addition to the cognitive services rendered.

If the physician admits the patient to the hospital from the emergency room, the appropriate level of initial hospital care should be billed. If significant services have been rendered in the emergency room prior to admission and are not considered part of admission, these services also should be billed. The billing should be accompanied by a copy of both the ER record (which should contain a notation of time spent in the emergency room prior to admission) and the hospital history and physical. If the services rendered in the emergency room are, indeed, critical care services, they should be billed at a critical care level rather than at the emergency room service level.

If a physician has been called to the emergency room by the ER physician to render an opinion or give advice about a specific problem, *it may be appropriate to charge for consultative services*. In addition, the physician also may bill the third party carrier for the process of coming to the emergency room, using codes 99062 through 99065. These codes state that the physician came to the emergency room from within the hospital or outside the hospital, either during or outside of office hours. These codes should be considered adjunct codes and used in addition to the office codes. Many carriers use modifiers to indicate when the care rendered was considered emergency treatment. The local HCPC directory should indicate whether such a modifier exists.

[6] **Immunization and Injections**

The codes for immunization and injections, 90701 to 90749, should be used in conjunction with medical service. Unfortu-

§ 17.04[7]   MANAGING YOUR MEDICAL PRACTICE   17–16

nately, many physicians miss the medical service charge when the patient comes in for an injection and does not see the physician. Physicians should be aware that a minimal level of service charge (90030) may be used as a compensatory charge in such cases.

[7] Preventive Medicine

Codes 90750 to 90778 are used to describe visits in which the patient has no specific complaints (e.g., routine physicals). Ironically, in an era when preventive medicine is touted as a potential method of lowering health care costs, most third parties will not cover preventive services. The exception to this is some HMO plans that provide patients with a certain amount of preventive care. If problems are discovered during preventive medicine procedures, the physician should avoid using the preventive medicine codes. The regular office visit codes and appropriate diagnostic codes should be used to explain the problem and procedures. This generally results in higher reimbursement.

[8] Psychiatry

Codes 90801 to 90899 are for psychiatric care. Physicians should read the notes preceding code 90801, as there are certain issues psychiatrists should be aware of pertaining to utilization of CPT codes for hospitalized patients. First, the psychiatrist should be aware that hospital visits can be billed in addition to psychotherapy for hospitalized patients. If the psychiatrist reviews patient activity reports, orders tests, discusses patient management with ancillary staff *and* provides psychotherapy or conducts a psychotherapy session, he or she should bill for both the psychotherapy and the hospital visit. On days when no psychotherapy services are provided but the physician reviews records, orders tests and the like, he or she should bill for the appropriate level of hospital service.

Psychiatrists asked by another physician asked to give an opinion regarding a patient's problem are likely to be providing that service on a consultative basis. In such situations, the psychiatrist will find that using consultative codes 90600 to 90654 results in a higher reimbursement. Other areas in which psychiatrists commonly lose billings include items such as telephone consultation (code 90831), environmental intervention (code 90882), interpretation or explanation of reports (code 90887), and preparation of report for another physician (code 90889).

[9] Ophthalmology

Ophthalmologists and their staff should use standard codes to report minimal, brief and limited office services, the same way other physicians do. There are unique definitions and codes for intermediate and comprehensive ophthalmology services (92002 to 92014).

Intermediate Ophthalmological Services. Intermediate ophthalmological services (92002) refer to a level of service where the patient either has two diagnostic problems or a complicated problem. The service would include history, general medical observation, internal ocular and adnexal exam and other diagnostic services or the use of mydriasis if needed. Intermediate services do not usually include determination of the refractive state, but may in an established patient (92012) who is under continuing active treatment.

Comprehensive Ophthalmological Services. Code 92004 should be used for comprehensive ophthalmological services, which constitute a single service entity but may not be performed at one session. This service includes the history, general medical observation, external and ophthalmoloscopic examination, gross visual fields and basic sensorimotor examination. Often comprehensive ophthalmological services include biomicrosopy, examination with cycloplegia or mydriasis, tonometry and usually determination of the refractive state unless known.

Ophthalmologists should be aware that under no circumstances are they to charge for prescribing lenses. The prescription of lenses is always included in the charge for intermediate or comprehensive ophthalmological services.

Ophthalmologists also should be aware that Medicare will not reimburse for determination of the refractive state. Medicare carriers generally assume that the ophthalmologist's charge for intermediate and comprehensive services includes the refraction and reduces the amount of reimbursement accordingly. In order to obtain maximum reimbursement, physicians need to communicate the refraction information to Medicare. Some Medicare carriers require use of an "X" or "Y" modifier with intermediate and comprehensive ophthalmological services. The "X" modifier indicates that a refraction has been performed, while a "Y" modifier indicates that a refraction was not performed. Other carriers require the use of the HCPC national modifier "AP" to communicate that the charge does not include refraction. If an appropriate modifier is not used for intermediate and comprehensive ophthalmological service codes, it is likely that the Medicare carrier will assume that the charge includes the determination of a refractive state and automatically reduces the reimbursement.

Ophthalmologists who prescribe and supply contact lenses should be aware that prescription of the lenses should be charged separately and is not part of the general ophthalmological services. The charge for fitting and supplying the lenses should be included in the charge for prescribing contacts. If a separate charge is used for the contact lenses, it should be coded 92391. The prescription and fitting codes, 92310 to 92313, should be used in conjunction with code modifier –26 to indicate that only the professional component is included in the fee.

[10] Echocardiography

Physicians performing echocardiographic procedures may be confused by two sets of CPT codes for the same procedure: one set of codes appears in the medicine section (93300 to 93320), while the other appears in the radiology section of the text (96620 to 96632).

In general, cardiologists, internists and other physicians should use the 93300 to 93320 codes. Radiologists should use the 76620 to 76632 codes. The exception is when carriers require all physicians, irrespective of their specialty, to use a particular set of codes. If claims in this area are rejected, an intermediary should be contacted to determine the requested procedure.

[11] Allergy and Clinical Immunology

A special medical conference code, 95105, should be used by the pulmonologist instead of conference codes 98900 to 98912 when the use of mechanical and electrical devices, climatotherapy, breathing exercises and/or postural drainage is applicable.

It should be noted that codes 95120 to 95134 include both professional services and allergenic extract. Physicians should not bill an additional charge for time spent by the physician or medical assistant who observes the patient immediately following the injection.

[12] Chemotherapy Injections

Physicians providing chemotherapy services should be aware that the injection codes (96400 to 96549) need to be charged "independent of the patient's office visit." In other words, when the physician provides services beyond the injection itself (an office visit), services should be billed in addition to the injection.

In addition, a separate charge generally is made for the chemotherapeutic agent. Chemotherapy agent code 96545 should be used for this coding; however, the specific HCPC chemotherapy drug code should be used for Medicaid and Medicare patients.

Sometimes the reimbursement for chemotherapeutic drugs may be less than the direct cost to the physician. There may be an additional collection loss as a result of rejected claims or bad debt. Thus, it is extremely important for the physician to pay close attention to the billing in this area.

[13] Case Management Services

Codes 98900 to 98922, which are new in the 1990 CPT text, are used when a physician is responsible for direct care of a patient and for coordinating and controlling access to or initiating and or supervising other health care services the patient needs. Since these codes are new at the time of this writing, it is uncertain how third parties will reimburse for them.

Codes 98920 and 98921 have replaced previous telephone consultation codes 99013 to 99015 (which have been deleted). Most third parties do not reimburse physicians for telephone consultations. Medicare regulations require that in order for a physician to charge a patient, he or she must be able to visualize a portion of the patient's body. This includes reading a radiograph, a scan, an EKG or some other test, but *does not* include providing test information to the patient over the phone.

[14] Handling Codes (99000, 99001 and 99002)

Currently these codes do not include obtaining specimens; rather, they apply to the handling and/or conveyance of a specimen from the physician's office to an outside laboratory. Except for blood drawing, there is no permitted code for specimen collection.

Venipuncture code 36415 should be used to code for a blood draw. Although Medicare and Medicaid programs usually do not reimburse for both the handling and drawing of blood, other third parties may. Medicare and Medicaid generally do not reimburse for blood-drawing charges when the test is performed in the office.

[15] Postoperative Follow-Up Visits

Code 99024, for postoperative follow-up visits, is an unusual code in that it is a no-charge code: It is not used when a service is provided but, rather, when that service is part of a global surgical package. In other words, the fee for that service already has been included in the surgery charges. As a practical matter, the code should be used to indicate that the service was in fact performed.

[16] After-Hours and Holiday Charges

If a physician sees a patient after normal office hours, late at night or on a Sunday or holiday, he or she may wish to make an additional charge for the inconvenience. In this case, code numbers 99050 to 99054 are used. Many carriers will not reimburse for these codes, and in some cases alternative methods of reporting may be used, such as modifier 22, for unusual services.

It should be noted that code 99050 is not appropriate when a physician behind schedule is seeing a patient at 6:00 p.m. and the physician's office normally closes at 5:00 p.m.

[17] Other Location

A physician may elect to perform services normally performed in the office at a location more convenient to the patient. In this circumstance, code number 99056, services provided at the request of the patient at a location other than the physician's office, is used. Although third parties may not reimburse for this, a physician providing this type of service generally does so because the patient is willing and able to pay for this additional service.

[18] Supplies

A general supply code, 99070, is available to indicate supplies. In the CPT text, this code is used for many different types of supplies; as such, it is appropriate to use 99070 more than once when describing specific supplies in the description section of the claim form.

HCPCs has expanded enormously on the supply code; thus it should be used for Medicare and Medicaid charges as well as for billing other carriers. Physicians who have not previously used supply codes and have included supplies in the salient fee code should be cautious when adopting a specific supply code, since Medicare may consider an additional charge for supplies as an illegal charge if the service was previously included with a fee and the prior fee was not correspondingly decreased.

Educational supplies (99071) includes specific materials such as books, videotapes or audiocassettes that were purchased by the physician and provided to the patient. Typically these items are not reimbursable. If special circumstances indicate the need for the supplies, a special report may be filed with the third party to explain the need. As a practical matter, many physicians view these materials as a promotional expense and do not charge the patient for them.

[19] Prolonged Services

Codes for prolonged services (99150 to 99155) should be used when the physician attends the patient (e.g., for operative stand-by monitoring ECG, EEG, etc.) for 30 minutes or more.

In addition, medical conference codes 99155 and 99156 are available when a physician spends 25 minutes or more with the patient and/or patient's family and guardian to discuss patient management issues. If carriers do not reimburse for codes 99155 and 99156, then appropriate intermediate visit codes should be used.[4]

---

[4] See § 17.04[1] supra.

[20] Critical Care

Unlike most other cognitive service codes in the CPT text, critical care codes are time-based. Initial critical care (99160, 99162) is used to describe the care of critically ill patients whose condition requires the constant attention of the physician (e.g., cardiac arrest, bleeding, respiratory failure, shock, postoperative complications, etc.). Critical care can be given in any location but is usually given in the emergency room or an intensive care unit (CCU, ICU, NICU). As it is a global service, it is intended to include a variety of services performed during this period (e.g., catheter placement, thoracostomy, intubation, ventilation management, blood gas monitoring, etc.). Other procedures not typically done in a critical care situation are included and can be billed separately, e.g., fracture care, laceration repair, peritoneal lavage, lumbar puncture, etc. The initial code is billed for the first hour of care. The second code is used for each additional 30 minutes. A two-hour critical care period would thus be billed using 99160 (1 unit) and 99162 (2 units).

Not all payers respond to the global nature of these codes the same way. Therefore, prior to billing critical care services, the payer should be asked which services it considers part of the critical care services and which can be billed separately, if any. If several extensive procedures were performed, greater reimbursement may be received by billing the procedures and a hospital admission or visit code rather than the global code. To make the decision regarding the best reimbursement, the physician should note the time excluding the procedures, and the total time required. In general, the longer the time it takes to stabilize the patient, the more appropriate the critical care code usage may be.

Codes 99171 to 99172 are used for subsequent visits to ICU-CCU patients. The same definitions of *brief, limited* and *extended* apply in these instances as they do to hospital visits.

§ 17.05 CPT: Surgery

The CPT "Surgery" section is coded for both individual surgical procedures and procedures performed as part of a surgical package. There are different codes for simple, intermediate and complex surgical repair. Different codes for injections, orthopedic surgery,

skin grafts and lesion incision vary with the extent of services rendered during these procedures.

The surgery section of the CPT text is difficult to use, since surgery coding requires an understanding of both the business aspects of coding and of the procedures actually being performed. As such, physicians should not depend exclusively on staff to code surgical procedures until the person(s) coding demonstrate extensive understanding of the surgeon's work. In addition, if the surgeon performs unusual services, he or she should take the time to review coding procedures with the coding person.

[1] Surgical Packages

Surgery charges include what is known as the surgical package. This includes:

- the operation itself;
- any local anesthetics, topical anesthetics or digital blocks used; and
- normal, uncomplicated postoperative follow-up care.

It is improper for a physician to itemize and charge separately for these items, and third parties will deny payment if they are itemized.

The CPT book does not indicate whether the surgical package includes or excludes preoperative procedures, and physicians vary with regard to how they bill for these procedures. Some physicians include them in their surgical packages, while others bill for them separately. As a result, some third parties will not reimburse for preoperative procedures performed a certain number of days prior to surgery, if the charge is listed with the same diagnosis or a related diagnosis.

Whether or not a physician will be paid for preoperative service also is determined by his or her historical practice of charging. If, historically, the physician has included preoperative procedures in the surgical package and he or she then changes to charging a separate fee for preoperative care and there is not a corresponding reduction in the surgical care fee, it will be considered an inappropriate price increase. As a result, the physician could face problems with Medicare and be in violation of the maximum allowable actual charge limitation (MAAC).

It is important to note that the surgical package includes normal and uncomplicated follow-up. Unusual or complicated follow-up may be billed for separately, using an appropriate diagnostic code to account for the additional charge.

Normal follow-up typically is includes procedures performed a number of days following surgery. The normal follow-up may vary from procedure to procedure. The Relative Value Index gives some guidelines as to how many postoperative days are to be included in the surgery package, and it is important that the physician know the length of normal follow-up periods so as to know when to begin billing for additional office calls.

[2] Separate Procedures

Surgeons should be aware that when a procedure has the words "separate procedure" listed next to it, that procedure should only be billed when performed as a separate procedure. For example, if a laparotomy, code 49000, was performed and a cancerous tumor was discovered and removed, the physician would bill for the incision and removal of the tumor but not for the exploratory laparotomy. On the other hand, if no cancer or other problems are discovered, the laparotomy would be considered a separate procedure and would be billed for.

[3] Nonpackage Surgical Procedures

Certain minor procedures do not require follow-up; as such, the surgery fee is not assumed to include the follow-up care. These procedures are indicated in the surgery section of the CPT text by an asterisk or star (*). When a procedure is shown in the surgery section with an asterisk, the pre- or postoperative procedures should be charged for separately. The surgery guidelines section of the CPT text outlines the following rules:

(1) The charge listed with any procedure that is starred should include only the surgery. It should not include any pre- or postoperative procedures.

(2) When a starred procedure is carried out at the time of an *initial* visit for a new patient and the procedure constitutes major service at the visit, code number 99025 should be listed in lieu of the usual initial visit to cover the administrative costs.

(3) When the starred procedure is carried out at the time of an initial or other visit involving significantly identifiable services, the appropriate visit is listed in addition to the starred procedure as follow-up care. If the starred procedure is carried out for an established patient as a follow-up visit, the procedure constitutes the major service and the service visit is not added.

(4) When a starred procedure requires hospitalization, an appropriate hospital visit charge should be utilized.

(5) All postoperative care should be added on according to the services provided.

(6) Any complication should be added on as provided.

[4] Incision of Lesions

Surgeons should note that the incision of lesions (11200 to 11646) may require additional reporting if maximum reimbursement is to be obtained. The salient codes include simple closure. If the procedure requires an intermediate or a complex closure, the closure can be listed in addition to the lesion incision code. On the other hand, if it is a simple, normal closure, an additional procedure and charge should not be listed.

[5] Repairs

Repair codes in the CPT text range from 12001 to 13300 and are broken down based on whether they are simple, intermediate or complex.

Simple Repair. This code is used when the wound is superficial and involves the suturing of superficial tissues. When adhesive tapes are used to close the wound, the repair code should not be listed. An appropriate service visit should be listed, however.

Intermediate Repair. This code includes the repair of wounds that require layer closure in addition to repair of superficial tissue. Such wounds usually involve deeper layers, including fascia or muscle, to the extent that at least one of the layers requires separate closure.

Complex Repair. This code is used for wounds requiring reconstructive surgery, complicated wound closures, skin grafts or unusual and time-consuming techniques to obtain maximum functional and cosmetic results.

A review of the codes 12001 to 13300 reveals that in addition to being broken down by the designations *simple, intermediate* and *complex,* repairs are broken down based on the location and size of the wound. Multiple wounds in the same category should be totaled to determine the code to be used. For example, simple repair of a wound on the cheek and nose is added together and listed as one charge rather than being listed as separate procedures, since these areas are included in the 12011-to-12018 group.

Unless gross contamination is present requiring prolonged cleansing, or appreciable amounts of devitalized or contaminated tissue are removed, or there is no primary closure, debridement is considered to be part of the wound repair codes. When extensive debridement is done, see codes 11040-11044. These codes specify the extent of debridement by noting the layers involved, e.g., partial skin, skin and subcutaneous, etc.

[6] Grafts and Flaps

Codes 15000 to 15776 cover skin grafts and flaps. Physicians should be alert to the fact that appropriate wound repairs or other related procedures can be listed in addition to a graft. There are notes in the CPT text that state, "Repair of donor site requiring skin graft or local flaps is to be added as an additional procedure."

Code 15000, excisional preparation or creation of recipient site by excision of essentially intact skin, should be used in addition to the graft charge when applicable. Grafts performed following major procedures, such as the removal of deep tumors, are not included in the charge made for the major procedure and should be listed and charged for separately.

[7] Orthopedic Services

Physicians performing orthopedic surgery should be aware of the following points:

- When a procedure being performed involves the application of casts and traction devices, the fee for the major procedure includes the first application of casts and traction. If a cast or strapping is reapplied either during or immediately after the normal period of follow-up, an additional charge for the casting or strapping procedure may be made.

- The charge for removing the cast is always included in the fee for applying the cast. A separate charge is submitted only when the cast is removed by a physician other than the one who originally applied it.
- An additional visit charge should not be used when billing for reapplication of a cast or strapping unless significant additional services beyond the cast or strapping were performed and documented.
- The fracture repair and cast application codes do not include casting supplies. These supplies can be billed using HCPC codes that specify either plaster or hexalite supplies.

[8] Vascular Injection Procedures

Physicians should use venipuncture code 36415 for the collection of blood when the specimen is sent to outside laboratories. They also should be aware that code 36410 should be used instead of 36415 when the physician's skill is needed for diagnostic or therapeutic purposes. Code 36410 should not be used for routine venipuncture.

Physicians giving vascular injections should note (depending upon the type of procedure being performed) that the fee should include local anesthetic, introduction of needle or catheter, injection of contrast media and pre- or postprocedure care related to the injection itself. The physician's charge should *not* include the charge for contrast media. The charge for these items provided by the physicians should be listed using supply code 99070 or the specific HCPC code.

[9] Maternity Care and Delivery

The delivery of most maternity care can be handled easily by the use of code number 59400, routine obstetric care. This code includes all the antepartum care, the normal vaginal delivery and postpartum care.

§ 17.06   MANAGING YOUR MEDICAL PRACTICE   17-28

Care for conditions not related to the pregnancy should be billed separately, using the appropriate procedure codes.

As the global obstetric code covers routine prenatal care with an uncomplicated labor and vaginal delivery, pregnancies in which complications arise may require additional resources. Amniocentesis, laboratory tests (other than the routine urinalysis) and ultrasounds, as well as other diagnostic or surgical procedures, should be billed separately. If the patient is hospitalized prior to delivery, hospital visits and procedures should also be billed.

For a pregnancy in which the high-risk condition of the patient results in a higher density or frequency of prenatal visits or a more difficult delivery, the global obstetric codes can be submitted with a −22 modifier. An explanation of the nature of the additional services should accompany the claim.

If more than one physician is involved in the obstetrical care process, separate codes for each portion of the process can be used (59420 — antepartum care only; 59410 — vaginal delivery and postpartum care only; 59515 — cesarean delivery only including postpartum care; and 59430 — postpartum care only.) If a subtotal or total hysterectomy is done following a cesarean delivery, the code 59525 should be submitted in addition to the c-section global or delivery only code (59510 or 59515). If a surgical assist is performed by the second physician, the c-section delivery only code can be used with the −80 or −81 modifier.

If a single physician provides a c-section delivery as well as the antepartum and postpartum care, the global c-section code (59410) can be used.

Code 58611 (ligation or transection of fallopian tubes, when done at the time of a c-section) or 58605 (ligation or transection of fallopian tubes during the same hospitalization) is also billed in addition to the global obstetric codes when appropriate.

§ 17.06 Radiology

CPT codes for diagnostic radiological procedures can present problems. If more than one physician participates in the procedure, or if the hospital supplies the technical radiological equipment or another physician is consulted to interpret the radiograph, separate

coding by each party may be necessary. **The physician must make sure that codes reflect the specific radiological modality employed.**

The radiology section of the CPT text is broken into four subsections: diagnostic radiology, diagnostic ultrasound, therapeutic radiology and nuclear medicine. The diagnostic radiology subsection, which is the most widely used portion of this part of the text, lists commonly performed radiology services, including x-rays and CAT scans. Each of the subsections is grouped by the following anatomic areas:

- Head and Neck
- Chest
- Spine and Pelvis
- Upper Extremities
- Lower Extremities
- Abdomen
- Gastrointestinal Tract
- Urinary Tract
- Gynecological and Obstetrical
- Vascular System
- Miscellaneous

[1] Complete Procedures

When contrast injections are given in conjunction with radiographs, a comprehensive code, 70011, is used. When the procedure is performed by two physicians, one giving the injection and the other supervising and interpreting, two codes are used: code

(Text continued on page 17–29)

70010 is used by the interpreting physician, and code 61055 or 62284 is used by the injecting physician.

In some circumstances radiologists obtain more reimbursement by separately coding, even though the procedure was performed by one radiologist. It is not recommended that physicians split their billing in order to achieve higher coding, since code 70011 clearly is to be used in those situations.

[2] Professional and Technical Component

Unlike regular cognitive services, which include the physician's equipment and staff, radiology services are thought of as having professional (i.e., the physician fee) and technical (i.e., the equipment, supplies and technical staff) components. When a radiology service is performed, the code is considered a global charge; that is, it includes both the professional and technical components. In the situation where a physician provides a service, such as a radiograph taken by the hospital that is interpreted by the radiologist, professional component modifier –26 should be used. Code modifier –26 indicates that the charge is for the physician's fee only and not the technical component of the procedure. In this particular case, the hospital bills for the technical component of the procedure.

Nonradiologists frequently are faced with practical problems regarding interpretation of radiographs. Since most states and hospitals require that a radiologist read all the radiographs, and since third parties generally pay only for the radiologist's interpretation of the radiograph if more than one physician interprets it, other physicians may be left unreimbursed when they need to interpret the radiograph as a result of an emergency or the need for another specialist's opinion. Since nonradiologists will probably not be paid for interpreting the radiograph in these circumstances, they should be careful to use the highest level of service applicable to the services performed. The interpretation of the radiograph may necessitate recording a higher code level.

[3] Miscellaneous

The miscellaneous heading at the end of the diagnostic radiology codes should not be overlooked, as it contains descriptions for fluoroscopy, bone age studies, joint surveys, CAT scans, cineradiography, consultations on x-rays made elsewhere, and magnetic resonance imaging (MRI). Failure to be aware of these codes or to use them may result in lost reimbursement.

§ 17.07 Pathology and Laboratory

> The CPT text codes for laboratory tests performed by the physician or referred to an outside laboratory. The physician should be aware that a third party may refuse full reimbursement for laboratory tests performed in the office if it is of the opinion that they could have been performed more cheaply through a reference lab that performs automated multichannel tests.

The pathology and laboratory section of the CPT text is organized in the following sections:

- Guidelines
- Automated, Multichannel Tests and Notes
- Therapeutic Drug Monitoring
- Organ or Disease Orientated Panels
- Consultations (Clinical Pathology)
- Urinalysis Procedures
- Chemistry and Toxicology Procedures and Notes
- Hematology Procedures
- Immunology Procedures
- Microbiology Procedures
- Anatomic Pathology Procedures
- Surgical Pathology Procedures and Notes
- Miscellaneous Pathology and Laboratory Procedures

When billing for lab services, a physician should use a −90 modifier if the laboratory services are performed by a reference (outside) laboratory. When a Medicare patient's specimen is sent to a reference laboratory, the ordering physician may not bill for those services; the reference lab must bill directly to Medicare for these services, accept assignment and accept Medicare reimbursement as payment in full. Effective January 1, 1987, all physicians must accept assignment on Medicare patients for laboratory services. Even a physician not participating with Medicare must accept assignment on laboratory charges. In many cases, nonparticipating physicians may prefer to send more tests to a reference lab, since they must accept assignment on those Medicare patients.

When a claim being filed for patients contains both lab and nonlab services and the physician is not willing to accept assignment, he or she should write "I accept assignment for clinical laboratory tests only" near the area in which he or she writes his or her name. Another way to handle this billing problem is to submit two separate claim forms, one for the assigned laboratory charges and another for the unassigned nonlaboratory charges.

Since the profit margin is low for laboratory procedures, physicians might consider using a reference lab as much as possible for Medicare patients or other parties who have poor reimbursement records. Frequently physicians are lured into a false sense of profit, thinking that they are generating "large charges" for laboratory procedures. As a practical matter, the primary physician's main reason for doing laboratory tests in-house should be service to the patient.

[1] Multichannel and Group Tests

Automated multichannel tests are listed in the first section of the pathology and laboratory section of the CPT text. These tests generally are performed by reference laboratories, although a large medical practice may employ the use of automated equipment.

When a physician performs a series of tests individually and each is reported separately, the use of the CPT codes listed in the chemistry and toxicology subsection may create reimbursement problems. Generally, the insurance carrier will believe that the tests could have been performed at a substantially lower expense by having an outside lab utilizing multichannel equipment perform the tests. They may therefore deny the individual lab charges or recode the individual chemistry tests under one multichannel code and reimburse at the same rate they would have paid an outside lab to perform the multichannel test.

[2] Individual Chemistry and Toxicology Test

Codes 82000 to 84999, used to report individual chemistry or toxicology tests, are listed in the CPT text alphabetically by the type of substance being analyzed. If a test being performed is not listed under the name of the substance, the physician should try to find a code for the method used to test the substance.

When trying to locate tests from chemistry and toxicology groups, the following guidelines should be followed:

(1) Look under the name of the substance.

(2) If the code is not listed alphabetically, check codes 84681 through 84810.

(3) Review the miscellaneous codes at the end of the laboratory and pathology section — codes 89051 through 89399.

(4) Look under the name of the technique used to analyze the substance.

(5) Unlisted procedures should be coded as 84999, and an explanation should be submitted with the claim.

[3] Surgical Pathology and Consultations

A pathologist may charge for a clinical pathology consultation in response to a request from an attending physician concerned with a test result requiring additional, interpretive medical judgment. Such consultation should include a written report, since reporting on a test result without medical interpretive judgment is not considered a clinical pathology consultation.

Codes 80500 and 80502 are used to bill for these services. Code 80500 is used for limited clinical pathology consultation without review of the patient's history and medical records. Code 80502 is the code for comprehensive clinical pathology consultation for a complex diagnostic problem, with a review of the patient's history and medical records.

Surgical pathology codes can be found in the range 88300 to 88399. Procedures outlined in this area of the text must include accession, handling and reporting. If these three services are not performed, code modifier –52 should be used to indicate a reduced level of service.

§ 17.08 Modifiers for CPT Codes

Appendix A of the CPT text lists the two-digit numbers of CPT modifiers and describes their application. Modifiers can be used to broaden the scope of a given CPT code or stretch existing codes to cover procedures or situations that fall outside the boundaries of commonly coded procedures. Use of a modifier may necessitate an accompanying letter of explanation for the third party.

Appendix A of the CPT text is a complete list of all the modifiers to the CPT codes in the preceding five sections. Modifiers are attached to the basic CPT code to indicate deviation from the standard description. In addition, modifiers applicable to a particular section of the CPT codes are listed in the guidelines area of each of the separate sections of the text.

Common modifiers are two digits long and are added on to the main CPT code. Alternative modifier numbers, originally developed to help third-party payers whose computers could not handle the add-on of additional two-digit codes, are not in common use today unless otherwise instructed by the third party.

Modifier Number: –20
(Alternative Modifier Number: –09920)
Microsurgery

When surgical services are performed using microsurgery techniques (i.e., requiring the use of an operating microscope), modifier number –20 may be added to the surgical procedure code. Alternatively, the separate five-digit modifier code 09920 may be used. This modifier should not be used when a magnifying surgical loupe is used. A special report may be necessary to document the necessity of the microsurgical approach.

Modifier Number: –22
(Alternative Modifier Number: –09922)
Unusual Services

The unusual service code should be used when the service(s) provided are greater than that usually required for the listed procedure. Generally, use of modifier –22 results in a higher fee. A special report should be submitted to explain the additional charge and why the unusual service code modifier is used.

Modifier Number: –23
(Alternative Modifier Number: –09923)
Unusual Anesthesia

This modifier is used in a circumstance in which a procedure generally performed under local anesthesia or with no anesthesia is seen to require general anesthesia. In order to procure reimbursement, it probably will be necessary to provide a special report indicating the reason for the general anesthesia.

Modifier Number: –26
(Alternative Modifier Number: –09926)
Professional Component

Certain procedures, such as radiological examination, are evaluated in terms of a technical component and a professional component. Generally, the codes in these cases represent the global fee, i.e., both the technical component and the professional component. In these circumstances, it is appropriate to use modifier –26 to indicate that only the professional component is included.

A specific example is a physician who reads a radiograph at the hospital. The physician's fee for this service includes only the professional component, since the technical component is billed for by the hospital. In this situation, modifier –26 is used to identify the fact that only the professional fee is being charged. If the procedure described is only for the interpretation, the –26 modifier would not be appropriate. An example of this is code 70010, which indicates clearly that the procedure is for interpretation only.

Modifier Number: –32
(Alternative Modifier Number: –09932)
Mandated Services

This modifier should be used when a consultation or related service is mandated (PRO, Third-Party Payer).

Modifier Number: –47
(Alternative Modifier Number: –09947)
Anesthesia by Surgeon

This code does not include local anesthesia but should be used when general anesthesia services, which normally are handled by an anesthesiologist, are provided by a surgeon. Presuming a surgeon provides both the procedure and anesthesia, the code is listed twice, once for the procedure and secondarily with code modifier –47 and an explanation that this was for anesthesia.

Modifier Number: –51
(Alternative Modifier Number: –09951)
Multiple Procedures

When a surgeon performs more than one procedure on the same patient in the same surgical session, the secondary or additional procedures should be billed by adding the modifier –51 to the procedure code. The major procedure should be listed without a modifier. However, prior to using the modifier, the physician needs to determine whether a different CPT code exists describing the combination of services performed; whether the additional procedures performed—but not included in the description of the primary surgery code—have separate procedure (SP) codes already established; or whether the additional services performed are incidental to the primary surgery and thus not separately billable. A closer examination of the section of the CPT book containing the primary surgical codes will assist in this decision.

In general, third party payers reduce the reimbursement level for the second and third procedures, citing that the intraoperative as well as the pre- and postoperative work of multiple procedures is reduced. As localities differ as to whether the physicians are required to submit prediscounted or full fees for additional procedures, the physician's office should explore the requirement of the specific third party payer involved and record the answer for future submissions. Starting in 1991, Medicare requires that nonparticipating physicians submit discounted Limiting Charges (50 percent) for additional procedures.

Modifier Number: –52
(Alternative Modifier Number: –09952)
Reduced Services

The reduced services modifier is used when the procedure performed was not completed as described in the CPT description of the code; instead, a portion of the service was reduced or eliminated at the physician's election. Again, prior to using the –52 reduced services modifier, the appropriate section of the CPT code book should be examined to determine whether another CPT code has been developed to address the procedure as it was done. As with the unusual services modifier, procedures done using the reduced services modifier should be submitted with the operating report, with the appropriate section highlighted.

Modifier Number: –54
(Alternative Modifier Number: –09954)
Surgical Care Only

When one physician performs a surgical procedure and another physician provides the preoperative and/or postoperative management, the surgical code performed by the first physician should be modified using the –54 modifier to indicate that only surgical services were being billed. It is not appropriate to use this modifier when both physicians are in a single practice.

Modifier Number: –55
(Alternative Modifier Number: –09955)
Postoperative Management Only

When a physician performs only postoperative management and another physician performs the surgical procedure, the postoperative component should be identified by adding the modifier –55.

Modifier Number: –56
(Alternative Modifier Number: –09956)
Preoperative Management Only

When a physician performs only the preoperative care and evaluation, and another physician performs the surgical procedure and postoperative care, the procedure code should be modified with a –56.

Modifier Number: –62
(Alternative Modifier Number: –09962)
Two Surgeons

When circumstances require the skills of two surgeons, the separate services should be identified by adding the modifier –62 to the procedure number used by each surgeon for reporting his or her service. To facilitate reimbursement, it is a good idea to provide information explaining the need for two surgeons.

Modifier Number: –66
(Alternative Modifier Number: –09966)
Surgical Team

Modifier –66 is used in the situation in which a highly complex surgical procedure requires several physicians, often of different specialties, plus other highly skilled, specially trained personnel and various types of complex equipment. An example of this is the implantation of an artificial heart. Under these circumstances, each physician should use the modifier –66 in addition to the basic procedure he or she is reporting.

Modifier Number: –75
(Alternative Modifier Number: –09975)
Concurrent Care

When a patient's condition requires the services of more than one physician, each physician should identify the services provided by adding the modifier –75 to the basic service or services he or she has performed. As a practical matter, in order to get reimbursed for concurrent care, the physician should include a special report explaining the need for more than one physician. In general, third parties feel that concurrent care is not necessary, i.e., the treatment could have been provided satisfactorily by one physician. Reimbursement for concurrent care will require that separate diagnosis and treatments are involved. An example is a complicated situation in which an infectious diseases physician is independently caring for a patient being treated by a cardiovascular surgeon.

Modifier Number: –76
(Alternative Modifier Number: –09976)
Repeat Procedure by the Same Physician

This code should be used to alert the third party to the fact that a procedure was, in fact, performed twice and that the physician's office is not erroneously rebilling for the same procedure. Since the third party will probably question the need for the repeat procedure, it is a good idea to provide a special report outlining the circumstances requiring the repeat procedure.

Modifier Number: –77
(Alternative Modifier Number: –09977)
Repeat Procedure by Another Physician

This code is used under the same circumstances as the –76 modifier when the repeat procedure is performed by another physician. As is the case with the use of modifier –76, in order to facilitate reimbursement when this code is used, an explanation of why the procedure needed to be repeated should be indicated in a special report.

Modifier Number: –80
(Alternative Modifier Number: –09980)
Assistant Surgeon

The –80 modifier is used to bill surgical assists. As of 1991, in addition to denying payment for cases in which a surgical assist was used less than 5 percent of the time, Medicare also requires that surgical assist limiting charges be capped at 16 percent of the global surgical service.

Modifier Number: –81
(Alternative Modifier Number: –09981)
Minimum Assistant Surgeon

This code would be used when a second assistant surgeon is involved in the surgery procedure.

Modifier Number: –82
(Alternative Modifier Number: –09982)
Assistant Surgeon (when qualified resident surgeon is not available)

See modifier –80, Assistant Surgeon.

Modifier Number: –90
(Alternative Modifier Number: –09990)
Reference (Outside) Laboratory

When a physician bills a patient for laboratory work that is performed by a reference lab, the modifier –90 should be used to indicate that the lab work was done outside the physician's office. Physicians should never bill Medicare or Medicaid patients for lab work done outside their office; the reference lab should bill Medicare directly for these services.

Modifier Number: –99
(Alternative Modifier Number: –09999)
Multiple Modifiers

Modifier –99 should be used if two or more different modifiers are added to the same procedure. This will alert the carrier to the fact that two or more modifiers are associated with the same procedure.

The modifier situation might look as follows:

- 33400–55 (postoperative care, provided separately)
- 33400–99 (indicating multiple modifiers)
- 33400–82 (for assistant surgeon, when qualified resident is not available)

§ 17.09 Other CPT Appendixes and Index

Additional appendixes to the CPT text inform the physician of which codes have been deleted or changed since the last edition and permit updating of computer data bases for CPT. The index provides multiple means for locating a specific code within the text.

Appendix B of the CPT text lists all the changes that have been made in the text since the previous year's volume. An explanation is given next to each code, indicating whether the code is new or changed or has been deleted. Codes that have been deleted from the CPT text will have a reference to the code that should be used in their place.

Appendix C of the CPT text can be used by users of the short procedure computer version of the CPT text to update their data without the need to purchase a new tape or diskette.

The CPT index is designed to facilitate the quick location of codes needed to complete the physician's billing. A review of the instructions for use of the index reveals that codes may be listed in one or more different ways:

- by the procedure or service;
- by the name of the organ or organ system;
- by the name of the condition being treated or diagnosed;
- by a synonym of the term being used;
- by an eponym; and
- by an abbreviation.

§ 17.10 HCPC Coding

HCPCs were designed to be more specific than CPT codes and to code for procedures not covered in the CPT text. Unlike CPT codes, HCPCs are organized alphanumerically. Like CPT codes, HCPCs have modifiers that permit greater flexibility in coding. In instances in which CPT and HCPCs codes are in conflict, third parties generally prefer HCPCs.

The Health Care Financing Administrations Common Procedure Coding System (HCPCs) was introduced by the Health Care Financing Administration in 1984. HCPCs were designed to be more specific than some of the CPT codes and to provide codes for items that were not CPT coded. The impact of HCPCs is greatest in the area of supply codes (CPT catchall supply code 99070 is no longer acceptable to Medicare and Medicaid) and injectable codes.

The different categories of procedures covered by HCPCs includes:

(1) general services, including miscellaneous medical procedures, cardiology, miscellaneous surgical procedures, lab and pathology, radiology, stand-by services and acupuncture;

(2) injections, drugs and solutions, including blood components, blood products, oral drugs and chemotherapy injections;

(3) miscellaneous providers and services, including nursing services, occupational therapy, speech therapy, physical therapy and osteopathic manipulative therapy; services by a social worker, an analyst, a counselor or an independently licensed psychologist; day treatment programs; and podiatry surgical procedures;

(4) chiropractic services;

(5) dental procedures;

(6) transportation services, including ambulance;

(7) dialysis supplies, equipment and procedures;

(8) durable medical equipment, including such items as chains, crutches, bathing equipment, hospital beds and oxygen-related respiratory equipment;

(9) orthotics;

(10) prosthetics;

(11) parenteral and enteral therapy, formulas and supplies;

(12) supply lists;

(13) hearing services and supplies; and

(14) ophthalmological services.

[1] Alphanumerical Coding

Unlike CPT codes, which are numerical, HCPC codes are alphanumerical. For example, the following references are used to code medical services:

- Injectable: J0220–J1999
- Medical and Surgical Supply: A4200–A4927
- Enteral and Parenteral Therapy: B4034–B9999
- Durable Medical Equipment: E0100–E1699
- Vision and Hearing Services: V2020–V5299
- Medical Service: M0005–M9999

- Surgery: T1000–T6999
- Rehabilitation Services: H5000–H5300
- Pathology and Laboratory: P0999–P9615
- Diagnostic Radiology Services: R0009–R0599
- Orthotic Procedures: L0100–L4210
- Prosthetic Procedures: L5000–L9999
- Ambulance and Transportation: A0010–A0999

[2] HCPC Modifiers

Like the CPT text, the HCPC text has modifiers that permit greater code specification. Where the CPT code modifiers are numerical, HCPC modifiers are alphabetical. Although there are approximately 50 modifiers (changes are made each year and, as with CPT, a new HCPC text must be obtained from a local carrier annually), some modifiers are more commonly used by physicians.

AP

Determination of a Refractive State Was Not Performed in the Course of a Diagnostic Ophthalmological Examination

It is assumed that the determination of the refractive state is included with CPT codes 92002 to 92014. If the fee does not include determination of the refractive state, it is important to use the HCPC modifier AP to alert the carrier. Certain local carriers may require other modifiers, such as X (indicating that the refraction has been performed) or Y (indicating that the refraction was not performed).

CC

Procedural Code Change

This modifier is not available for physician use. It is instead meant for the third party payer to use in indicating to the physician that the third party payer has changed the CPT or HCPC code originally submitted by the physician's office. As the change may have been a result of an erroneous assumption on the part of the payer, the individual in your office responsible for reviewing the third party payment reimbursement records should note these changes and determine whether the change was indeed warranted. For example, the third party payer may determine that the hospital visit code reflected a higher level of service than would have been expected. They could indeed have reduced the level of care of the visit code as well as the associated payment and notified the physician simply by using the CC code. As that assumption was made based on an expected pattern of code usage rather than based on the circumstances of your patient's stay, an appeal may be in order. A pattern of changed codes for inappropriate code usage that has not been responded to by the physician's practice is likely to result in a third party audit. Third party audits are to be avoided whenever possible.

MP

Multiple Patients Seen

This code is used in conjunction with CPT procedural codes 90300 to 90470 to alert the third party that multiple patients were seen during the nursing home visit. This presumably would lower the relative value of the procedure and result in a lower reimbursement. Nevertheless, not using this modifier may result in a claim being rejected.

SP

Single Patient

While the MP modifier should be used when multiple patients are seen, the SP modifier should be used in connection with the nursing home codes 90300 to 90470 to indicate that only a single patient was seen. Presumably this maintains a higher relative value than the MP modifier. Again, failure to use these modifiers may result in rejection of a claim, since the third party will not be able to conclude whether it is a multiple-patient visit or a single-patient visit.

TC

Technical Component

The TC modifier should be used when the physician bills only for the technical component of a diagnostic procedure. For example, the primary care physician uses his or her office equipment to take x-rays and has an outside radiologist read the results. The primary care physician bills the process of taking the x-rays or ultrasounds using the TC modifier; the radiologist bills the process of reading the films using the –26 modifier. In the absence of a modifier, the code is presumed to represent global services.

XB

Medical Unnecessary Advance Notice Obtained (Medicare Only)

Medicare has developed a listing of procedures it considers to be medically unnecessary or medically unnecessary under specific circumstances, e.g., vitamin B^{12} injections are only considered to be medically necessary for pernicious anemia. These services are therefore considered to be outside the contracting arrangement with Medicare. Medicare's regulations state that if the patient has been informed prior to the service being performed that Medicare is likely to deny payment for these services, and the patient has signed a notice stating he or she is willing to pay for the services outside the Medicare contract, the services can be submitted to the patient for payment. The XB is used when submitting the claim to Medicare. When the XB is used, the Medicare intermediary will not generate the mandatory paperwork informing physicians they have performed a medically unnecessary procedure and requiring them to respond, but will instead let that portion of the claim go directly to the patient for payment.

§ 17.11 Levels of Service

The level of service involved in performing various cognitive procedures can affect physician reimbursement. Level of service is coded on the basis of whether the patient is new or established and whether the service involved was minimal, brief, limited, extended, comprehensive or complex.

Levels of service pertain to various cognitive procedures, such as office visits, hospital visits, nursing home visits and consultations. It is extremely important that physicians understand them, as they are defined for coding purposes. Levels of service have very specific definitions and criteria that must be met in order to bill for them.

[1] New Versus Established Patients

A number of procedures are distinguished only by whether the physician is seeing a new or an established patient. As such, the definitions of new and established patients are helpful.

Although each carrier may have an individual derived definition, in general, a new patient is one who has not been seen in the practice during the last three years. An established patient is one whose recent medical history is known to the practice and who has established medical and billing records within the practice. All carriers pay more for new-patient cognitive services than they do for established-patient services, since new patients require creating medical and billing records as well as a slightly more thorough examination.

A review of procedures 90000 to 90580 illustrates a number of cognitive procedures that distinguish between a new patient and an established patient.

(Text continued on page 17-45)

[2] Defining Services

The introduction section of the CPT text discusses the different levels of service and should be studied by all physicians and billers. Unfortunately, many physicians do not take the time to learn, memorize and use the various levels of services for procedures they are performing and instead fall into the habit of picking their favorite code and using it consistently. Physicians who make an effort to use codes properly should make it a point to re-evaluate their code utilization every few months to make certain that they do not fall back into old patterns. Improper use of the level of service codes is one of the biggest areas of exposure when physicians are receiving an audit. Thus, physicians should make certain that medical records support the CPT or other code being used to bill the third party.

[a] Minimal Service

Code 90030 is used to describe a minimal service, which refers to a service supervised by the physician but not requiring his or her presence. This code should not be used when billing for a physician service. An example of a service for which this code is appropriate is a patient receiving an injection from a nurse.

[b] Brief Services

Brief service (code 90040) should be used only for established patients. It refers to a physician-rendered service, requiring only an abbreviated history and examination (e.g., otitis media pediatric follow-up visit; examination of acute tonsillitis).

[c] Limited Services

Code 90010 is used to describe limited services for new patients, while code 90050 is used to describe limited services for an established patient. Limited services are services rendered by the physician, including an evaluation of a circumscribed acute illness or re-evaluation of a problem on a periodic basis. It should include an interval history and examination, review of past medical management, ordering of diagnostic testing, adjustment of therapeutic management and discussion of findings and/or medical management. An example is the diagnosis and treatment of acute respiratory infection.

[d] Intermediate Services

CPT code 90015 is used for new patients receiving intermediate services, while CPT code 90060 is used for established patients receiving intermediate services. Intermediate services include evaluation of a new condition or an existing condition complicated with a new diagnostic or management problem (not necessarily related to the primary diagnosis) that necessitates obtaining and evaluating pertinent history and physical or mental status findings; diagnostic testing procedures; and ordering therapeutic management or formal patient, family or hospital staff conferences regarding the patient medical management and progress. This code can be used for any situation in which two or more body systems or diagnostic or management problems exist (co-morbidity). Examples of intermediate services might include the evaluation of a patient with a specific disease (e.g., arteriosclerotic heart disease) diagnosed previously but complicated by recent onset of new symptomotology (e.g., unstable angina). This service involves a detailed interval history, physical examination, ordering of diagnostic tests and discussion of new therapeutic management.

[e] Extended Services

CPT code 90017 is used for new patients receiving extended services, while CPT code 90070 is used for established patients receiving extended services. Extended services are defined as cognitive services that entail an unusual amount of effort or judgment, with a detailed history; review of medical records; examination and formal conference with patient, family or staff or a comparable medical diagnostic or therapeutic service.

On the service continuum, an extended service falls between an intermediate and a full comprehensive service. An example is a review of results of diagnostic evaluation, followed by performance of a detailed examination and thorough discussion of physical findings, laboratory studies, x-ray examinations, diagnostic conclusions and recommendations for the treatment of complicated chronic pulmonary disease.

[f] Comprehensive Services

CPT code 90020 is used for new patients receiving comprehensive services, while CPT code 90080 is used for established patients receiving comprehensive services. Comprehensive services involve an in-depth evaluation of a patient with a new or an existing problem requiring the development or complete re-evaluation of medical data, including recording of chief complaints and present illness, family history, past medical history, personal history, systems review, complete physical examination and the ordering of appropriate medical diagnostic tests and procedures.

§ 17.12 Consultations

> Codes for physician consultation services differ based on whether the consultant simply rendered an opinion, assumed responsibility for the patient management afterward or participated in concurrent care of the patient. Consultations differ with regard to whether they are just visits, intermediate, extended, comprehensive, complex or for follow-up.

CPT codes 90600 to 90654 describe various levels of service in the consultation area. Consultative services carry a higher relative value than ordinary cognitive services; thus care should be taken to use these codes properly. Failure to use consultative codes when appropriate will result in underreimbursement, while abuse of consultative codes may result in accusations of fraud and an audit.

A consultation can be billed when one physician gives another physician or another appropriate source his or her opinion or advice regarding the further evaluation and/or management of a patient. The consultant must document that he or she has recommended a course of action to the attending physician and is initiating treatment at his or her request.

Consultant services can be delivered in the office, in the hospital or in the emergency room. After the initial consultation, if the consultant physician takes over active management of the patient's care, the services should then be billed using the appropriate medical or hospital service code. For example, when the physician is asked to see a hospitalized patient on another service regarding a problem in his or her area of specialty, the first visit is billed as a consultation and a subsequent visit could be billed either as a follow-up consultation or a standard hospital visit, depending on whether the consultant has taken over active management of the patient's care.

It is important to remember that the decision to use hospital or follow-up consultation codes will depend on whether the consulting physician assumes active management of a portion of the patient's care or continues simply to render consultative advice. If the physician assumes responsibility for a portion of the patient's care, he or she will then be rendering concurrent care, in which case the concurrent care modifier (–75) should then be added to the hospital visit. (If the physician takes over complete care of the patient, the concurrent care modifier is not required.) The diagnosis used for the consultation and for all follow-up visits should relate to the problem about which the physician was consulted rather than the initial reason for hospitalization.

Written documentation for all consultations must be provided in the patient's chart or sent to the referring physician. If a physician is audited by a third party, the auditor will ask to see the patient's medical records. After comparing the level of services against the information in the medical record, the auditor can request a refund if the appropriate information is not adequately documented. In addition, financial penalties may be implemented by Medicare.

In writing a consultation report, the physician should avoid using the word "refer." Some insurance carriers state that they routinely deny consultant charges when the word "refer" is used, as it indicates transfer of care rather than consultation. As an alternative, the opening statement could refer to "the opportunity to render an opinion on behalf of this patient." In addition to chart documentation, it is important to acknowledge the physician or organization who requested the consultation.

Consultation codes have been expanded to include the follow-up consultation and confirmatory or second- or third-opinion consultation. The confirmatory consultation codes have better reimbursement rates than the initial consultation codes and should be used accordingly. The basic definition of levels of services (i.e., limited, extended and comprehensive) are valid for all forms of consultation. When billing a Medicare patient for a second opinion consultation, the physician should check not only for the appropriate definition but also the MAAC rate for the code. As some offices have not billed a full range of codes, the existing MAAC fees are not always appropriate to the level of services delivered. When a lower level code reimburses at a more appropriate rate than the higher level of code, down-coding the service should be considered.

[1] Consultant Visits

A limited consultation (code 90600) is an examination or an evaluation of a single organ system. It includes documentation of the complete complaint, present illness, pertinent examination, review of medical data and establishment of a plan of management related to the specific problem. An example is a dermatological opinion about an uncomplicated skin lesion.

[2] Intermediate Consultation

Intermediate consultation (code 90605) refers to an examination or evaluation of an organ system, a partial review of the general history, recommendations and preparation of a report. An example of an intermediate consultation is the evaluation of the abdomen for possible surgery that did not proceed to surgery.

[3] Extended Consultation

An extended consultation (code 90610) is an evaluation of problems that do not require a comprehensive evaluation of the patient as a whole. It includes documentation of the history of the chief complaint, past medical history and pertinent physical examination, review and evaluation of the past medical data, establishment of a plan of investigative and/or therapeutic management and the preparation of an appropriate report. An example of an extended consultation is an examination of a cardiac patient who needs assessment before undergoing a major surgical procedure and/or general anesthesia.

[4] Comprehensive Consultation

A comprehensive consultation (code 90620) is an in-depth evaluation of a patient with a problem that requires the development and documentation of medical data, establishment or verification of a plan for further investigative and/or therapeutic management and the preparation of a report. The documentation of medical data would include documenting the chief complaint, present illness, family history, past medical history, personal history, system review and a review of all the diagnostic tests and procedures. An example of a comprehensive consultation is the evaluation of a young person with a fever, arthritis or anemia.

[5] Complex Consultation

The complex consultation (code 90630) is used for an uncommonly performed service involving in-depth evaluation of a critical problem that calls for unusual knowledge, skill and judgment on the part of the consulting physician as well as the preparation of an appropriate report. An example of a complex consultation is one for a patient with acute myocardial infarction with major complications.

[6] Follow-up Consultations

The following codes should be used when the consultant revisits a patient who has been consulted upon previously but for whom the consultant has not taken responsibility in terms of patient care and management:

- Follow-up Consultation, Brief: 90640
- Follow-up Consultation, Limited: 90641
- Follow-up Consultation, Intermediate: 90642
- Follow-up Consultation, Complex: 90643

§ 17.13 Relative Value Indexes

The relative value index takes into account the amount of effort, physician expertise and risk to the patient and physician a given procedure entails. With the help of the relative value index, the physician can develop a billing schedule and spot discrepancies in billing in specific service areas.

Relative value indexes are a coded listing of physician services assigning unit values to indicate the relative effort each procedure entails. Important elements to determine the relative value of each procedure would include the following:

- time involved in providing the service;
- skill required to deliver the service;
- severity of the condition generally involved in the service;

- risk to the patient inherent in the service;
- risk to the physician (medical/legal) in providing the service; and
- cross-specialty comparisons.

In order for a physician to use a relative value index effectively, he or she must first calculate a "conversion" factor (a multiplier or link between the relative value and the fee to be charged). The conversion factor is multiplied by the relative value to determine the fee. Before a physician computes the conversion factor, he or she should realize that each section of the relative value index—surgery, anesthesia, radiology, pathology and medicine—was developed independently, and thus a separate conversion factor is used for each section.

To compute an initial conversion factor, the following steps should be followed:

(1) List 20 to 30 basic procedures (those procedures most commonly performed) for each of the five sections of the index. The procedures should be separated according to the section of the index into which they fall. In column 1 of the worksheet, list the procedure code; in column 2 list the description.

(2) In column 3 of the worksheet, list the relative value assigned to the procedure, from the relative value index.

(3) In column 4, list the current fee for the procedure.

(4) Add the sum of the relative values for each section. Divide these by the number of procedures that are listed in the section to determine the "average" relative value.

(5) Add the column of fees for each section and divide by the number of procedures in that section to determine the "average" fee.

(6) Divide the average fee by the average relative value to determine the average conversion factor.

Once this conversion factor has been determined, it can be used to develop an entire fee schedule simply by multiplying the specific relative value of each procedure by the consistent conversion factor. Comparing this new "relative value" fee schedule to the current fee schedule should reveal any peculiarities in a physician's current fee schedule. For example, if the current fee schedule has any areas in which the fee is particularly high or low, this should quickly become evident.

Physicians starting practice can use the relative value index to develop an entire fee schedule. Both new and established practitioners will find use of the relative value index helpful to determine a fee for procedures that are commonly performed. The relative value index can also be useful in helping a physician determine what a potential reimbursement will be for a particular procedure.

§ 17.14 ICD-9-CM Diagnostic Coding

> The three-volume ICD-9-CM provides diagnostic codes for 17 different areas of injury and disease, with numerous subheadings and sub-subheadings. The physician uses the second volume of the ICD-9-CM to locate the specific diagnostic entity, then refers back to the first volume to locate the full description of that entity and determine whether it is appropriate. Proper use of the ICD-9-CM entails familiarity with use of modifying symbols, abbreviations and notations.

Diagnostic coding is beginning to play a bigger and bigger role in determining how much the physician will be reimbursed for services. Third parties have developed computer programs to cross-reference the appropriateness of a procedure based on the diagnosis. Casual use of diagnostic codes will ultimately lead to lower reimbursement and possibly flag a physician for an audit.

Today diagnostic coding is taken from the ICD-9-CM manual, the International Classification of Disease, 9th Edition, Clinical Modification, which describes diagnosis and treatment of patients in both inpatient and outpatient settings. Although the history of this text goes back several decades, in 1979, in the interests of making its system more usable in the hospital setting, the U.S. Public Health Service completed an updated version of the ICD with more detail and specific coding.

The ICD-9-CM has become well known in the medical setting and is put to much greater use there. The Catastrophic Coverage Act of 1988 mandated that effective April 1, 1989, physicians must use ICD-9-CM codes on all claims for Medicare services provided under Part B. It was expected that most, if not all, parties will require utilization of the ICD-9-CM coding in the future.

[1] The ICD-9-CM Text

The ICD-9-CM system is organized into three volumes:
- Volume One, Diseases: Tabular List
- Volume Two, Diseases: Alphabetical List
- Volume Three, Procedures: Tabular List and Alphabetical Index

[a] Volume Three

The third volume of the ICD-9-CM is generally not used in the physician's office, since procedure coding is accomplished through CPT codes and HCPCs. Hospitals, outpatient facilities and other settings use the ICD-9-CM procedural coding extensively.

[b] Volume Two, Section One

Volume Two of the ICD-9-CM includes an alphabetical index to diseases, a table of drugs and chemicals and an index to external causes of injuries.

The first section of Volume Two is the alphabetical index to diseases and injuries. This section should be used as the key to finding the appropriate diseases listed in Volume One. When using Volume Two to locate a diagnostic code, the physician should refer directly to the general diagnosis as opposed to the location of the problem or the seriousness of the problem.

In reviewing a particular diagnosis, there may be subheadings or sub-subheadings that can be used to further specify the diagnosis. For example, in looking for an acute bone abscess diagnosis, one would look under "abscess." A review of page seven, Volume Two, shows "abscess" in bold print, indicating that it is a main heading. After the main heading come indented subheadings. Following them down, one finds "bone." Further indented under "bone" is the sub-subheading "acute." When looking at subheadings and sub-subheadings, the physician must be careful not to drift into another category of subheadings or headings. After the specific sub-subheading has been located, it should be traced back

§ 17.14[1]   MANAGING YOUR MEDICAL PRACTICE   17-54

to make sure that it is still under the appropriate subheading and heading.

Once the appropriate heading, subheading, and sub-subheading have been identified, they should be looked up in Volume One, where more specific information and identification of the proper heading is available. The physician should never code a procedure directly from Volume Two, as failure to follow the diagnostic code back to Volume One can lead to error.

[c] **Volume Two, Section Two**

Section two of Volume Two, which runs from page 762 to page 763, provides an alphabetical index to poisoning and internal causes of adverse effects of drugs and other chemical substances. It is a table of drugs and chemicals that contains a classification of drugs and other chemical substances to identify poisoning states and external causes of adverse effects. Each of the substances in the table is assigned a code according to poisoning classification. The table also contains a listing of external causes of adverse effects.

Table headings pertaining to external causes are defined as follows:

Accidental Poisoning (E850–E869). These codes are used to indicate an accidental overdose given or taken.

Therapeutic Use (E930–E949). These codes are used to indicate substances that, when properly administered in therapeutic or prophylactic dosages, cause any adverse effects.

Suicide Attempt (E950–E952). These codes are used in instances of self-inflicted injuries or poisoning.

Assault (E961–E962). These codes are used when another person has inflicted injury or poisoning with the intent to injure or kill.

Undetermined (E980–E982). These codes are used when it cannot be determined whether the poisoning or injury was intentionally or accidentally inflicted.

[d] **Volume Two, Section Three**

Section three of Volume Two is the alphabetical index to external causes of injury and poisoning. It contains an index to the codes that classify environmental events, circumstances and other conditions as the cause of injury or other adverse effects. These are referred to as E Codes, and it is intended that the E code be used in addition to a code from the main body of the classifications. The alphabetical index to the E codes is organized by main terms that describe the accident, circumstance, event or specific agent that caused the injury or adverse effect.

Section three of Volume Two ranges from page 864 through page 910. Pages 906 through 910 cover a four-digit subdivision for external cause, railway accidents, motor vehicle traffic and nontraffic, other road vehicle accidents, water transport accidents, and air and space transport accidents.

[e] Volume One

Volume Two of the ICD-9-CM will be used mainly in a medical office as a guide or key to Volume One. Diagnostic selections for the medical office should be made from Volume One. Ignoring the Forward, Preface and Acknowledgments, ICD-9-CM Volume One consists of the following areas:

- Introduction
- Conventions Used in the Tabular List
- Guidance to the Use of the ICD-9-CM
- Classification of Diseases and Injuries (17 chapters)
- Supplementary Classifications (Classification of Factors Influencing Health Status, Contact with Health Service and Classification of External Cause of Injury and Poisoning)
- Appendixes

The 17 chapters of the Classification of Diseases and Injuries describe anatomical systems or types of conditions. Chapter One, "Infectious and Parasitic Diseases," for example, is concerned with a type of condition. Chapter Six, "Diseases of the Nervous System and Sense Organs," refers to an anatomical system. Within each of the chapters, codes are broken down into sections or related groups. For example, Intestinal Infectious Disease, in Chapter One, "Infectious and Parasitic Diseases," is a subheading for related group codes ranging from 001 to 018. This is followed by Zoonotic Bacterial Diseases.

The diagnostic codes in each of the sections of the ICD-9-CM have at least three digits. Two more codes may be added to the right of the principal code following a decimal point. For example, while code 003 is Other Salmonella Infections, Code 003.21 is Salmonella Meningitis. The three-digit code is referred to as the category code (Other Salmonella Infections). The fourth digit is added to provide specificity in anatomical site and is considered a subheading code (003.2 localizes salmonella infection). The fifth digit is designed to provide more information about the disease process, such as complications, health status factors or other information (003.21 salmonella meningitis).

The use of the four- and five-digit code is not optional. If the code exists, it must be used. As such, the list must be read carefully to ensure that the appropriate category, subcategory and subclassification are being used.

As with the CPT text, the physician, medical assistants and physician's insurance staff should take the time to read the introduction, tabular list and sections on conventions and guidance in the use of the ICD-9-CM information. More often than not, this information is improperly used. (*See Figures 17-3* and *17-4.*)

[2] Alphabetical Index

The alphabetical index uses a letter-by-letter system or order, in accordance with the University of Chicago *Manual of Style*. Single spaces and hyphens are ignored, and terms are alphabetized as though they were one continuous word.

NEC: Not Elsewhere Classifiable. The abbreviation NEC appears in the alphabetical index and the tabular list. In the alphabetical index, the NEC abbreviation indicates that more specific codes exist and that the code with NEC designation should only be used if more specific information is not available. The NEC designation also is used to indicate that the diagnostic statement contains more information than can be classified in the ICD system.

In the tabular list, the NEC designation should be used to indicate that the coder lacks the information necessary to code the term to a more specific category.

FIG. 17-3. Example of health insurance claim form with poorly specified diagnostic codes.

§ 17.14[2] MANAGING YOUR MEDICAL PRACTICE 17-58

HEALTH INSURANCE CLAIM FORM
(CHECK APPLICABLE PROGRAM BLOCK BELOW) FORM APPROVED OMB NO. 0938-0008

☐ MEDICARE (MEDICARE NO.) ☐ MEDICAID (MEDICAID NO.) ☐ CHAMPUS (SPONSOR'S SSN) ☐ CHAMPVA (VA FILE NO.) ☐ FECA BLACK LUNG (SSN) ☒ OTHER (CERTIFICATE SSN)

PATIENT AND INSURED (SUBSCRIBER) INFORMATION

1. PATIENT'S NAME: Patient Name	2. PATIENT'S DATE OF BIRTH: 08 08 38	3. INSURED'S NAME: Patient Name
4. PATIENT'S ADDRESS: Address, Address	5. PATIENT'S SEX: ☒ FEMALE	6. INSURED'S I.D. NO.: 1234567890
	7. PATIENT'S RELATIONSHIP TO INSURED: ☒ SELF	8. INSURED'S GROUP NO.
9. OTHER HEALTH INSURANCE COVERAGE: Blue Cross Blue Shield Medicare ###-##-####B	10. WAS CONDITION RELATED TO: A. PATIENT'S EMPLOYMENT: ☒ NO B. ACCIDENT:	11. INSURED'S ADDRESS: Address, Address 11a. CHAMPUS SPONSOR'S STATUS: ☒ RETIRED
12. PATIENT'S SIGNATURE: Signature On File		13. Signature On File

PHYSICIAN OR SUPPLIER INFORMATION

21. NAME & ADDRESS OF FACILITY WHERE SERVICES RENDERED: Abbott Northwestern Hospital — Mpls., MN

22. WAS LABORATORY WORK PERFORMED OUTSIDE YOUR OFFICE? ☒ NO

23. DIAGNOSIS OR NATURE OF ILLNESS OR INJURY:
1. 682.4 Hand, Wrist Infection
2. 786.2 Bronchial Cough
3. 992.0 Pyrexia

EPSDT: ☒ NO   FAMILY PLANNING: ☒ NO

DATE OF SERVICE FROM	TO	PLACE OF SERVICE	PROCEDURE CODE	DESCRIBE PROCEDURES	DIAGNOSIS CODE	CHARGES	DAYS OR UNITS	T.O.S.
7/24/90		3	90060	Intermediate Office	1	32 00	1	1
7/24/90		3	36415	Venipuncture	3	6 00	1	5
7/24/90		3	85022	Blood Count Hemogram Differn	3	28 00	1	5
7/24/90		3	71020	X-Ray Chest Bilateral	2	72 00	1	4

25. SIGNATURE OF PHYSICIAN: Dr. Signature

26. ACCEPT ASSIGNMENT: ☒ YES

27. TOTAL CHARGE: 138 00   28. AMOUNT PAID: 56.00   29. BALANCE DUE: 82.00

30. YOUR SOCIAL SECURITY NO.: ###-##-####

31. PHYSICIAN'S SUPPLIERS AND OR GROUP NAME:
Infectious Disease Consultants, P.A.
2545 Chicago Ave. S., Suite 211
Minneapolis, MN 55404
Telephone: (612) 687-9815

32. YOUR PATIENT'S ACCOUNT NO: Account Number
33. YOUR EMPLOYER ID NO: 41-1594275

ID NO BS 22769 IN

Form HCFA-1500 (1-84). Form OWCP-1500. Form CHAMPUS-501 (1-84) Form RRB-1500
#19385 - MEDICAL ARTS PRESS, MPLS., MN 55427

FIG. 17-4. Example of health insurance claim form with properly specified diagnostic codes.

NOS: Not Otherwise Specified. The NOS abbreviation should be used if the diagnostic statement does not contain enough information to assign a more specific code. This abbreviation is the equivalent of saying "unspecified." Since the ICD-9-CM must provide a place for every disease or condition, the NOS abbreviation allows a particular disease, not otherwise specified, to be categorized in the main category. As such, it will be possible to retrieve and compute statistics on a particular category of diseases.

[3] **Punctuations**

Brackets [ ]. Brackets are used to enclose synonyms, alternate wordings or explanatory phrases.

Parentheses ( ). Parentheses are used to enclose supplementary words that may be present or absent in the statement of a disease or procedure without affecting the code number to which it is assigned. It is not mandatory that terms exist in the diagnostic statement in order for the code to be used; rather, the terms enclosed in the parentheses are to serve as guides.

Colons :. Colons are used in the tabular list after an incomplete term that requires one or more of the modifiers that follow in order to make it assignable to a given category.

Braces { }. Braces are used to enclose a series of terms, each of which is modified by the statement appearing at the right of the brace. For example, on page 71 of Volume One, code 123.8, Other Specified Cestode Infection, the entities Diplogonoporus (grandis) and the Dipylidium (caninum) are modified by "infection."

[4] **Symbols**

The Lozenge Symbol ■. This symbol, when printed in the left margin preceding the disease code, denotes a four-digit rubric unique to the ICD-9-CM. The contents of these rubrics in the ICD-9-CM are not the same as those in the earlier ICD-9. This symbol is used only in Volume One in Diseases: Tabular List. Since the lozenge symbol does not affect physician coding, medical office coders may ignore it.

The Section Mark §. This symbol preceding a code denotes placement of a footnote at the bottom of the page that is applicable to all subdivisions in that code. It also serves as a reminder that all five digits should be used.

Typeface. **A bold typeface** is used for all codes and titles in the tabular list. *Italic typeface* is used for all exclusion notes and to identify those rubrics that are not to be used for the primary tabulation of diseases.

Indentations. An indented format is used to indicate subheadings and sub-subheading categories.

[5] **Instructional Notations**

Includes. This note appears immediately under a three-digit code title to further define or give examples of the contents of the category.

Excludes. Terms following the word "excludes" are to be coded elsewhere, as indicated in each case.

§ 17.15 Checklist for a Coding Library

Sources for the texts described in the chapter and additional guides to using them are provided.

Physician's Current Procedural Terminology (CPT Text). All physicians' offices should have a current copy. The text is updated each year, so a copy should be ordered annually. The text is published by the American Medical Association and can be ordered at the following address:

Book and Pamphlet Fulfillment:
OPO54190 American Medical Association
P.O. Box 10946
Chicago, IL 60610

HCPCS Code Book. The national HCPC book can be ordered at the following address:

Superintendent of Documents
U.S. Government Printing Office
Washington, DC 20402

As a practical matter, physicians should contact their local Medicare carrier to obtain a local copy of the local HCPC codes, since local codes supersede the national codes. (The local codes are based on the national codes and, typically, additional items are modifiers.)

ICD-9-CM, International Classification of Diseases, 9th Revision, Clinical Modification, Volumes One, Two and Three. As mentioned elsewhere, physicians should code from Volume One and use Volume Two as an index. The ICD-9-CM manual may be ordered from the Superintendent of Documents (listed before) or from:

ICD-9-CM
P.O. Box 911
Ann Arbor, MI 48106-0991
(313)-769-1000

Relative Value Index. This book may be ordered from:

McGraw-Hill Book Company
P.O. Box 400
Hightstown, NJ 08520

[1] **Ancillary Texts**

Getting Paid for What You Do: CPT and HCPC Coding for Optimum Reimbursement, by Gary M. Knaus. This book may be ordered from:

Medical Administration Publications
671 Executive Drive
Willow Brook, IL 60521
1-800-624-6994

CPT Coding Made Easy: A Technical Guide to CPT, by Gabriell M. Kotoski, R.N. This text may be ordered from Medical Administration Publications at the address and phone number just described.

ICD-9-CM Coding Handbook for Physician Practices, by Theresa M. Jorwic, R.R.A. This book may be purchased through Medical Administration Publications, at the address and phone number described earlier.

Medicare Regulations. Larger clinics, consultants or attorneys and accountants specializing in the medical area should have access to current Medicare regulations. These regulations may be ordered from the following:

Commerce Clearing House, Inc.
4025 W. Peterson Ave.
Chicago, IL 60646

[2] Third-Party Manuals

Every physician's office should have a third-party manual in which all the coding and billing procedures received directly from the third parties, including Medicare and Medicaid, are assembled. This information should be obtained directly from the third parties with which the physician participates. All bulletins and updates should be photocopied and circulated among the physicians and billing staff. The original material should be kept with the office third party contract. It also is recommended that a copy of current contracts be kept on hand in a separate section of each manual.

§ 17.16 Tips for Proper Coding

Tips are provided on on how to establish a good relationship with staff and third parties with regard to coding.

(1) Take coding seriously. The first step in achieving proper coding in the medical office is for the physician and medical staff to take the issue seriously. Failure on the part of the physician to do so can have many ramifications. Ultimately, it is the physician who will be responsible for what is coded. Lack of interest or discounting of the matter by the physician will lead the coding staff to believe that coding is not a serious issue.

(2) Proper training and development. Both the physician and the staff must be properly trained in the area of coding and must be up to date on coding issues. There are a number of ways to achieve this. Building a coding library for the office is one. Be sure to read all the bulletins that come in from your Medicare and Blue Cross carriers, and other third parties with whom you participate. Make sure your billing staff has read the procedural manuals for each of those third parties.

Training can be achieved though seminars, a number of which are held periodically throughout the United States. These seminars will not only help train your staff and keep them up to date but will generally leave your staff with a more positive feeling knowing that you are willing to help them obtain coding skills and that others share the same type of problems.

(3) Take the time to identify the procedures, services and supplies provided. While this may sound elementary, it cannot be emphasized enough. There are still many offices in which the physicians do not use a charge slip or routing slip of any type. They rely on the staff to do the billing, based on the staff's interpretation of the medical record or, perhaps worse yet, on the appointment schedule. This can only put the physician in a losing situation. Loss of reimbursement when procedures are undercoded or not coded, and charges of fraud and abuse in situations in which a higher level of service is coded than has been provided for, are likely to result.

When the physician and other medical professionals take the time to identify the procedures that have been performed and properly record them in the medical records, the chances of coding errors are greatly reduced. This applies to both procedural and diagnostic coding. A frequently updated routing slip, including both common procedural codes and diagnostic codes, is fundamental. So, too, is having the CPT text, HCPC text and ICD-9 text readily available to those people coding. When the medical staff or physician do not have time to look up an unusual code or set of codes, they should indicate so on the routing slip so that the time can be taken later for the coder to discuss this problem with the medical staff and ensure that the correct code or codes are selected.

(4) Be aware of the possibility that unusual coding situations may arise and know how to deal with them. For example, compare time-based critical care charges against the procedure code to make an evaluation based on the relative values of the different codes that might be used.

(5) On the billing invoice, be sure to list procedures by order of importance: The service with the highest relative value or fee should be listed first. When listing procedures that have been performed on different days, the procedures should first be grouped by date of service, ranking the most important at the top for the day. Since

some third parties will reduce the secondary charges or pay only for one service per day, it would be foolish not to receive full fee for the highest service, if possible.

(6) Remember to use modifiers as necessary. Failure to use the appropriate modifiers can quickly lead to a rejected claim.

(7) Match the diagnosis with the procedures being performed. Frequently a physician may be treating more than one problem. If the bill only shows one diagnostic code or applies the wrong diagnostic code to the wrong procedure, the claim may be denied as inappropriate.

Use special reports and letters as necessary. (*See Figure 17–5.*) In a situation in which the care provided is unusual, be sure to include a report explaining the circumstances. Although all carriers have a procedure for appealing rejected claims, in most cases it will be far easier to head the problem off at the pass by anticipating it and submitting a letter with the initial claim.

Physicians who frequently find themselves in unusual, complex situations may develop a standard letter to submit to third parties when the claim is filed. In other cases it may be beneficial to submit a claim to the carrier explaining the procedures the physician commonly performs, to avoid the need for an ongoing special report or letter submission with each claim.

(8) Make direct attempts to establish good working relationships with the third parties, and encourage your staff to do the same. The doctor's office may be correct but end up "shooting itself in the foot" by becoming angry or belittling the employees of the third parties. On the other hand, if a physician and the physician's staff have a good working relationship with the third party, problems can be solved quickly and more often to the physician's benefit. Consider funding some public relations expenses, such as having staff invite some key third party representatives to talk shop over lunch.

(9) Document problems. If a simple phone call doesn't get the claim processing procedure initiated, start documenting the situation with a letter or series of letters.

Infectious Disease Consultants, P.A.

Kathryn R. Love, M.D. Daniel J. Anderson, M.D.

January 10, 1990

Insurance Company
Claim Division
P.O. Box XYZ
Minneapolis, Minnesota 55440

RE: Jane Doe

To Whom it May Concern:

This patient has been under my care since December 1988, when she received a heart transplant. She subsequently contracted cytomegalovirus enteritis by acquiring the virus with the transplanted heart. After two long courses of treatment she had an apparent second relapse in the summer of 1989 and was retreated.

Her treatments consisted of four weeks of intravenous Ganciclovir, the only effective therapy available in the USA for serious CMV infections. Most of this therapy was given at home which greatly reduced the cost to her insurance company, and gave good quality of life to her.

There should be no question of the relationship of this infection to transplantation nor of the need for treatment and certainly not of the indication for home therapy in this case.

Yours,

Kathryn R. Love, M.D.

ABBOTT NORTHWESTERN HOSPITAL (11136)
800 E. 28TH ST. AT CHICAGO AVENUE • MINNEAPOLIS, MN 55407-3799
BUSINESS OFFICE: 750 S. PLAZA DR. • SUITE 321• MENDOTA HEIGHTS, MN 55120
(612) 687-9815

FIG. 17-5. Sample letter to third party explaining prcoedure that would necessitate use of a modifying code.

This way, if in four months there is still a problem, you will have documented your efforts to solve the problem. If there is any question of the physician's disclosure of facts and circumstances, having the information outlined in a written format will be helpful.

When writing a letter, be sure to restate any promises or comments made by the carrier over the phone. If there is any lack of communication or misunderstanding at that point, the third party should immediately respond.

(10) Enlist the patient's help when necessary. Try to get the patient on your side as quickly as possible when a problem situation arises. Since the patient is the customer of both the physician and the third party, maintaining a good relationship with the patient is important to both the third party and the physician. Third parties have taken the approach of making the physician look like the "bad guy." This is particularly true when an insurance company is attempting to support its reasons for refusing to pay a claim. Medicare has made numerous attempts to imply that any out-of-pocket costs to the patient are attributable to the physician rather than the program.

The physician should work with the patient on the patient's behalf in order to bond the physician-patient relationship and to be able to weather any unfounded attacks any third party may attempt.

§ 17.17 Coding Checklist

A comprehensive checklist of points described in this chapter is provided.

__ Physician and staff training and development
　　__ In-office library
　　　　__ CPT text
　　　　__ HCPC text
　　　　__ ICD-9-CM text
　　　　__ Relative Value Index

- Third-party manuals
- Other educational texts
- Third-party seminars and seminars given by consulting groups and schools
— In-office protocol
  - Develop comprehensive routing slip, including commonly used procedural and diagnostic codes
  - Systematize documentation to ensure that medical records support what codes designate
  - Ensure that both physician and medical staff understand, discuss and monitor the codes being used
— General coding practices
  - Select diagnostic or procedural codes that most specifically describes situation
  - Use proper modifiers to specify procedures
  - List procedures by order of importance and/or expense
  - Match appropriate diagnostic code to applicable procedure
  - If more than one code can be used for a given situation, select code that will yield the greatest reimbursement
  - Use letters and supporting reports when unusual circumstances occur, explaining reason for charges
— Using the CPT text
  - General information to know
    - Uses five-digit code numbers
    - Arranged by headings, specified by subheadings
    - Meaning of modifying symbols
    - Deleted codes
    - Notations
  - Major procedural headings
    - Medicine
    - Anesthesia

- Surgery
    - Surgical package vs. single procedures
- Radiology
    - Technical vs. professional component
    - One or more physicians interpret findings
    - Specify radiological modality
- Pathology and laboratory
    - In-house or outside lab referral
    - Refer Medicare procedures to outside lab
- Appendix A: two-digit code modifiers
- Appendix B: changes since last edition
- Appendix C: computer database update
- Index: multiple means for locating specific code entity

— Using HCPCs Text
- Generally takes priority over CPT codes when in conflict
- Organized alphanumerically
- Two-letter modifier codes

— Consultations; know differences between and proper coding for
- Consultant visits
- Intermediate consultation
- Extended consultation
- Comprehensive consultation
- Complex consultation
- Follow-up consultations

Levels of Service; know differences between and proper coding for
- New versus established patients
- Minimal service
- Brief service
- Limited service

- — Intermediate service
- — Extended service
- — Comprehensive service
— Using ICD–9–CM text
  - — Three volumes
    - — Volume One, Diseases: Tabular List
    - — Volume Two, Diseases: Alphabetical List
    - — Volume Three, Procedures: Tabular List and Alphabetical Index
  - — Alphanumeric organization
  - — Three-, four- and five-digit codes (higher number of digits takes priority)

Always consult alphabetical index (Volume Two) for main diagnosis, specified by subeadings

  - — Refer from Volume Two back to Volume One, locating selective code; do not code from Volume Two
  - — Pay attention to modifying symbols
— Relative Value Index
  - — Compute average conversion factor
  - — Multiply specific relative value by conversion factor

CHAPTER 18

Managing Professional Liability Risk

by Kathleen Moghadas

> **SCOPE**
>
> Professional liability risk can be divided into two basic areas: clinical and administrative. In the clinical sphere, a well organized medical record is crucial to minimizing liability. Records should be chronologically ordered, legibly written and contain the patient history and physical. All outside consultations, communications and treatments should be documented, and any alterations in the record initialed and dated. Before any medication is prescribed for the patient, the drug history should be known. Prescriptions should be written clearly so that they cannot be altered, and they should be periodically reviewed. Refills should never be given over the phone, nor should unlicensed office personnel be allowed to administer drugs. When treatment is to be rendered, the physician must obtain informed consent from the patient. Every effort should be made to supply the patient with preoperative and postoperative educational materials. Patient failure to keep appointments should be documented in the record. In the administrative sphere, effort should be made to keep the office experience satisfying. The physician should develop good rapport with the patient, the patient's family and office staff. Patients should find it easy to communicate with the office, and their diagnostic test results and treatments should be explained in detail. Office staff should be kept up to date about systems and equipment used in the office, and only licensed staff should be allowed to perform tests that warrant such licensing. Patients should have their bills fully explained to them. If patients are noncompliant

> about their medical care or paying their bills, procedures must be established to show that the physician made every effort to sustain the physician/patient relationship and that he or she is not negligent in discharging them from medical care.

SYNOPSIS

§ 18.01 Overview of the Malpractice Climate
§ 18.02 Medical Records
　　[1] Organization
　　[2] Legibility
　　[3] Documentation
　　[4] Altering the Medical Record
　　[5] Abbreviations
　　[6] History and Physical
　　[7] Presenting Complaints and Treatment Rendered
　　[8] Clinical Findings
　　[9] Consultations
　　[10] Records Release
　　[11] Confidentiality
　　[12] Vital Signs
　　[13] Test Results
§ 18.03 Communication
　　[1] Oral
　　[2] With Patients
　　[3] With the Family
　　[4] Written
　　[5] With Staff Members
　　[6] With Other Members of the Health Care Team
　　[7] Handling Patients Who Are Hostile or Complain
§ 18.04 Medication
　　[1] Allergy Documentation
　　[2] Explanation of Side Effects
　　[3] Follow-up Review of Medications
　　[4] Refill Policies
　　[5] Administration of Medication by Office Personnel
　　[6] Written Prescriptions
§ 18.05 Treatment and Procedures
　　[1] Informed Consent
　　[2] Contributory Negligence and Comparative Negligence
　　[3] Treatment Provided
　　[4] Preoperative Teaching
　　[5] Postoperative Teaching
　　[6] Discharge Instructions

MANAGING PROFESSIONAL LIABILITY RISK

   [7] Medication
   [8] Diagnostic Procedures
    [a] Guidelines
    [b] Radiological Studies
    [c] Diagnostic Log

§ 18.06 Patient Rapport and Risk Management
   [1] Office Schedules
   [2] Waiting Area
   [3] Patient Flow
   [4] Educational Materials
   [5] Refreshments
   [6] Entertainment
   [7] Information Packets
   [8] Recall System
   [9] Releasing Patients from Medical Care

§ 18.07 The Telephone and Risk Management
   [1] Conveying First Impressions
   [2] Telephone Advice and Treatment
   [3] Classifying Calls
   [4] Establishing Telephone Hours
   [5] Answering Service

§ 18.08 Accounts Receivable and Risk Management
   [1] Policy for Billing and Collection of Patients Accounts
   [2] Method of Payments Accepted
   [3] Explanation of Fees
   [4] Insurance Processing Policy
   [5] When the Patient Refuses to Pay the Bill
   [6] Discharging a Patient for Nonpayment

§ 18.09 Personnel
   [1] Policy Manual
   [2] Training Programs
   [3] Professional Licensure
   [4] CPR Certification
   [5] Personnel Manual and Job Descriptions
   [6] Staff Meetings

§ 18.10 Equipment
   [1] Maintenance Records
   [2] Calibration Records
   [3] Staff In-Service Records
   [4] Cleaning and Disinfecting Equipment

§ 18.11 General Quality Assurance Recommendations

§ 18.12 Handling Potential Litigation
   [1] Actions to Take When a Claim Is Pending
   [2] Actions to Take When a Claim Is Filed

§ 18.01   MANAGING YOUR MEDICAL PRACTICE   18–4

    [3] Selecting a Defense Attorney
    [4] Helping the Attorney
    [5] What to Expect from the Attorney
    [6] Making a Settlement
 § 18.13 Managing Professional Liability Checklist
 § 18.100 Bibliography

Appendix 18-A Policy Proposal for Prescription Refills

Appendix 18-B Medication Supplies Control Form

Appendix 18-C Outline for Policy Manual

Appendix 18-D Equipment Records

§ 18.01 Overview of the Malpractice Climate

Malpractice claims arise from real or perceived negligence brought about by professional failure in the clinical or administrative sphere.

Malpractice claims arise from both real and perceived negligence in the areas of legal obligations, patient relations and standards of care. Although there are thousands of causes of malpractice claims, the foundation for each is professional failure. Minimizing liability in the medical practice involves a commitment on the part of the physician, his or her staff and the patient.

There is currently no national center to receive and analyze medical liability data, although plans are being made to develop such a clearinghouse. From the data that is available, though, trends emerge regarding the types of problems for which physicians are being sued. This chapter outlines some common problem areas in their order of frequency and identifies ways for physicians to decrease their risks. Specifically, it examines two spheres into which these problems fall: the clinical sphere, which includes keeping medical records, communication between the patient or the patient's family and the physician and office staff, dispensing medication, and educating the patient about treatment and diagnostic procedures; and the administrative sphere, which includes techniques used to forge the physician/patient relationship, office protocols for giving information over the telephone, billing patients, training office personnel and maintaining office equipment.

§ 18.02 Medical Records

An organized, legible medical record is the best defense against liability. The record should be kept in chronological order and typed rather than handwritten. It should document all communications between the physician and patient, outside treatment and consultations. It should be jargon free and document the patient's medical history, current condition and vital signs. Diagnostic test results should be recorded and a system implemented for informing the patient whether results are positive or negative and whether follow-up is necessary. The record should always reflect the complexity of the condition for which the patient is being treated. If the medical record is to be released, the physician must obtain informed consent from the patient.

Liability experts estimate that 35 to 40 percent of all suits alleging medical malpractice are indefensible because of problems with the medical record. Thus, every physician should take to heart the axiom, "If it is not written down or otherwise recorded, it never happened."

A well-written, legible record conveys the impression of proper medical care. A poorly organized, incomplete or indecipherable record suggests indifference on the part of the physician and staff. In a medical malpractice trial, the record constitutes the most important piece of evidence.

[1]—Organization

Medical records that fail to substantiate proper care are many times simply the result of information not being accessible. Thus, medical records should be organized to help the doctor and staff locate information quickly. This can be achieved easily if documents are consistently placed in the patient's chart.

The use of dividers in the medical record to separate information and of flags for proper placement of information is encouraged. Information should be inserted chronologically, with the most current information on top. All records should be organized in this fashion.

Personnel should never use scraps of paper to transmit information from one person to another. Rather, the practice should implement a procedure for the transmittal of information. A form specifically designed for this purpose virtually eliminates the possibility of information getting lost. If a malpractice suit is brought against a physician who is unable to provide the medical record because it was lost or destroyed, then the physician's defense is markedly compromised if not untenable.

It is essential that medical records be kept for at least the time period prescribed by state law. The physician needs to be cognizant of these limitations.

[2]—Legibility

All entries made in the chart should be legible and preferably typed. Documentation within the record should be clear and legible, so that laypersons can understand the content. The physician can be held liable if only he or she can decipher the record. The significance of legible records is best appreciated when one realizes that malpractice suits sometimes come to trial two to ten years after the incident, of which the participants may have poor memory.

Documentation in the record should be made in black ink to facilitate the highest quality of photocopying. All members of the treatment team should adopt the same format for documenting information. Standardized forms should be used whenever possible.

[3]—Documentation

The medical record should demonstrate the physician's application of his or her education and expertise. It should document the diagnostic and therapeutic plan and the rationale behind it, and should also include the patient's response to treatment and any modifications to or deviations from the original treatment plan.

The medical record should reflect the complexity of the problem being treated. Courts have found liability in malpractice cases when records were sparse and failed to adequately record complaints, history, symptomatology and findings of the examination.

Treatment provided outside the office should also be documented. For example, it is imperative that telephone conversations are documented in the medical record in the interest of limiting physician liability.

[4]—Altering the Medical Record

A special type of malpractice bungler is the physician who alters medical records, for whatever reason, *after* receiving notice of a malpractice claim. Acceding to the temptation to alter records when one is sued can be disastrous.

Sometimes, however, an entry might need to be corrected after it has been made in the natural course of keeping the record accurate and up to date. When errors need correction, the method of revision should be a simple line through the original, next to which the initials of the individual making the change and the date and time of the change are noted. The original entry must remain legible. At the next available spot in the record, a new note, with the same date and time, should be written to explain the need for the adjustment. Adherence to these guidelines eliminates any question as to why and when the change was made and who made it.

[5]—Abbreviations

Although certain abbreviations are commonly used within the medical community, caution should be exercised when additional shorthand notations are made in the medical record. A list of sanctioned abbreviations should be developed and displayed in a location that is accessible to the staff. To facilitate compliance with this procedure, a list of these abbreviations should be included in each medical record. The use of "cute" abbreviations can become embarrassing at best and incriminating at worst if the medical record is examined in court.

[6]—History and Physical

No health care provider should initiate immediate treatment in a non-life-threatening situation without first obtaining a complete and comprehensive patient history. The history and physical findings should be retained in a separate section of the record. Valuable information such as history of disease, surgical history, medications the patient is currently taking and allergies, should be extracted from the history and physical and indicated in a separate area of the chart.

[7]—Presenting Complaints and Treatment Rendered

In reflecting the complexity of a case, the medical record must include a differential diagnosis that attempts to pinpoint the source of the patient's problem (or symptoms) and determine the best way to manage it or at least control it, if that is the only reasonable alternative.

It is crucial to document whatever advice the physician or staff gives to a patient, and any medication that is prescribed. Response to treatment is an area that is often overlooked, but that should be documented as well.

[8]—Clinical Findings

Although it is necessary that the physician review the available diagnostic information, it is also necessary that he or she record the clinical findings. It is inadequate for the physician to merely initial diagnostic findings without referencing them within the written summary.

The law demands that a physician use all available and relevant information to reach a diagnosis and formulate an appropriate treatment plan. This includes not only the history the patient provides but also data accumulated by means of a complete physical examination and laboratory, x-ray and other tests or procedures that are appropriate and indicated.

No physician is held liable for an error in judgment when a similarly trained, prudent physician might well have reached the same conclusion. Rather, the physician is held responsible for error when he or she relies on inadequate or incomplete data, interprets the data inappropriately or uses the data to build an unsupported conclusion with respect to diagnosis or treatment.

[9]—Consultations

When consultations are requested, a note should be included in the chart to this effect. A tracking system should be implemented to assist the office in follow-up on consultations.

In situations where outside consultants were used, it is important to note whether their recommendations were followed. If a consultant's advice was not followed, then the physician should

§ 18.02[10] MANAGING PROFESSIONAL LIABILITY RISK

be able to give a reason. It is not mandatory to follow a consultant's recommendations slavishly, but if a health care provider chooses to ignore the consultant, an explanation for this decision must be stated in the record.

The physician should have a good relationship with fellow physicians, especially those called in as consultants, who deserve the courtesy of complete clinical data. Consultants may include radiologists or other imaging specialists, laboratory consultants and other clinicians. Whenever a complex case is to be treated by both the consultant and the referring physician, there must be specific and complete understanding and delineation of whose responsibility it is to follow particular aspects of the patient care.

[10]—Records Release

Written consent should be obtained from the patient whenever information about the patient is to be released to anyone.[1] In cases when a patient is being referred to another physician, it is necessary to obtain a release. If information needs to be released to an insurance carrier, then it is necessary to obtain a written release. It is not a wise practice to relinquish information via the telephone, unless the office personnel has a written release on record. Written consents must be kept on the patient's chart.[2]

Patients should be asked to provide the office with a list of people who have their consent to have their medical information. When consent is obtained over the telephone, as in an emergency, it should be witnessed by two licensed professionals. The release of records to individuals designated by the patient over the telephone may be a convenience to the patient; however, it puts the medical office in a position of legal liability.

The physical record belongs to the physician or the hospital, but the information it contains belongs to the patient. The patient has both the right to view the record and the right to obtain a copy of the record, provided he or she pays for the cost of duplication. Release of information to another practitioner

---

[1] See also ch. 12.

[2] See also J. Taraska, Legal Guide for Physicians, ch. 3 (Matthew Bender 1988) for physician obligations to respect patient confidentiality.

should be done as a courtesy to the patient, providing it is not excessive.[3]

[11]—Confidentiality

Protecting the patient's right to privacy is a critical concern of the medical office. Patients should be provided with an atmosphere that allows them to express their concerns and needs. When they enter the medical practice, they should do so with the reassurance that their privacy will be protected.

Although the medical record must be accessible, it should be maintained in such a way as to prevent other people from having access to it. Both the staff and the physician should be cautioned about discussing patients in front of other patients. In telephone conversations with patients, permission should be asked before repeating the patient's name.

The front office should be designed in such a way as to reduce the sound in the reception area.

[12]—Vital Signs

Complete and accurate recording of vital signs is an essential component of each medical examination. Inclusion of the vital signs during the dictation of the visit indicates that care has been comprehensive. Most medical records have an area in which to list vital signs. Having a specific vital sign sheet assists the physician in observing trends and patterns.

[13]—Test Results

When tests are ordered, a note should be made in the patient's chart and a log should be generated to prevent the test results from 'falling through the cracks.' When a lab result has not been returned in a timely fashion, a log serves as a rapid reminder to institute a tracking of that result. If a separate section of the chart is to be used to include test results, then the physician should initial that he or she saw the results before they are filed in the chart.

---

[3] *See also* J. Taraska, Legal Guide for Physicians, ch. 5 (Matthew Bender 1988) regarding proper disposition of medical records.

The practice must have a system for notifying patients of test results. Failure to notify patients of normal test results is poor practice management and poor public relations. A simple method of notification is the use of fold-over postcards. Normal test results can be indicated on the card, which is signed by the doctor.

The use of postcards is not recommended for reporting abnormal results unless there is a fail-safe method of follow-up. Without such a system in place, the medical office will never know if the patient was properly notified, and there will be no certainty that proper medical attention has been given to the problem.

The office should maintain a log for the control of all tests and verification that the patient has been notified and properly advised as to follow-up on abnormal test results. It should also maintain a policy to ensure that the problem has been followed up on.

Consider the following example: A physician receives a Pap smear report describing "severe inflammation and dysplasia." Proceeding on the assumption that the dysplasia was due to inflammation, the physician treats the woman with antibiotics and recommends a repeat Pap smear in one year. The patient returns in one year with invasive cancer that necessitates a hysterectomy. By failing to have the patient come in for an earlier follow-up visit after the recommended treatment, the physician has subjected her to poor patient care and is liable for malpractice. The same negative result—i.e., the manifestation of invasive cancer in the interval before the follow-up examination—could occur when a postcard notifying the patient of an abnormal Pap smear and recommending a follow-up smear only six months later is lost in the mail and not followed up on by the physician's staff.

§ 18.03 Communication

Essential communication in the medical office includes establishing rapport with the patient and his or her family, communication with office staff and instruction in the limitations of their responsibilities. Oral communication or communication over the telephone should be witnessed or otherwise documented and included in the medical record.

Communication with patients, family and staff is essential to preventing misunderstanding that can lead to claims of malpractice. Whenever possible, communication should be documented and included in the patient record.

[1]—Oral

The basis for a healthy physician-patient relationship is good rapport and communication. It is important that the lines of communication remain open with the patient's family as well.[4] Communication should also extend to fellow physicians, office staff, nurses and other health care personnel.

The telephone may be a convenient way to save time, but in the hands of an untrained employee, it may become a risk-laden substitute for a face-to-face visit with the physician. Strict guidelines must be established when instructing office personnel to screen calls for the physician. Staff need to know the limits of their responsibility.

The staff should exercise extreme caution when making appointments, particularly when the front office opens to the reception area. This is important to protect the confidentiality of the patient on the telephone. Patients should be asked to spell their name, but this should not be repeated out loud if other patients can hear. This is especially true when the patient has been asked questions about symptoms that may alert others in the waiting room to the nature of his or her condition.

The physician should not acknowledge a patient as his or hers to another patient without being given permission by the first patient. Similarly, the physician should secure permission from the second patient to thank the referral source. This can be done by incorporating the question "Whom may we thank for referring you to our practice?" on the new-patient information form.

[2]—With Patients

A decreased level of patient satisfaction is the underlying reason for the increased number of legal suits. A number of reasons account for most complaints brought by patients to attorneys, but

---

[4] *See also* ch. 15.

poor communication between the physician and the patient is primary among them.

Typical complaints include the following:

- My doctor doesn't seem really concerned about me.
- They never tell me what they are doing and why.
- The doctor's staff seems so inconsiderate.
- My doctor always talks down to me.
- I don't know if I can afford the treatment I am getting.
- I always have to wait so long.
- Everyone in the waiting room can hear the personal questions they ask.

If the patient does not understand the physician's diagnosis, or if the patient believes the physician has not dealt honestly and forthrightly with him or her, then the lines of communication can break down. Maintaining good rapport, assuring that questions are answered, resolving misconceptions and repeating instructions when appropriate will often prevent problems.

Whenever possible, the physician should strive to communicate as honestly as possible with the patient. To that end, it is recommended that the physician dictate in front of the patient, while he or she is in the examining room.

In some instances firm or forceful warning may be an appropriate response to a noncompliant patient. However, harshness, excessive criticism, profanity and verbal abuse go far beyond professional boundaries and do more than interfere with the rapport the physician strives to create.

[3]—With the Family

When the patient is elderly or has a terminal illness, it is essential that the physician communicate with the patient's family. This strengthens the bonds among all those involved and promotes a deeper respect for the physician.

It is often necessary, especially in the case of an elderly patient or a child, for a family member to be present during the examination or consultation. At this point, the physician has the opportunity to develop rapport and to communicate verbal instructions that can be retained.

§ 18.03[4] MANAGING YOUR MEDICAL PRACTICE

[4]—Written

Information that is written can have a great impact on the reader.[5] Thus, caution is appropriate for comments entered into the record. Irrelevant or derogatory information about the patient, the family or members of the treatment team do not belong in the medical record. Information that other people must read and act upon should be objective. Whenever possible, such information should be dictated for transcription rather than written in longhand.

[5]—With Staff Members

Communication with the physician's own office staff is critical. This starts with the selection of competent individuals whose duties are specifically delineated according to their training and demonstrated ability within statutory or local regulations. Employees need to be informed of the limits of their duties and authority. A nurse or receptionist can place a physician in jeopardy by offering inaccurate, incomplete or inappropriate advice to a patient.

The staff should never undermine the doctor by making comments to the patient about the doctor's advice, instructions or treatments. They should be instructed to ask questions regarding treatment or medication in private. Lack of communication with personnel may lead to errors on their part, for which the patient ultimately pays the price.

It is inappropriate for a health care provider to openly admonish a member of the staff in front of others. If criticism or correction is due, the responsible or involved individual should be counseled privately. Should a patient or family member overhear criticism or insult when the outcome has been less than optimal, confidence and trust may erode.

[6]—With Other Members of the Health Care Team

Nothing will get the attention of a patient or family member more quickly than a physician's negative comment regarding the skills of another physician. Likewise, the physician should not put himself or herself in the position of either verbally or nonverbally

---

[5] *See also* ch. 15.

reinforcing a patient's opinion of mistreatment at the hands of another physician.

During information exchanges with another health care provider, discussion should not deviate from the patient and his or her condition. This reduces the chance of prejudicing the new doctor with the first doctor's impression.

The physician and staff should always be judicious in making remarks in a nonclinical setting. Medical people are looked on with great respect by many members of the lay population. People love to hear stories of medical experiences, especially the more dramatic ones, and care should be taken to avoid relating "war stories" for the entertainment of others, especially when the subject of those remarks may be identifiable. Such statements are a gross violation of the unspoken assurance of patient privacy and confidentiality.

[7]—Handling Patients Who Are Hostile or Complain

When the medical office receives a complaint, the calls should be handled in a specified manner. The patient should be allowed to vent his or her anger, and the staff should be receptive to these remarks. Many times patients just want to be heard. The staff should be instructed not to interrupt, escalate the dialogue or be defensive. More often than not, patients will calm down after speaking their piece.

At no time should the staff's emotions interfere. Staff should be trained not to take patients' remarks personally, to take notes on what patients say and to convey sympathy. They should use phrases such as, "I understand how unhappy you are. I am sorry you feel that way." But they should be instructed never to accept blame or incriminate themselves unless it is an obvious error on their part. They should ask what it would take to resolve the problem. The next step is to refer the call to the physician or the office manager.

The office manager or the doctor should not offer a refund automatically. Usually an apology or an explanation will suffice. The goal is to move the conversation from anger to finding a solution.

§ 18.04 Medication

A good medication protocol involves taking a detailed drug history before prescribing medications. Patients should be educated by the physician and patient-information sheets about the drugs they are taking and any potential side effects. Patients should be evaluated periodically to ensure that their medication regimen is appropriate. Prescriptions should be written legibly and in such a way that they cannot be altered or duplicated without physician consent. Prescriptions should never be renewed over the phone. Staff should follow the office medication protocol and never be allowed to prescribe. Any data regarding medication should be documented in the patient record.

Nothing the physician does will cause problems faster than having a poor medication protocol. A physician should never prescribe medication for anyone without proper medical indication. Frequently physicians are called upon to write prescriptions for patients or other health care members as a favor. Problems occur when the medication is incompatible with another medication the patient is currently using or when the patient proves sensitive to the drug prescribed.

The physician should be aware of possible contraindications to the use of any particular drug because of medical problems or allergies the patient has or because of the drug's incompatibility with other medications. Before prescribing medication, a detailed history should be taken along with a drug history that notes possible adverse reactions to any medications in the past.

When prescribing medication, care should be taken to elucidate whether the patient has been under the care of another physician since the last visit. A phone call to the other physician, with the patient's permission, might be indicated if follow-up is necessary.

[1]—Allergy Documentation

The medical record should provide a designated area for drug allergy documentation. The preferred practice is to mark the allergies in red, to reduce the chance of missing this information. Drug allergies should also be documented on the medication records. Any adverse reactions should be noted.

[2]—Explanation of Side Effects

Patient education with regard to both proper administration and potential side effects is another area of risk management that frequently does not receive the attention it should. Physicians should not delegate medication education to one of their employees. Patients should be instructed on both the administration of the medication and its potential side effects.

Physicians also must be aware of the rate of absorption of medication. They must be aware of the potential of absorption, i.e., when the medication is taken with something other than water or on an empty stomach. Many offices provide patient information sheets produced by pharmaceutical companies and medical societies that explain the characteristics, administration and potential adverse reactions to the medication in easy-to-read language.

It is important to enter a note into the medical record indicating that the patient has received instruction on the use of a particular medication and its potential side effects. If pharmaceutical samples are given to the patient, then a note to that effect should be made in the medical record.

[3]—Follow-up Review of Medications

Timely follow-up regarding a particular medication is important for assuring optimal results. This should be done in a quick medication review appointment. Vital signs should be taken and documented along with the patient's stated affect.

[4]—Refill Policies

Patients often will attempt to take advantage of a medication refill policy. Many times the medical practice will attempt to assist the patient by refilling a prescription over the telephone. This practice is unwise, as it does not provide adequate follow-up. Patients who attempt to avoid going to the physician often abuse this service, to their own detriment. These are often the same patients who will later suffer complications and blame the physician's office.

Every medical office should adopt a standard protocol for prescription refills. Drug enforcement regulations are available by request from many state medical societies to assist practices in developing their policies. (*See Appendix 18-A.*) The following items should be considered when establishing a medication policy: the date of last refill, the date the patient was last seen, the number of refills permitted between visits, and the best time to call the office for refills. The office should never refill a prescription for a medication that was not prescribed by the physician. Office personnel should not be permitted to okay medication without the written permission of the physician. Patients should be instructed to call for prescription refills when they have less than one week's supply left.

[5]—Administration of Medication by Office Personnel

If medications are stored in the office, care must be taken to maintain an accurate record of the quantities on hand. (*See Appendix 18-B.*) Medication administration standards and policies should be established and available for personnel. All persons responsible for the administration of medication should be required to participate annually in a training session dealing with medication administration procedures. Their participation and training should be documented in their employee record. The physician should routinely observe employee technique to ensure compliance with office standards. An injection site chart should be available wherever medications are administered.

[6]—Written Prescriptions

Alteration of prescriptions is becoming a problem for physicians. The best way to guarantee that a prescription is not altered is to use security paper and two-part prescription pads. Prescription pads should always be kept locked in a special place that is inaccessible to patients.

Physicians who write prescriptions in script also face potential risks. Instances have been reported in which a physician wrote a prescription for a medication, only to have the office clerk misread the handwriting and call in the wrong prescription to the pharmacy, with adverse consequences to the patient. All medication prescriptions should be carefully printed. The office staff should be instructed to question the physician about what he or she wrote when in doubt.

§ 18.05 Treatment and Procedures

Liability can result from treatment that is rendered and that is not rendered. Informed consent must be obtained from any patient who is to undergo treatment. When patients elect to cancel appointments for procedures important for their treatment, this should be noted in the medical record.

Proper treatment procedures entail informing the patient of what may happen when he or she elects to undergo treatment or to do without it. Only properly trained personnel should be allowed to run laboratory studies.

[1]—Informed Consent

The requirements of informed consent are intended to give the patient the information and power to accept or reject the physician's recommendations before a treatment or procedure is initiated. These requirements obligate the doctor to assure the patient a choice from among a range of available treatments as well to decline treatment if desired.

The legal standard for obtaining informed consent is much more complex than simply having the patient sign an informed consent form. A lawsuit for failure to obtain informed consent may allege that the patient did not understand enough about the therapy for the consent to be effective. Communication between physician and patient must be effective and convey the following:

- the diagnosis;
- the nature and purpose of the treatment plan;
- the possible alternatives; and
- the prognosis if treatment is not provided.

The content of this communication should be documented in the medical record.

The physician cannot delegate responsibility for obtaining informed consent. Informed consent needs to be presented by the physician and should include a statement indicating the role he or she played in the process of obtaining it.[6]

---

[6] *See also* J. Taraska, Legal Guide for Physicians, ch. 6 (Matthew Bender 1988) for further discussion on the proper means of obtaining informed consent.

[2]—Contributory Negligence and Comparative Negligence

Documentation of possible contributory negligence is necessary in today's medical practice. Steps can be taken to protect the office from claims on the part of patients that they were not informed or were not given the opportunity for adequate follow-up. One of the areas in which simple record keeping can prevent any claims of medical negligence is appointment cancellations. When a patient cancels an appointment, it is important that the appointment not be erased from the book. This may become important evidence in a malpractice case in which it is argued that the patient was not given an opportunity for treatment.

Before filing charts back into the records, all canceled, failed missed or rescheduled appointments should be stamped or otherwise documented. This is very important when attempting to show possible contributory negligence on the part of the patient. A prepared stamp that notes the patient altered the appointment date is an efficient way to accomplish this.

Recall reminders[7] to follow-up on patients and assure that they are offered a chance for consultation offer additional benefits besides filling the appointment book and regulating patient flow: they help reinforce a defense against accusations of failure to diagnose, treat and refer claims.

[3]—Treatment Provided

The patient account history provides further documentation of services rendered. Having appropriate information on services previously rendered provides the physician with a format for making an informed diagnosis. When other physicians have provided services to the patient, having that information further assists the attending physician.

[4]—Preoperative Teaching

All too often, the physician's staff is delegated the responsibility of explaining preoperative instructions to the patient. To minimize liability risk, the physician should explain all preoperative instructions and, if possible, supplement them with additional

---

[7] *See also* ch. 4.

information in the form of written material or brochures created by hospitals and surgical societies specifically to address these issues. During the preoperative period, patients typically experience a great deal of anxiety and stress that makes communication difficult. If they have been given pertinent written material to read at home, this creates an atmosphere conducive to instruction and affords every opportunity for the patient to have a clear understanding of what he or she will encounter during surgery. Any material that is given to the patient should be documented in the preoperative teaching section of the medical record.

[5]—Postoperative Teaching

Prior to the patient's discharge after surgery, any printed information that is provided should be noted, not just in the hospital record but also in the medical record back at the office. Many times physicians make the mistake of assuming that the hospital record is sufficient proof that postoperative instructions were provided. It is important that office personnel be advised that the patient has been given specific instructions, especially when there is a need for follow-up in the office.

[6]—Discharge Instructions

Copies of all discharge instructions provided in the hospital should also be included in the medical record in the office. Providing the patient and family with written discharge information promotes a clearer understanding of postoperative instructions.

[7]—Medication

If prescriptions were provided for the patient, copies should be retained for the office's medical record.[8]

[8]—Diagnostic Procedures

Special regard should be given to the management of the medical office laboratory. Without accurate diagnostic data, the doctor is unable to reach reliable conclusions. Many practices

---

[8] See § 18.04 *infra* for information regarding the documentation of medication.

choose to perform simple tests in their offices; however, the tests are usually performed by medical assistants who have not been properly trained in laboratory procedures. Further, employees may drift away from salient procedures without consistent reinforcement. A number of problems can occur as a result of using inadequately trained personnel. Remedying this problem requires periodic continuing education for the personnel responsible for diagnostic studies. It is important to document participation in continuing education programs in the employee records.

[a]—Guidelines

The medical office should provide guidelines on correct test procedures as recommended by their licensing agency. Legislation regarding this issue is being generated on the federal level. Currently, medical office laboratories are governed by the Clinical Laboratory Impact Act (CLIA) of 1988. Information on this subject is available through most medical and dental management consultants, the American Medical Association or the Commission on Office Laboratory Assessment (COLA).

The following recommendations will be helpful in developing sound laboratory practices:

- The laboratory must have an operations manual available.
- A quality control program should be established and well documented.
- Periodic reviews of all protocols should be performed and documented.
- All maintenance and service of laboratory equipment should be documented.
- Recommendations of the manufacturer should be followed precisely when using any supplies in the performance of tests.

[b]—Radiological Studies

Any medical office that chooses to perform radiological studies should follow the recommendations of the licensing agency. Whenever possible, more than one individual should read the x-ray. The Radiation Control Department of the Department of Health and Human Services provides guidelines to assist medical offices seeking to offer these services.

[c]—Diagnostic Log

An effective method to prevent diagnostic test results from falling through the cracks is the maintenance of a diagnostic log. Patients for whom studies are requested are entered into the log, and when the results come back to the office, those items are checked off as completed.

§ 18.06 Patient Rapport and Risk Management

> To minimize patient dissatisfaction and guarantee patient compliance, it is necessary for the medical office to have convenient office hours and organized patient flow. Refreshments, instructional materials, entertainment and information packets in the waiting room can have a positive impact on the patient's impression of the practice's concern. Systems should be implemented for contacting patients who fail to keep follow-up appointments and who must be discharged from medical care for noncompliance.

Highest among the reasons patients sue their physicians is dissatisfaction with the way they are treated. In addition to providing patients with benefits of their education and experience, physicians must communicate that they care about the welfare of theirs.

In situations where a patient may not feel completely confident about the care being provided, attention to the way the practice assists the patient is evaluated. First impressions are often lasting impressions in the area of patient relations.[9] The physical layout of the office, the speed with which the patient is seen and the rapport that is developed by office personnel are all areas where the physician can provide the opportunity to make an enduring positive impression. Just as the medical record provides the backbone of patient care, so can the delivery of care and the establishment of positive patient relations be a determining factor if the patient chooses to seek legal counsel.

[1]—Office Schedules

Office hours need to be convenient for patients and their families. When a patient calls the doctor's office, he or she is comforted knowing that there is someone there who can assist. Information on a number of factors are important for developing

---

[9] *See also* ch. 16.

the office schedule: appointment times, patient arrival time, the time the patient is seen by the assistant, the time the physician enters and exits the room and the patient's checkout time.

Studies are available to assist the practice in establishing the best hours of operation. More and more practices are choosing to offer appointments in the evenings and on weekends. With the success of urgent care centers, more offices are beginning to realize that patients need medical treatment outside normal business hours.

[2]—Waiting Area

The waiting area should be set up with enough space to accommodate waiting patients. It should be comfortably laid out and should contain material to occupy their attention while they are waiting. Soft music is often recommended to soothe anxieties. The waiting room is an excellent place to provide patients with educational material.

[3]—Patient Flow

Patients who are seen on time and given ample opportunity to discuss their medical concerns with their doctor are happy patients. Expedient patient flow leaves the patient with the impression that the office is well organized. Patients who are delayed and inconvenienced have time to ponder—often adversely—the competence of their physician.

[4]—Educational Materials

Providing educational material in the waiting room affords the patient an opportunity to become an intelligent, active participant in the care he or she receives. The informed patient is more likely to make rational decisions regarding his or her health care. These patients also tend to be more medically compliant and will be less likely to resist recommendations.[10]

---

[10] *See also* ch. 16 for further discussion of the various types of educational material available, as well as where they can be obtained.

[5]—Refreshments

Refreshments should be available for patients in the waiting room. However, they should be limited to fresh bottled water or decaffeinated beverages. This both serves as an act of courtesy and also reinforces some positive health habits. The refreshment area needs to be maintained periodically throughout the day to avoid an unkempt appearance.

[6]—Entertainment

While patients are in the waiting area, soft music can be provided to reduce their anxieties. Some medical offices prefer to have a television available. Depending on the specialty and type of patient population, a television can be an excellent source of education. Educational videotaped material can be provided for patient viewing.

[7]—Information Packets

Information packets detailing the medical practices and policies should be provided for the patient. The greater the understanding patients have about office policies, the less likely they are to have confrontations over policy issues later on. Office policies can be communicated in the form of a patient information packet.

[8]—Recall System

A recall system is an integral part of practicing good medicine. A well-organized recall system will enable the medical office to keep track of patients. Additionally, it provides the medical office with valuable information on patients who are not complying with treatment recommendations.

[9]—Releasing Patients from Medical Care

Canceled appointments pose one of the most difficult obstacles to providing satisfactory patient care. When patients have to cancel their appointments, attempts should be made to reschedule them while they are available by phone. Patients who repeatedly cancel their appointments need to be contacted by the medical office to determine the problem. All attempts to reschedule appointments should be documented. After repeated unsuccessful attempts to arrange follow-up care for the patient, the physician should make a decision about discharging the patient.[11]

The process of releasing a patient from medical care usually involves a phone call from the physician followed by a certified letter advising the patient of his or her release from medical care. The patient should be informed of an interval of time during which the physician will continue to provide emergency services and recommendations of where the patient can call to find a new physician.[12]

§ 18.07 The Telephone and Risk Management

A routing system should be established for telephone calls, and an answering service used when personnel are not available. Treatment never should be administered over the phone, and staff should be instructed as to limits on information they can release over the phone.

The telephone is commonly the area of office policy over which the physician has the least control. Because physicians and staff exchange information over the telephone, proper protocols and documentation of such communication is important. Otherwise, the physician can be held liable for incorrect, inappropriate or incomplete information.

[1]—Conveying First Impressions

How the patient views the doctor depends a great deal on how personnel answer the telephone and handle patient calls. The greeting should include the name of the medical office and the name of the individual answering the phone. Patients should always be given the opportunity to have a moment to speak before they are asked to be placed on hold.

---

[11] *See also* ch. 12 for a sample letter to release patient from medical care.

[12] *See also* J. Taraska, Legal Guide for Physicians, ch. 2 (Matthew Bender 1988) for additional information regarding procedures for releasing a patient from your medical care.

[2]—Telephone Advice and Treatment

The medical office should have a policy that limits how much advice is given over the telephone. Symptoms that the patient describes and what the person taking the message transcribes are not always the same. Therefore, providing medical advice over the telephone is strongly discouraged. However, patients should always be provided with an opportunity to thoroughly explain their problem and instructed that the physician will return their call.

The office staff should not give any advice over the telephone that is not dictated by the physician. This is especially true when a patient asks for advice regarding a medication or treatment. Furthermore, the staff should never reassure a patient about the seriousness of his or her condition, as this could result in a patient not coming in for an examination or a follow-up visit. Instead, the staff should be instructed to explain to patients that the doctor wants to give them the best care possible, and that to do so requires an office visit. It is impossible to diagnose the cause of symptoms accurately over the telephone.

When the physician is giving advice over the telephone, the medical record should be available for review and documentation. Treatment over the telephone is a risky situation for anyone. When the physician has to respond to patient calls when he or she is away from the office, a small printed note pad can be used to document the call. The note should then be transferred to the patient's medical record.

[3]—Classifying Calls

When a patient calls the medical office, routing the call to the appropriate person expedites the information-gathering process. This practice also frees the receptionist to handle other calls.

[4]—Establishing Telephone Hours

The physician should establish precise telephone hours for the staff, giving them explicit direction as to when it is acceptable to turn the phone over to the answering service.

Determining the peak and slow phone times will allow the physician to staff the phone accordingly. It may be unreasonable to expect one person to adequately handle all the incoming calls at peak periods; alternatively, it may not be necessary to have more than one person covering the phone during slower periods. By keeping track of the volume of phone calls during various periods of the day, patterns of use can be easily discerned.

One tip in establishing phone hours is to avoid turning the telephones over to the answering service during lunch hours. Although this practice may be convenient for the office staff, it can be bothersome for the patient and translate as poor public relations. Many patients find the lunch hour the only time during the business day when they can confidentially and appropriately handle personal business. Having their call referred to an answering service can be frustrating and annoying. The physician should consider implementing a rotating lunch hour for the staff, so that someone will be present to take incoming calls during the lunch period. Another tip is to consider establishing specific times for patients to call in and speak with the physician.

[5]—Answering Service

The answering service is perceived as an extension of the medical office, and as such, it is important that care is given to selecting a quality answering service. In addition, it is important to monitor the answering service to make sure that they are courteously and efficiently handling calls. The answering service is best checked by the physician calling the number, identifying himself or herself as a patient with a problem and evaluating how the call is dealt with.

Specific protocols and directions on how you desire your calls to be handled should be given to the answering service. Typically, answering services retain their records for 90 days. The physician should request copies of all messages to keep in his or her files and review them to ensure that all calls were properly followed up on.

§ 18.08 Accounts Receivable and Risk Management

> To ensure that patients pay their fees, billing procedures should be spelled out in detail. Patients should be informed in advance of the cost of outside diagnostic pr ̱edures or consultations. Consent should be secured to release necessary records to the

> patient's insurance company. Every effort should be made to collect the bill from nonpaying patients before they are discharged from medical care.

Many people perceive the cost of medical services to be unreasonably high. The more ambiguous the office payment policy, the greater the chances the physician will not be compensated for his or her services. This puts the patient and the physician in an awkward relationship and can only increase the chances of poor compliance with medical treatment.

A patient's fulfillment of his or her financial obligation to the medical office should be viewed as part of his or her commitment to sustaining the physician-patient relationship. In developing a strong, clear policy to provide financial restitution for the provision of medical service, the medical office removes an obstacle to this relationship.[13]

[1]—Policy for Billing and Collection of Patients Accounts

A patient information brochure that explains the billing policies assists the patient in developing a clear understanding of his or her responsibilities. This policy should be developed with the physician's values taken into consideration.[14] Included in the development of any financial policy is the patient's right to confidentiality, which extends to medical bills. For this reason, the patient should be asked to sign a release that allows the practice to discuss the patient's account with the insurance carrier.

[2]—Method of Payments Accepted

Many medical offices now accept payment by credit cards. If the physician's office offers this service, this information should be included in the patient information brochure.

[3]—Explanation of Fees

The billing policy should address the fees for services provided. When diagnostic services are arranged, it is a courtesy to notify

---

[13] *See also* chs. 7 and 10 for further information on accounts receivable management, credit and collections.

[14] *See also* ch. 7 for instructions on how a medical office should develop its billing policy.

the patient in advance of the cost for those services. This goes along with informed consent of alternatives available.

[4]—Insurance Processing Policy

The establishment of a third-party policy is an integral part of the billing policy. If the medical office agrees to accept assignment for medical services, it must bear in mind that it will need an experienced person to process the insurance information. Most insurance forms contain a 'release of confidential information' line that the patient must sign to facilitate processing of the claim. In the case of electronic claims transmission, a release must be kept on file and updated regularly.

[5]—When the Patient Refuses to Pay the Bill

Many physicians are uncomfortable with the financial side of their medical practice and prefer to stay remote from it. However, a patient's refusal to pay a bill may indicate a disgruntled patient who is contemplating filing a malpractice suit against the doctor. Collection policies should include a requirement for physicians to review all records of patients who refuse to pay their bill. The physician at that time can make the decision as to the next action needed. It would be prudent for the physician to review the medical record at that time to make sure proper documentation regarding the case is included in the chart.

[6]—Discharging a Patient for Nonpayment

Prior to discharging a patient from the practice for nonpayment for services, the collection policy must be utilized. Documentation is needed to establish that attempts were made to work with the patient to remedy the past-due account. Prior to discharge from the practice, a certified letter contact should be attempted. If no response is obtained, the physician should review the patient record and then dictate a letter informing the patient of his or her intention to discharge the patient from medical care based on noncompliance with billing agreements.

§ 18.09 Personnel

An office policy manual should be created, and employees should be instructed to refer to it. Job descriptions should be written so employees know the full scope of the duties expected of them. Employees should be licensed for the type of duties they perform, and all office staff should be instructed in CPR technique. Personnel training can be reinforced through continuing education classes and office meetings.

Professional liability extends to the employees within the organization.[15] A common mistake physicians make is placing greater importance on the cost of an employee than on the skills and licensure the employee offers. An inexpensive, unskilled, improperly trained or disgruntled employee can create liability for a medical practice. In the long run, this will cost the medical practice substantially.[16]

There are a number of areas related to personnel issues where physicians can reduce their medical liability.

[1] — Policy Manual

Very few physicians have the time to train their employees in proper procedures. The well-organized office has a policy manual that identifies key policies for the employee. New employees should be required to study the policy manual and subsequently offered the opportunity to ask any questions.

Preparing the policy manual can be time consuming and expensive, as it may necessitate the employment of many medical management consultants. However, although the initial cost of the manual may be high, it is reduced with each use. Once the office establishes an office policy manual, it should be reviewed annually or at least on a regular basis.[17] (*See Appendix 18-C.*)

[2] — Training Programs

Once the medical practice has developed its policy manual, the practice needs to offer a training program to assure that the policies will be implemented. The office manager is usually assigned this task. Care should be taken to ensure that whoever

---

[15] *See also* J. Taraska, Legal Guide for Physicians, ch. 4 (Matthew Bender 1988) for additional information regarding the physician's vicarious liability for acts committed by those in the physician's employ.

[16] *See also* J. Taraska, Legal Guide for Physicians, ch. 15 (Matthew Bender 1991) for a legal guide for the physician's office staff.

[17] *See also* ch. 2.

offers the training is familiar with the policies of the practice and that he or she has the necessary hands-on experience.

[3] — Professional Licensure

The better trained the personnel, the less the medical office needs to expend energy training employees. Medical offices often hire licensed personnel to assist the physicians. It should be required that they maintain proper licensure as part of their employment agreement.

[4] — CPR Certification

All medical office employees should maintain CPR certification. Most professional licensing agencies require that CPR certification be current as a prerequisite to renewing a practice's license. However, administrative personnel are many times overlooked. Since patients who might develop a cardiac or respiratory crisis frequently appear in the office, it is sound practice to require that all personnel be certified. The American Heart Association and the Red Cross both offer classes regularly and will provide group certification for the office.

[5] — Personnel Manual and Job Descriptions

The medical office should have a personnel manual available for employees that includes a job description for each position. When developing the manual, the office should consult a professional who is knowledgeable in the areas of personnel laws and regulations. Employees need to understand not only the scope of the policies in the medical office but also their own position.

Having a manual reduces poor job performance and misunderstandings. Having job definitions assures that all the tasks in the office are completed because someone is accountable for performing these tasks.[18]

[6] — Staff Meetings

Every organization, regardless of size, needs to have time set aside for the employees to come together to discuss the practice. Staff meetings should follow the protocol of standard business

---

[18] *See also* ch. 2.

meetings to prevent them from deteriorating into gripe or gossip sessions.

Staff meetings are an excellent opportunity to evaluate the operations of the organization and come up with solutions to problems that may arise. A copy of both the personnel manual and the office policy manual should be present at all meetings.

§ 18.10 Equipment

> **Employees should be trained to operate office equipment by manufacturer's representatives and checked periodically to ensure that they follow manufacturer's guidelines. Records of equipment maintenance, servicing and cleaning should be kept in the office for updating.**

All equipment must kept current and operational. Diagnostic equipment needs to be kept in tiptop condition, since proper diagnosis depends on accurate test results. The requirements of the Clinical Laboratory Improvement Act require that a log be kept for all equipment to ensure that it is tested periodically. Medical staff should be familiar with the proper use of the equipment as recommended by the manufacturer.

[1]—Maintenance Records

Maintenance contracts on equipment should be retained in the office files. Maintenance agreements should include timely inspections of the equipment by a trained manufacturer's representative. Allowing anyone other than a trained representative of the manufacturer to service the equipment is highly discouraged.

Maintenance records need to be kept at the office in the event any questions arise. Regular maintenance should include the proper cleaning of machines. Any equipment that has parts that are subject to excessive wear and tear should be replaced regularly. Cleaning should include dusting the areas around the machine. No practice wants to be sued because a patient received an electrical shock due to damaged or faulty wiring. (*See Appendix 18-D.*)

[2]—Calibration Records

Diagnostic equipment needs to be calibrated at regular intervals as specified by the manufacturer and governing agency. Run controls daily to guarantee that equipment is properly calibrated. The service and calibration records should be kept near the machine.

[3]—Staff In-Service Records

When equipment is installed in the office, all personnel who will use the equipment should receive proper training. When determining the equipment to purchase, it is important to secure "in-service"—manufacturer representative training of employees—as part of the purchase agreement.

In-services should be carried out in such a way that employees understand the full operation of the equipment. Periodic reviews are necessary to ensure that employees do not stray from the manufacturer's recommend procedures. Routine evaluation of employees assures that any breaks in proper procedure will be corrected in a timely fashion.

[4]—Cleaning and Disinfecting Equipment

Equipment should be cleaned frequently, using the manufacturer's recommended cleaning agents. Chemicals or cleaning agents other than those recommended by the manufacturer can cause damage to the equipment. Disinfection of the equipment should follow infection control standards. Records documenting cleaning should be maintained with the repair and maintenance records.

§ 18.11 General Quality Assurance Recommendations

The following guidelines are offered to the physician as general recommendations for minimizing liability risk in the medical office:

(1) Be sure that every procedure you perform falls well within the standard of care. Remember that specialty procedures require specialty education, specialty training and specialty experience and are measured against the national specialty standard.

(2) If you are not experienced in a necessary procedure, refer the patient to someone else in the office with the

appropriate experience, even if it is another physician within your own specialty.

(3) Accurate and complete records are a must.

(4) A good peer review system should be in place in your office to ensure that all staff members are up to date and performing at acceptable levels.

(5) Make sure all staff members report adverse incidents. You must determine the underlying causes and take corrective action.

(6) Whenever possible, try to arrange office visits. It is very difficult to communicate accurately and completely with a patient over the telephone.

(7) Make your prescriptions clear. Pharmacist's questions are normally intended to help, not hinder, good patient care.

(8) Stress can lead to physical, psychological or chemical impairment. This is a threat to your performance and that of your colleagues and staff. It should be assessed and controlled.

(9) Refresh your memory on the operation of complex and seldom-used equipment.

(10) Make sure you have a backup for vital equipment, supplies and people.

(11) Frequent and serious injuries occur regularly from improperly administered injections. Make sure you have teaching aids available to staff and visual charts for patients to see.

(12) Even good aseptic techniques during medical procedures cannot always prevent infection. However, failure to properly diagnose and treat those infections may make you liable.

(13) It takes very little effort to prevent the indefensible errors of writing on the wrong chart, reading wrong tests and treating the wrong patient. Whenever possible, implement a backup system.

(14) A third person should be present when examining a patient of the opposite sex, except in an emergency.[19]

§ 18.12 Handling Potential Litigation

No matter what steps a physician takes and no matter how competent and well run the office, he or she may be charged with professional malpractice. There are many documented cases of unwarranted charges of malpractice. Therefore, it is prudent to know what steps to take should you be officially charged with malpractice.

In order for the litigation process to begin, an incident must occur, attempts to remedy the situation must fail and the patient must contact an attorney. The following are often a prelude to litigation:

- patient complications;
- patient dissatisfaction;
- contact by an attorney;
- a formal request to obtain medical records;
- patient failure to keep scheduled follow-up visits; and
- patient failure to pay the bill.[20]

[1]—Actions to Take When a Claim Is Pending

If a liability claim seems imminent, you should take the following actions:

- Notify the insurance carrier.
- Avoid any direct contact or negotiation with the plaintiff (patient) or the plaintiff's attorney.
- Make contemporaneous written notes of all oral communications with the patient or the patient's family concerning the incident.
- Avoid casual discussion of the treatment of the patient with anyone except your attorney, who has a privileged

---

[19] *See also* ch. 8, Appendix 8–A, for further suggestions on how to avoid malpractice suits.

[20] *See also* J. Taraska, Legal Guide for Physicians, ch. 7 (Matthew Bender 1991) for a discussion of the anatomy of a malpractice suit.

client-attorney relationship. The attorney will advise you regarding contact with the professional liability insurance carrier.

- Review the details of the patient's records without making any changes in them. Any additional notes on the records should be indicated as such, with no attempt to make them appear as part of the original records.
- If records are requested, check with your attorney. If you must provide the records, always send copies, never originals, and then only after securing proper authorization for release of information.
- Save all correspondence regarding the incident in a separate file from the patient's medical record. You should include a list of all records that have been provided and all notes of oral communications concerning the incident.

[2]—Actions to Take When a Claim Is Filed

If a claim is actually filed against you, you should take the following steps:

- Immediately notify your insurance company.
- Deliver the summons.
- Prepare a thorough analysis of the case for your attorney, keeping in mind that materials used by the attorney in preparation for litigation are not subject to discovery by the plaintiff's counsel and are privileged information.
- Do not alter records in any way.
- Never send originals of records; always send copies, but only after appropriate releases have been prepared.
- Be a medical education resource for the defense team, since you are probably the most knowledgeable medical professional involved in the case.
- Cooperate with your insurance representative and attorney.
- Stay calm and level-headed.

[3]—Selecting a Defense Attorney

It is important that the physician do his or her best in selecting a competent attorney in the event of a malpractice claim. You should ponder the following questions before selecting a particular defense attorney:

- Has the attorney demonstrated competence?
- Does the attorney understand the medicine involved?
- Has the attorney handled malpractice cases successfully before?
- What type of reputation does the attorney have?
- Will the attorney be personally handling all the important aspects of the case?
- Does the attorney have a defense plan?
- Do you communicate well and feel comfortable with the attorney, and is he or she comfortable with you?
- Does the attorney have a possible conflict of interest?
- Is the attorney more concerned with the insurance carrier's interest or with your interest?
- Is this attorney's representation sufficient?

[4]—Helping the Attorney

You can help the defense attorney strengthen your defense by remembering the following points:

- Cooperate fully with the attorney and participate in your defense.
- Provide medical input; remember that the attorney is a layperson, not a physician.
- Provide the attorney with a written chronological summary of the incident.
- Review your treatment rationale with your attorney and compare it with alternative treatments. Discuss the pros and cons of the various possible treatments.
- Review with your attorney the possible need for visual aids and exhibits and provide assistance in obtaining them.

- Act as a resource in identifying noted experts, when requested.
- Never withhold any pertinent information from your attorney. If you are not certain whether something is pertinent, discuss it with your attorney.
- Assist with the jury selection if asked.[21]

[5]—What to Expect from the Attorney

There are certain things you should expect from a defense attorney. He or she should:

- Keep you informed about litigation procedures.
- Explain the significance of each stage of the proceedings.
- Thoroughly prepare you for your role in the proceedings.
- Carefully investigate and prepare the case by deciding strategy, tactics and means to defend you.
- Evaluate all the factors that could win or lose the case for the defense, for example:

    (1) status of medical records;

    (2) gravity of the injury and potential loss;

    (3) appearance and credibility of the plaintiff, defendant and expert witnesses;

    (4) ability and experience of the plaintiff's attorney;

    (5) trial judge assigned to the case;

    (6) locale in which the case is to be tried;

    (7) caliber of the jurors; and

    (8) track record of similar cases in your jurisdiction;

- Advise you on matters such as court appearance and manner as well as the importance of dress, demeanor and communication skills.

---

[21] *See also* J. Taraska, Legal Guide for Physicians, ch. 15 (Matthew Bender 1991) for tips on how to help your attorney prepare your defense.

[6]—Making a Settlement

If a potential fore-settlement comes into play, you will need to determine whether it is in your best overall interest to make a settlement. Do not allow emotions to affect your thinking process.

Settling a case has benefits for everyone, such as the following:

- The judge wants to clear the calendar and dispose of cases quickly. He or she may require the parties to participate in a pretrial settlement conference.
- The insurance carriers are eager to settle the claim in order to limit defense costs, establish a fixed sum for payment and avoid the uncertainty of a jury verdict.
- The plaintiff's attorney considers a settlement a victory. It assures compensation for the client and for his or her time and effort.
- The plaintiff benefits from a settlement because it assures compensation for any damages and avoids further delay and the uncertainty of a verdict.
- The physician and defense attorney may appreciate a settlement because it avoids the uncertainty of a jury verdict, avoids the potential of the verdict exceeding insurance coverage and eliminates a further commitment of time and energy to a litigation process.

In making the decision whether to settle, you should consider the evidence of the case:

- Are there any missing medical records or unavailable witnesses?
- Are the records illegible or altered?
- What is the opinion of the expert witnesses?
- Will the expert witnesses in the aggregate support the physician or the plaintiff?
- What are the amount of damages the plaintiff has sustained and the potential amount of the verdict?
- How much money is required to reach the settlement?
- What is the physician's willingness to go to trial and what is the attitude of the plaintiff?

Settlement will depend on all the parties coming together and assessing the incident. If you are found to be at fault, settlement is recommended to expedite the process. If you, your insurance company and your defense attorney decide to fight the claim, the final outcome will be decided by the trial.

§ 18.13 Managing Professional Liability Checklist

A comprehensive checklist is provided for items to consider when safeguarding against professional liability.

____Medical Records

    ____Organized chronologically

    ____Legible

    ____Alterations initialed and dated

    ____Documentation

        ____History and physical

        ____Presenting complaints and treatment rendered

        ____Clinical findings

        ____Current vital signs

        ____Consultations

        ____Outside communications

        ____Diagnostic test results

    ____Follow-up system

        ____Patient test results

        ____Future appointments

    ____Records release

        ____Informed consent form

____Communication

    ____With patient

        ____Explanation of treatment

        ____Avoiding being abusive

        ____Restraint in criticism of staff or colleagues

    ____With family

____With staff or health care team members:

    ____Protocol for listening to patient complaints

    ____Instruction of staff in limitations of their duties

____Medication Procedures

    ____Patient record

        ____Patient drug history

        ____Drug allergy documentation

        ____Explanation of side effects

        ____Follow-up reviews of medications

    ____Office procedures

        ____Protocol for refill policies

        ____Legible, unalterable prescriptions

        ____No prescription refills by telephone

        ____Inventory of medications on supply

        ____Rule that unlicensed staff cannot prescribe medications

____Treatment and Procedures

    ____Informed Consent

        ____Diagnosis

        ____Nature and purpose of treatment plan

        ____Possible alternatives

        ____Prognosis if treatment is not provided

    ____Contributory Negligence

        ____Record of appointments canceled by patient

    ____Record of treatment provided

    ____Duty to supply patient with preoperative and postoperative information

    ____Documentation of discharge instructions and medications prescribed

    ____Diagnostic Procedures

    ____Attendance to sanctioned guidelines for specific procedures

____Qualified personnel only permitted to perform diagnostic procedures

____Continuing education classes for office staff

____Periodic checkup to ascertain that correct protocols are followed

____Record of all procedures in diagnostic log

____Patient Rapport

____The following areas should be considered as means for improving patient satisfaction with medical care:

____Office hours

____Patient flow

____Waiting area

____Educational materials

____Refreshments

____Entertainment

____Information packets

____Recall systems

____Releasing noncompliant patients from medical care

____Telephone

____Fixed staff phone hours

____Routing system for calls

____Answering service for off-hour calls

____Avoidance of treatment over telephone

____Clear instruction to staff limiting advice that can be given over the telephone

____Financial Management

____Policy for billing and collection of patient accounts

____Procedure for explaining fees and acceptable methods of payment

____Informed consent to release patient records to insurers

____System for collecting bills

____System for discharging patients for noncompliance

§ 18.100 MANAGING YOUR MEDICAL PRACTICE

____Personnel
    ____Office policy manual
    ____Written job descriptions and duties
    ____Confirmation of professional licensure
    ____Training of office staff in CPR techniques
    ____Continuing education classes for staff
    ____Office meetings to discuss and reinforce office policy
____Equipment
    ____Maintenance records
    ____Calibration records
    ____Staff in-service records
    ____Cleaning and disinfecting records

§ 18.100 Bibliography

Ankerholtz, Donald L.: Patient Recalls: Are You Overlooking Your Most Valuable Asset? Physician's Management Magazine, October 1988, pp. 59–68.

Brooten, Kenneth E., Jr., and Chapman, Stu: Establishing Effective Patient Relationships. Physician's Management Magazine, May 1987, pp. 203–237.

Committee on Professional Liability, American College of Surgeons: Professional Liability: A Blueprint for Reform. American College of Surgeons Bulletin 71(3), March 1986.

DeKornfeld, Thomas J.: Medical Records: Backbone of Malpractice Prevention. Physician's Management Magazine, Feb. 1987, pp. 163–170.

Department of Professional Liability of the College of Obstetricians and Gynecologists: Litigation Assistant. American College of Surgeons Bulletin 72(5), May 1987.

Garr, David Ross, et al.: Medical Malpractice and the Primary Care Physician. Southern Medical Journal 79(10): 1280–1284, Oct. 1986.

Gregory, Dorothy Rasinski: Risk Management in Practice. American Society of Internal Medicine, ASIM Publication No. 353, R12/90:5M.

Lancaster, Ralph I.: How to Minimize Your Malpractice Risks. Physician's Management Magazine. June 1988, pp. 75–89.

Practice and Liability Consultants and Professional Management Concepts: Improving Telephone Skills, Scheduling Techniques and Patient Relations. Seminar, Alameda Contra Costa Medical Association, Practice and Liability Consultants, 1990.

Smith, Jeannie: Client's Malpractice. Speech, Society of Medical/Dental Management Consultants, Charleston, SC. Dec. 2, 1988.

Wright, Richard E., and Gaudiosi, Thomas S.: A Management-Oriented Program Implemented Through the Medical Director's Office. Quality Review Bulletin 7:10–12, July 1981.

APPENDIX 18-A
Policy Proposal for Prescription Refills

Issue:

Medication refills without benefit of office visit.

Recommendation:

Require periodic office visits to monitor the patient's condition. This approach addresses case management issues, quality assurance needs and cost/care issues and reduces potential for liability concerns.

Steps for Resolution:

(1) When patients request a refill for medication that was ordered by a physician who is not a member of this practice, refer them back to the prescribing physician.

(2) Keep two-part prescription pads in nurses' office and with doctors. (Avoid leaving them in exam rooms.) Place the second part of the prescription in the patients' chart.

(3) Plan refills to last until the next scheduled visit.

(4) A canceled appointment can prompt a refill call-in. Provided that the appointment is rescheduled, the refill should last only until the next appointment. The patient should understand that additional refills will not be made available until the next appointment.

(5) An office examination is required to refill a prescription for patients not seen in the last six months.

(6) Patients on pain medications, especially narcotics, should be assessed every three months.

(7) Patients who are being followed as a result of work-related injury or auto accident should be seen every six weeks until the case is resolved.

(8) Patients suspected of abusing medication qualify as high risk and should be monitored every four weeks.

(9) Call-in requests for refills act as a prompt to check the patient's chart for a scheduled appointment time. Schedule an appointment if this has not already been

done. Note the scheduled appointment on the front of the chart for prescribing doctor's review.

(10) Inform patients that the office practice is to call refills in to the pharmacy by the day's end. Suggest that the patient contact the pharmacy to confirm readiness of medication before pickup. Secure the patient's daytime phone number in the event a question should arise.

(11) After-hours refill requests are to be assessed for level of emergency by the on-call doctor. Emergency refills can be ordered to cover a 48-hour (72-hour for weekends) period. Redirect nonemergency calls by requesting that the patient contact the office the next business day. Inform all patients that the office contact will allow for a chart and appointment check. Note instructions given in the telephone log for office follow-up.

(12) Patients should understand that continued care is dependent upon compliance with the prescribed medical regimen.

APPENDIX 18-B

Medication Supplies Control Form

This form, or one similar to it, is designed to be used both as a checklist and as a way to measure monthly supply usage and cost. Minimums and maximums should be set by the person responsible for stocking and ordering. This same stocking form may be used for the central supply closet. It should be turned in periodically to the administrator, who will review the minimums and maximums and assess monthly supply costs. The administrator will report monthly to the physician regarding supply cost and usage.

Monthly Medication Supplies Control Form

Date: _____

Room # _____

Vendor Name _____

Total Supply	Unit	Minimum	Maximum	Number	Needed
Tylenol	250 mg/tab	Company A 5	10	126643088	*21*
Advil	200 mg/tab	Company B 20/box	1 bx.	5678	*1 bx.*
Aspirin	250 mg	Company C 1 box	2 bx.	012345678	*1 bx.*
Penicillin	250 mg/box	Company D 20 tabs/box	10 bxs.	987654321	*2 bxs.*
Ampicillin	500 mg/tab	Company E 20 tabs/box	10 bxs.	012345678	*1 bx.*

APPENDIX 18-C

Outline for Policy Manual

Daily Policies and Procedures

    Procedures for Opening the Office
    Daily Medical Office Tasks
    Daily Maintenance of the Waiting Room
    Daily Preparation of Exam Rooms
    Exam Room Clean-up
    Patient Registration
    Daily Sign-in Sheet
    Patient Registration
    Consent for Treatment
    Medical Consent Form
    Patient Exit
    Handling Telephone Calls
    Telephone Call Action Chart
    Front Desk Coverage
    Handling Patients' Complaints
    Patient Complaint Form
    Medical Records
    Release of Medical Records
    Medical Records Release Form
    Filing System for Medical Records
    Inactive Medical Files
    Processing Prescriptions
    Patient Referral for Specialty Care
    Patient Referral for Specialty Care Form
    Reporting Lab and Test Results to Patients
    Laboratory Records
    Laboratory Records Form
    Stocking Medical Supplies
    Medical Supplies Control Form
    Equipment Records
    Visitors
    Alarm System
    Closing Office Procedure
    Appointment Scheduling
    Appointment Scheduling by Physician
    Hospital Admission and Scheduling

App. 18-C MANAGING YOUR MEDICAL PRACTICE 18–50

Surgical Posting
Surgical Posting Form
Dictation
Call-Back Recall/Tickler File

Front Office Patient Accounting Policies

General Cash Controls—Front Office
Cash Drawer at Front Office
Petty Cash Fund
Petty Cash Receipt
Handling of Mail and Deposits by the Receptionist
Deposit Transaction Sheet
Mail Log
Use of Check As Payment
Handling of Returned Checks
Sample Letter When Check Bounces
Use of Credit Cards As Payment
When No Cash Is Received
Patient Without Means of Paying
Collection Agency of Legal Collection Accounts
Collection Activity Summary
Policy Regarding Authorization for Write-offs
Form for Authorization of Write-offs
Obtaining Hospital Billing Information
Posting of Hospital Charges
Form for Posting Hospital Charges (front)
Form for Posting Hospital Charges (back)
Physicians' Weekly Report
Patient Account Statistics
Patient Account Statistics—Patient Census
Patient Account Statistical Report (Charges and Collections by Payor Class)
Patient Account Statistical Report—Aged Accounts
Payment Policy upon Patient Discharge
Treatment of Workers' Compensation Cases at the Practice
Workers' Compensation Form for Treatment at Physician's Office

APPENDIX 18-D

Equipment Records

Records on practice equipment must be maintained to keep up with maintenance schedules, to avoid paying for repairs when a machine is still under warranty and to help identify equipment in case of loss or theft. This information should be recorded regularly; sample forms for this purpose are provided here. Attach any warranty information to these forms.

Repair Record

Warranty Date and Parts Covered: _____

Date	Problem	Repair Performed	Other

A label containing an internal identification number should be attached to each piece of equipment. The administrator should maintain these records, and the physician should review them periodically.

Equipment Record Number: _____

Type of equipment_____
Vendor Name_____
Vendor Address_____
Telephone Number_____

App. 18-D   MANAGING YOUR MEDICAL PRACTICE   18–52

Manufacturer's Name_____
Trade Name_____
Date purchased ____/____/____   Cost $_____

SUPPLEMENTAL INDEX

Managing Your Medical Practice

Prepared by
Publisher's Indexing Staff

[This index pamphlet covers material in chapters 13, 14, 15, 16, 17 and 18.
Please consult main index for references to all other material.]

JANUARY 1992

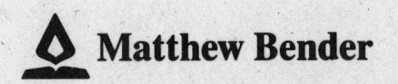

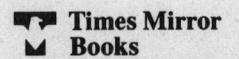

▲ Matthew Bender

Times Mirror Books

Copyright © 1987, 1988, 1989, 1990, 1991, 1992
By Matthew Bender & Company
Incorporated

All Rights Reserved
Printed in United States of America

MATTHEW BENDER & CO., INC.
EDITORIAL OFFICES
11 PEN PLAZA, NEW YORK, NY 10001-2006 (212) 967-7707
2101 WEBSTER ST., OAKLAND, CA 94612-3027 (510) 446-7100

(Matthew Bender & Co., Inc.) (Rel.6–Supp.Ind. Pub.372)

SUPPLEMENTAL INDEX

[References are to Sections and Appendices.]

A

ACCOUNTANTS
Affiliated medical practices, role in (See AFFILIATED MEDICAL PRACTICES)

ACCOUNTING PRACTICES
Affiliated medical practices (See AFFILIATED MEDICAL PRACTICES)
Prepaid health care programs . . . 14.07[1]; Fig. 14-3

ACCOUNTS PAYABLE
Affiliated medical practices (See AFFILIATED MEDICAL PRACTICES)

ACCOUNTS RECEIVABLE
Affiliated medical practices (See AFFILIATED MEDICAL PRACTICES)
Front office accounting policies for . . App. 18-C
Professional liability arising from
    Acceptance of payment, methods of . . . 18.08[2]
    Billing policy as grounds . . . 18.08[1]
    Collection policy as grounds . . . . . . 18.08[1]
    Discharge of patient for nonpayment . . . 18.05[6]; 18.08[6]
    Fees, inadequate explanation of . . . . 18.08[3]
    Generally . . . 18.08
    Insurance policy processing . . . . 18.08[4]
    Payment policy, ambiguity of . . 18.08
    Refusal to pay, implications of . . . . . 18.08[5]

ADVERTISING AND MARKETING
Affiliated medical practices (See AFFILIATED MEDICAL PRACTICES)
Budget planning . . . 16.05[2]; Fig. 16-6
Checklist . . . 16.17
Communications between physician and patient . . . 16.15[1][b]
Coupons, use of . . . 16.12[4]
De-marketing, elements of
    Communications . . . 16.15[1][b]
    Generally . . . 16.15[1]
    Office environment . . . 16.15[1][c]
    Staff attitude . . . 16.15[1][c]
    Waiting periods . . . 16.15[1][a]

ADVERTISING AND MARKETING—Cont.
Development of marketing plan (See subhead: Planning)
Direct mail campaigns
    Efficacy of . . . 16.13
    Launching of campaign, guidelines for . . . 16.13[1]
    Preparation, guidelines for . . . 16.13
External marketing . . . 16.02
Generally . . . 16.01; 16.02; 16.12
Internal marketing . . . 16.02
Logos
    Elements of . . . 16.11[1]
    Generally . . . 16.11
    Preparation, guidelines for . . 16.11[1]
    Purpose of . . . 16.11[1]
Media analysis
    Generally . . . 16.05
    Goals and objectives, consideration of . . . Fig. 16-5
    Guidelines for choosing media . . . . . 16.05[1]
Negative marketing (See subhead: De-marketing, elements of)
Newsletters
    Content, guidelines for . . . 16.07
    Described . . . 16.07
    Format . . . 16.07; Fig. 16-7
Newspaper advertisements . . . 16.12[1]
Office environment . . . 16.15[1][c]
Patient education
    Audio tapes . . . 16.14[5]
    Consultations, guidelines for . . . . . . 16.14[1]
    Generally . . . 16.14
    Information cards . . . 16.14[2], [3]
    Instruction cards . . . 16.14[4]
    Note pads and pencils, distribution of . . . 16.14[5]
    Staff education, importance of . . . . . 16.14[7]
    Standardized materials . . . 16.14[3]
Physician-patient relationship
    De-marketing (See subhead: De-marketing, elements of)
    Education of patient (See subhead: Patient education)
    Follow-up visits, encouraging . . . . . . 16.15[3]
    Generally . . . 16.15
    Internal prospecting . . . 16.15[2]

[References are to Sections and Appendices.]

ADVERTISING AND MARKETING—Cont.
Physician-patient relationship—Cont.
    Waiting room resume, use of . . . . . .
      16.15[4]
Planning
    Budget planning . . . 16.05[2]; Fig.
      16-6
    Evaluation of marketing plan, methods
      for . . . 16.03[4]
    Generally . . . 16.03
    Goals and objectives, formulation of
      . . . 16.03[2]
    Implementation of protocol . . . . . .
      16.03[3]
    Media analysis (See subhead: Media
      analysis)
    Practice analysis . . . 16.03[1]; 16.03[2]
    Sample outline . . . Fig. 16-1
    Strategies, development of (See subhead:
      Strategies, formulation of)
    Targeting of market (See subhead: Tar-
      geting of market)
Practice brochure
    Described . . . 16.06
    Production guidelines . . . 16.06
Prepaid health care programs
    Restrictions on advertising of programs
      . . . 14.05[2]
    Sales presentation vs. actual contract
      terms . . . 14.06[6][e]
Professional relations, development of
    Complementary practices, referrals from
      . . . 16.16[1]
    Generally . . . 16.16
    Networking strategies . . . 16.16[2]
Public relations
    Feature articles
      Generally . . . 16.08[5]
      New developments in specialty, on
        . . . 16.08[5][a]
      Success stories . . . 16.08[5][b]
    Generally . . . 16.08
    Interviews . . . 16.08[3]
    News releases
      Content of . . . 16.08[2]; Fig. 16-9
      Generally . . . 16.08[2]; Fig. 16-8
      Preparation of, guidelines for . . .
        16.08[2]; Fig. 16-9
    Photographs . . . 16.08[4]
    Press kits . . . 16.08[1]
    Purpose of . . . 16.08
    Targets for . . . 16.08
Public speaking
    Booking of speaking engagements . . .
      16.09

ADVERTISING AND MARKETING—Cont.
Public speaking—Cont.
    Generally . . . 16.09
    Presentation guidelines . . . 16.09
    Speakers' kits . . . 16.09
    Targeting of audience . . . 16.09
    Visual aids, use of . . . 16.09
Purpose of . . . 16.01; 16.12
Radio advertising . . . 16.12[3]
Research
    Media analysis (See subhead: Media
      analysis)
    Practice analysis . . . 16.03[1], [2]
    Targeting research (See subhead: Target-
      ing of market)
Resources . . . App. 16-A
Signs . . . 16.11, [2]
Special events . . . 16.10; Fig. 16-10
Staff attitude, relevance of . . . 16.15[1][c]
Staff education . . . 16.14[7]
Strategies, formulation of
    Budget planning . . . 16.05[2]; Fig.
      16-6
    Channel of communication, choices re-
      garding (See subhead: Media analysis)
    Generally . . . 16.04
    Targeting (See subhead: Targeting of
      market)
    Type of practice, relevance of
      Generally . . . 16.05[1]
      Referral methods, differences in
        . . . 16.05[1]; Fig. 16-2
      Specialties . . . 16.05[1]; Fig. 16-3
Targeting of market
    Community analysis . . . 16.04[3]
    Generally . . . 16.04
    Identification of desired market . . . .
      16.05
    Patient profiles . . . 16.04[2]
    Service analysis . . . 16.04[1]
Television advertising . . . 16.12[3]
Waiting periods, shortening of . . . .
    16.15[1][a]
Yellow Pages advertising . . . 16.12[2]

AFFILIATED MEDICAL PRACTICES
Accountants
    Advisory team, working with . . . . . .
      13.07, [2], [7]
    Budgeting projections made by . . . . .
      13.07[4]
    Current practices
      Hidden assets and liabilities . . .
        13.09[6]
      Valuation, formula for . . . .
        13.07[8]

SUPPLEMENTAL INDEX

[References are to Sections and Appendices.]

AFFILIATED MEDICAL PRACTICES—
Cont.
Accountants—Cont.
  Economic benefits of services of . . . . 13.02[3], [7]
  Experience, effect of lack of . . . . 13.03[4]
  Qualifications of . . . 13.07[2]
  Reorganization, role in
    Additional costs, detecting . . . . 13.07[4]
    Advisory team, working with . . . 13.07[2], [7]
    Insurance coverage, assessing . . . 13.12
    Tax liability, avoiding . . . . 13.07[7]
    Type of organization, determination of . . . 13.07[5]
  Schedule, keeping to . . . 13.07
  Selection of . . . 13.01
Accounting practices
  Balance sheet (See subhead: Balance sheet)
  Cash flow . . . 13.07[3]
  Checkbook disbursements . . . 13.07
  Expenses and costs (See subhead: Expenses and costs)
  Initial considerations . . . 13.07[3]
  Purchases and purchasing (See subhead: Purchases and purchasing)
Accounts payable
  Check-writing system, establishing . . . 13.07, [3]
  Contributions of physicians . . . 13.07
  Current practices of candidates . . . . . 13.07, [8]
  Hidden assets in current practices, disposing of . . . 13.07
Accounts receivable
  Current practice accounts
    Access to . . . 13.07[9]
    Age . . . 13.07[6]
    Expense reports . . . 13.05[3]
    Third party accounts . . 13.07[6]
    True value, formula determining . . . 13.07
    Valuation of . . . 13.07, [6], [8]
  Reorganization
    Control, methods for . . 13.02[4]
    Standardizing bookkeeping methods . . . 13.07[6]
Advertising and marketing
  Advisory boards, agency executives serving on . . . 13.10[1]

AFFILIATED MEDICAL PRACTICES—
Cont.
Advertising and marketing—Cont.
  Attitudes of physicians toward . . . . . 13.03[7]; 13.04[1]
  Benefits of . . . 13.02[3]
  Business cards and letterheads, standardizing . . . 13.10[5]
  Generally . . . 13.03[3]
  Health care community, prior notice of opening to . . . 13.11
  Marketing executive as appropriate advisory board member . . . 13.10[1]
  Public relations, need for . . . 13.11
  Reputation of new group expanded by . . . 13.02[3]
  Resources for . . . 13.02[3], [9]
  Secrecy of negotiations conflicting with . . . 13.11
Antitrust regulations . . . 13.06[3]
Appointment scheduling
  Advisory board meetings, detailed schedules for . . . 13.10[1]
  Management controlling, attitude of physician toward . . . 13.04[1]
  Rotation of physicians
    Advertising and . . . 13.02[3]
    Attitude of physicians toward . . 13.10[2]
    Generally . . . 13.10
  Time management . . . 13.10[5]
Attorneys
  Advisory board of new entity, as member of . . . 13.10[1]
  Antitrust regulations, familiarity with . . . 13.06[3]
  Budgets, aiding in preparation of . . . 13.07[4]
  Business contracts of members, reviewing . . . 13.06[1]
  Claims against members, checking . . . 13.06[1]
  Contingent liabilities of old entities, evaluating . . . 13.06[1]
  Experience, effect of lack of . . . . 13.03[4]
  Generally . . . 13.01
  New members, assessing liabilities of . . . 13.06[1]
  Scheduling deadlines for . . . 13.07
  Tax liabilities of new entity, avoiding . . . 13.07[7]
  Valuation of current practices by . . . 13.07[8]

SUPPLEMENTAL INDEX

[References are to Sections and Appendices.]

AFFILIATED MEDICAL PRACTICES—Cont.
Balance sheet
    Budget projections, use in . . 13.07[4]
    Current practices, of
        Access to . . . 13.07[9]
        Accounts payable . . . 13.07
        Contingent liabilities . . 13.06[1]
Banks and banking
    Advisory board, bank president serving on . . . 13.10[1]
    Check writing systems, establishing . . . 13.07, [3]
    Loans of potential entities, investigating . . . 13.06[1]
Billing systems
    Pre-merger systems, evaluation of . . . 13.06[4]
    Standardizing . . . 13.10[6]
Bookkeeping systems
    Balance sheet (See subhead: Balance sheet)
    Budgeting (See subhead: Budgeting)
    Cash flow (See subhead: Accounting practices)
    Computerizing . . . 13.10[5]
    Current practices of candidates, evaluation of . . . 13.06[4]
    Purchases and purchasing (See subhead: Purchases and purchasing)
Budgeting
    Ancillary services, frequency of use of . . . 13.02[6]
    HMO contracts . . . 13.02
    Initial insurance expenses . . . 13.12
    Overhead budget . . . 13.03[3]
    Reorganized group, projections for . . 13.07[4]
Bureaucratic inefficiencies . . . 13.03, [3]
Buy-out agreements . . . 13.09
Buy-sell agreements . . . 13.09
Checklist . . . 13.14
Compensation or fee arrangement (See subhead: Fees)
Competition
    Critical care centers, competing with . . . 13.02[3]
    Emergency rooms, competing with . . 13.02[3]
Computer systems
    Assessing equipment of current practices . . . 13.06, [4]
    Bookkeeping systems . . . 13.10[5]
    Lease with computer company, potential liability of . . . 13.06[2]

AFFILIATED MEDICAL PRACTICES—Cont.
Confidentiality, provisions for . . . 13.07[9]
Consultants
    Accountants (See subhead: Accountants)
    Advisory board
        Function of . . . 13.10
        Sources of . . . 13.10[1]
    Attorneys (See subhead: Attorneys)
    Benefit consultant . . . 13.10[3]
    Business consultants . . . 13.10[1]
    Insurance advisor . . . 13.10[3]
    Justice Department and Federal Trade Commission as . . . 13.06[3]
    Management consultant . . . 13.07[8]
Contracts
    Binding agreement, premerger agreement as . . . 13.09
    Business contracts of current practices . . . 13.06[1]
    Buy-out agreements . . . 13.09
    Buy-sell agreements . . . 13.09
    Confidentiality, provisions protecting . . . 13.07[9]
    HMO contracts . . . 13.02
    Incorporated practice, employee agreements in . . . 13.10
    IRS scrutiny of . . . 13.09
    Noncorporate legal agreements 13.09
    Restrictive covenants . . . 13.08
    Shares and shareholders . . . 13.09
Control of individual physician
    Appointments, management control of . . . 13.04[1]
    Frustration, loss of control resulting in . . . 13.03[2]
    Initial consideration, as . . . 13.07[1]
    Joint ventures, in . . . 13.01[1]
    Membership in group, as factor in . . . 13.02[1]; 13.03[2]
    Risk, loss of control as . . . 13.03, [2]
Cost sharing
    Advantages of . . . 13.02, [9]
    Advertising and marketing campaigns, for . . . 13.02[9]
    Checking accounts . . . 13.07, [3]
    Equipment purchases, for . . . . 13.01; 13.02[9]
    Expenses, reducing . . . . . . 13.01[1]; 13.02[9]
    Generally . . . 13.01
    Initial considerations as to . . . 13.07
    Joint ventures, in . . . 13.01[1]
    Reorganization costs . . . 13.07[9]

SUPPLEMENTAL INDEX

[References are to Sections and Appendices.]

AFFILIATED MEDICAL PRACTICES— Cont.
Cost sharing—Cont.
    Unsuccessful merger . . . 13.07[9]
Credibility of organization . . . 13.02[2]
Credit and collection
    Contract provisions for . . . 13.07[9]
    Credit philosophy of physician . . . . . 13.04[1]
    Insurance companies, collecting from . . . 13.02[4]
    Liabilities of prior practice, entity responsible for . . . 13.07[9]
    Reorganization standardizing policies of . . . 13.10[4]
Employees
    Appointment to positions . . 13.10[4]
    Business professionals, selecting 13.01
    Chain of command, explaining . . . . . 13.10[4]
    Cost of living increases, implementing . . . 13.10[3]
    Duties of
        Redundant or overlapping duties, remedying . . . 13.06[4]
        Reorganization, following . . . . . 13.10, [4]
    Employee agreements . . . 13.10
    Expenses and costs . . . 13.05[3]
    Fringe benefits for . . . 13.10[3]
    Hiring and firing, as to . . . 13.03[2]
    Incorporated practice, employee agreements in . . . 13.10
    Job descriptions, drafting . . 13.06[4]; 13.10[3]
    Joint venture participation extended to non-medical personnel . . . 13.01[1]
    Performance evaluations, new systems for . . . 13.10
    Personnel policy, establishing . . . . . 13.10, [4]
    Selection of personnel . . . 13.01
    Terminating or reassigning redundant positions . . . 13.06[4]; 13.10[4]
    Valued employees of prior practice, protecting . . . 13.06[4]
    Wage scales
        Generally . . . 13.05[3]
        Maximum salary, promotions increasing . . . 13.10[3]
        Range of salaries, implementing . . . 13.10[3]
        Reorganization, adjusting levels following . . . 13.10

AFFILIATED MEDICAL PRACTICES— Cont.
Equipment
    Cost-sharing, benefits of . . . 13.01
    Generally . . . 13.03[3]
    Reduction of cost of . . . 13.02[3]
Expenses and costs
    Advisory board members, compensation of . . . 13.10[1]
    Ancillary services, of . . . 13.02[6]
    Arrangements for sharing (See subhead: Cost sharing)
    Benefits of affiliated practices, generally . . . 13.02, [6]
    Bureaucratic inefficiencies affecting . . 13.03[3]
    Compensation or fee arrangement (See subhead: Fees)
    Cost containment techniques . . . . . . 13.02[6]
    Cost sharing (See subhead: Cost sharing)
    Employee and staff wages . . 13.05[3]
    Equipment costs . . . 13.03[3]
    Excess expenses and costs . . 13.03[4]
    Facility cost . . . 13.02[3]
    Joint venture with hospital . . 13.02[1]
    Outside services
        Monitoring . . . 13.02[6]
        Research by outside advisers, effect of . . . 13.03[4]
    Overhead control, attitudes toward . . 13.04[1]l 13.05[3]
    Plan development, in . . . 13.05[3]
Fees
    Additional compensation, deriving . . 13.05[6]; 13.07[10]
    Advisory board members, compensation of . . . 13.10[1]
    Capitated fees
        Affiliated practices, meeting needs of . . . 13.07[10]
        Attitude of physicians toward . . 13.04[2]; 13.05[4]
        Evaluation of . . . 13.06[1]
        Fees for service compared . . . . 13.04[2]; 13.05[4]
    Distribution of profits . . . 13.07[10]; 13.09
    Extended hours, compensation for . . . 13.05[6]
    Generally . . . 13.01
    Incentive compensation, disadvantages of . . . 13.07[10]
    Insurance reimbursement laws . . . . . 13.03[5]

SUPPLEMENTAL INDEX

[References are to Sections and Appendices.]

AFFILIATED MEDICAL PRACTICES— Cont.
Fees—Cont.
    Management duties, compensation for undertaking . . . 13.07[10]
    Personal earnings, members' attitudes toward . . . 13.04[1]; 13.05[4]
    Planning for . . . 13.05[3]
    Primary care physician fees . . . . 13.05[3]
    Reimbursement systems . . . . 13.03[5]; 13.04[1]
    Specialist fees . . . 13.05[3]
    Uniform fee schedule, establishing . . . 13.05[3]
Financing
    Generally . . . 13.06[5]
    Joint ventures . . . 13.01[1]
    Office systems, current needs of 13.06
Health Maintenance Organizations (HMOs) (See subhead: HMOs)
HMOs
    Control of physician, loss of . . . . . . 13.03[1]
    Initial dealing with . . . 13.04[3]
    Pooling resources to establish HMO plan . . . 13.02[9]
    Self-insurers in . . . 13.02[4]
Hospitals and nursing homes
    Costs of, monitoring . . . 13.02[6]
    Direct employment of physician . . . . 13.03[1]
    Limitation of privileges as recent trend . . . 13.06[4]
    Privileges for all members at . . . . . . 13.06[4]
    Takeovers by . . . 13.03[1]
Incorporated practices, reorganizing as . . . 13.10
Indemnification of new entity . . . 13.07[9]
Initial considerations
    Attitudes of individual members . . . . 13.04[3]
    Compatibility of new members . . . . 13.04[1]
    Federal and state regulations, compliance with . . . 13.06[3]
    Specialties required . . . 13.07
Insurance companies
    Beneficiary in key person coverage, affiliated practice as . . . 13.12
    Credibility of affiliated entity . . 13.02
    Duplicate coverage, avoiding . . . . . . 13.10[3]

AFFILIATED MEDICAL PRACTICES— Cont.
Insurance companies—Cont.
    Joint venture with hospital establishing . . . 13.02[4]
    Malpractice insurance (See subhead: Malpractice insurance)
    PPGs, enhanced credibility of . . . . . 13.01[2]
    Premiums, obtaining control of . . . . 13.02[4]
    Professional liability insurance 13.12
    Profile changes . . . 13.10[6]
    Regulations imposed by, effect of . . . 13.03
    Reorganized entity, coverage of 13.12
    Self-insurers, affiliated members as . . 13.02[4]
Internists, joint ventures advantageous to . . . 13.01[1]
Joint ventures
    Advantages of . . . 13.01, [1]
    Binder limited to specific projects as benefit . . . 13.01[1]
    Expansion of practice as benefit of . . . 13.01[1]
    Generally . . . 13.01
    Hospital-physician venture, example of benefits for . . . 13.01[1]
    Involvement with more than one venture . . . 13.01[1]
    PPG as . . . 13.10
    Scope of . . . 13.01[1]
Malpractice insurance
    Access to policy of candidate . . . . . . 13.07[9]
    Assessment against previous practice, new entity liable for . . . 13.07[9]
    Disposal of candidate's paid insurance . . . 13.07[6]
    Hidden assets, prepaid malpractice insurance as . . . 13.07[6]
    Reorganized entity, coverage under . . 13.12
Management and management techniques
    Administration by in-house administrator, advantages of . . . 13.02[8]
    Attorneys, effect of inexperience of . . 13.03[4]
    Bureaucratic inefficiencies in large groups . . . 13.03, [3]
    Chain of command . . . 13.10[4]

SUPPLEMENTAL INDEX

[References are to Sections and Appendices.]

AFFILIATED MEDICAL PRACTICES—Cont.
Management and management techniques—Cont.
  Changes in, participants adjusting to . . . 13.01; 13.03[4]
  Delegating authority
    Advantages of . . . 13.02
    Business management, delegating . . . 13.02, [8]
    Compensation of physician undertaking managerial responsibilities . . . 13.07[10]
    Purchases and purchasing, for . . 13.10[7]
  Job descriptions, drafting . . . 13.06[4]
  Personnel policy, establishing . . . . . 13.10, [4]
  Productivity
    Meetings impeding . . . 13.03[3]
    Rotating physician/patient meetings . . . 13.02[3]
    Salary formula for increasing . . . 13.07[10]
  Risk, mismanagement as . . . 13.03[4]
Medicare and Medicaid regulations
  Control of individual physician (See subhead: Control of individual physician)
  Effect of, generally . . . 13.03
  Legality of affiliated practice, need to determine . . . 13.03[5]
  Reimbursement laws, need for review of . . . 13.03[5]
  Risk factor created by . . . 13.06[1]
Membership
  Attitudes of candidates for
    Affiliation, as to . . . 13.04[3]
    Compatibility with other members . . . 14.04[1]
    Control, loss of (See subhead: Control of individual physician)
    Generally . . . 13.05
    Goals of candidates . . . 13.05[5]
    Hours of work, number of . . . . 13.04[1]
    Life, attitudes toward . . . 13.05
    Personal attitudes . . . 13.05[7]
    Professional attitudes . . 13.04, [3]
    Quality of care . . . 13.05[1]
    Ratio of staff to physicians, attitude toward . . . 13.04[1]
    Work, attitudes toward . . . . . . 13.05[6]

AFFILIATED MEDICAL PRACTICES—Cont.
Membership—Cont.
  Commitment to group, restrictive covenants increasing . . . 13.08
  Future associate members, signed restrictive covenants influencing 13.08
  Generally . . . 13.05
  Liabilities of member . . . 13.04[1]
  Physician considerations, generally . . 13.02[1]
  Recruitment of members
    Business entanglements . . . . . . 13.06[2]
    Contingent liabilities . . 13.06[1]
    Issues to explore . . . 13.03
    Job descriptions . . . 13.06[4]
    Questionnaire . . . 13.06[1]
    Specialists . . . 13.07
  Selection of, basis for . . . 13.05
  Termination of employment in group . . . 13.09
Name of new entity
  Initial considerations as to . . . 13.07
  Reorganization, after . . . 13.10
Office systems
  Appointment schedules (See subhead: Appointment scheduling)
  Bookkeeping systems (See subhead: Bookkeeping systems)
  Generally . . . 13.01
  Reorganization, following (See subhead: Reorganization)
  Telephone systems (See subhead: Telephones and telephone use)
  Unification of . . . 13.07; 13.10[5]
Patients
  Announcement of merger by letter . . 13.11
  Charts and records of patients . . . . . 13.02[5]; 13.10[5]
  Confidence in new group, advertising fostering . . . 13.02[3]
  Costs and expenses per person, estimating . . . 13.02[6]
  Coverage arrangements of new entity . . . 13.06[4]
  Insurance plans
    Choices restricted by . . 13.02[1]
    Cost savings of . . . 13.02[1]
  Loyalty of
    Group loyalty, attempt to gain . . . 13.08; 13.10[2]
    Physician, to . . . 13.08

SUPPLEMENTAL INDEX
[References are to Sections and Appendices.]

AFFILIATED MEDICAL PRACTICES— Cont.
Patients—Cont.
    Patient relationships, changes in . . . . 13.02[1]
Payroll system and records
    Individual earnings of employees
        Generally . . . 13.10[3]
        Profit distribution . . . 13.07[10]
    Profit distribution . . 13.07[10]; 13.09
    Reorganized entity, needs of . . . . . . 13.07[10]
Physician practice groups (PPG's)
    Advantages of . . . 13.01[2]
    Case example . . . 13.01[2]
    Control of physician affected by patient surrender to . . . 13.03[1]; 13.03[1]
    Defined . . . 13.01[2]
    Generally . . . 13.01
Pooling resources (See subhead: Cost sharing)
Premises and facilities
    Duplicate facilities, eliminating . . . . 13.02[7]
    Equipment
        Cost-sharing, benefits of . . 13.01
        Generally . . . 13.03[3]
        Reduction of cost of . . 13.02[3]
    Space, reducing cost of . . . 13.02[3]
Profit
    Joint venture, potential profit increase in . . . 13.01[1]
    Reorganized entity, distribution of profits in
        Generally . . . 13.07[10]
        IRS scrutiny of . . . 13.09
Purchases and purchasing
    Bulk ordering . . . 13.02[7]
    Centralized purchasing
        Authorized member overseeing . . . 13.10[7]
        Cost savings, proper systems leading to . . . 13.10[7]
    Cost efficiency as primary goal of . . . 13.07[6]
    Discounts, vendors allowing . . . . . . 13.02[7]
    Disposing of pre-merger purchases . . 13.07[6]
Quality control
    Generally . . . 13.01
    Plan goals . . . 13.05[1]
    Potential members, attitudes of 13.05
Records and reports
    Accounts receivable records . . . . . . 13.07[9]

AFFILIATED MEDICAL PRACTICES— Cont.
Records and reports—Cont.
    Business records . . . 13.09[7]
    Contractual provisions . . . 13.09[7]
    Corporate records, reviewing . . . . . . 13.06[1]
    Dictation process, standardizing . . . . 13.10[5]
    Documents, availability of . . . 13.09
    Patient records . . . 13.02[5]; 13.10[5]
    Recall systems, standardizing . . . . . . 13.10[5]
    Routing slips, standardizing . . . . . . 13.10[5]
Reorganization
    Advisory boards, duties of . . 13.10[1]
    Agreements and contracts (See subhead: Contracts)
    Antitrust regulations . . . 13.06[3]
    Assessments against previous owner . . . 13.07[9]
    Incorporated practice, as . . . 13.10
    Initial problems . . . 13.06[3]
    Liabilities . . . 13.07[9]
    Plan, development of . . . 13.05 *et seq.*
    Profile changes . . . 13.10[6]
    Secretary of State, approval by 13.10
    Steering committee
        Appointment of . . . 13.07, [1]
        Valuating current practices . . . . 13.07[8]
    Tax liabilities . . . 13.07[9]
Retirement and pension plans
    Death of member
        Insurance coverage, absorbing cost of . . . 13.12
        Sale or transfer of stock . . 13.09
    Disabled member, providing for equitable sale or transfer of stock . . 13.09
    Fringe benefits . . . 13.10[3]
    Group life insurance . . . 13.02[7]
    Pension and profit sharing plans . . . . 13.02[7]
    Personnel benefits, integrating . . . . . 13.10[3]
    Reduced rates for group members . . . 13.02[7]
Risk factors
    Accountability of non-associated physician . . . 13.03[2]
    Bureaucratic inefficiencies . . 13.03[3]
    Business entanglements of new members . . . 13.06[2]

SUPPLEMENTAL INDEX

[References are to Sections and Appendices.]

AFFILIATED MEDICAL PRACTICES— Cont.
Risk factors—Cont.
    Contingent liabilities . . . 13.06[1]
    Control of individual physician, loss of . . . 13.03[2]
    Direct competition from hospitals . . . 13.02
    Generally . . . 13.01; 13.03
    Hospital takeovers . . . 13.03[1]
    Insurance regulations, effect of 13.03
    Mismanagement as . . . 13.03[4]
Risk management and insurance
    Claims against new members . . . . . . 13.06[1]
    Contingent liabilities of new members . . . 13.06[1]
    Diversification of risk . . . 13.01[1]
    Insurance coverage . . . 13.02[4]
    Loans from previous entity, divesting . . . 13.09
    Loss of member, absorbing costs of insurance coverage for . . . 13.12
    Malpractice insurance (See subhead: Malpractice insurance)
    Risk prevention
        Antitrust regulations, complying with . . . 13.06[3]; 13.10
        Joint ventures . . . 13.01[1]
        No-action letters, obtaining . . . . 13.10[2]
        Private or government lawsuits, avoiding . . . 13.10[3]
    Sale of stock, restrictions on . . 13.09
Shares and shareholders . . . 13.09
Specialists, care by
    Fees for . . . 13.05[3]
    Planning . . . 13.05[2]
    Referrals, insurance prohibitions on . . . 13.03[5]
    Required specialties . . . 13.07
    Type of specialty offered . . . 13.05
Taxation
    Advisors lacking experience, IRS and . . . 13.03[4]
    Contingent liabilities of new members . . . 13.06[1]
    Fiscal year, adopting
        Incorporated practice, in . . 13.10
        Initial considerations as to 13.07
    Liabilities resulting from reorganization . . . 13.07[9]

AFFILIATED MEDICAL PRACTICES— Cont.
Taxation—Cont.
    Noncorporate legal agreements, of . . . 13.09
Telephones and telephone use
    Current entities, belonging to . . 13.07
    Generally . . . 13.10
    Service contracts for . . . 13.10[8]
Type of affiliation
    Generally . . . 13.01
    Incorporated practice
    Joint venture (See subhead: Joint ventures)
    Physician practice group (PPG) (See subhead: Physician practice group (PPG))

AMERICAN MEDICAL ASSOCIATION (AMA)
Physicians Current Procedure Terminology (CPT) (See CPT)

APPOINTMENT SCHEDULING
Affiliated medical practices (See AFFILIATED MEDICAL PRACTICES)
Appointment cancellation, documentation of . . . 18.06[9]
Waiting periods, shortening of . . . . 16.15[1][a]

ATTORNEYS
Affiliated medical practices, role in (See AFFILIATED MEDICAL PRACTICES)
Prepaid health care programs, consultation prior to signing contract for 14.05; 14.06

AUDIT
Third party payer, by
    Coding patterns, deviations in 17.02
    Consultative services . . . 17.12
    Documentation required . . 17.02; Fig. 17-2
    Level of service, misuse of . . 17.11[2]

B

BANKS AND BANKING
Affiliated medical practices (See AFFILIATED MEDICAL PRACTICES)

BILLING SYSTEMS
Affiliated medical practices (See AFFILIATED MEDICAL PRACTICES)

SUPPLEMENTAL INDEX

[References are to Sections and Appendices.]

BOOKKEEPING SYSTEMS
Affiliated medical practices (See AFFILIATED MEDICAL PRACTICES)

BUDGETING
Advertising and marketing, budget planning for . . . 16.05[2]; Fig. 16-6
Affiliated medical practices (See AFFILIATED MEDICAL PRACTICES)

BUSINESS PLANNING
Prepaid health care programs . . . 14.02[2]; 14.04[6][a]

C

CODING SYSTEMS
Changes, proposals for . . . 17.01
CPT coding (See CPT)
Current Procedure Terminology (See CPT)
Determination as to use of . . . 17.01[2]
Generally . . . 17.01
HCPCS coding (See HCPCS)
Health Care Financing and Administrations Common Procedural Coding Systems (See HCPCS)
ICD-9-CM (See ICD-9-CM)
International Classification of Disease, 9th Edition, Clinical Modifications (See ICD-9-CM)
Sources of publications . . . 17.15 *et seq.*
Training and education in use of codes . . . 12.16

COMMUNICATION SKILLS (See OFFICE COMMUNICATION)

COMPUTER SYSTEMS
Affiliated medical practices (See AFFILIATED MEDICAL PRACTICES)
Prepaid health care programs, use in . . . 14.07[4]

CONFIDENTIALITY
Affiliated medical practices . . . 13.07[9]
Insurance company, release of information to . . . 18.02[10]; 18.08[4]
Medical bills, applicability to . . . 18.08[1]
Medical records
    Doctor-patient privilege . . . 18.02[10]
    Generally . . . 18.02[11]
    Patient's rights concerning . . . . 18.02[10]
    Release of records, guidelines for . . . 18.02[10]; 18.08[4]
Oral communication and . . . 18.03[1]

CONFIDENTIALITY—Cont.
Prepaid health care programs . . . . 14.06[6][d], [i]

CONSULTANTS
Affiliated medical practices (See AFFILIATED MEDICAL PRACTICES)
CPT coding for services
    Complex consultation . . . 17.12[5]
    Comprehensive consultation . . . . . . 17.12[4]
    Determination of code . . . 17.12
    Documentation, requirements for . . . 17.12
    Emergency room consultation . . . . . 17.04[5]
    Extended consultation . . . 17.12[3]
    Follow-up consultation . . . 17.12[6]
    Intermediate consultation . . 17.12[2]
    Level of service . . . 17.12
    Pathology consultation . . . 17.04[2]
    Psychiatric services . . . 17.04[8]
    Violation of . . . 17.12
    Visit by consultant . . . 17.12[1]
Prepaid health care programs
    Arrangements for consultants . . . . . . 14.04[7]
    Restriction of consultant services . . . 14.06[2][d]

CONTRACTS
Affiliated medical practices (See AFFILIATED MEDICAL PRACTICES)
Prepaid health care programs (See PREPAID HEALTH CARE PROGRAMS)

CPT
(See also HCPCS)
After-hours and holiday charges . . . . 17.04[16]
Allergy and clinical immunology . . . . . . 17.04[11]
Ancillary texts . . . 17.15[1]
Appendixes, content of . . . 17.09
Assistant surgeon modifier . . . 17.08
Case management services . . . 17.04[13]
Checklist . . . 17.17
Chemotherapy services . . . 17.04[12]
Claim forms; illustrative example . . . Fig. 17-3; 17-4
Concurrent care modifier . . . 17.08
Consulting services (See CONSULTANTS)
Critical care, codes for . . . 17.04[20]
Deleted codes . . . 17.03[3]
Echocardiography . . . 17.04[10]
Emergency room services . . . 17.04[5]

SUPPLEMENTAL INDEX

[References are to Sections and Appendices.]

CPT—Cont.
Format . . . 17.03[1]
Fraud and abuse allegations, prevention of . . . 17.02; 17.11[2]
Generally . . . 17.01; Fig. 17-1
Handling of specimen . . . 17.04[14]
Hospital care, codes for (See HOSPITALS AND NURSING HOMES)
Immunization . . . 17.04[6]
Indexes
    Purpose of . . . 17.09
    Relative value index (See subhead: Relative value index)
Injections
    Medical services, in conjunction with . . . 17.04[6]
    Surgical procedures, in conjunction with . . . 17.05[8]
Introduction to . . . 17.03[5]
Laboratory services (See subhead: Pathology and laboratory services)
Level of service
    Abuse of . . . 17.11[2]
    Brief service
        Generally . . . 17.11[2][b]
        Hospital charges . . . 17.04[1]
    Comprehensive service
        Generally . . . 17.11[2][f]
        Hospital charges . . . 17.04[1]
    Determination of . . . 17.11[2]
    Established patient defined . . 17.11[1]
    Extended service . . . 17.11[2][e]
    Generally . . . 17.11
    Intermediate service
        Generally . . . 17.11[2][d]
        Hospital charges . . . 17.04[1]
    Limited service . . . 17.11[2][c]
    Minimal service . . . 17.11[2][a]
    New patient defined . . . 17.11[1]
Location other than office, service provided at . . . 17.04[17]
Maternity care and delivery
    Generally . . . 17.05[9]
    Hospital charges . . . 17.04[1]
    Modifiers . . . 17.05[9]
    Unrelated conditions, care for . . . . . 17.05[9]
Modifiers, application of
    Explained . . . 17.08
    Letter to third party regarding . . Fig. 17-5
Multiple procedure modifier . . . 17.08
Notations, use of . . . 17.03[4]
Nursing home services (See HOSPITALS AND NURSING HOMES)

CPT—Cont.
Ophthalmology
    Comprehensive services . . . 17.04[9]
    Intermediate services . . . 17.04[9]
Organization of . . . 17.03
Orthopedic surgery . . . 17.05[7]
Pathology and laboratory services
    Generally . . . 17.07
    Individual chemistry and toxicology test . . . 17.07[2]
    Modifiers, application of . . . 17.08
    Multichannel tests . . . 17.07[1]
    Organization of sections . . . 17.07
    Surgical pathology and consultations . . . 17.07[3]
Preventive medicine . . . 17.04[7]
Professional component modifier . . 17.08
Prolonged services . . . 17.04[19]
Psychiatric care . . . 17.04[8]
Radiology services
    Anatomic groupings . . . 17.06
    Complete procedures . . . 17.06[1]
    Components of . . . 17.06[2]
    Interpretation of radiographs . . . . . . 17.06[1], [2]
    Miscellaneous procedures . . 17.06[6]
    Modifiers for . . . 17.08
    Types of . . . 17.06
Reduced services modifier . . . 17.08
Relative value index
    Conversion factor, computation of . . 17.13
    Development of . . . 17.01[1]
    Procedure, elements of . . . 17.13
Repeat procedure modifier . . . 17.08
Resource Based Relative Value Scale (RBRVS), importance of . . . 17.01[3]
Scope of cognitive services . . . 17.04
Sources of publication . . . 17.15
Supplies . . . 17.04[18]
Surgery
    Anesthesia by surgeon modifier 17.08
    Assistant surgeon modifier . . . 17.08
    Complex repairs . . . 17.05[5]
    Difficulties in coding . . . 17.05
    Grafts and flaps . . . 17.05[6]
    Incision of lesions . . . 17.05[4]
    Intermediate repairs . . . 17.05[5]
    Maternity care and delivery, surgery related to (See subhead: Maternity care and delivery)
    Microsurgery modifier . . . 17.08
    Minor procedures . . . 17.05[3]
    Modifiers, use of . . . 17.08

SUPPLEMENTAL INDEX

[References are to Sections and Appendices.]

CPT—Cont.
Surgery—Cont.
    Orthopedic surgery . . . 17.05[7]
    Preoperative procedures . . . 17.05[1]
    Repairs, categories of . . . 17.05[5]
    Separate procedure, what constitutes . . . 17.05[2]
    Simple repairs . . . 17.05[5]
    Surgical package . . . 17.05[1]
    Vascular injection procedures . . . . . 17.05[8]
Symbols used in . . . 17.03[2]
Third-party manuals, need for . . . 17.15[2]
Training and education, guidelines for . . . 17.16
Update of . . . 17.01[2]
X-rays (See subhead: Radiology services)

CREDIT AND COLLECTION
Affiliated medical practices (See AFFILIATED MEDICAL PRACTICES)
Inter-office communication affecting 15.01
Third parties, collecting from
    CPT coding (See CPT)
    Current Procedure Terminology (See CPT)
    HCPCS (See HCPCS)
    Health Care Financing and Administrations Common Procedural Coding Systems (See HCPCS)
    ICD-9-CM (See ICD-9-CM)
    International Classification of Disease, 9th Edition, Clinical Modifications (See ICD-9-CM)

CURRENT PROCEDURE TERMINOLOGY (See CPT)

D

DIAGNOSTIC PROCEDURES
Professional liability, avoidance of
    Checklist for laboratory practices . . . 18.05[8][a]
    Clinical Laboratory Impact Act (CLIA) of 1988 . . . 18.05[8][a]
    Diagnostic log . . . 18.05[8][c]
    Equipment
        Calibration records . . . 18.10[2]
        Clinical Laboratory Impact Act (CLIA) of 1988 . . . 18.05[8][a]
        Maintenance and maintenance records . . . 18.10[1]
        Sample forms for equipment records . . . App. 18-D

DIAGNOSTIC PROCEDURES—Cont.
Professional liability, avoidance of—Cont.
    Generally . . . 18.05[8]
    Guidelines for correct test procedures . . . 18.05[8][a]
    Radiological studies . . . 18.05[8][b]

DRUGS
Professional liability, avoidance of
    Allergy documentation . . . 18.04[1]
    Follow-up review of medications . . . 18.04[3]
    Generally . . . 18.04
    Instruction on use of medication . . . . 18.04[2]
    Patient response to medication, documentation of . . . 18.02[7]; 18.04[3]
    Prescriptions
        Difficulties arising from . . . . . . 18.04[5]
        Documentation of . . 18.02[3], [7]; 18.04[3]; 18.05[7]
        Policy proposal for prescription refills . . . App. 18-A
        Refill policies, adoption of protocol for . . . 18.04[4]
        Side effects, warnings as to . . . . 18.04[2]
    Side effects, warnings as to . . 18.04[2]
    Staff, administration of drugs by . . . . 18.04[5]
    Supplies control form . . . App. 18-B
    Vital signs and patient's stated affect, documentation of . . . 18.04[3]

E

EMPLOYEES
Affiliated medical practices (See AFFILIATED MEDICAL PRACTICES)
Coding systems, education and training concerning . . . 17.16
Communication with (See OFFICE COMMUNICATION)
Consolidated Omnibus Budget Reconciliation Act of 1986, applicability of . . 2.09
Education and training of
    Coding systems, use of . . . 17.16
Patient's relationship with staff (See PATIENT-STAFF RELATIONS)
Policy manual, outline for
    Daily policy and procedures . . . App. 18-C
    Front office accounting policies . . . . App. 18-C

SUPPLEMENTAL INDEX

[References are to Sections and Appendices.]

EMPLOYEES—Cont.
Policy manual, outline for—Cont.
    Generally . . . 2.04; Fig. 2-4; 18.09[1]
    Modification of policy, reservation of rights regarding . . . 2.04
    Prescription refills, policy proposal for . . . App. 18-A
    Termination, reservation of rights regarding . . . 2.04
Professional liability, avoidance of
    CPR certification, importance of maintaining . . . 18.09[4]
    Generally . . . 18.09
    Personnel manual, job descriptions contained in . . . 18.09[5]
    Policy manual, outline for (See subhead: Policy manual, outline for)
    Professional licensure, maintenance of . . . 18.09[3]
    Staff
        Meetings with, benefits of . . . . . 18.09[6]
        Preoperative information given by, supplementation of . . 18.05[4]
    Training programs . . . 18.09[2]
Staff, preoperative information given by, supplementation of . . . 18.05[4]
Telephones and telephone use (See TELEPHONES AND TELEPHONE USE)

EXPENSES AND COSTS
Affiliated medical practices (See AFFILIATED MEDICAL PRACTICES)

F

FEES
Affiliated medical practices (See AFFILIATED MEDICAL PRACTICES)
Explanation to patient, importance of . . . . 18.08[3]
Prepaid health care programs
    Anti-trust concerns in fee-setting . . . . 14.06[5]
    Change of fees, unilateral, by third party . . . 14.06[6][1]
    Fee-for-service practice, effect on . . . 14.01[1]
    Negotiated fees, cost reduction through . . . 14.07[4]

FINANCING
Affiliated medical practices (See AFFILIATED MEDICAL PRACTICES)

FORMS OF PRACTICE
Affiliated medical practices (See AFFILIATED MEDICAL PRACTICES)

FRINGE BENEFITS
Affiliated medical practices (See AFFILIATED MEDICAL PRACTICES, subhead: Employees)
Consolidated Omnibus Budget Reconciliation Act of 1986, under . . . 2.09

G

GROUP PRACTICES
Affiliated medical practices (See AFFILIATED MEDICAL PRACTICES)
Prepaid program established by group as alternative to third party . . . 14.04[1]

H

HCPCS
(See also CPT)
Ancillary texts . . . 17.15[1]
Checklist . . . 17.17
Claim forms; illustrative example . . . Fig. 17-3; 17-4
Coverage . . . 17.10
Described . . . 17.10[1]
Design of . . . 17.10
Generally . . . 17.01; Fig. 17-1
Modifiers
    Described . . . 17.10[2]
    Letter to third party regarding . . Fig. 17-5
Multiple patients, modifier used for . . . . . 17.10[2]
Procedural code change, modifier used for . . . 17.10[2]
Refractive state determination modifier . . . 17.10[2]
Single patient, modifier used for . . . . 17.10[2]
Sources of publication . . . 17.15
Technical component modifier . . 17.10[2]
Third-party manuals, need for . . . 17.15[2]
Training and education, guidelines for . . . 17.16

HEALTH CARE FINANCING AND ADMINISTRATIONS COMMON PROCEDURAL CODING SYSTEMS (See (HCPCS)

HEALTH MAINTENANCE ORGANIZATIONS (See HMOs)

[References are to Sections and Appendices.]

HIRING AND FIRING
Affiliated medical practices (See AFFILIATED MEDICAL PRACTICES, subhead: Employees)

HMOs
Affiliated medical practices (See AFFILIATED MEDICAL PRACTICES)
Capitated payments . . . 14.01[2][a]
Defined . . . 14.09
Economics of . . . 14.01[2][a]
Federal laws regulating . . . 14.05[1]
Fee-for-service practice, comparison with . . . 14.01[2][a]
Insurance replaced by . . . 14.01[2][b]
Limited liability of . . . 14.06[2][a]
Positive selection procedure . . . 14.09
Types of HMOs
    Exclusive contract . . . 14.01[2][a]
    Group model . . . 14.01[2][a]
    Independent practice model . . . . . . 14.01[2][a]
    Mixed models . . . 14.01[2][a]
    Nonexclusive contract . . . 14.01[2][a]
    Staff model . . . 14.01[2][a]

HOSPITALIZATION
CPT codes (See CPT)
Prepaid health care programs
    Arrangements for hospitalization . . . 14.04[7]
    Responsibility for hospital services . . 14.04[3][a]

HOSPITALS AND NURSING HOMES
Affiliated medical practices (See AFFILIATED MEDICAL PRACTICES)
CPT codes for services rendered by
    Brief service defined . . . 17.04[1]
    Comprehensive service defined . . . . . 17.04[1]
    Critical care . . . 17.04[20]
    Discharge from hospital, services related to . . . 17.04[3]
    Emergency room care . . . 17.04[5]
    Grouping of services . . . 17.04[4]
    Initial hospital care . . . 17.04[1]
    Intermediate service defined . . . . . . 17.04[1]
    Labor and delivery . . . . . . 17.04[1]; 17.05[9]
    Neonatal care . . . 17.04[1]; 17.05[9]
    Post-operative follow-up visits . . . . . 17.04[15]
    Psychotherapy . . . 17.04[8]
    Subsequent hospital care . . . 17.04[2]

HOSPITALS AND NURSING HOMES—Cont.
CPT codes for services rendered by—Cont.
    Visits by physician to nursing home (See subhead: Visits by physician to nursing home)
Diagnostic-Related Groups (DRGs), significance of . . . 17.01
HCPCS codes
    Visits by physician to nursing home . . . 17.10[2]
ICD-9-CM (See ICD-9-CM)
Visits by physician to nursing home
    CPT code for . . . 17.04[4]
    HCPCS code for . . . 17.10[2]
    Intermediate care facility, visits to . . . 17.04[4]
    Limitations on . . . 17.04[4]
    Nursing home, visits to . . . 17.04[4]
    Skilled nursing facility, visits to . . . . 17.04[4]
    Transitional care unit, visits to . . . . . 17.04[4]

I

ICD-9-CM
Adverse drug effects, causes of . . . . 17.14[1][c]
Ancillary texts . . . 17.15[1]
Checklist . . . 17.17
Claim forms; illustrative example . . . Fig. 17-3; 17-4
Digital characteristics of . . . 17.14[1][e]
Diseases and injuries . . . 17.14[1][b]
E Codes . . . 17.14[1][d]
Generally . . . 17.01; Fig. 17-1
Indexes
    Abbreviations used in . . . 17.14[2]
    Adverse drug effects, causes of . . . . . 17.14[1][c]
    Diseases and injuries, to . . 17.14[1][b]
    Injury and poisoning, external causes of . . . 17.14[1][d]
    Structure of . . . 17.14[1][b]
    Style of . . . 17.14[2]
    Use of . . . 17.14[1][b]
Injury and poisoning, external causes of . . 17.14[1][d]
Instructional notations . . . 17.14[5]
Organization of . . . 17.14[1]
Punctuation . . . 17.14[3]
Role of . . . 17.14
Selection of code . . . 17.14[1][e]
Sources of publication . . . 17.15

SUPPLEMENTAL INDEX 17

[References are to Sections and Appendices.]

ICD-9-CM—Cont.
Symbols . . . 17.14[4]
Third-party manuals, need for . . . 17.15[2]
Training and education, guidelines for . . . 17.16

INCORPORATED PRACTICES
Affiliated medical practices (See AFFILIATED MEDICAL PRACTICES)

INFORMED CONSENT
Requirements of . . . 18.05[1]
Staff, preoperative information given by, supplementation of . . . 18.05[4]

INSURANCE PLANS
Affiliated medical practices (See AFFILIATED MEDICAL PRACTICES)
CPT coding (See CPT)
Current Procedure Terminology (See CPT)
Diagnostic evaluations
    International Classification of Disease, 9th Edition, Clinical Modifications (See ICD-9-CM)
    HCPCS (See HCPCS)
Health Care Financing and Administrations Common Procedural Coding Systems (See HCPCS)
ICD-9-CM (See ICD-9-CM)
International Classification of Disease, 9th Edition, Clinical Modifications (See ICD-9-CM)
Procedural evaluations
    CPT coding (See CPT)
    HCPCS (See HCPCS)

INTERNATIONAL CLASSIFICATION OF DISEASE, 9th EDITION, CLINICAL MODIFICATIONS (See ICD-9-CM)

J

JOINT VENTURES
Affiliated medical practices (See AFFILIATED MEDICAL PRACTICES)

M

MALPRACTICE ACTIONS
Administrative failure giving rise to 18.01
Affiliated medical practices (See AFFILIATED MEDICAL PRACTICES, subhead: Malpractice insurance)
Clerical failure giving rise to . . . 18.01

MALPRACTICE ACTIONS—Cont.
Diagnostic procedures, liability arising from (See DIAGNOSTIC PROCEDURES, subhead: Professional liability, avoidance of)
Generally . . . 18.01
Litigation guidelines
    Attorney for defense
        Physician's expectations . . . . . . 18.12[5]
        Selection of . . . 18.12[3]
    Defense, physician's strengthening of . . . 18.12[4]
    Filing of claim, measures subsequent to . . . 18.12[2]
    Generally . . . 18.12
    Pending claim, handling of . . 18.12[1]
    Settlements
        Benefits of . . . 18.12[6]
        Evidence, review of . . . 18.12[6]
Medication, liability arising from (See DRUGS)
Prepaid health care plans
    Malpractice insurance, limitations on . . . 14.06[2][a], [3]
    Peer review causing action . . . . 14.06[3], [6][j]
Treatment, liability arising from (See TREATMENT)

MANAGEMENT AND MANAGEMENT TECHNIQUES
Affiliated medical practices (See AFFILIATED MEDICAL PRACTICES)
Communication skills (See OFFICE COMMUNICATION)

MARKETING (See ADVERTISING AND MARKETING)

MEDICAID
Affiliated medical practices (See AFFILIATED MEDICAL PRACTICES)
Blood drawing, reimbursement for . . . . . 17.04[14]

MEDICAL EQUIPMENT
Maintenance, records pertaining to (See RECORDS AND REPORTS)
Professional liability, avoidance of (See RECORDS AND REPORTS)

MEDICAL RECORDS
Confidentiality of (See CONFIDENTIALITY)
Defense against professional liability, records as
    Abbreviations, standardization of . . . 18.02[5]

(Matthew Bender & Co., Inc.)   (Rel.6–Supp.Ind. Pub.372)

SUPPLEMENTAL INDEX

[References are to Sections and Appendices.]

MEDICAL RECORDS—Cont.
Defense against professional liability, records as—Cont.
    Advice to patient, documentation of . . . 18.02[7]
    Allergies, documentation of . . . . 18.04[1]
    Alterations, prescribed methods for . . . 18.02[4]
    Clinical findings, recording of . . . . . 18.02[8]
    Complaints from patient, documentation of . . . 18.02[7]
    Confidentiality of records (See CONFIDENTIALITY)
    Consultants, coordination and documentation of . . . 18.02[9]
    Discharge instructions, documentation of . . . 18.05[6]
    Doctor-patient privilege . . . 18.02[10]
    Examination findings, documentation of . . . 18.02[3]
    Generally . . . 18.02
    Legibility of records . . . 18.02[2]
    Medical history of patient, documentation of . . . 18.02[6]; 18.05[3]
    Medication, records pertaining to (See DRUGS, subhead: Professional liability, avoidance of)
    Organization of records . . . 18.02[1]
    Procedures and treatment, documentation of (See TREATMENT, subhead: Professional liability, avoidance of)
    Release of, guidelines governing the . . . 18.02[10]
    Symptoms, documentation of . . . . . 18.02[7]
    Test results, documentation . . . . . . 18.02[13]
    Treatment rendered and response, documentation of (See TREATMENT)
    Vital signs, documentation of . . . . . 18.02[12]; 18.04[3]
Professional liability arising from
    Alteration of records . . . 18.02[4]
    Defense against (See subhead: Defense against professional liability, records as)
    Doctor-patient privilege, breach of . . 18.02[10]
    Inadequate documentation
        Allergies of patient, of . . . . 18.04[1]
        Examination findings, of . . . . . 18.02[3]

MEDICAL RECORDS—Cont.
Professional liability arising from—Cont.
    Inadequate documentation—Cont.
        Response to medication and treatment of . . . . . . 18.02[3], [7]; 18.04[3]; 18.05[3]; [7]
    Legibility of records . . . 18.02[2]
    Organization of records . . . 18.02[1]
    Patient's rights concerning medical records . . . 18.02[10]
    Release of records . . . 18.02[10]

MEDICARE
Accounts receivable
    Sample surgical disclosure letter . . . . Fig. 10-3A
Affiliated medical practices (See AFFILIATED MEDICAL PRACTICES)
Blood drawing, reimbursement for . . . . . 17.04[14]
Diagnostic coding of claims (See ICD-9-CM)
Elective procedures, HCPCS modifier used for . . . 17.08[2]
HCPCS modifier, use of . . . 17.10[2]
ICD-9-CM (See ICD-9-CM)
International Classification of Disease, 9th Edition, Clinical Modifications (See ICD-9-CM)
Laboratory services, payment for . . 17.07
Ophthalmological services, reimbursement for . . . 17.04[9]
Prepaid health care programs
    Federal laws on Medicare provisions . . . 14.05[1]
    Use of programs by Medicare . . . . . 14.01[1]
Resource Based Relative Value Scale (RBRVS), importance of . . . 17.01[3]
Second opinion consultation, billing for . . 17.12
Supplemental plan, defined . . . 14.09

MEDICATION (See DRUGS)

N

NURSING HOMES (See HOSPITALS AND NURSING HOMES)

O

OFFICE COMMUNICATION
Audience, analysis of
    Factors to be considered . . . 15.05
    Memory curve, effect of . . . 15.06

SUPPLEMENTAL INDEX

[References are to Sections and Appendices.]

OFFICE COMMUNICATION—Cont.
Audience, analysis of—Cont.
    Personality types, characteristics of
        Feeling personality . . . 15.05[5]
        Generally . . . 15.05[1]
        Intuitive personality . . . 15.05[3]
        Sensing personality . . . 15.05[4]
        Thinking personality . . 15.05[2]
Collection policies, effect on . . . 15.01
Consultative meeting (See subhead: Meetings)
Correspondence, formats of . . . 15.07[2]
Daily report; illustrative example . . . App. 15-A
Delegation meeting (See subhead: Meetings)
Efficiency, effect on . . . 15.01
Information meeting (See subhead: Meetings)
Instructional meeting (See subhead: Meetings)
Inter-office communications, failure to establish . . . 15.01
Managerial styles, description of
    Consult style . . . 15.04[3]
    Generally . . . 15.04
    Joint style . . . 15.04[4]
    Sell style . . . 15.04[2]
    Tell style . . . 15.04[1]
Marketing, importance in . . . 16.15[1][b]
Meetings
    Agenda
        Adherence to . . . 15.09[7][b]
        Items of . . . 15.09[6]
    Consultative meeting, purpose of . . . 15.09[2][a]
    Delegation meeting, organization and purpose of . . . 15.09[2][c]
    Duration of . . . 15.09[4]
    Environment, effect of . . . 15.09[4]
    Generally . . . 15.09
    Information meeting, form of . . . . . 15.09[2][d]
    Instructional meeting, organization of . . . 15.09[2][e]
    Leader, guidelines for
        Agenda, adherence to . . . . 15.09[7][b]
        Conclusion, scheduling of . . . . . 15.09[7][e]
        Conflicts, avoidance of . . . . . . 15.09[7][c]
        Consensus, directing toward . . . 15.09[7][d]
        Generalizations, evaluation of . . 15.09[7][c]
        Minority opinions, protection of . . . 15.09[7][c]

OFFICE COMMUNICATION—Cont.
Meetings—Cont.
    Leader, guidelines for—Cont.
        Minutes, recording of . . . . 15.09[7][f]
        Participation, means of insuring . . . 15.09[7][c]
        Productivity, means increasing . . . 15.09[7][a]
        Recorder, appointment of . . . . . 15.09[7][b]
        Vague statements, clarification of . . . 15.09[7][c]
    Notification of; illustrative example . . . App.15-C
    Participants
        Briefing of . . . 15.09[5]
        Involvement of . . . 15.09[7][c]
        Reporting back to . . 15.09[7][a]
        Selection of . . . 15.09[3]
    Planning for . . . 15.09[1]
    Presentation at (See subhead: Presentation)
    Purpose and objective of . . . 15.09[1]
    Recommendation meeting, organization of . . . 15.09[2][b]
    Time of . . . 15.09[4]
Memorandum; illustrative example . . App. 15-B
Message, structure of
    Direct approach . . . 15.06
    Indirect approach . . . 15.06
Objectives, formulation of . . . 15.03
Oral communications
    Forms of . . . 15.02[1]
    Memory curve, effect of . . . 15.06
Presentation
    Humor, introduction of . . . 15.08[3]
    Introduction to . . . 15.08[3]
    Issues to be considered . . . 15.08
    Memory curve, effect of . . . 15.06
    Objectives, outline of . . . 15.08[2]
    Planning for . . . 15.08[1]
    Stress, dealing with . . . 15.08[3]
    Subject, selection of . . . 15.08[1]
    Visual aids, use of . . . 15.08[2]
Professional liability, avoidance of
    Complaints, handling of . . . 18.03[7]
    Family, guidelines for communications with . . . 18.03[2]
    Generally . . . 18.03
    Hostile patient . . . 18.03[7]
    Oral communication, limitations on . . . 18.03[1]

SUPPLEMENTAL INDEX

[References are to Sections and Appendices.]

OFFICE COMMUNICATION—Cont.
    Patients, guidelines for communications with . . . 18.03[2], [5]
    Physicians, communication between . . . 18.03[6]
    Staff members, communication with . . . 18.03[5]
    Test results, notification of patient as to . . . 18.02[13]
    Written communication, guidelines for . . . 18.03[4]
  Receptivity, heightening of . . . 15.05
  Recommendation meeting (See subhead: Meetings)
  Referring physician, letter to . . . 15.07[2]; 16.16
  Telephones and telephone use (See TELEPHONES AND TELEPHONE USE)
  Written communications
    Advantages of . . . 15.07
    Editing of . . . 15.07[3]
    Format of . . . 15.07[2]
    Forms of . . . 15.02[2]
    Planning for . . . 15.07[1]
    Word processor, use of . . . 15.07[3]

OFFICE SYSTEMS
  Affiliated medical practices (See AFFILIATED MEDICAL PRACTICES)
  Prepaid health care programs . . . 14.04[4], [6][a]

P

PATIENTS (GENERALLY)
  Affiliated medical practices (See AFFILIATED MEDICAL PRACTICES)
  Education of patient, importance of (See ADVERTISING AND MARKETING)
  Marketing concerns (See ADVERTISING AND MARKETING)

PATIENT-STAFF RELATIONS
  Professional liability, avoidance of
    Appointment cancellation, documentation of . . . 18.06[9]
    Generally . . . 18.06
    Guidelines for communications with patients . . . 18.03[2], [5]
    Information packets, providing patients with . . . 18.06[7]
    Office schedules, convenience of . . . . 18.06[1]
    Patient flow, expedience of . . 18.06[3]
    Recall system, patient tracking through . . . 18.06[8]

PATIENT-STAFF RELATIONS—Cont.
  Professional liability, avoidance of—Cont.
    Release of patient from medical care . . . 18.06[9]
    Waiting area, contents of
      Educational materials . . 18.06[4]
      Entertainment . . . 18.06[6]
      Generally . . . 18.06[2]
      Information packets . . . 18.06[7]
      Refreshments . . . 18.06[5]
  Telephones and telephone use (See TELEPHONES AND TELEPHONE USE)

PAYROLL SYSTEM AND RECORDS
  Affiliated medical practices (See AFFILIATED MEDICAL PRACTICES)

PERSONNEL (See EMPLOYEES)

PHYSICIAN-PATIENT RELATIONSHIP
  Marketing, importance in (See ADVERTISING AND MARKETING)

PHYSICIAN PRACTICE GROUPS (PPG'S)
  Affiliated medical practices (See AFFILIATED MEDICAL PRACTICES)

PREFERRED PROVIDER ORGANIZATIONS (PPOs)
  Defined . . . 14.01[2][b]; 14.09

PREMISES AND FACILITIES
  Affiliated medical practices (See AFFILIATED MEDICAL PRACTICES)
  Prepaid health care programs
    Cost reduction through maximum use of facilities . . . 14.07[4]
    Expansion for rapid growth . . . . 14.04[6][a]

PREPAID HEALTH CARE PROGRAMS
  Accounting methods, accrual vs. cash basis
    Financial management, accuracy of . . . 14.07[1]
    Generally . . . 14.07[1]
    Tax benefits . . . 14.07[1]; Fig. 14-3
  Actuarial soundness of program . . . . 14.04[2][d]
  Administrative burdens increased by open-ended utilization review of contract . . . 14.06[6][a]
  Advantages for employers . . . 14.01[1]
  Advertising, limitations on . . . 14.05[2]
  Alternative delivery system, defined 14.09
  Anti-trust concerns
    Fee-setting policies . . . 14.06[5]

SUPPLEMENTAL INDEX

[References are to Sections and Appendices.]

PREPAID HEALTH CARE PROGRAMS—
Cont.
Anti-trust concerns—Cont.
    Unreasonable restraint of competition, example of . . . 14.06[5]
Arbitration in third-party-physician dispute . . . 14.06[6][b]
Attitudes of physicians . . . 14.03[2]
Attorney, consultation with prior to signing of contract . . . 14.05; 14.06
Bookkeeping and reporting requirements
    Charges from outside providers, review of . . . 14.04[4]
    Claims processing, responsibility for . . . 14.04[4]
    Costs of new office systems . . . . 14.04[4]
Budget preparation . . . 14.07[2]; Fig. 14-4
Business staff productivity . . . 14.04[6][a]
Capitation
    Defined . . . 14.09
    Distribution of money to physician . . . 14.04[3][a]
    Outside services, for . . . 14.04[7]
Certificate of need requirements . . 14.05[2]
Checklist for evaluation of program viability . . . 14.08
Competitive Medical Plan
    Defined . . . 14.09
    Medicare providers, use of plan by . . 14.01[1]
    TEFRA legislation, creation by . . . . 14.05[1]
Computer use in data management . . . . . 14.07[4]
Confidentiality of records . . 14.06[6][d], [i]
Consultants
    Arrangements for . . . 14.04[7]
    Restriction of services by contract . . . 14.06[2][d]
Contract provisions, evaluation of
    Anti-trust concerns
        Fee-setting policies . . . 14.06[5]
        Unreasonable restraint of competition, example of . . . 14.06[5]
    Arbitration in third-party-physician dispute . . . 14.06[6][b]
    Assignability of contract . . 14.06[6][k]
    Attorney, consultation with prior to signing contract . . . 14.06
    Cash flow problems from untimely payment by third party . . . 14.06[6][m]
    Confidentiality of records . . . . 14.06[6][d], [i]
    Cross-liability . . . 14.06[4]

PREPAID HEALTH CARE PROGRAMS—
Cont.
Contract provisions, evaluation of—Cont.
    Defensive medicine, practice of . . . . 14.06[1]
    Dispute settlement, disadvantages of arbitration provisions in . . . . 14.06[6][b]
    Fee schedule, unilateral third-party change of . . . 14.06[6][1]
    Grievance procedures, open-ended nature of . . . 14.06[6][f]
    Insurer, third party as additional . . . . 14.06[6][h]
    Joint and several liability
        Consultant services, restriction on . . . 14.06[2][d]
        Cost containment, effects on medical judgment . . . 14.06[2][a]
        Defined . . . 14.06[2]
        HMO, limited liability of . . . . . 14.06[2][a]
        Hold harmless clause . . . . 14.06[2][a]
        Implied indemnification clause . . . 14.06[2][a]
        Liability insurance limitations in peer review . . . 14.06[3]
        Malpractice insurance limitations . . . 14.06[2][a]; 14.06[3]
        Non-covered services, extra expense to patient for . . . . 14.06[2][d]
        Peer review, liability in . . . . . . 14.06[3]
        Quality of care, contractual restrictions on . . . 14.06[2][b]
        Referral restrictions . . . . 14.06[2][d]
        Treatment not authorized by third party . . . 14.06[2][c]
    Malpractice action in peer review . . . 14.06[6][j]
    Modification of contract by third party, unilateral . . . 14.06[6][1]
    Open-ended utilization review of contract
        Administrative burdens . . . . . . 14.06[6][a]
        Liability risk . . . 14.06[6][a]
        Restrictions on physician services . . . 14.06[6][a]
    Payment schedule . . . 14.06[6][m]
    Peer review systems . . . 14.06[6][j]

[References are to Sections and Appendices.]

PREPAID HEALTH CARE PROGRAMS— Cont.
Contract provisions, evaluation of—Cont.
  Physician, liability of
    Costs of referrals outside third-party network, for . . . . 14.06[6][g]
    Insurance requirements . . . . . . 14.06[6][h]
    Peer review, in . . . 14.06[6][j]
    Unwarranted disclosure of records . . . 14.06[6][i]
  Records, confidentiality of . . . . 14.06[6][d][i]
  Referrals restricted to third-party network . . . 14.06[6][g]
  Renewal of contract, automatic . . . . 14.06[6][c]
  Sales presentation vs. actual contract terms . . . 14.06[6][e]
  Standard of care . . . 14.06[1]
  Termination agreement . . 14.06[6][c]
Co-payment, defined . . . 14.09
Corporate practice of medicine, limitations on . . . 14.05[2]
Cost containment
  (See also subhead: Features of program, pros and cons)
  Growth anticipation . . . 14.07[2]; Fig. 14-4
  Incentives . . . 14.07[3]
  Medical judgment affected by cost control . . . 14.06[2][a]
Cost monitoring (See subhead: Profitability, monitoring of)
Costs of services, increase in . . 14.04[3][a]
Dangers of inadequate program evaluation
  Financially unstable programs 14.04
  Multiple programs, entry into 14.04
  Patient loss after program termination . . . 14.04
Discounts on supplies, cost reduction through . . . 14.07[4]
Disputes
  Physician and outside provider . . . . 14.04[5]
  Physician and third party, arbitration provisions . . . 14.06[6][b]
Dual-choice option, defined . . . 14.09
Economic considerations (See subhead: Evaluation of program viability)
Employers, advantages to . . . 14.01[1]

PREPAID HEALTH CARE PROGRAMS— Cont.
Enrollment of patients
  Minimum necessary for program success . . . 14.04[6][b]
  Prediction of number . . . 14.04[6][b]
Equipment, adequacy of in rapid expansion of patient base . . . 14.04[6][a]
Ethical considerations . . . 14.03
Evaluation of program viability
  Bookkeeping and reporting requirements
    Charges from outside providers, review of . . . 14.04[4]
    Claims processing, responsibility for . . . 14.04[4]
    Office systems . . . 14.04[4]
    Pre-admission screening . . . . . 14.04[4]
    Referral documentation . . . . . . 14.04[4]; Fig. 14-2
  Capitation for outside services . . . . . 14.04[7]
  Checklist . . . 14.08
  Consultants, arrangements for . . . . . 14.04[7]
  Dangers of inadequate evaluation
    Financially unstable program . . . 14.04
    Multiple programs, entry into . . 14.04
    Patient loss after program termination . . . 14.04
  Disputes between physician and outside provider, resolution of . . . 14.04[5]
  Economic considerations
    Capitated dollar, distribution of . . . 14.04[3][a]
    Capitation, basis for . . 14.04[3]; Fig. 14-1
    Costs of services, increase in . . . 14.04[3][a]
    Generally . . . 14.02[1]
    Hospital services, responsibility for . . . 14.04[3][a]
    Outside vendor services, contract for . . . 14.04[3][a]
    Payment to physician, timeliness of . . . 14.04[3][b]
    Premium, services included in . . . 14.04[3]; Fig. 14-1
    Services, responsibility of practice for . . . 14.04[3][a]
  Stability of program . . . 14.04

[References are to Sections and Appendices.]

PREPAID HEALTH CARE PROGRAMS—Cont.
Evaluation of program viability—Cont.
  Expansion for rapid growth in patient base
    Business staff productivity . . . . 14.04[6][a]
    Equipment, adequacy of . . . . . . 14.04[6][a]
    Facility planning . . . 14.04[6][a]
    Furniture evaluation . . . . 14.04[6][a]
    Generally . . . 14.04[6]
    New patients, initial heavy use of services by . . . 14.04[6][b]
    Non-physician staff productivity . . . 14.04[6][a]
    Office hours, possible increase in . . . 14.04[6][a]
    Office space, adequacy of . . . . . 14.04[6][a]
    Patient enrollment, prediction of . . . 14.04[6][b]
    Patient use of services, projected vs. historical . . . 14.04[6][b]
    Physician staff productivity . . . . 14.04[6][a]
    Program goals, consideration of . . . 14.04[6][a]
    Specialties of physicians, evaluation of . . . 14.04[6][a]
  Hospitalization, arrangements for . . . 14.04[7]
  Needs of practice vs. program features
    Actuarial soundness of program . . . 14.04[2][d]
    Assignment of patients by program . . . 14.04[2][d]
    Experience of program . . . . 14.04[2][a]
    Financial strength of program . . 14.04[2][b]
    High-risk patients, proportion of . . . 14.04[2][d]
    Inexperienced programs, avoidance of . . . 14.04[2][a]
    Market share of program . . . . . 14.04[2][d]
    New patients, ability of program to attract . . . 14.04[2][d]
    Patients following physician into program . . . 14.04[2][d]
    Patients lost if physician leaves program . . . 14.04[2][d]

PREPAID HEALTH CARE PROGRAMS—Cont.
Evaluation of program viability—Cont.
  Needs of practice vs. program features—Cont.
    Patient type served by program . . . 14.04[2][c], [d]
    Premiums, adequacy of . . . . . . 14.04[2][b], [d]
    References about program from other physicians . . 14.04[2][a]
    Reputation of program . . . . . . 14.04[2][c]
  Outside services, arrangements for . . . 14.04[7]
  Prepaid program established by physicians' group as alternative to third party . . . 14.04[1]
  Reputation of program . . . 14.04
  Strengths of practice, review of . . . . 14.04[1]
Exclusive Provider Organization . . . . 14.01[2][b]
Expansion for rapid growth in patient base (See subhead: Evaluation of program viability)
Experience of program . . . 14.04[2][a]
Facilities
  Expansion, planning for . . 14.04[6][a]
  Maximum use of facilities, cost reduction through . . . 14.07[4]
Failure of program, physicians' attitudes toward . . . 14.03
Features of program, pros and cons
  Cost containment, pressure for
    Preference for healthy patients . . . 14.03[1]
    Profitability vs. quality of service . . . 14.03[1]
  Ethical considerations . . . 14.03
  Failure of program, physicians' attitudes toward . . . 14.03
  Incentives offered to physicians
    Attitudes of physicians toward programs . . . 14.03[2]
    Minimum patient enrollment . . . 14.03[2]
    Risk categories of patients . . . . 14.03[2]
Federal statutes applicable to
  Competitive Medical Plan created by TEFRA legislation . . . 14.05[1]
  Health Maintenance Organizations defined under . . . 14.05[1]
  Medicare provisions . . . 14.05[1]

SUPPLEMENTAL INDEX

[References are to Sections and Appendices.]

PREPAID HEALTH CARE PROGRAMS—Cont.
Fee-for-service practice
    Prepaid program, effect on practice . . 14.01[1]
Fee-for-service/prepaid medical group, defined . . . 14.09
Fee setting policies
    Change of, unilateral, by third party . . . 14.06[6][1]
    Cost reduction through negotiation . . 14.07[4]
    Generally . . . 14.06[5]
Financial considerations
    Report system for program . . . 14.07
    Reserve requirements . . . 14.05[2]
    Strength of program . . . 14.04[2][b]
    Unstable program . . . 14.04
Furniture requirements in rapid expansion of patient base . . . 14.04[6][a]
Goals of program . . . 14.04[6][a]
Grievance procedures, open-ended nature of . . . 14.06[6][f]
Growth, anticipation of (See subhead: Evaluation of program viability)
Health Maintenance Organizations (See HMOs)
Historical aspects . . . 14.01[1]
HMOs (See HMOs)
Hold harmless clause . . . 14.06[2][a]
Hospital services, arrangements for payment of . . . 14.04[3][a]; 14.04[7]
Implied indemnification clause . . . . 14.06[2][a]
Incentives offered to physicians . . 14.03[2]
Income increase by decreasing cost per patient . . . 14.07[4]
Independent Practice Association, defined . . . 14.09
Inexperienced programs, avoidance of . . . 14.04[2][a]
Insolvency laws . . . 14.05[2]
Insurance
    Contractual requirements . . . . 14.06[6][h]
    Limitations on . . . 14.06[2][a], [3]
    Patients, insurance programs for . . . . 14.01[2][b]
    Peer review, coverage for . . . 14.06[3]
    Self-insurance . . . 14.09
    Third party as additional insurer . . . . 14.06[6][h]
Joint venture, defined . . . 14.09
Legislation pertaining to
    Attorney specializing in health care, advice by . . . 14.05

PREPAID HEALTH CARE PROGRAMS—Cont.
Legislation pertaining to—Cont.
    Federal laws (See subhead: Federal statutes applicable to)
    State laws (See subhead: State statutes governing)
Liability of physician
    (See also subhead: Contract provisions, evaluation of)
    Contractual requirements . . . 14.06
    Costs of referrals outside third-party network, for . . . 14.06[6][g]
    Cross-liability . . . 14.06[4]
    Peer review . . . 14.06[6][j]
    Risk of liability in open-ended utilization review of contract . . . . 14.06[6][a]
    Unwarranted disclosure of record, for . . . 14.06[6][i]
Licensing requirements . . . 14.05[2]
Malpractice action in peer review . . . . . . 14.06[6][j]
Malpractice insurance, limitations on . . . . 14.06[2][a], [3]
Managed health care, defined . . . 14.09
Market share of program . . . 14.02
Medicaid prepaid plan, defined . . . 14.09
Medical group, defined
    Participating group . . . 14.09
    Prepaid only group . . . 14.09
Medicare supplemental plan, defined 14.09
Member months, defined . . . 14.09
Multiple programs, entry into . . . 14.04
Negative selection, defined . . . 14.09
Noncovered charges, defined . . . 14.09
Office considerations
    Costs of additional systems . . . . 14.04[4]
    Hours, expansion of . . . 14.04[6][a]
    New procedures . . . 14.04[4]
    Space, adequacy of . . . 14.04[6][a]
Open-ended utilization review of contract . . . 14.06[6][a]
Para-professionals, limitations on use of . . 14.05[2]
Participation in programs, reasons for
    Competition of large groups with small groups . . . 14.02[2]
    Control over business, protection of . . . 14.02[2]
    Economic benefits . . . 14.02[1]
    Fee-for-service practice within prepaid program . . . 14.02[2]

SUPPLEMENTAL INDEX 25

[References are to Sections and Appendices.]

PREPAID HEALTH CARE PROGRAMS—Cont.
Participation in programs, reasons for—Cont.
    Market share, expansion of . . . 14.02
    Patient base, protection of . . . 14.02
Patient base
    Assignment by program . . 14.04[2][d]
    Following physician into program . . . 14.04[2][d]
    Loss of patients if physician leaves program . . . 14.04[2][d]
    Minimum number for viable program . . . 14.03[2]
    New patients attracted by program . . 14.04[2][d]
    Projected vs. historical patient load . . . 14.04[6][b]
    Protection of base . . . 14.02
    Risk categories of patients . . 14.03[2]; 14.04[2][d]
    Type of patients served by program . . . 14.04[2][c], [d]
    Updated list of . . . 14.04[3][b]
Payment to physician
    Schedule for payment . . . 14.06[6][m]
    Timeliness of payment . . 14.04[3][b]
    Withholding payment . . . 14.06[6][m]
Peer review
    Generally . . . 14.06[6][j]
    Insurance limitations . . . 14.06[3]
    Liability for damages . . . 14.06[3], [j]
Physicians' group establishing prepaid program . . . 14.04[1]
Pre-admission screening . . . 14.04[4]
Preferred Provider Organization . . . . 14.01[2][b]; 14.09
Premiums
    Adequacy of . . . 14.04[2][b][d]
    Defined . . . 14.09
    Services included in . . . 14.04[3]; Fig. 14-1
Productivity evaluation
    Business staff . . . 14.04[6][a]
    Non-physician staff . . . 14.04[6][a]
    Physicians . . . 14.04[6][a]; 14.07[3]
Profitability, monitoring of
    Accounting methods; accrual vs. cash basis
        Financial management, accuracy of . . . 14.07[1]
        Generally . . . 14.07[1]; Fig. 14-3
        Tax benefits . . 14.07[1]; Fig. 14-3
    Cost monitoring
        Computer use in data management . . . 14.07[4]

PREPAID HEALTH CARE PROGRAMS—Cont.
Profitability, monitoring of—Cont.
    Cost monitoring—Cont.
        Cost reduction . . . 14.07[4]
        Discounts on supplies, cost reduction through . . . 14.07[4]
        Fixed expense per patient, decrease in . . . 14.07[4]
        Income increase by decreasing cost per patient . . . 14.07[4]
        Maximum use of facilities, cost reduction through . . . 14.07[4]
        Negotiated fees, cost reduction through . . . 14.07[4]
        Net income per patient, increase in . . . 14.07[4]
        Per-diagnosis basis, on . . . . . . 14.07[4]
        Per-physician basis, on . . . . . . 14.07[4]
    Financial report system . . . 14.07
    Growth, anticipation of
        Budget preparation . . . 14.07[2]; Fig. 14-4
        Cost control methods . . . . 14.07[2]; Fig. 14-4
        Expense allocation among responsibility centers . . . 14.07[2]
        Responsibility center, defined . . . 14.07[2]
    Profit distribution to participants
        Cost control incentives . . . . . . 14.07[3]
        Cost of treatment per patient in physician evaluation . . . . . . 14.07[3]
        Generally . . . 14.07[3]
        Productivity of physicians, evaluation of . . . 14.07[3]
        Salary structure in prepaid plan vs. production-oriented system . . . 14.07[3]
Public health care, impact on . . . 14.01[1]
Quality of care, contractual restrictions on . . . 14.06[2][b]
Records and reports
    Charges from outside providers, review of . . . 14.04[4]
    Claims processing, responsibility for . . . 14.04[4]
    Confidentiality of records . . . . 14.06[6][d], [i]
    Liability for unwarranted record disclosure . . . 14.06[6][i]

[References are to Sections and Appendices.]

PREPAID HEALTH CARE PROGRAMS—Cont.
Records and reports—Cont.
    Office systems, new . . . 14.04[4]
    Pre-admission screening . . . 14.04[4]
    Referral documentation . . . 14.04[4]; Fig. 14-2
    Third-party access to records . . . . . . 14.06[6][i]
References from other physicians about program features . . . 14.04[2][a]
Referrals to consultants
    Costs of referral, liability for . . . . . . 14.06[6][g]
    Documentation . . . 14.04[4]; Fig. 14-2
    Restrictions on . . . 14.06[2][d], [g]
Reports (See subhead: Records and reports)
Reputation of program . . . 14.04[2][c]
Responsibility centers, expense allocation among . . . 14.07[2]
Risk management and insurance (See subhead: Insurance)
Salary structure in prepaid plan vs. production-oriented system . . . 14.07[3]
Self-insurance prepaid plan, defined 14.09
Services
    Cost of . . . 14.04[3][a]
    Covered services . . . 14.09
    Fully covered services . . . 14.09
    Insured services . . . 14.09
    Outside vendor, services contracted to . . . 14.04[3][a], [7]
    Premium covering services . . 14.04[3]
    Responsibility of practice for . . . . . . 14.04[3][a]
    Restriction of services by open-ended utilization review of contract . . . . 14.06[6][a]
    Shared-risk services . . . 14.09
Shadow pricing, defined . . . 14.09
Staff productivity . . . 14.04[6][a]
Standard of care, established vs. contractual . . . 14.06[1]
State statutes governing
    Advertising, limitations on . . 14.05[2]
    Certificate of need requirements . . . . 14.05[2]
    Corporate practice of medicine . . . . . 14.05[2]
    Financial reserve requirements . . . . . 14.05[2]
    Insolvency laws . . . 14.05[2]
    Licensing . . . 14.05[2]

PREPAID HEALTH CARE PROGRAMS—Cont.
State statutes governing—Cont.
    Para-professionals, limitations on use of . . . 14.05[2]
Stop-loss limit, defined . . . 14.09
Strengths of practice, review of . . 14.04[1]
Termination of contract . . . 14.06[6][c]
Treatment
    Cost per patient in physician evaluation . . . 14.07[3]
    Unauthorized by third party
        Generally . . . 14.06[2][c]
        Patient responsibility for payment . . . 14.06[2][d]
Triple-choice option, defined . . . 14.09
Types of programs
    Exclusive Provider Organization . . . . 14.01[2][b]
    HMOs (See HMOs)
    Insurance programs . . . 14.01[2][b]
    Preferred Provider Organization . . . . 14.01[2][b]

PROFESSIONAL LIABILITY
Accounts receivable, liability arising from (See ACCOUNTS RECEIVABLE)
Administrative failure giving rise to 18.01
Checklist for managing professional liability . . . 18.13
Clerical failure giving rise to . . . 18.01
Confidentiality (See CONFIDENTIALITY)
Defense against, medical records as (See MEDICAL RECORDS, subhead: Defense against professional liability, records as)
Diagnostic procedures giving rise to (See DIAGNOSTIC PROCEDURES)
Equipment maintenance, records pertaining to (See RECORDS AND REPORTS)
Generally . . . 18.01
Maintenance of equipment, records pertaining to (See RECORDS AND REPORTS)
Malpractice actions (See MALPRACTICE ACTIONS)
Medical records as defense against (See MEDICAL RECORDS, subhead: Defense against professional liability, records as)
Medication protocol minimizing (See DRUGS, subhead: Professional liability, avoidance of)
Patient-staff relations minimizing (See PATIENT-STAFF RELATIONS)
Policy manual, outline for
    Daily policy and procedures . . . App. 18-C

SUPPLEMENTAL INDEX

[References are to Sections and Appendices.]

PROFESSIONAL LIABILITY—Cont.
Policy manual, outline for—Cont.
    Front office accounting policies . . . . App. 18-C
    Generally . . . 18.09[1]
    Modification of policy, reservation of rights regarding . . . 2.04
    Prescription refills, policy proposal for . . . App. 18-A
    Termination, reservation of rights regarding . . . 2.04
Quality assurance recommendations; list . . . 18.11
Telephones and telephone use (See TELEPHONES AND TELEPHONE USE)
Treatment and procedures, liability arising from (See TREATMENT)

PURCHASES AND PURCHASING
Affiliated medical practices (See AFFILIATED MEDICAL PRACTICES)

R

RAPPORT WITH PATIENT
Staff, patient's relationship with (See PATIENT-STAFF RELATIONS)
Telephones and telephone use (See TELEPHONES AND TELEPHONE USE)

RECORDS AND REPORTS
Affiliated medical practices (See AFFILIATED MEDICAL PRACTICES)
Audit by third party payer (See AUDIT)
Equipment maintenance, records pertaining to
    Calibration records . . . 18.10[2]
    Cleaning and disinfecting, documentation of . . . 18.10[4]
    Clinical Laboratory Impact Act (CLIA) of 1988 . . . 18.05[8][a]
    Generally . . . 18.10
    In-service records . . . 18.10[3]
    Maintenance and maintenance records . . . 18.10[1]
    Sample forms for equipment records . . . App. 18-D
    Staff in-service records . . . 18.10[3]
    Training of personnel . . . 18.10[3]
Medical records (See MEDICAL RECORDS)
Prepaid health care programs (See PREPAID HEALTH CARE PROGRAMS)

RETIREMENT AND PENSION PLANS
Affiliated medical practices (See AFFILIATED MEDICAL PRACTICES)

RETIREMENT AND PENSION PLANS—Cont.
Individual Retirement Plans (IRA)
    Maximum deductible contribution . . . 11.05
    Simplified Employee Pension Plan, deduction for . . . 11.05
Profit sharing plans
    Benefits
        Distribution penalties . . 11.08[2]

RISK MANAGEMENT AND INSURANCE
Affiliated medical practices (See AFFILIATED MEDICAL PRACTICES)
Prepaid health care programs (See PREPAID HEALTH CARE PROGRAMS, subhead: Insurance)

S

SPECIALISTS
Affiliated medical practices (See AFFILIATED MEDICAL PRACTICES)
Consultants (See CONSULTANTS)

STAFF (See EMPLOYEES)

T

TAXATION
Accounting methods for prepaid health care program, tax benefits of . . 14.07[1]; Fig. 14-3
Affiliated medical practices (See AFFILIATED MEDICAL PRACTICES)

TELEPHONES AND TELEPHONE USE
Advice given over telephone . . . 18.07[2]
Affiliated medical practices (See AFFILIATED MEDICAL PRACTICES)
Answering service, importance of . . . . . . 18.07[5]
Classification of calls . . . 18.07[3]
First impressions . . . 18.07[1]
Generally . . . 18.07
Prescription refills, telephone use for . . . . 18.04[4]
Professional liability, avoidance of
    Advice given over telephone . . . . . . 18.07[2]
    Answering service, importance of . . . 18.07[5]
    Classification of calls . . . 18.07[3]
    First impressions . . . 18.07[1]
    Generally . . . 18.07

SUPPLEMENTAL INDEX

[References are to Sections and Appendices.]

TELEPHONES AND TELEPHONE USE—Cont.
Professional liability, avoidance of—Cont.
   Prescription refills, telephone use for . . . 18.04[4]
   Telephone hours, establishment of . . . 18.07[4]
Telephone hours, establishment of . . . . . 18.07[4]

TREATMENT
Medication, administration of (See DRUGS)
Professional liability, avoidance of
   Comparative negligence . . . 18.05[2]
   Contributory negligence . . . 18.05[2]
   Diagnostic procedures (See DIAGNOSTIC PROCEDURES)
   Discharge instructions, documentation of . . . 18.05[6]
   Documentation of treatment and medication . . . . . 18.02[3], [7]; 18.04[3]; 18.05[3], [7]
   Generally . . . 18.05
   Medication, documentation of . . . . . 18.02[7]; 18.04[3]; 18.05[7]
   Medication, liability arising from (See DRUGS)

TREATMENT—Cont.
Professional liability, avoidance of—Cont.
   Postoperative information, availability of . . . 18.05[5]
   Preoperative information, availability of . . . 18.05[4]
   Response to medication and treatment, documentation of . . . . . 18.02[7]; 18.04[3]
   Symptoms, documentation of . . . . . 18.02[7]
   Telephone, treatment given over . . . . 18.07[2]
   Vital signs and patient's stated effect of treatment, documentation of . . . . . 18.04[3]

W

WAGES AND SALARIES
Affiliated medical practices (See AFFILIATED MEDICAL PRACTICES, subhead: Employees)
Prepaid health care programs vs. production-oriented system . . . 14.07[3]

INDEX

(References are to sections.)

A

ACCOUNTANTS
Credentials of. . . . .6.06[2]
Group practice consulting. . . . .3.01[3][a]
IRS audit, representation at. . . . .6.06[1]
Management consultant, as. . . . .9.07[3]
Need for. 6.06
Productivity, increasing. 9.07
Professional organizations
    Membership in. 6.06
    Names of. . . . .6.06[2]
Selection of, criteria for. . . . .6.06[1]
Unincorporated accounts, advising. 3.02

ACCOUNTING PRACTICES
Banks and banking, concerning (See BANKS AND BANKING)
Billing systems (See BILLING SYSTEMS)
Bookkeeping systems
    Accounts receivable forms. App.10-A: Figs.10-11, 10-12, 10-13
    Balance sheet, sample of. . . . .App. Fig.6-3
    Computer systems (See COMPUTER SYSTEMS)
    Double-entry system. . . . .10.01[2]
    EOB, bookkeeper's need to understand. . . . .10.03[1][c]
    Generally. 10.01
    Journal sheets. 10.07
    Ledger cards
        Accounts receivable. . . . .10.01[1]; 10.07; Fig.10-1
        Embezzlement, balancing cards avoiding. 8.02
    Manual systems
        Generally. . . . .10.01 *et seq.*
        Ledger compared to manual ledger. 6.08
        Monitoring collections. . . . .7.04[2]
        Pegboard system (See subhead: Pegboard system)
    Preservation of documents, requirements as to. . . . .5.06[1]
    Single-entry sytem. . . . .10.01[1]
    Third party coverage. . . . .4.03[1]
    Types of. 10.01
    Unincorporated practices. 3.02

I-1

(References are to sections.)

ACCOUNTING PRACTICES—Cont.
Budgeting
    Forecasting, generally. . . . .6.01[4]
    Group practice, need in. 6.01
Cash flow, methods for. . . . .6.02[3]
Chart of accounts. 6.08
Computer systems (See COMPUTER SYSTEMS)
Embezzlement by employees, avoiding
    Accounts receivable practices. . . . .10.01[2]; 10.07
    Banking documents review. 8.02
    Insurance for. . . . .8.01[1][a]
Expenses and costs
    Actual income and expenses, forecast compared to. . . . .App: Fig.6-2
    Capital expenditures. . . . .6.02[3]
    Depreciation. . . . .6.02[3]
    Forecasting. . . . .6.01[1]
    Group practice sharing. . . . .3.01[3]
    Listings of. . . . .6.02[1][b]
    Loans. . . . .6.02[3]
    Methods for reducing. 9.01
    Premises and facilities (See PREMISES AND FACILITIES)
    Professional corporations, of. . . . .3.01[1]
    Self-employed physicians, advantages of incorporating. . . . .3.01[1]
    Starting practice
        Sample spreadsheet. . . . .App: Fig. 6-1
        Operating costs, initial ability to pay. 1.01
General ledger
    Balance sheet, sample of. . . . .App. Fig.6-3
    Bank deposits (See: BANKS AND BANKING)
    Chart of accounts. 6.08
    Checkbook disbursements. . . . .6.05[2], [a], [b]
    Computerized ledger, manual ledger compared to. 6.08
    Generally. 6.05
    Group practice, customized system for. . . . .5.02[5]
    Records
        Form for. . . . .App: Fig. 6-21
        Preservation of, legal requirements as to. . . . .5.06[1]
        Reconciling. . . . .6.05[3]
Income
    Determination of. . . . .3.01[1]
    Computer system analyzing. . . . .5.02[5]

INDEX

(References are to sections.)

ACCOUNTING PRACTICES—Cont.
Income—Cont.
    Expenses compared. . . . .5.02[5]
    Fees (See FEES)
    Group practice, allocation of income in. . . . .3.01[3][a]; 3.04[2]
Pegboard system
    Automation of. . . . .5.03[1]
    Balancing concepts of, computer utilizing. . . . .5.01[1][g][ii]
    Computerized billing services compared. . . . .5.03[1][2]
    Generally. . . . .10.01[3]
    Illustration. . . . .App: Fig.10-1
    Ledger cards
        Accounts receivable. . . . .10.01[1]; 10.07; Fig.10-1
        Embezzlement, balancing cards avoiding. 8.02

ACCOUNTS PAYABLE
Account control log, computer monitor. . . . .5.02[7]
Bill paying. . . . .6.03[3]
Capital assets, separate file for. . . . .6.03[4]
Checklist. 6.08
Check writing system. . . . .6.03[3], [5]
Clerks, duties of. . . . .9.07[1]
Filing system. . . . .6.03[4]
Generally. 6.03
Invoices
    Computer program for. . . . .5.02[7]
    Filing of. . . . .6.03[2][b], [4]
    Packing invoices, receipt controls for. . . . .6.03[2][b]
    Shipping invoice, sample of. . . . .App. Fig.6-9
Mistakes to avoid. 6.03
Paid statements. . . . .6.04[4]; App.6-11
Petty cash
    Embezzlement from, prevention of. 8.02
    Expenditures. . . . .6.03[6]
    Main checkbook as funding for. . . . .6.03[6]
    Sample of. . . . .App. Fig. 6-11
Premises and facilities, billing systems for. 1.11
Purchases and purchasing
    Centralized system for. . . . .6.03[1]
    Computer system (See COMPUTER SYSTEMS)
    Receipts for (See subhead: Receipt controls)
    Sample order. . . . .App. Fig.6-8
    Starting practice, ability to pay costs of. 1.01
    Supplier statements. . . . .6.03[2][c]

(References are to sections.)

ACCOUNTS PAYABLE—Cont.
Receipt controls
    Notices and statements, filing of. . . . .6.03[2]
    Packing invoices. . . . .6.03[2][b]
    Preservation of receipts, requirements as to. . . . .5.06[1]
    Purchasing
        Centralized system for. . . . .6.03[1]
        Orders. . . . .6.03[2][a]
        Supplier statements. . . . .6.03[2][c]

ACCOUNTS RECEIVABLE
Age reports, computer system for. . . . .5.02[1][f]
Bank deposits
    Clerks, delegating duties to. . . . .9.07[1]
    Deposit slips, postings compared. . . . .10.01[2]; 10.07
Billing systems (See BILLING SYSTEMS)
Blue Cross/Blue Shield. . . . .1.02[3]; 7.01[3]; 10.03[4][a]
Bookkeeping systems (See ACCOUNTING PRACTICES)
Checklist. 10.07
Clerks, delegating duties to. . . . .9.07[1]
Control of, methods for
    Adjustments of debits and credits. . . . .10.01[3]
    Balancing accounts. . . . .10.02[4]
    Bank statements as third party control. . . . .10.01[2]; 10.07
    Bookkeeping forms. App.10-A: Figs.10-11, 10-12, 10-13
    Charge slips. . . . .10.01[1]; 10.07; Fig. 10-10
    Currency used as payment, listing types of. . . . .10.01[2]; 10.07
    Employees (See EMPLOYEES)
    Payments. . . . .10.02[1]
    Routing slips. . . . .10.02[1]; 10.07; Fig. 10-10
    Welfare agency checks, reviewing. . . . .10.01[2]; 10.07
Credit and collection (See CREDIT AND COLLECTION)
Embezzlement, avoiding. . . . .10.01[2], [5]; 10.07
EOB
    Patient, to. Fig.10-4
    Remittance advice. Fig.10-5
Health Maintenance Organizations (HMO)
    Preventive care, emphasis on. . . . .10.03[5]
    Regular accounts, HMO accounts separated from. . . . .10.03[5]
Hospitals (See HOSPITALS AND NURSING HOMES)
House calls, recording charges and payment for. . . . .10.05[2]
Initial considerations as to. 1.01

INDEX

(References are to sections.)

ACCOUNTS RECEIVABLE—Cont.
Insurance forms (See INSURANCE PLANS)
Medicaid (See MEDICAID)
Medicare (See MEDICARE)
Medicare/Medicaid
    Generally. . . . .10.03[3]
    Standard form used by. . . . .Fig. 10-6
Miscellaneous charges. . . . .10.05 *et seq.*
Miscellaneous income. . . . .10.05[3]
New patients. 10.04
Non-participating physicians
    Medicare payment to. . . . .10.03[1][b]
    PPO, approval of referrals by. . . . .10.03[4][b]
Nursing homes (See HOSPITALS AND NURSING HOMES)
Outstanding accounts. . . . .10.06[1]
Preferred Provider Organizations (See PREFERRED PROVIDER ORGANIZATIONS PPO)
Private accounts receivable, evaluation of. . . . .3.07[1]
Private insurance. . . . .10.03[6]
Records and reports
    Adjustment log, physician reviewing. . . . .10.02[3]; 10.07
    Aging accounts. . . . .10.06[1][a]
    Bookkeeping forms. App.10-A: Figs.10-11, 10-12, 10-13
    Coverage for other physicians, fees from. . . . .10.05[3]
    Depositions, fees from. . . . .10.05[3]
    EOB, bookkeeper's need to understand. . . . .10.03[1][c]
    Expenses for, sharing. . . . .1.08[1]
    Expert witness fees, record of. . . . .10.05[3]
    Fees, record of. . . . .10.05[3]
    HMO accounts separated from regular accounts. . . . .10.03[5]
    Hospital log, establishing. . . . .10.04[1]; Fig.10-9
    Journal sheets. 10.07
    Ledger cards. . . . .10.01[1]; 10.07; Fig.10-1
    Loss of, insurance coverage for. . . . .8.01[1][a]
    Management reports, generally. 10.06
    Medicare, importance of recordkeeping for. . . . .10.03[1][c]
    Monthly charge slip. . . . .Fig. 10-10
    Nursing home log, establishing and maintaining. . . . .10.05[1]
    Pocket notebook or charge tablet, physician's use of. Fig.10-10
    Summaries. . . . .10.06[1][b]
Statements to patient
    Computer-generated
        Generally. . . . .10.01[2]; Fig. 10-2

(Pub 372)

(References are to sections.)

ACCOUNTS RECEIVABLE—Cont.
Statements to patient—Cont.
    Computer-generated—Cont.
        Payments, for collection of. . . . .7.04[2][b]
        Professional look of. . . . .10.01[2]
    CPT codes. . . . .Fig. 10-2
    ICD/9 codes. . . . .Fig. 10-2
    Manual system. . . . .7.04[2][b]; 10.01[3]
    Preservation of, requirements as to. . . . .5.06[1]
    Procedures for issuing. . . . .7.04[2]
    Providing. . . . .10.01[1]
    Sequence. . . . .7.04[2][a]
Welfare agencies, check-writing system of
    One check for multiple patients seen, EOB showing. . . . . Fig. 10-5
    Review by physician, need for. . . . .10.01[2]; 10.07
Worker's compensation
    Insurance forms, worker's compensation forms treated as. . . . . 10.03[7]

ADVERTISING AND MARKETING
Business cards. . . . .1.11[6]
Costs and expenses
    Financial planning for. . . . .6.01[2][b]
    Sharing of. . . . .1.08[1]
Employee recruitment, newspaper ads as source. . . . .2.02[1][a]
Generally. . . . .1.11[1]
Group practice, new physicians in, policy applicable to. 3.06
Internal marketing. . . . .1.12 et seq.
Office manager, role of. . . . .2.01[1]
One-to-one contact. . . . .1.11[5]
Promotional or financial assistance
    Banks, special arrangements for physicians with. . . . .1.02[4]
    Chamber of commerce . . . . .1.02[2]
    Community groups as source. . . . .1.02[1]
    Hospital administrators, meetings with. . . . .1.02[1]
    Industrial employers as source. . . . .1.02[2]
    Third party health coverage, availability of. . . . .1.02[3]
Public relations
    Community events, participation in. . . . .1.11[3]
    Hospitals, affiliation with. . . . .9.11, [1]
    Patient contacts
        Consultant or hospital, as to. . . . .1.11[2]
        Courtesy, extending. . . . .1.12[1]

(Pub 372)

INDEX

(References are to sections.)

ADVERTISING AND MARKETING—Cont.
Public relations—Cont.
    Patient contacts—Cont.
        Follow-ups. . . . .1.12[3]
        Free drug samples, dispensing. . . . .1.11[6]
        Initial contact. . . . .1.12[1]
        Psychological and personality needs, catering to. . . . .1.12[2]
        Visits to patients. . . . .1.12[2]
    Recall and reminder systems. . . . .1.12[3]; 5.02; 5.07
    School programs. . . . .1.11[6]
    Thanking referral sources as. 4.06
Public speaking. . . . .1.11[2]
Publishing. . . . .1.11[4]
Radio. . . . .1.12[2]
Seminars. . . . .1.11[2]
Third parties
    Advantages of participating with. 1.01
    Business consultants. 1.01
    Hospitals
        Administrators, meetings with. . . . .1.02[1]
        Affiliation with. . . . .9.11, [1]

APPOINTMENT SYSTEMS
Appointment books
    Computers, compared to. 4.09
    Examinations, physician's notations as to. . . . .4.03[4]
    Types of. . . . .4.02[1]
Broken appointments, charging for, legal factors in. . . . .7.01[3]
Checklist. 4.09
Computerized systems
    Advantages of. . . . .4.02[2]
    Appointment books, compared to. 4.09
    ARM computer system, capabilities of. . . . .5.02[2]], [3]
    Back-up printouts, need for. . . . .4.02[2]
    Down time, dealing with. . . . .4.02[2]
Clerks
    Coordinating appointments with. . . . .4.02[3]
    Delegating duties to. . . . .9.07[1]
Delays
    Checklist. 4.09
    Methods for handling. . . . .4.02[5]
Diagnosis at initial consultation. . . . .4.03[2]; 4.09
Emergencies causing delays, methods of handling. . . . .4.02[5]; 4.09

(Pub 372)

(References are to sections.)

APPOINTMENT SYSTEMS—Cont.
Examination of patient, factors in
    Additional tests. . . . .4.03[2]; 4.09
    Completion of examination, routines following. . . . .4.03[4]
    Diagnosis at initial consultation. . . . .4.03[2]; 4.09
    Discharge of patients. . . . .4.03[3]
    Medical history. . . . .4.03[2]; 4.09
    Payment
        Insurance forms, signing of. . . . .4.03[4]
        Receptionist dealing with. . . . .4.03[4]
    Questions of patients, careful answering of. . . . .4.03[2]
    Routine procedures, informing office staff of. . . . .4.03[2]
    Routing slip (See RECORDS AND REPORTS)
    Treatment at initial consultation. . . . .4.03[2]; 4.09
Flow chart illustrating routine. . . . .4.03[4]: Fig: 4-2; 4.09
Follow-up systems
    Appointment book, notations following examinations. . . . . 4.03[4]
    Appointment scheduling, for. 4.08; 4.09
    ARM computer system, capabilities of. . . . .5.02[3]
    Computer sytems. . . . .5.02, [3]; 5.07
    Consulting physician. 4.08; 4.09
    Malpractice actions, adequate systems avoiding. . . . .8.02[2]
    Reports
        Consulting physicians, reports to and from. 4.08
        Generally. . . . .App.5-B, C
    Telephone calls insuring. 4.07
    Test results
        Post-cards to patients informing of. 4.08
        Scheduling future appointments following. 4.08; 4.09
Forms, scheduling time for completion of. . . . .4.02[5]
Generally. 4.01
Initial consultation. . . . .4.03[2]; 4.09
New physician in group practice. 3.06
Office manager, role of. . . . .2.01[1]
Open time, scheduling. . . . .4.02[5]
Patient convenience and comfort, planning for. . . . .4.02[3]
Productivity, increasing. . . . .9.05; 9.07[1]
Review of schedule, preparation of. . . . .4.03[1]
Third party coverage, bookkeeping tasks for. . . . .4.03[1]
Timing appointments, factors in. . . . .4.02[3]
Treatment at initial consultation. . . . .4.03[2]; 4.09
Walk-in patients, dealing with. . . . .4.02[5]; 4.09

INDEX

(References are to sections.)

APPOINTMENT SYSTEMS—Cont.
Wave system
    Attitudes of patients toward. . . . .4.02[4]
    Modified system. 4.09
    Productivity and. 9.01
Work schedules
    Computer print out of. . . . .4.02[2]
    Customizing schedule according to patient flow. 4.09

ATTORNEYS
Corporation, role in forming. . . . .3.01[3][b]
Credit and collection, using for. . . . .12.07 *et seq.*
Employment contracts, handling. 3.06
Malpractice, as to. . . . .8.02[2]
Productivity of office, aiding. 9.07
Purchasing computers, consulting for. 5.06; 5.07
Records and reports, consulting as to preservation or destruction of. 12.06
Taxation, attorney advising as to. . . . .3.01[3][a]

(References are to sections.)

B

BANKS AND BANKING
Bank deposits
    Clerks splitting duties as to. . . . .9.07[1]
    Disbursements. . . . .6.05[2], [a], [b]
    Duplicate records. . . . .6.08; 8.02; 12.06[1]
    Generally. . . . .6.05[1]
    Postings compared to. . . . .10.01[2]; 10.07
    Prenumbered documents, use of. 8.02
    Preservation of duplicate slips. . . . .12.06[1]
    Productivity as to, increasing. . . . .9.07[1]
    Revenue sources of. 6.08
Checks and check writing
    Accounts payable. . . . .6.03[3], [5]
    Balancing checks, time for. . . . .6.03[3]
    Check writing system. . . . .6.03[5]
    Computerized checks
        Generally. . . . .6.03[5]
        Printing checks, computer system reducing costs of. . . . . 5.02[6]
    Disbursements by check
        General disbursements. . . . .6.05[2][a]
        Generally. . . . .6.05[2]
        Payroll check disbursements. . . . .6.05[2][b]
    Embezzlement, avoiding. 8.02
    Hand writing checks, advantages of. 8.02
    Management of. . . . .6.07[1]
    Minimum balance. 6.08
    Payroll, for
        One-write payroll check. . . . .App. 6-17
        Systems for. . . . .6.04[6]
    Petty cash, main checkbook as funding for. . . . .6.03[6]
    Printing checks, reducing costs of. . . . .5.02[6]
    Savings accounts, management of. 6.08
    Types of checks. . . . .6.03[5]
    Welfare agencies, need for review of checks from. . . . .10.02[2]; 10.07
Embezzlement, avoiding. 8.02
Financing
    Depreciation. 1.09
    Equipment. . . . .1.09[1]
    Forecasting as tool for obtaining. . . . .6.01[4]
    Loans, interest on. . . . .1.09[2]

(References are to sections.)

BANKS AND BANKING—Cont.
Financing—Cont.
    Special arrangements for physicians as to. . . . .1.02[4]
    Variable rate financing. . . . .1.09[1]

BILLING SYSTEMS
Accounts receivable (See ACCOUNTS RECEIVABLE)
Accounts Receivable Management (ARM). . . . .5.02[1][e]
Blue Cross/Blue Shield. . . . .7.01[3]; 10.03[4][a]
Collection of payment
    Generally (See CREDIT AND COLLECTION)
    Methods for. . . . .7.01[2]
    Requirements for coverage, complying with. . . . .App: Fig. 10-3
    Time lag between. . . . .6.01[3]
Computers used for
    Batch/mail-in service bureaus. . . . .5.03[2]; 10.01[2][b]]
    Generally (See COMPUTER SYSTEMS)
    Third party handling of. . . . .5.03[1], [2]
Hospital business office as source of information. 10.04
Insurance, requirements of. 10.03: Fig.10-3
Medicaid. . . . .10.02[2]; 10.03[2]
Medicare (See MEDICARE)
Medicare/Medicaid. . . . .10.03[3]
New patient information form entered into. . . . .4.04[1]
PPO procedures. . . . .10.03[4][b]
Third party billing (See specific heading, i.e. MEDICARE)

BLUE CROSS/BLUE SHIELD
Billing system
    Generally. . . . .10.03[4][a]
    Monies owed, billing patient for. . . . .7.01[3]
Credit and collection. . . . .7.01[3]
Described. . . . .1.02[3]
Provider numbers, securing. 1.13

BUSINESS PLANNING
Advertising and marketing (See ADVERTISING AND MARKETING)
Initial considerations. 1.01
Insurance plans (See INSURANCE PLANS)
Lease arrangements (See PREMISES AND FACILITIES)
Location of practice (See PREMISES AND FACILITIES)
New patients (See PATIENTS, GENERALLY)
Third party coverage (See INSURANCE PLANS)

(Pub 372)

(References are to sections.)

C

COMPUTER SYSTEMS
Access requirements, contract provisions for. . . . .5.04[4][a]
Accounts payable system. . . . .5.02[7]
Accounts Receivable Management (ARM)
    Billing practices. . . . .5.02[1][e]
    Batch processing. . . . .10.01[2][b]
    Cash flow, effect of cycle billing on. . . . .5.02[1][e]
    Collection management. . . . .5.02[1][f]
    Components of. . . . .5.02[1]
    Data transaction entry. . . . .5.02[1][c]
    Generally. . . . .5.02[1]
    Insurance processing
        Computer submission of forms, capacity of system for. . . . .5.02[1][d]
        Forms for claims. . . . .5.02[1][d]
    Master file maintenance. . . . .5.02[1][b]
    Medicare billing and reimbursement systems. . . . .10.03[1][c]
    Outstanding accounts, advantages as to. . . . .10.06[1]
    Patient maintenance functions. . . . .5.02[1][a]
    Recall of patient. . . . .5.02[3]
    Reporting needs, evaluating system's capability to meet. . . . .5.02[1][g] *et seq.*
    Statements. . . . .5.02[1]
    Systems utilities. . . . .5.02[1][j]
Appointment scheduling. . . . .5.02[2]; App.5-A
Assignment and subcontract rights. . . . .5.04[4][a]
Back-up systems
    Advantages and disadvantages. Fig.5-3
    Choice of procedures, criteria for. . . . .5.04[2][c][ii]
    Disk copy. . . . .5.04[2][c][i]
    Facilitating. . . . .5.01[1][j]
    File back-up. . . . .5.04[2][c][i]
    Loss of files, liability for. . . . .8.02[3]
    Methods and procedures. . . . .5.04[2][c]
    Microfiche records for down time. . . . .4.04[6]
    Removal of data, liability for. . . . .8.02[3]
    Table of options. Fig.5-3
    Types of. . . . .Fig. 5-3
Billing systems
    Batch/mail-in service bureaus. . . . .5.03[2]; 10.01[2][b]
    Third party handling of. . . . .5.03[1], [2]
Checklist. 5.07

INDEX

(References are to sections.)

COMPUTER SYSTEMS—Cont.
Computer consultant
    Client, interaction with. Fig.5-2
    Costs of. . . . .5.04[2][b]
    Disadvantages of using. . . . .5.04[2][b]
    Matching systems for referrals to and from. . . . .5.02[1][i]
    Role of. . . . .5.04[2]; App. Fig.5-2
    Selecting. . . . .5.04[2][g]
Costs
    Computer consultant. . . . .5.04[2][b]
    Cost-efficient service, computer as. . . . .5.01, [1]
    Price increases, written notice of. . . . .5.04[4][a]
    Word processing capacity. . . . .5.02[4]
Credit and collection (See CREDIT AND COLLECTION)
Data processing
    Alternatives to. . . . .5.03 *et seq.*
    Batch/mail-in service bureau for. . . . .5.03[2]
    Batch processing. . . . .10.01[2][b]
    Entries of transactions, integrity of. . . . .5.02[1][c]
    Information retrieval. . . . .10.01[2][c]
    In-house computer system. . . . .5.03[4]; 10.01[2][d], [ii]
    On-line/real time service bureau. . . . .5.03[3]; 10.01[2]
    Operating expenses. . . . .5.01[2]
    Pegboard system, automation of. . . . .5.03[1]
    Purchasing alternative systems, sources of. . . . .5.03[5]
Employee records, monitoring. . . . .5.02[8][c]
Errors of computer, evaluation of. . . . .5.02[1][g][ii]
Flow chart for planning. Fig.5-1
General accounting ledger. . . . .5.02[5]
Generally. . . . .10.01[2]
Glossary of computer terminology. App.5-D
Hardware
    Bytes, access and retrieval of. . . . .5.04[3][b]
    Checklist. 5.07
    Contract provisions. 5.06
    Demonstrations, factors in viewing. . . . .5.04[3][c]
    Educational training of employees, ongoing. . . . .5.04[4][d], [f]
    Errors in selecting. . . . .5.04[3][c]
    Expandability. . . . .5.04[3][b]
    Generally. . . . .5.04[3]
    Maintenance contracts for. . . . .5.04[4]
    Multiuser/multiprocessing concept. . . . .5.04[3][b]
    Operating system. . . . .5.04[3][a]

(References are to sections.)

COMPUTER SYSTEMS—Cont.
Hardware—Cont.
    Service and maintenance, vendor supplying. . . . .5.04[4]
    Single user concept. . . . .5.04[3][b]
    Software choice made prior to. . . . .5.04[3][c]
    Special deals, avoiding. . . . .5.04[3][c]
    Technical abilities and limitations of persons using. . . . . 5.04[3][c]
    Vocabulary generally. . . . .5.04[3][b]
Installation of system. . . . .5.04[4][f]
Insurance forms, submission of. . . . .5.02[1][d]
Legal considerations as to. 5.06
Maintenance contracts
    Cost of. . . . .5.04[4]
    Hardware, for. . . . .5.04[4][a]
    Preventive maintenance. . . . .5.04[4][a]
    System, for. . . . .5.04[4]
Management, systems for
    Accounts Receivable Management (See subhead: ARM)
    Benefits of. . . . .5.01[2]
    Business needs, resolving. . . . .5.01[1]
    Finances, control of. . . . .5.01[2]
    Flow chart for planning. Fig.5-1
    Operating expenses. . . . .5.01[2]
    Reports of (See subhead: Records and reports)
    RFP, using. 5.05
    Selection of
        Company or vendor, factors in selecting. . . . .5.05[1]
        Generally. 5.05
        Goals and objectives, assessing. . . . .5.04[1]
        Planning, schematic illustration of. . . . .5.04: Fig. 5-1
        Software (See subhead: Software)
Microfiche records. . . . .4.04[6]
Patient records
    Accounts Receivable Management (ARM) system for. . . . . 5.02[1][a]
    Availability of equipment for. 5.02
    Confidentiality, insuring. . . . .5.02[8][a]
    Defining, problems in. . . . .5.02[8][b]
    Filing. . . . .4.04[6]
    Generally. . . . .5.02[8] *et seq.*
    Mass data, ability of system to handle. . . . .5.02[8][a]

INDEX

(References are to sections.)

COMPUTER SYSTEMS—Cont.
Patient records—Cont.
    Medical history profiles, availability of software for. . . . .5.02, [8][b]
    Subfunctions related to, system's capacity for. . . . .5.02[8][c]
Planning for automation. . . . .5.03[5]
Print functions
    Mailing labels. . . . .5.02[1][h]
    Purchasing or leasing, factors in. . . . .5.02; 10.01[2][d][ii]
    Statement preparations. . . . .5.02[1][j]
Purchasing
    Attorney, consulting. 5.06; 5.07
    Confidentiality, considerations of. . . . .5.04[2][b]
    Group practice, payment shared by. . . . .3.04[2]
    Leasing compared. . . . .10.01[2][d][ii]
    On-site visits to vendor's clients. . . . .5.04[2][b]
    Print functions, need for. . . . .5.02; 10.01[2][d][ii]
    Request for proposal (See subhead: Request for Proposal)
    Software of vendor as criteria for selecting. 5.05
    Turnkey vendor. . . . .5.03[5]
Recall and reminder systems
    Accounts Receivable Management (ARM) system, capabilities of. . . . .5.02[3]
    Patient recall. . . . .5.02[3]
    Searching. . . . .5.01[2]
    Software storing. 4.07
Referral information, facilitating. 4.06
Request for proposal (RFP)
    Cost of preparing. . . . .5.04[2][b]
    Model RFP. . . . .App. 5- *et seq.*
    Problems associated with. . . . .5.04[2][a]
    Selection process, use in. . . . .5.04[2][b]
    Specifications. . . . .5.04[2]
    Vendor, development of RFP for. . . . .5.04[2][b]
Reports
    Accessibility of information. . . . .5.02[1][g][i]
    Accounts Receivable Management (ARM) system, capabilities of. . . . .5.02[1][g] *et seq.*
    Back-up of records, facilitating. . . . .5.02[1][j]
    Comparative analyses. . . . .5.02[1][g][iii]
    Custom reports, generating. . . . .5.02[1]
    Financial management
        Errors of computer, evaluating. . . . .5.02[1][g][ii]

(Pub 372)

(References are to sections.)

COMPUTER SYSTEMS—Cont.
Reports—Cont.
    Financial management—Cont.
        Financial integrity, maintaining. . . . .5.02[1][g][iii]
      Generating. . . . .5.02[1][g][i]
      Hard copies, screen viewing compared. . . . .5.02[1][g][iii]
      Management by exception basis. . . . .5.02[1][g][iii], [h]
      Miscellaneous factors. . . . .5.02[1][g][iii], [iv]
      Specific entry, system's ability to search for. . . . .5.02[1][g][iii], [h]
      Standard reports. . . . .5.02[1][g][i]
      Work processing capacity. . . . .5.02[4]
Security system
    Back-up system (See subhead: Back-up system)
    Generally. . . . .5.01[1][j]
    Software, for. . . . .5.04[2][b]
Service contracts
    Hardware. . . . .5.04[4][a]
    System, for. . . . .5.04[4]
    Type of service provided. . . . .5.04[4][a]
Software
    Back-up systems (See subhead: Back-up systems)
    Choice of procedures, criteria for. . . . .5.04[2][c][ii]
    Compatibility considerations. . . . .5.04[2][a]
    Documentation of programs. . . . .5.04[4][e]
    Editing, full-screen. . . . .5.04[2][a]
    Generally. . . . .5.02[1][j]
    Labeling media. . . . .5.02[2][c][ii]
    Language of. . . . .5.04[2][a]; App. 5-D
    Maintenance of. . . . .5.04[4][b]
    Random data access. . . . .5.04[2][a]
    Security, levels of. . . . .5.04[2][b]
    Selection of, generally. . . . .5.04[2]
    Storing, environmental conditions for. . . . .5.04[2][c][ii]
Terminology for, glossary of. . . . .App. 5-D
Third parties, collecting from. . . . .7.03, [1]
Third party handling
    Batch/mail-in service bureaus. . . . .5.03[2]
    Billing systems. . . . .5.03[1], [2]
    Computer service bureaus. . . . .10.01[2][d], [i]
    Hard copies, reliance on. . . . .5.01[1], [2]
Word processing, criteria for evaluating. . . . .5.02[4]

(Pub 372)

INDEX

(References are to sections.)

CONFIDENTIALITY
Attorney, consulting. . . . .12.02[1]
Computer systems and
    Medical records. . . . .5.02[8], [a]
    Purchasing, consideration in. . . . .5.04[2][b]
Financial information about patients, requesting and revealing. . . . .
    12.07[1][b]
Generally. . . . .12.01[2]
Insurance company
    Appending statement as to. . . . .4.04[1]
    Release form for, signed. . . . .12.01[2]; App: Fig.12-4
    Sample form. . . . .4.04[2]; App. Fig.4-4
Employees, delegating duties to. . . . .9.01; 12.07[1][b]
Revocation of license, disclosure of confidential information leading
    to. . . . .12.01[2]

CONSULTANTS
Group practice, availability of consultants at. . . . .3.04[2]
Non-participating physicians, PPO referrals to. . . . .10.03[4][b]
Physician-patient relationship, basis of. 12.01
Referrals to
    Appointment schedules and. 4.08; 4.09
    Checklists. 4.09
    Clerks, delegating duties to. . . . .9.07[1]
    Compensation. . . . .6.04[9]
    Follow-up appointments and. 4.08; 4.09
    Identification numbers, filing of. . . . .6.04[9]
    Insurance benefits. . . . .4.03[5]
    Location of consulting physician. . . . .4.03[5]
    Medical insurance form, patient bringing. . . . .4.03[5]
    Non-participating physicians, PPO referrals to. . . . .10.03[4][b]
    Preparation for. . . . .4.03[5]
Records and reports sent to
    Dictated transcription. 4.05
    Tests results. 4.09
Self-employed physician's access to. 3.04
Sources of. App.1-A

CONTRACTS
Buy-sell agreements
    Disability buy-out. . . . .8.04[3][c]
    Group practice. . . . .3.07[3]
    Incorporated practice. . . . .3.01[3][b]
Computer systems
    Hardware. . . . .5.04[4][a]; 5.06

(References are to sections.)

CONTRACTS—Cont.
Computer systems—Cont.
    Maintenance contracts. . . . .5.04[4], [a]
    Service contracts. . . . .5.04[4][a]
Corporate practice, forming. . . . .3.01[3][b]
Disability income. . . . .8.04[2][c], [d]
Employment contracts
    Group practice, new physicians in. 3.06
    Incorporated practices. . . . .3.01[3][b]
    Wage-continuation agreements. . . . .3.01[3][b]
Sale of practice (See subhead: Buy-sell agreements)

CORPORATE PRACTICE (See INCORPORATED PRACTICE)

CREDIT AND COLLECTIONS
Appointments broken, legal factors involving. . . . .7.01[3]
Billing systems
    Generally. . . . .7.01[2]
    Third party coverage requirements, complying with. . . . .App: Fig. 10-3
Cash only policies. . . . .7.01[2]
Checklist for. 7.06
Collection agencies
    Computer systems, cost-effective methods of. . . . .5.02[1][f]
    Letters to, computer generating. . . . .5.02[1][f]
    Generally. . . . .7.04[6]
    Malpractice actions arising from actions of. . . . .8.02[2]
    Monitoring. . . . .5.02[1][f]; 7.04[6][b], [c]
    Sources of. . . . .7.04[6][a]
Collection letters
    Collection letter services. . . . .7.04[4]
    Computer generating. . . . .5.02[1][f]
    Credit arrangements. . . . .7.04[3][b]
    Generally. . . . .7.04[3]
    Procedure for. . . . .7.04[3][a]
    Special circumstances. . . . .7.04[3][c]
Computer systems
    ARM system, capabilities of. . . . .5.02[1][f]
    Batch/mail-in service bureaus. . . . .5.03[2]
    Cost-effective methods of. . . . .5.02[1][f]
    Data processing equipment for. . . . .5.01[2]
    Management, ARM system facilititating. . . . .5.02[1][f]
    Monitoring agencies and bureaus. . . . .7.04[2]
    Statements, issuing. . . . .7.04[2][b]
    Third parties, collecting from. . . . .7.03 *et seq.*

(References are to sections.)

CREDIT AND COLLECTIONS—Cont.
Computer systems—Cont.
    Third party handling of. . . . .5.03[1], [2]
Conciliation court
    Advantages and disadvantages. . . . .7.04[8][a]
    Generally. . . . .7.04[8]
    Procedures. . . . .7.04[8][b]
Credit bureaus. . . . .7.04[7]; App.12-C[6]
Creditor defined. . . . .App.12-C[5]
Current Procedure Terminology. . . . .7.03[1]
Delinquent accounts
    Chart flags for. . . . .4.03[1]: Fig.4-1; 4.09
    Computer management of
        Evaluating need for. . . . .5.04[1]
        Letters to, computer generating. . . . .5.02[1][f]
Discrimination in credit, laws applicable to. . . . .7.01[3]; App. 12-C[5]
Equal Credit Opportunity Act. . . . .App.12-C[5]
Fair Debt Collection Practices Act. . . . .7.01[3]; 12.07[1], [a]
Fees, determination of. . . . .7.03[4]
Freedom of Information Act. . . . .App.12-C[3]
Insurance companies, collecting from (See subhead: Third parties, collecting from)
Interest, charging. . . . .App.12-C [4]
Monitoring collections
    Computerized systems. . . . .5.02[1][f]; 7.04[2]
    Generally. 7.05
    Lost charges, routing slips providing control for. . . . .4.04[3]
    Manual systems. . . . .7.04[2]
    Review by physician. . . . .7.05[1]
Patients, collecting from
    Broken appointments, for. . . . .7.01[3]
    Collection agencies (See subhead: Collection agencies)
    Collection letters (See subhead: Collection letters)
    Computer systems (See subhead: Computer systems)
    Fair Debt Collection Practices Act. . . . .7.01[3]; 12.07[1], [a]
    Financial information about patients, requesting and revealing. 12.07[1][b]
    Garnishment, federal requirements as to. . . . .12.07[3]
    Generally. 7.04
    Legal proceedings. . . . .12.07 *et seq.*
    New patients. . . . .7.01[3]

(References are to sections.)

CREDIT AND COLLECTIONS—Cont.
Patients, collecting from—Cont.
    Statements (See subhead: Statements to patient)
    Telephone calls (See subhead: Telephone calls)
    Time of service, payment at. . . . .7.04[1]
Policy of physician
    Credit philosophy. . . . .7.01[1]
    Guidelines for establishing. . . . .7.01 *et seq.*
    Legalities of physician-patient relationship. . . . .7.01[3]
    Marketing considerations. . . . .7.01[2]
Personal information about patient, physician entitled to receive. . . . 12.04; Figs.12-5, 12-6
Statements to patient
    Computer generated
        Automatic collection notices printed on statement. . . . . 5.02[1][f]
        Batch/mail-in service bureau. . . . .5.03[2]
        Cycle billing function, effect of. . . . .5.02[1][e]
        Generally. . . . .7.04[2][b]
        Printing function. . . . .5.02[1][e]
        Third party handling of. . . . .5.03[1], [2]
    Manual issuing of. . . . .7.04[2][b]
    Procedures for issuing. . . . .7.04[2]
    Sequence. . . . .7.04[2][a]
Telephone calls
    Commitment from patient, obtaining. . . . .7.04[5][b]
    Generally. . . . .7.04[5]
    Illustration. . . . .7.04[5][a]
Third parties, collecting from
    Appointment scheduling. . . . .4.03[1]
    Assignment of benefits. . . . .7.03[7]
    Bookkeeping tasks for. . . . .4.03[1]
    Current Procedure Terminology (CPT codes). . . . .7.03[1]
    Diagnostic codes. . . . .7.03[2]
    Fees, determination of. . . . .7.03[4]
    Generally. 7.03
    Health Care Financing Procedure Codes (HCPCS). . . . .7.03[3]
    International Classification of Diseases. . . . .7.03[2]
    Participation agreements
        Advantages and disadvantages. . . . .7.03[6][a]
        Evaluation of contracts. . . . .7.03[6][b]
    Profiles. . . . .7.03[5]
    Relative values. . . . .7.03[4]

(References are to sections.)

CREDIT AND COLLECTIONS—Cont.
Time of payment, defining. . . . .7.01[3]
Truth-in Lending Act. . . . .7.01[3]; App. 12-C [2], [4]

(References are to sections.)

E

EMERGENCIES
Employee handling calls. . . . .4.01[2]
Good Samaritan laws, applicability of. 12.03
Scheduled appointments, delay in. . . . .4.02[5]; 4.09

EMPLOYEES
Absenteeism, policy applicable to. 2.04
Age Discrimination in Employment Act of 1967. . . . .2.09
Attitude of, policy applicable to. . . . .2.04: Fig. 2-4
Back-up personnel
    Generally. 2.08
    Nurses. . . . .2.08[3]
    Part-time employees. . . . .2.08[2]
    Temporary agencies. . . . .2.08[1]
Breaks, policy applicable to. . . . .2.04: Fig. 2-4
Chain of command, establishing. 2.06
Civil Rights Act of 1866, applicability of. 2.09
Civil Rights Act of 1964, Title VII, applicability of. 2.09
Clerks (See subhead: Receptionist/clerk)
Confidentiality
    Policy applicable to. . . . .2.04: Fig. 2-4
    Violations of, penalties for. . . . .8.02[2]
Disciplinary actions, policy applicable to. 2.04: Fig.2-4
Discrimination in employment
    Age as basis of, statute prohibiting. 2.09
    Dismissal, federal legislation against discrimination in. 2.09
    Interview, avoiding discriminatory questions at. . . . .2.02[4]
    Policy applicable to. 2.04
    Protection from accusations of. . . . .2.07[1]
Duties of
    Ancillary services. . . . .4.03[3]
    Blood work-ups. . . . .4.03[3]; 9.07[2]
    Bookkeeping duties
        Payments, splitting duties as to. . . . .8.02; 10.01[5]; 10.02[2]; 10.07
        Routing slips (See RECORDS AND REPORTS)
    Delegation of, productivity increasing through. . . . .9.07, [1]
    Flow chart illustrating routine. . . . .4.03[4]: Fig: 4-2; 4.09
    Group practice, in. 3.06
    Laboratory tests. . . . .4.03[3]
    Medical assistant (See subhead: Medical assistant, duties of)
    Pre-examination procedures. . . . .9.07[2]
    Procedures and diagnosis, checking. . . . .4.03[2]

INDEX

(References are to sections.)

EMPLOYEES—Cont.
Duties of—Cont.
    Productivity, increasing. . . . .9.07[3]
    Technicians, duties of. . . . .4.03[3]
    X-rays. . . . .4.03[3]
Education and training of
    Computer processing, desire and ability to learn. . . . .5.04[1]
    Fringe benefit, as. 2.04
    Safety procedures. . . . .8.01[3]
Embezzlement by
    Accounts receivable practices avoiding. . . . .10.01[2]; 10.07
    Computer security preventing. . . . .5.04[2][b]
    Honesty and reliability deterring. . . . .2.02[7]; 8.02; 10.02[5]
    Insurance for. . . . .8.01[1][a]
    Payments, splitting duties as to. . . . .8.02; 10.01[5]; 10.02[2]; 10.07
    Warning signals as to. . . . .8.02; App. Fig. 8-1
Equal Employment Opportunity Act of 1972, applicability of. 2.09
Equal Pay Act. 2.09
Evaluation of performance (See subhead: Performance evaluation)
Fair Labor Standards Act
    Provisions of. 2.09
    Record keeping requirements of. . . . .5.06[6]
Family emergencies. 2.04: Fig.2-4
Federal laws
    Checklist for. 2.10
    Compliance with. 2.09
    Voluntary termination, statutory requirements as to. . . . .2.07[2]
Fringe benefits (See FRINGE BENEFITS)
Generally. 2.01
Hiring procedures (See HIRING AND RECRUITMENT PROCEDURES)
Hours
    Compensatory time. . . . .2.03[3]
    Fair Labor Standards Act, provisions of. . . . .2.09; 5.06[6]
    Federal and state laws limiting. . . . .2.03[3]
    Overtime pay
        Exemptions from wage and hour laws. . . . .2.03[3]
        Mandatory nature of. . . . .2.03[3]
        Manual explaining policy. 2.04: Fig.2-4
    Time sheets
        Purpose of. . . . .2.03[3]

(References are to sections.)

EMPLOYEES—Cont.
Hours—Cont.
    Time sheets—Cont.
        Sample of. . . . .2.03[3]: Fig.2-3
    Wage and hour laws, provisions of. . . . .2.03[3]
Interview process (See HIRING AND RECRUITMENT PROCEDURES)
Jury duty. 2.04: Fig.2-4
Management of (See MANAGEMENT AND MANAGEMENT TECHNIQUES)
Manual of procedure
    Checklist for. 2.10
    Creation of. 2.05
    Generally. 2.05
    Job descriptions. . . . .2.05[1]
    Specific duties. . . . .2.05[2]
    Voluntary termination. . . . .2.07[2]
Medical assistant, duties of
    Accompanying patients to technicians. . . . .4.03[3]; 9.07[2]
    Consultants, arranging for referrals to. . . . .4.03[5]
    Delegation of duties to. . . . .9.07[2]
    Flagging room. . . . .4.03[3]; 4.09
    Hospitalization, arranging for. . . . .4.03[5]
    Large practice, duties in. . . . .4.03[3]
    Part-time hours. . . . .2.01[2]
New employees interviewed by office manager. . . . .2.01[2]
Nurse
    Delegating duties to. 9.07
    Part-time employment of. . . . .2.01[2]
Office manager (See MANAGEMENT AND MANAGEMENT TECHNICQUES)
Part-time employees, vacation time for. 2.04
Performance evaluation
    Policy applicable to. 2.04
    Procedure. . . . .2.03[4][a]
    Retaining records of. . . . .12.02[2]
    Salary adjustment as part of. . . . .2.03[4][b]
    Written evaluations. 2.04
Personal appearance
    Name tags, wearing. . . . .4.03[1]
    Policy applicable to. . . . .2.04: Fig. 2-4
Physicians' assistants, duties of. . . . .9.07[2], [3]

INDEX

(References are to sections.)

EMPLOYEES—Cont.
Policy
    Amendments and addenda to. 2.04
    Checklist for. 2.10
    Development of. 2.04
    Disciplinary action. 2.04: Fig.2-4
    Job descriptions
        Illustration. . . . .App: Fig. 2-B
        Manual outlining. . . . .2.05[1]
    Group practice, factors in hiring new physicians for. 3.06
    Holidays. . . . .2.03[2]; 2.04
    Manual for personnel policy, sample. 2.04: Fig.2-4
    Performance review. 2.04
    Salary review. 2.04: Fig.2-4
    Sample manual. 2.04: Fig.2-4
    Statement of acknowledgment. 2.04; 2.10
    Telephone use, policy applicable to. . . . .2.04: Fig. 2-4
    Termination
        Procedure for (See subhead: Termination of employment)
        Voluntary termination. . . . .2.07[2]
    Written copies, distribution of. 2.04
Probationary period served by
    Manual explaining policy. 2.04: Fig.2-4
    Purpose of. . . . .2.02[3]
Productivity, incentives increasing
    Clerks, delegation of duties to. . . . .9.07[1]
    Group practice, in. 9.09
    Incentive programs. 9.09
    Merit bonuses for. 9.08
Receptionist/clerk
    ARM system, usefulness of. . . . .5.02[2]
    Delegation of duties to. . . . .9.07[1]
    Duties of. . . . .4.03[1]
Recruitment (See HIRING AND RECRUITMENT PROCEDURES)
Salary (See WAGES AND SALARIES)
Screening applicants (See HIRING AND RECRUITMENT PROCEDURES)
Security, policy applicable to. . . . .2.04: Fig. 2-4
Termination of employment
    Checklist for. 2.10
    Confidentiality violations as grounds for. . . . .8.02[2]
    Discrimination
        Discharge notices. App.12A-Fig. 12-1, 12-2

(Pub 372)

(References are to sections.)

EMPLOYEES—Cont.
Termination of employment—Cont.
    Discrimination—Cont.
        EEO guidelines. App.12-3
        Federal legislation against. 2.09
        Pre-employment inquiries. App.12-B
        Protection from accusations of. . . . .2.07[1]
    Generally. 2.07
    Personnel folders, using. . . . .2.07[1]
    Policy applicable to. 2.04
    Procedure for firing. . . . .2.07[1]
    Retaining records of. . . . .12.02[2]
    Voluntary termination. . . . .2.07[2]
Types of. 2.01
Wages and salary (See WAGES AND SALARY)

(Pub 372)

INDEX

(References are to sections.)

F

FEES
Collection of (See CREDIT AND COLLECTION)
Depositions, fees from. . . . .10.05[3]
Determination of
    Insurance plans, by. . . . .7.03[4]
    Profiles used in. . . . .7.03[4]; 10.03[1][a]
    Relative value index. . . . .7.03[4]
Expert witness fees. . . . .10.05[3]
Hospital charges. 10.04; 10.05
Malpractice actions and. . . . .8.02[2]
Office manager handling. . . . .2.01[1]

FINANCIAL MANAGEMENT
Accountants (See ACCOUNTANTS)
Accounting practices (See ACCOUNTING PRACTICES)
Accounts payable (See ACCOUNTS PAYABLE)
Accounts receivable (See ACCOUNTS RECEIVABLE)
Advertising and marketing costs (See ADVERTISING AND MARKETING)
Banks and banking (See BANKS AND BANKING)
Billing systems (See BILLING SYSTEMS)
Budgeting (See ACCOUNTING PRACTICES)
Capital expenditures. . . . .6.02[3]
Cash flow
    Basic accounting methods. . . . .6.02[3]
    Billing and collecting, time lag between. . . . .6.01[3]
    Comparative reports, computer developing. . . . .5.02[5]
    Computer functions, effect of. . . . .5.02[1][e]
    Cycle billing system, advantages of. . . . .5.02[1][e]
    Forecasting of. . . . .6.01[3]
    Management of
        Bonuses, periodic distribution of. . . . .6.07[3]
        Checking accounts. . . . .6.07[1]
        Early pay discounts. . . . .6.07[4]
        Minimum balance. 6.08
        Money markets. . . . .6.06[1]
        Pension and profit sharing plans, early contribution to. . . . 6.07[2]
        Savings accounts. 6.08
    Principal payments. . . . .6.02[3]
    Reports. . . . .6.02[3]; 6.08
    Salaries. . . . .6.02[3]
    Simplified statement, example of. App.6-7

(References are to sections.)

FINANCIAL MANAGEMENT—Cont.
Checklist. 6.08
Checks and check writing (See BANKS AND BANKING)
Depreciation. . . . .6.02[3]
Earnings of individual employees (See PAYROLL, subhead: Individual earnings of employees)
Expenses and costs (See ACCOUNTING PRACTICES)
Filing system
    Accounts payable. . . . .6.03[4]
    Alphabetized expandable file, sample of. App.6-11
    Notices and statements, for. . . . .6.03[2]
Forecasting revenue
    Actual income and expenses, forecast compared. . . . .App. Fig.6-2
    Budget, generally. . . . .6.01[4]
    Cash flow. . . . .6.01[3]
    Data, obtaining. . . . .6.01[1]
    Generally. 6.01
    Profits, anticipation of. . . . .6.01[4]
General ledger (See ACCOUNTING PRACTICES)
Income statement
    Automobile expenses. . . . .6.01[1][b]
    Business expenses. . . . .6.02[1][b]
    Cash receipts, keeping separate accounts for. . . . .6.02[1][a]
    Depreciation expenses. . . . .6.02[1][b]
    Equipment lease payments. . . . .6.02[1][b]
    Expenses, lists of. . . . .6.02[1][b]
    Fringe benefit expenses. . . . .6.02[1][b]
    Generally. 6.02
    Insurance expenses, types of. . . . .6.02[1][b]
    Interest. . . . .6.02[1][a]
    Itemization of. . . . .6.02[1][c]; App: Fig.6-3
    Laboratory work, fees of. . . . .6.01[1][b]
    Medical supplies, expenses of. . . . .6.02[1][b]
    Miscellaneous income. . . . .6.02[1][a]
    Office supplies, costs of. . . . .6.02[1][b]
    Patients, income from. . . . .6.02[1][a]
    Payroll tax expenses. . . . .6.02[1][b]
    Pension and profit sharing plans, employer contributions to. . . . 6.02[1][b]
    Rent and utility expenses. . . . .6.02[1][b]
    Staff salaries. . . . .6.02[1][b]

(References are to sections.)

FINANCIAL MANAGEMENT—Cont.
Income statement—Cont.
    Supplemental accounts receivable report.. . . .6.02[1][d]; App. Fig.6-4
    Telephone charges. . . . .6.01[1][b]
    Third party reimbursement. . . . .6.02[1][a]
    Total income. . . . .6.02[1][a]
    Trend analysis report. . . . .6.02[1][e]; App. 6-5
Individual earnings of employees (See PAYROLL) SYSTEM AND RECORDS)
Invoices (See ACCOUNTS PAYABLE)
Loans. . . . .6.02[3]
Payroll system and records (See PAYROLL SYSTEM AND RECORDS)
Petty cash
    Embezzlement from, prevention of. 8.02
    Expenditures. . . . .6.03[6]
    Main checkbook as funding for. . . . .6.03[6]
    Sample of. . . . .App. Fig. 6-11
Professional dues and journals, fees for. . . . .6.02[1][b]
Purchases and purchasing (See ACCOUNTS PAYABLE)
Reports
    Cash flow (See subhead: Cash flow)
    Income statement (See subhead: Income statement)
    Payroll tax reports. . . . .6.04[8]
    Practices, comparisons between types of. . . . .6.02[2]
    Preparation of, need for. 6.08
Retirement and benefit plans (See RETIREMENT AND BENEFIT PLANS)
Shipping invoice, sample of. . . . .App. Fig.6-9
Specialty practices
    Comparison reports. . . . .6.02[2]
    Statistical data relevant to. . . . .6.01[1]
    Taxes. . . . .6.04[7][a], [b], [8]
Taxation (See TAXATION)
Valuation of practice, factors in
    Assets. . . . .3.07[1]
    Buy-sell agreements. . . . .3.07[3]
    Liabilities. . . . .3.07[2]

FORMS OF PRACTICE
Checklist. 3.08

(References are to sections.)

FORMS OF PRACTICE—Cont.
Corporate practice (See CORPORATE PRACTICE)
Group practice (See GROUP PRACTICE)
Partnerships (See GROUP PRACTICE)
Single practice (See SELF-EMPLOYED PHYSICIANS)
Types of, generally. . . . .3.01 *et seq.*
Unincorporated practice. 3.03
Valuation of practice
    Assets, factors in evaluating. . . . .3.07[1]
    Buy-sell agreements. . . . .3.07[3]
    Generally. 3.07
    Liability limitations. . . . .3.07[2]

FRINGE BENEFITS
Bonuses. 2.04
Computer monitoring of. . . . .5.02[8][c]
Education. 2.04
Equal Employment Opportunity Act of 1972. . . . .2.09
Family emergencies. 2.04: Fig.2-4
Funeral leave. 2.04: Fig.2-4
Health insurance. . . . .2.03[2]; 2.04: Fig. 2-4; 5.01, [1]
Holidays. . . . .2.03[2]; 2.04
Insurance. 2.04
Life insurance. . . . .3.03[6]
Local customs and. . . . .2.03[2]
Maternity
    Equal Employment Opportunity Act of 1972, applicability of. . . 2.09
    Leave for, policy as to. . . . .2.04: Fig. 2-4
Part-time employees, provisions for. . . . .2.03[2]
Pension plans. 2.04
Personal days. . . . .2.03[2]
Physician preferences affecting. . . . .2.03[2]
Policy applicable to, written. 2.04
Profit sharing plans. 2.04
Proportioning benefits. . . . .2.03[2]
Sick days. . . . .2.03[2]; 5.02[8][c]
Sick pay. 2.04: Fig.2-4
Temporary employees. . . . .2.03[2]
Vacations. . . . .2.03[2]; 2.04, Fig. 2-4; 5.02[8][c]
Worker's compensation. 2.04: Fig.2-4

(References are to sections.)

G

GROUP PRACTICE
Advantages of. . . . .3.01[3]
Budgeting, need for. 6.01
Consultants, availability of. . . . .3.04[2]
Coverage of patients, availability of. . . . .3.04[2]
Delegation of duties in. 9.09
Disability of associate, effect of. 3.07
Disadvantages of. . . . .3.04,[1]
Malpractice insurance, sharing. . . . .3.01[3]
Membership
    Changes in affecting valuation of practice. 3.07
    New physicians, policy applicable to. 3.06
New physicians in. 3.06
Profits
    Criteria for. . . . .3.05[2]
    Distribution of, generally. 3.05
    Productivity, distribution of profits based on
        Equity compared to. . . . .3.05[1]
        Formula for. . . . .App. Fig.3-4
Retirement from, effect of. 3.07
Sale of practice, effect of. 3.07
Simple partnerships. . . . .3.01[3][a]

(References are to sections.)

H

HEALTH MAINTENANCE ORGANIZATIONS (See HEALTH MAINTENANCE ORGANIZATIONS HMO)

HIRING AND RECRUITMENT PROCEDURES
Application form
    Assessment of applicant. . . . .2.02[7]
    Civil rights laws and. 12.08
    Discriminatory questions on, avoiding. 12.08
    Evaluation of. . . . .2.02[2][a]
    Filing of. . . . .2.02[8]
    Illustration. . . . .2.02[2][a]: Fig.2-1
    Skill testing. . . . .2.02[2][b]
Character of applicant
    Attitude. . . . .2.02[2]
    Determining. . . . .2.02[4]
    Generally. 2.02
    Interview questions establishing. . . . .2.02[4]
Checklist for. 2.10
Compatibility with staff, determining. . . . .2.02[2]
Competence and efficiency, determining. . . . .2.02, [1][f]
Discrimination
    Applications, avoiding on. 12.08
    Precautions as to. . . . .2.02[4]
    Statutory provisions. 2.09
Educational experience. . . . .2.02[2][a]
Employment agencies, applicants from. . . . .2.02[1][b], [c]
Experience and expertise, screening for. . . . .2.02, [1][f], [2]
Graduates of specialized schools, screening. . . . .2.02[1][d]
Interview process
    Application form (See subhead: Application form)
    Bonding, attitude toward. . . . .2.02[7]
    Generally. . . . .2.02[3]
    Initial interview, timing. . . . .2.02[3]
    Office manager, role of. . . . .2.01[2]
    Physician excluded from. . . . .2.02[3]
    Questions (See subhead: Questions)
    Rapport, establishing. . . . .2.02[4]
    Review of applicants. . . . .2.02[5]
    Second interview
        Preparing applicants for. . . . .2.02]7]
        Purpose of. . . . .2.02[6]
    Skills (See subhead: Tests)
    Structuring. 2.02

INDEX

(References are to sections.)

HIRING AND RECRUITMENT PROCEDURES—Cont.
Interview process—Cont.
    Tests (See subhead: Tests)
    Timing of interview. . . . .2.02[3]
Job functions
    Analysis of. 2.02
    Descriptions. . . . .2.05[1]
    Illustration. . . . .App: Fig. 2-B
    Test, relationship to. . . . .2.02[2][b]
Notice of acceptance. . . . .2.02[8]
Nurses or technicians, on-the-job testing required for. . . . .2.02[2][b]
Office manager, role of. . . . .2.01[2]; 2.02[2]
Personality problems
    Forestalling. . . . .2.02, [2]
    Reference checks screening for. . . . .2.02[7]
Policies, formulation of. . . . .2.01[2]
Pre-interview planning. 2.02
Probationary period, conditions of. . . . .2.03[8]
Questions
    Extracurricular activities. . . . .2.02[2][a]
    Job performance, relevant to. 12.08
    Open-ended questions. . . . .2.02[4]
    Overtime, feelings toward. . . . .2.02[2]
    Preparation of. . . . .2.02[2]
    Salary. . . . .2.02[4]
    Sample questions. . . . .2.02[4]
    Second interview, informing applicants of. . . . .2.02[7]
    Skills, testing for (See subhead: Testing)
    Transportation. . . . .2.02[2][a]: Fig.2-1
Recruitment
    Advertisement in newspapers. . . . .2.02[1][a]
    Employment agencies
        Fees of, clarifying. . . . .2.02[1][b]
        Government supported agencies. . . . .2.02[1][c]
        Private. . . . .2.02[1][b]
    Family or friends, problems created by hiring. . . . .2.02[1][e]
    Generally. . . . .2.02[1]
    Graduates of specialized schools. . . . .2.02[1][d]
    Pirating from other doctors. . . . .2.01[1][f]
    Schools, placement services of. . . . .2.02[1][d]
    Standards for, generally. 2.02
    Unemployment office as source. . . . .2.02[1][c]
    Welfare office as source. . . . .2.02[1][c]

(Pub 372)

(References are to sections.)

HIRING AND RECRUITMENT PROCEDURES—Cont.
Reference checks
    Application forms, comparing. . . . .2.02[7]
    Guide to. . . . .2.02[7]: Fig.2-2
    Money handling and bonding. . . . .2.02[7]
    Personal references, value of. . . . .2.02[7]
    Selection of finalists. . . . .2.02[5]
    Women returning to job market, alternative checks for. . . . . 2.02[7]
Rejected applicants, written notice to. . . . .2.02[5], [8]
Screening applicants
    Pirating from other doctors, screening process for. . . . . 2.01[1][f]
    Reference checks (See subhead: Reference checks)
    Salary expectations. . . . .2.02[2]
    Skills, testing of (See subhead: Tests)
    Team, compatibility with. 2.02
Technicians, on-the-job testing required for. . . . .2.02[2][b]
Telephone screening
    Preparation for interview, as. . . . .2.02[2]
    Reference checks. . . . .2.02[7]
    Response to ads. . . . .2.02[1][a]
Tests
    Bookeeping skills. . . . .2.02[2][b]; App: Fig. 2-A
    Clerk, spelling test for. App.2-A
    Job, relationship to. . . . .2.02[2][b]
    Legal measurement of skills, as. . . . .2.02[2][b]
    Receptionist position, for. . . .App. 2-A
    Role playing. . . . .2.02[2][b]
    Sample tests. . . . .2.02[2][b]: App. A
    Technical ability. 2.02
    Transcriber-types. . . . .App. 2-A
    Validity of. . . . .2.02[2][b]
    Writing skills. . . . .2.02[2][a]

HMO (HEALTH MAINTENANCE ORGANIZATIONS)
Billing and filing claims for. . . . .5.01[1]
Computers used by
    Cost-efficiency of. . . . .5.01[1]
    Patient population, monitoring. . . . .5.02[1][i]
Described. . . . .1.02[3]
Preventive care, emphasis on. . . . .10.03[5]
Provider numbers secured from. 1.13
Regular accounts, HMO accounts separated from. . . . .10.03[5]

INDEX

(References are to sections.)

HOSPITALS AND NURSING HOMES
Accounts receivable
- Business office of hospital, billing information obtained from. . . 10.04
- Fees for services at. 10.04; 10.05
- Hospital log. . . . .4.03[5]; 10.04[1]; Fig.10-9
- Nursing home log, establishing and maintaining. . . . .10.05[1]
- Recording charges, methods for. . . . .10.04[2]

Admission to
- Hospital log entries. . . . .4.03[5]
- PPO approval prior to. . . . .10.03[4][b]
- Pre-admissions information. . . . .4.03[5]

Affiliation of physician with. . . . .9.11[1]; 9.12

Checklist. 4.09

Dictation services available for private physicians. . . . .4.05[2]

Financial aid from. . . . .1.01[1]

Referrals to
- Medical insurance coverage form, need for patient bringing. . . . . 4.03[5]
- Pre-admissions information. . . . .4.03[5]

(Pub 372)

(References are to sections.)

I

INCORPORATED PRACTICE
Advantages of. 3.03
Articles of Incorporation, filing. . . . .3.01[3][b]
Benefit plans
    Documentation of. . . . .3.01[3][b]
    Generally. . . . .3.03[5]
Budget management. . . . .3.03[1]
Buy-sell agreements. . . . .3.01[3][b]
By-laws, creating. . . . .3.02[3][b]
Cafeteria plans. . . . .3.03[5]
Checklist. 3.08
Control of finances. . . . .3.03[7]
Documents
    Formation of corporation, filing of. . . . .3.01[3][b]
    Preserving, requirements of types of documents needing. . . . .5.06[1]
Fiscal year, scheduling of. . . . .3.03[2]
Flexible benefit plans. . . . .3.03[5]
Insurance benefits. . . . .3.03[6]
Limited liability. . . . .3.03[4]
Malpractice, liability for. . . . .3.03[4]
Minutes of meetings, preservation of. . . . .5.06[1]
Partnership, compared. . . . .3.01[3][b]
Profits of, retaining. . . . .3.03[3]
Taxation, advantages as to. . . . .3.03[3]

INFORMED CONSENT
Battery, treatment of minor without as. . . . .12.02[1]
Divorced couple, child of. . . . .12.02[3]
Emergency treatment. . . . .12.02[1];[4]
Forms for. 12.09
Generally. 12.02
Mentally incompetent person, consent of. . . . .12.02[2]
Minors. . . . .12.02[1] *et seq.*
Third party consent, as to. . . . .12.02[4]
Types of. 12.02
Written consent. 12.02

INSURANCE PLANS
Appointment scheduling. . . . .4.03[1]
Assignment of benefits
    Advantages to patient. . . . .4.04[1]
    Checklist. 4.09

(Pub 372)

(References are to sections.)

INSURANCE PLANS—Cont.
Assignment of benefits—Cont.
    Computer service bureaus handling. . . . .5.03[1], [2]
    Double payment, importance of prompt refunding. . . . .4.04[1]
    Generally. 4.04
    Payment
        Requirements as to. . . . .7.03[7]
        Signing of form for. . . . .4.03[4]
    Release of information to third party
        Appending statement as to. . . . .4.04[1]
        Sample form. . . . .4.04[2]; App. Fig. 4-4
        Signed release form for. . . . .12.01[2]; App: Fig.12-4
    Third party handling of. . . . .5.03[1], [2]
Billing requirements, data processing for. . . . .5.01[2]
Closed and open panels. . . . .1.02[3]
Collecting payment, requirements for
    Assignment of benefits (See subhead: Assignment of benefits)
    Bookkeeping tasks
        Billing requirements, complying with. . . . .Fig. 10-3
        Diagnosis, indicating (See subhead: Diagnostic evaluations)
        Generally. . . . .4.03[1]
    Current Procedure Terminology. . . . .7.03[1]
    Fees
        Profiles as basis of. . . . .7.03[5]
        Relative value indexes determining reimbursement of. . . . .7.03[4]
        Generally. 7.03
    Health Care Financing Procedure Coding System, requirements of. . . . .7.03[3]
    Reimbursement policies. . . . .4.03[5]; 7.03[2], [4]
    Treatment, specifying. . . . .4.03[5]
Consulting physicians
    Location of consulting physician. . . . .4.03[5]
    PPO approving referrals to. . . . .10.03[4][b]
Coverage by
    Availability of, initial considerations as to. . . . .1.02[3]
    Physical examination, company requirements as to. . . . .10.03[8]
    Physicians, coverage for (See RISK MANAGEMENT AND INSURANCE)
Diagnostic evaluations
    Codes for
        Computer, use of. . . . .7.03[2]
        Current Procedure Terminology (CPT). . . . .7.03[1]

(Pub 372)

(References are to sections.)

INSURANCE PLANS—Cont.
Diagnostic evaluations—Cont.
    Codes for—Cont.
        Health Care Financing Procedure Coding System (HCPCS). . . . .7.03[3]
        International Classification of Diseases (ICDA or ICD-9 codes). . . . .7.03[2]; App.4-5
        Sample codes. App.4-5, 4-9
    Specification of. . . . .4.03[5]; 7.03[2]
    Standard codes. . . . .7.03[2]
Dictated transcriptions for reports. 4.05
Forms for claims
    Assignment of benefit forms (See subhead: Assignment of benefits)
    Bookkeeping tasks for. . . . .4.03[1]
    Computer submission of, capacity of system for. . . . .5.02[1][d], [e]
    Confidential information, release of
        Appending statement as to. . . . .4.04[1]
        Release form for, signed. . . . .12.01[2]; App: Fig.12-4
        Sample form. . . . .4.04[2]; App. Fig. 4-4
    Diagnosis, indicating (See subhead: Diagnostic evaluations)
    Patient identifying number. 12.04
    Regular accounts, HMO accounts separated from. . . . .10.03[5]
    Requirements for. . . . .4.03[5]
    Standard forms, availability in office of. . . . .10.03[6]
    Treatment plan, indicating. . . . .4.03[5]
    Worker's compensation forms. . . . .10.03[7]
Medicare (See MEDICARE)
Non-participating physicians
    Consulting physician, location of. . . . .4.03[5]
    Medicare payment to. . . . .10.03[1][b]
    PPO, approval of referrals by. . . . .10.03[4][b]
Participation agreements
    Advantages and disadvantages. . . . .7.03[6][a]
    Evaluation of contracts. . . . .7.03[6][b]
    Profiles as basis of fees. . . . .7.03[5]
Personal information, refusal of patient to divulge. 12.04
Physicians and physician-employees, coverage for (See RISK MANAGEMENT AND INSURANCE)
Private insurance. . . . .1.02[3]; 10.03[6]
Starting practice, considerations for. . . . .1.02[3]

(References are to sections.)

M

MALPRACTICE ACTIONS
Avoiding. . . . .8.02[2]
Checklist. 8.05; 8-A

MANAGEMENT AND MANAGEMENT TECHNIQUES
By-laws, participation in. 4.09
Chain of command, establishing. 2.06
Checklist for. 2.10
Computer systems assisting (See COMPUTER SYSTEMS)
Delegation of duties, productivity increasing through. 9.07
Feedback, need for. 2.06
Financial management
    Accounts receivable (See ACCOUNTS RECEIVABLE)
    Generally (See FINANCIAL MANAGEMENT)
Flow chart, use of. 2.06
Listening, methods for. 2.06
Meetings, regular scheduling of. 2.06
Office manager
    Fee collection. . . . .2.01[1]
    Initial benefits. . . . .2.01[1]
    Lay person in charge, as. . . . .2.01[2]
    Performance evaluation by. . . . .2.03[4][a]
    Responsibilities of. . . . .2.01[1]
    Third party insurance reimbursement, experience with. . . . . 2.01[1]
Productivity
    Ancillary services, use of. 9.10
    Checklist. 9.12
    Delegation of duties. . . . .9.07 *et seq.*
    Employees, delegation of duties to. . . . .9.07 *et seq.*
    Equipment (See PREMISES AND FACILITIES)
    Generally. 9.01
    Goals, basis of. 9.04
    Hospital affiliations. . . . .9.11, [1]
    Incentive programs, effect of. 9.09
    Merit bonuses increasing. 9.08
    Patient needs, coordinating schedule with. 9.01
    Profit distribution based on. Fig.3-4
    Self-employed practitioners, incentives for. 9.09
    Wave scheduling. 9.01
    Time management
        Apportioning. 9.05
        Earnings and time, formula for. 9.02

(References are to sections.)

MANAGEMENT AND MANAGEMENT TECHNIQUES—Cont.
Productivity—Cont.
 Time management—Cont.
  Planning for. 9.05
  Value of, generally. 9.01
  Work hours. 9.03

MEDICAID
Accounts receivable
 Copies of forms, preservation of. . . . .10.03[2]
 Generally. . . . .10.03[2]
 Personal information, refusal of patient to divulge. 12.04
 Social security number, identification of patient through. 12.04
 Welfare agencies paying one check for multiple patients seen, EOB showing. . . . .Fig. 10-5

MEDICARE
Accounts receivable
 Billing system. . . . .10.03[1][c]
 Delays in payment, handling. . . . .10.03[1][c]
 EOB, bookkeeper's need to understand. . . . .10.03[1][c]
 Fees, basis of. . . . .10.03[1][a]
 Generally. . . . .10.03[1]
 Non-participating physicians, payment to. . . . .10.03[1][b]
 Profiles of communities, purpose of. . . . .10.03[1][a]
 Provider numbers secured from. 1.13
 Recordkeeping for, importance of. . . . .10.03[1][c]
 Reimbursement. . . . .10.03[1][a]
 Terms of coverage. . . . .10.03[1][b]

MEDICARE/MEDICAID
Accounts receivable
 Generally. . . . .10.03[3]
 Standard form. . . . .Fig. 10-6

(References are to sections.)

N

NURSING HOMES (See HOSPITALS AND NURSING HOMES)

(References are to sections.)

O

OFFICE SYSTEMS
Appointments (See APPOINTMENT SCHEDULING)
Checklists for. 4.09
Equipment (See PREMISES AND FACILITIES)
Follow-up systems (See APPOINTMENT SCHEDULING)
Generally. 4.03
Layout of office (See PREMISES AND FACILITIES)
New patients (See PATIENTS, (GENERALLY))
Patient records (See RECORDS AND REPORTS)
Personnel (See EMPLOYEES; MANAGEMENT AND MANAGEMENT TECHNIQUES)
Telephone system (See TELEPHONES AND TELEPHONE USE)

(References are to sections.)

P

PATIENTS (GENERALLY)
Abandonment, procedures for avoiding charges of. . . . .8.02[2]
Confidentiality (See CONFIDENTIALITY)
Concern for, recall and reminder systems showing. 4.07; 4.09
Good Samaritan laws, applicability of. 12.03
Informed consent (See INFORMED CONSENT)
Legal duties to, generally. . . . .8.02[2]
Medical services, physician's right to deny. 12.04
New patients
    Accounts receivable, generally. 10.04
    Accounts Receivable Management (ARM) computer system, capabilities of. . . . .5.02[3]
    Billing information. . . . .4.04[1]
    Cash payments required from. . . . .7.01[3]
    Hospital consultations, charges for. 10.04
    Initial office consultation. . . . .4.01[2]; App: Fig. 4-2
    Insurance plans. . . . .7.01[3]
    Payment by. . . . .7.01[3]
    Preparation for. . . . .4.03[1]
    Records of
        Addresses or third party coverage, changes in. . . . .4.03[1]
        Charts, new patient information form kept with. . . . . 4.04[5]
        Generally. 4.04
        Items included on. . . . .4.04[1]
        Medical history. . . . .4.04[4]
        Referral of patient, names of. 4.06; 4.09
        Sample form. . . . .4.04[1]; App: Fig. 4-3
        Time for entering and completing. . . . .4.03[1]; 4.04
        Updating. . . . .4.04[1]
    Scheduling time for. 4.09
    Sources of
        Advertising and marketing for. . . . .1.12[1], [2], [3]
        Generally. 1.01
Physician-patient relationship
    Confidentiality (See CONFIDENTIALITY)
    Contract as basis. 12.01
    Good Samaritan laws, applicability of. 12.03
    Informed consent (See INFORMED CONSENT)
    Medical records, ownership of. 12.05
    Medical services, physician's right to deny. 12.04
        Obligation to patient. . . . .12.01[1]

(References are to sections.)

PATIENTS (GENERALLY)—Cont.
Physician-patient relationship—Cont.
    Property loss and. . . . .8.01[1][b]
    Release of information to third party (See CONFIDENTIALITY)
    Rejection of patients, right of. . . . .12.01[1]
Revocation of license, disclosure of confidential information leading to. . . . .12.01[2]
Survey of. App.1-B
Termination of patient
    Forms for. 12.09
    Generally. . . . .8.02[2]; 12.01[1]
Witness for procedures and examinations, need for. . . . .8.02[2]

PAYROLL SYSTEM AND RECORDS
Checklist. 6.08
Check-writing. . . . .6.04[6]; App: Fig. 6-17
Clerks, delegating duties to. . . . .9.07[1]
Computer systems
    Cost-effectiveness of. . . . .5.02[6]
    Security. . . . .5.04[2][b]
    Purchase of. 5.02
Consultants, compensation to. . . . .6.04[9]
Earnings of individual employees (See subhead: Individual earnings of employees)
Fair Labor Practices Standards Act, complying with. . . . .6.04; 12.02[2]
Generally. 6.04
Individual earnings of employees
    Breakdown by paycheck and quarterly totals. . . . .App: Fig.6-16
    Data included on. . . . .6.04[2]
    Records, generally. . . . .6.04[2]
    Reports to employees. . . . .6.04[5]
    W2 forms, records used to prepare. . . . .6.04[2]
Maintenance workers, compensation to. . . . .6.04[9]
Non-employee compensation. . . . .6.04[9]
Outside consultants, payments to. . . . .6.04[9]
Policy applicable to. . . . .2.04: Fig. 2-4
Records
    Fair Labor Standard Practices Act, applicability of. . . . .6.04; 12.02[2]
    Preservation of records
        Legal requirements as to. 12.06
        Permanent records. 6.04

INDEX

(References are to sections.)

PAYROLL SYSTEM AND RECORDS—Cont.
Records—Cont.
    Sick pay records. . . . .6.04[4]; App: Fig.6-15
    Taxes. . . . .6.02[3]; 6.04[7][a], [b], [8]
    Time cards. . . . .6.04[1]; App. Fig.6-13; 12.06[1]
    Unemployment taxes. . . . .6.04[7][a]
    Vacation records. . . . .6.04[3]; App: Fig.6-15

PERSONNEL (See EMPLOYEES; MANAGEMENT AND MANAGEMENT TECHNIQUES)

PREFERRED PROVIDER ORGANIZATIONS (PPO)
Accounts receivable processing. . . . .10.03[4][b]
Advantages of. . . . .10.03[4]
Billing procedures. . . . .5.01[1]; 10.03[4][b]
Blue Cross/Blue Shield compared to. . . . .10.03[4][a]
Computers aiding in cost-effective services of. . . . .5.01[1]
Described. . . . .1.02[3]
Filing claims. . . . .5.01[1]
Forms used by. Fig.10-7
Generally. . . . .10.03[4]
Hospital admission, approval prior to. . . . .10.03[4][b]
Non-participating physician, approval of referrals to. . . . .10.03[4][b]
Provider numbers secured from. 1.13

PREMISES AND FACILITIES
Bathrooms. 1.04
Business office. 1.04
Changing room, assessing need for. 1.04
Checklist. . . . .Fig: 1-6
Computer room
    Generally. 1.04
    Large practice, advantages of computers for. . . . .4.02[2]
Consultation room. 1.04
Drugs and narcotics, storage room for. 1.04
Employees
    New physicians in group practice, factors in hiring. 3.06
    Space for. 1.04
Equipment
    Acquisition of. 9.10
    Assets, as. . . . .5.07[1]
    Costs of. . . . .1.08[2]; 1.09
    Determining need for. . . . .9.10[1]
    Fire safety. . . . .8.02[2], [3]
    Electrocardiogram equipment. . . . .9.10[2]
    Leasing or purchasing, considerations as to. 1.01; 1.09

(References are to sections.)

PREMISES AND FACILITIES—Cont.
Equipment—Cont.
    Malpractice actions caused by malfunctions in. . . . .8.02[2]
    Productivity of practice, effect on. . . . .9.10, [1], [2]
    Records as to. . . . .8.02[2]; Fig.3-6
    Smoke detectors. . . . .8.01[3]
    Starting practice, considerations as to. 1.01
    Types of. . . . .1.01; 9.10[2]
    Ultrasound, need for. . . . .9.10[2]
    Valuation of. . . . .8.02[3]
    X-ray
        Need for. . . . .9.10[2]
        Rooms, requirements for. 1.03
Examination rooms
    Productivity affected by. 9.06
    Size and number of. 1.04
    Status of examining room, signal system on. . . . .4.03[2]
Expenses for
    Overhead. Fig.1-8
    Sharing. . . . .1.08[1]
File space. 1.04
Fire, liability for. . . . .8.02[3]
Furniture (See subhead: Equipment)
Hallways. 1.04
Hospital
    Distance from. 1.03
    Interaction of physicians with. 1.02
Laboratories
    Allocation of space for. 1.04
    Medicare regulations as to charges for outside procedures. . . . .
        9.10[2]
Layout of office
    Charts, location in examining room for. . . . .4.03[2]
    Initial preparation of. 1.05
    Model layout. Fig.1-3, 1-3, 1-5
    Receptionist's ability to see arriving patients, planning for. . . . .
        4.03[1]
    Signal systems on doors. . . . .4.03[2]
    Wheelchairs, accomodating. 1.03
Lease arrangements
    Attorney, need for review by. 1.06
    Checklist for office lease. . . . .1.06: Fig. 1-6
    Death or disability, termination of lease upon. 1.06

INDEX

(References are to sections.)

PREMISES AND FACILITIES—Cont.
Lease arrangements—Cont.
    Leasehold improvements. 1.06; 3.07
    Length of lease. 1.06
    Options, securing. . . . .1.04[2]
    Sharing space. 1.08
    Tax credits for. . . . .1.09[1]
Location of
    Community demographics. 1.02
    Considerations as to. 1.01
    Generally. 1.01
    Industry, considerations as to. . . . .1.02[2]
    Initial considerations as to. 1.02
    Patient population
        Accessibility to. 1.03
        Demographics as to. 1.02
    Physician-patient ratio of community, guide to. . . . .1.02; App: Fig.1-1
    Profile of community. Fig.1-1
    Signs, erection of. 1.03
    Source materials, researching. 1.02
    Specialties of community physicians, ascertaining. 1.02
    Visibility as factor. 1.03
    Worksheet as guide to selection of. . . . .1.02[4]
Maintenance of, liability for. . . . .8.02[3]
Name of facility. . . . .1.08[1]
Operation I.D., participating in. . . . .8.02[3]
Overhead, sharing expenses for. Fig.1-7
Parking facilities, accessibility to. 1.03
Physicians practicing, number of. . . . .1.04[2]
Public transportation, accessibility to. 1.03
Reception areas. 1.03
Rental charge
    Basis of. 1.06
    Space sharing and. 1.08
    Special provisions. 1.06
    Sublets. 1.06
    Tenant rights and responsibilities. 1.06
Security of, liability for. . . . .8.02[3]
Space
    Assessment of physician's needs. 1.04
    Computer printers and terminals, available space for. . . . .5.04[1]

(References are to sections.)

PREMISES AND FACILITIES—Cont.
Space—Cont.
    Contractors, preparation prior to meeting with. . . . .1.05: Fig 1-3, 1-4, 1-5
    Costs
        Fixed space sharing. 1.08: Fig.1-7
        Initial practice. . . . .1.04[2]
        Space sharing, allocation of costs in. 1.08
        Variable space sharing. 1.08: Fig.1-8
    Dimensions of rooms. . . . .1.04[1]: Fig. 1-2
    Future space, planning for. . . . .1.04[2]
    Generally. 1.03
    Group practice, arrangements in. . . . .3.01[3]
    Initial considerations. 1.01
    Leases of premises, restrictions on use of space. 1.06
Specialists, list of rooms required by. . . . .1.03[1]
Storage space. 1.03
Telephones (See TELEPHONES AND TELEPHONE USE)
Termination agreement, provisions of. . . . .1.08[2]
Valuation of practice as factor in. . . . .3.07[1], [2], [3]
    Third-party providers. 1.02

PRIVILEGED COMMUNICATIONS (See CONFIDENTIALITY)

(References are to sections.)

R

RECORDS AND REPORTS
Accounts receivable, for (See ACCOUNTS RECEIVABLE)
Adjustment log, physician reviewing. . . . .10.02[3]; 10.07
Billing system (See ACCOUNTS RECEIVABLE)
Business records, preservation of. . . . .12.06[1]
Checklist for. 4.09
Color coded systems. . . . .4.04[6]
Computer
    Coding, lack of standardized system for. . . . .5.02[8][a]
    Employee records monitored by. . . . .5.02[8][c]
    Medical records, problems as to. . . . .5.02[8][a]
    Monitoring systems, availability of. . . . .5.02[7]
Corporate meetings, preservation of minutes of. . . . .3.01[3][b]
Diagnostic codes (See INSURANCE PLANS)
Dictation processing
    Advantages and disadvantages. . . . .4.04[5]
    Clerks, delegating duties to. . . . .9.07[1]
    Desktop equipment. . . . .4.05[1]
    Financial information. 4.05
    Generally. 4.05
    Outside transcribing services. . . . .4.05[2]
    Patient charts
        Advantages and disadvantages. . . . .4.04[5]
        Generally. 4.05
    Photocopied transcribed notes, physician reviewing. . . . .4.04[5]
    Portable equipment. . . . .4.05[1]
    Secretarial services, availability of. . . . .4.05[2]
    Spelling errors, effect of. . . . .4.05[2]
    Staff, messages to. 4.05
    Transcribing equipment, review of. . . . .4.05[2]
Employee records
    Computer monitoring. . . . .5.02[8][c]
    Retaining. . . . .12.02[2]
Filing
    Alphabetical or numerical filing. . . . .4.04, [6]
    Patient charts and records. . . . .4.04[6]
    Prescription refill file, checking. . . . .4.01[2]
    Updating of records, importance of. . . . .10.02[1]
    X-rays, separate filing of. . . . .4.04[4]
Hospital log, establishing. . . . .10.04[1]; Fig.10-9
Insurance forms (See INSURANCE PLANS)
Journal sheets. 10.07

(References are to sections.)

RECORDS AND REPORTS—Cont.
Ledger cards. . . . .10.01[1]; 10.07; Fig.10-1
Loss of, liability for. . . . .8.02[3]
Malpractice actions, maintenance of records avoiding. . . . .8.02[2]
Medical chart (See subhead: Patient charts and records)
Medical history
    Forms. 4.09
    New patient information form. . . . .4.04[1], [4]
    Size of. . . . .4.04[4]
    Standard questionnaire forms, suppliers of. . . . .4.04[4]
Nursing home log, establishing and maintaining. . . . .10.05[1]
Ownership of. 12.05
Patient charts and records
    ARM system, evaluating need for. . . . .5.02[2]
    Assignment of benefit forms (See INSURANCE)
    Clerks, delegating duties to. . . . .9.07[1]
    Computer systems and
        Patient profiles, availability of software for. . . . .5.02[8][b]
        Problems. . . . .5.02[8], [a]
        Remote data bases, access to. . . . .5.02[8][b]
    Dictation processing (See subhead: Dictation processing)
    Efficiency and organization, need for. 4.04
    Examination, recording following. . . . .4.04, [5]
    Flags on medical charts
        ARM system automatically supplying. . . . .5.02[1][f]
        Physician acting on. . . . .4.03[1]; 4.09
    Generally. 4.04
    Forms for. 12.09
    Handwritten notes. . . . .4.04[5]
    Location of. . . . .4.03[2]
    Medical history (See subhead: Medical history)
    New patient information (See PATIENTS, GENERALLY)
    Office staff, duties of. . . . .4.03[1]
    Ownership of. 12.05
    Physician's notations. 4.04
    Preservation of, legal requirements as to. 12.06
    Referral of patient, notations on. 4.09
    Routing slips (See subhead: Routing slips)
    Size of office determining type of system. . . . .4.04[6]
    Standardization of. 4.04
    Systematic filing of. . . . .4.04[6]
    Typed notes. . . . .4.04[5]
Pocket notebook or charge tablet, physician's use of. . . . .Fig. 10.10

INDEX

I-51

(References are to sections.)

RECORDS AND REPORTS—Cont.
Preservation of
    Federal Tax Law requirements. . . . .5.06[1]
    Legal requirements as to. 12.06
    Permanent preservation, types of documents requiring. . . . . 5.06[1]
    Statutes of limitations and. 12.06
Recall and reminder systems
    ARM computer system, capabilities of. . . . .5.02[3]
    Index cards, salient information recorded on. 4.07; 4.09
Referrals
    Information systems for. 4.06
    Master sheet, preparation of. 4.06; 4.09
    Patients, recording referral by. 4.06
Routing slips
    Accounts receivable. . . . .10.02[1]; 10.07; Fig. 10-10
    ARM system, evaluating need for. . . . .5.02[2]
    Billing records, entering into. . . . .4.04[3]
    Clerks, delegating duties to. . . . .9.07[1]
    Diagnoses
        Checking, physician's duties as to. . . . .4.03[2]
        Codes for insurance benefits, sample slip listing. . . . . App. 4-9
        Generally. . . . .4.04[3]
        ICDA or ICD-9 codes, sample slips showing. App.4-5
    Financial information. . . . .4.04[3]
    Numerical sequence by appointment, daily organizing by. . . . . 4.04[3]
    Outstanding accounts, flagging charts for. . . . .App. 4-1
    Patient charts and records. 4.04; 4.09
    Procedures performed
        Charges for. . . . .4.04[3]
        Checking, physician's duties as to. . . . .4.03[2]
    Purpose of. . . . .4.04[3]
    Sample routing slips. . . . .App.4-5 *et seq.*
    Third parties, as documentation for. . . . .4.04[3]
Thank you letters
    Clerks, delegating duties to. . . . .9.07[1]
    Mailing list for. 4.06; 4.09

RETIREMENT AND PENSION PLANS
Checklists for. 11.09
Contributions by employer, tax benefits for. . . . .3.01[3][a]

(Pub 372)

(References are to sections.)

RETIREMENT AND PENSION PLANS—Cont.
Corporate practice
    Contributions of physician. . . . .3.03[6]
    Documentation of. . . . .3.01[3][b]
    Generally. . . . .3.03[5]
Defined benefit plans
    Checklist for. 11.09
    Contributions
        Illustration of. . . . .11.03[3]: Fig.11-4
        Limitations on. 11.09
    Defined contribution plan compared. . . . .11.03[3]
    Described. . . . .11.03, [2]
    Social Security benefits and. . . . .11.06: Fig. 11-7
Defined contribution plan
    Defined benefit plan compared. . . . .11.03[3]
    Limitations on contributions and benefits. . . . .11.03[4]
Disbursement of funds and benefits
    Loans. . . . .11.08[1]
    Options available. 11.08
    Payment of benefits. . . . .11.08[2]
401(k) plan
    Advantages and disadvantages. 11.04
    Deduction limitations. . . . .11.04[2]: Fig. 11-6
    Deferral percentages. . . . .11.04[1]
    Defined benefit plan, deductions compared to. . . . .11.03[2]: Fig. 11-4
    Disadvantages of. . . . .11.04[1]
    Generally. 11.04
    Matching contributions. . . . .11.04[1]: Fig. 11-5
    Limitations on contributions and benefits. 11.09
    Profit-sharing. . . . .11.03[1]
    Salary reduction agreements. . . . .11.04[1]
Generally. 11.01
Individual Retirement Plans (IRA)
    Generally. 11.05
    Limitations on contributions and benefits. 11.09
Joint and survivor annuities. . . . .11.08[2]
Keogh plans
    Contributions and benefits, limitations on. 11.09
    Generally. 11.07
    Partnerships, benefits for. 11.07
    Self-employed physicians. 3.03; 11.07

(References are to sections.)

RETIREMENT AND PENSION PLANS—Cont.
Money purchase plans
    Cash flow, management of. . . . .6.06[1]
    Contributions
        Basis of. . . . .11.03[3]: Fig.11-3
        Limitations on. 11.09
    Payment of benefits. . . . .11.08[2]
    Retirement plan, as. 11.03
Payment of benefits. . . . .11.08[2]; 11.09
Pension plans
    Administration of. . . . .3.01[2]; App. Fig.3-2
    Contributions
        Early contribution to. . . . .6.07[2]
        Tax benefits of. . . . .3.01[3][a]
    Corporate practice. 3.03
    Documentation of. . . . .3.01[3][b]
    Generally. 11.01
    Qualifications for, generally. . . . .11.01[2]
    Selection of, generally. . . . .11.01[1]
Profit sharing plans
    Administration of. . . . .3.01[2]; App. Fig.3-2
    Benefits
        Limitations on. 11.09
        Payment of. . . . .11.08[2]
    Contributions
        Basis of. . . . .11.03[3]: Fig.11-2
        Early contribution. . . . .6.07[2]
        Limitations on. 11.09
    Corporate practice. 3.03
    Documentation of. . . . .3.01[3][b]
    401-k plan (See subhead: 401-k plan)
    Retirement plan, comparison to. . . . .11.02[1]; App. Fig. 11-2
Qualifications for
    Checklist for. 11.09
    Generally. . . . .11.01[2]
Qualified plans
    Defined benefit plans (See subhead: Defined benefit plans)
    Generally. 11.02
    Money purchase plans (See subhead: Money purchase plans)
    Retirement trusts. . . . .11.02[2]
    Target benefit plans. 11.02; 11.09
    Tax-deductible plans, provisions for. . . . .11.02[2]
    Trust, establishing. . . . .11.02[1]

(References are to sections.)

RETIREMENT AND PENSION PLANS—Cont.
Selection of, generally. . . . .11.01[1]; 11.09
Social Security plans
    Contributions and benefits, limitations on. 11.09
    Generally. 11.06

RISK MANAGEMENT AND INSURANCE
Accounts receivable, coverage for. . . . .8.03[1][a]
Burglaries. . . . .8.02[3]
Checklist. 8.05
Contributions by employer, tax benefits for. . . . .3.01[3][a]
Disability insurance
    Contract provisions. . . . .8.04[2][c], [d]
    Documentation of. . . . .3.01[3][b]
    Exclusions. . . . .8.04[2][f]
    Generally. . . . .8.04[2]
    Group practice. 3.07
    Initial policy. . . . .8.04[2][a]
    Sick pay plan. . . . .8.04[2][b]
    Non-smoker discounts. . . . .8.03[1][e]
Embezzlement, coverage for. . . . .8.03[1][a]
Employee benefits, liability for. . . . .8.03[1][f]
ERISA. . . . .8.03[1][f]
Financial risks (See subhead: Property loss)
Group practices
    Contributions by employer, tax benefits for. . . . .3.01[3][a]
    Coverage, availability of. . . . .8.04[3][a]
    Overhead expenses. . . . .8.04[3][b]
    Property loss
        Disability buyout. . . . .8.04[3][c]
        Generally. . . . .8.04[3]
        Medical insurance. . . . .8.04[3]
        Overhead expense. . . . .8.04[3][b]
        Questions. . . . .8.04[3][a]
Identification of risks. 8.01
Liability loss
    Automobile liability. . . . .8.03[2][b]
    Disclosure to patients of insurance for. . . . .8.02[2]
    Employer's liability. . . . .8.03[2][c]
    Fiduciary liability. . . . .8.03[2][f]
    Fire, tenant's legal liability for. . . . .8.03[2][e]
    Generally. . . . .8.01[2]
    Professional liability, coverage for. . . . .8.03[2][a]
    Public liability, coverage for. . . . .8.03[2][b]

(References are to sections.)

RISK MANAGEMENT AND INSURANCE—Cont.

Malpractice, avoidance of
    Checklist. . . . .App: Fig. 8-A
    Generally. . . . .8.02[2]

Physician-employee, coverage for
    Cost of living increases. . . . .8.03[2][e]
    Disability income (See subhead: Disability income)
    Life insurance. . . . .8.04[1]

Practice loss. . . . .8.01[3]

Property loss
    Consequential losses. . . . .8.01[1][b]
    Direct losses. . . . .8.01[1][a]
    Furniture and equipment. . . . .8.01[1][a]
    Generally. . . . .8.01[1]
    Group practice (See subhead: Group practice)
    Insurance for. . . . .8.03, [1]et seq.
    Leasehold improvement. . . . .8.01[1][a]

Risk prevention
    Generally. 8.02
    General risks, avoidance of. . . . .8.05[3]
    Internal control. . . . .8.02[1]
    Malpractice actions, avoiding. . . . .8.02[2]

Slips and falls, coverage for. . . . .8.03[1][b]

Umbrella policies. . . . .8.03[1][g]

Worker's compensation, coverage for. . . . .8.03[1][c]

(References are to sections.)

S

SALARIES (See WAGES AND SALARIES)

SELF-EMPLOYED PHYSICIANS
Business expenses. . . . .3.01[1]
Coverage of patients, lack of back-up for. 3.04
Disadvantages of self-employment. . . . .3.04,[1]
Fee-for-service patients, reduction in. . . . .5.01[1]
Financial management, control of decisions as to. . . . .3.04[1]
Keogh plans for. 3.03; 11.07
Productivity, incentives for increasing. 9.09
Professional corporation
    Advantages of changing to. . . . .3.01[1]
    Methods of incorporating practice. . . . .3.01[2]
    Structure of; illustration. . . . .App: Fig.3-1
Sole responsibility. . . . .3.01[1]
Taxation, effect of self-employment on. . . . .3.01[1]
Time and cost sharing plans, lack of. 3.04

INDEX

(References are to sections.)

T

TAXATION
Clerks, delegation of duties. . . . .9.07[1]
Corporate practice
    Contributions by. 3.03
    Dividends, profits as. . . . .3.03[2]
    FICA. . . . .3.03[1]
    Fiscal year, scheduling. . . . .3.03[2]
    Investment earnings of, taxability of. . . . .3.03, [1]
    Pension and profit sharing. 3.03
Depreciation on equipment. 3.02
Federal tax deposit. . . . .App: Fig. 6-20
FICA
    Corporate practice. . . . .3.03[1]
    Family members as employees. 3.02
    Generally. . . . .6.04[7][a]
    Self-employment, effect of. . . . .3.01[2]
    Unincorporated practice. 3.02
Income tax returns
    Filing of. . . . .3.01[2]
    Personal income tax returns. . . . .3.01[3][a]
    Schedule K-1. . . . .App.3-3
Investment tax credits
    Self-employment, as to. 3.02
Leasing, tax credits for. . . . .1.09[1]
Payroll taxes
    Management of. . . . .6.02[3]
    Reports. . . . .6.04[8]
    Unincorporated practice. 3.02
Penalties. . . . .6.04[7][b]
Record keeping. . . . .3.01[2]
Schedule of tax deposits. App:6-21
Self-employment, effect of. . . . .3.01[1]
Specialty practices. . . . .6.04[7][a], [b], [8]
State and local taxes. . . . .6.04[7][a]
Tax identification numbers, obtaining. 1.13
Withholding tax
    Federal withholding. . . . .6.04[7][a]
    Self-employment, effect of. . . . .3.01[1]
W2 form; sample. . . . .App: Fig. 6-19
W4 form; sample. . . . .App: Fig.6-18

(References are to sections.)

TELEPHONES AND TELEPHONE USE
Answering devices and services
    Answering machines
        Appropriate messages for. . . . .4.01[3][a]
        Checklist. 4.09
        Generally. . . . .4.01[3]
        Purpose of. . . . .4.01[3]
    Services
        Evaluating. . . . .4.01[3][b]
        Pick-up policy. 4.09
        Sources of. . . . .4.01[3][b]
ARM computer system, capabilities of. . . . .5.02[3]
Buying or leasing
    Checklist. 4.09
    Options as to. . . . .4.01[4]
Checklist for. 4.09
Credit and collection, for
    Commitment from patient, obtaining. . . . .7.04[5][b]
    Generally. . . . .7.04[5]
    Illustration. . . . .7.04[5][a]
Dependability of system, importance of. . . . .4.01[4]
Emergency calls, employee handling. . . . .4.01, [2]
Family and friends, calls from. . . . .4.01[2]
Generally. 4.01
Hiring, use of telephone in. . . . .2.02[2]
Initial patient-physician contact, telephone as instrument for. 4.01
Policy
    Checklist for. 4.09
    Implementation of. 4.01
    Low priority calls, employee handling. . . . .4.01[2]
    Message slips, essential information on. . . . .4.01[1]; 4.09
    Number of rings prior to answering. 4.09
    Telephone use, policy applicable to. . . . .2.04: Fig. 2-4
Priority routing
    Checklist. 4.09
    Employee's knowledge of. . . . .4.01[2]
Prescription refills, pharmacy calls for. . . . .4.01[2]
Sales representatives
    Generally. . . . .4.01[2]
    Purpose of. . . . .4.01[3]
    Services, obtaining and evaluating. . . . .4.01[3][b]

(Pub 372)

INDEX

(References are to sections.)

TELEPHONES AND TELEPHONE USE—Cont.
Starting practice, importance of contacting telephone company. 1.11
Yellow pages, listing in. 1.11

(References are to sections.)

W

WAGES AND SALARIES
Adjustment of salary. . . . .2.03[4][b]
Application form and. . . . .2.02[2][a]
Computer monitoring of. . . . .5.02[8][c]
Equal Pay Act, applicability of. 2.09
Expectations of applicant. . . . .2.02[2]
Forms for. 12.09
Generally. 2.03
Gross receipts as basis of. . . . .2.03[1]
Hospitals, availability of wage surveys from. . . . .2.03[1]
Increase as motivation. . . . .2.03[4]
Insurance for loss of. . . . .8.01[1][a]
Interview, discussion at. . . . .2.02[4]
Miscellaneous factors. . . . .2.03[1]
Payroll (See PAYROLL SYSTEM AND RECORDS)
Performance evaluation. . . . .2.03[4][a]
Physician's authority as to. . . . .2.02[4]
Policy applicable to, written. 2.04
Quality employees, retaining. 2.03
Records of, Fair Labor Standards Act applicable to. . . . .5.06[6]
Regional differences in wage scales. . . . .2.03[1]
Telephone screening. . . . .2.02[2]

Index written by DOROTHY SILVER